Emerging Programs for Autism Spectrum Disorder

Emerging Programs for Autism Spectrum Disorder

Improving Communication, Behavior, and Family Dynamics

Edited by

Neophytos L. Papaneophytou
Psychotherapist, Magic Always Happens, Inc., NJ, United States

Undurti N. Das
UND Life Sciences, Battle ground, WA, United States

ELSEVIER

ACADEMIC PRESS
An imprint of Elsevier

Academic Press is an imprint of Elsevier
125 London Wall, London EC2Y 5AS, United Kingdom
525 B Street, Suite 1650, San Diego, CA 92101, United States
50 Hampshire Street, 5th Floor, Cambridge, MA 02139, United States
The Boulevard, Langford Lane, Kidlington, Oxford OX5 1GB, United Kingdom

Notices
Knowledge and best practice in this field are constantly changing. As new research and experience broaden our understanding, changes in research methods, professional practices, or medical treatment may become necessary.

Practitioners and researchers must always rely on their own experience and knowledge in evaluating and using any information, methods, compounds, or experiments described herein. In using such information or methods they should be mindful of their own safety and the safety of others, including parties for whom they have a professional responsibility.

To the fullest extent of the law, neither the Publisher nor the authors, contributors, or editors, assume any liability for any injury and/or damage to persons or property as a matter of products liability, negligence or otherwise, or from any use or operation of any methods, products, instructions, or ideas contained in the material herein.

British Library Cataloguing-in-Publication Data
A catalogue record for this book is available from the British Library

Library of Congress Cataloging-in-Publication Data
A catalog record for this book is available from the Library of Congress

ISBN: 978-0-323-85031-5

For Information on all Academic Press publications
visit our website at https://www.elsevier.com/books-and-journals

Publisher: Nikki Levy
Acquisitions Editor: Melanie Tucker
Editorial Project Manager: Billie Jean Fernandez
Production Project Manager: Selvaraj Raviraj
Cover Designer: Limbert Matthew

Typeset by MPS Limited, Chennai, India

Contents

List of contributors

Eric C. Alcera Department of Psychiatry and Behavioral Health, Hackensack Meridian School of Medicine, Nutley, NJ, United States; Department of Psychiatry, Riverview Medical Center, Red Bank, NJ, United States

H.A. Alonim The Mifne Center, Treatment, Research, Training, Rosh Pinna, Israel; School of Social Science, Bar Ilan University, Ramat Gan, Israel

María Astorga Imagine Academy for Autism, New York, NY, United States; Profectum Foundation Professional Membership, United States

Tatyana Batysheva Clinical and Research Center of Children Psycho-Neurology, Moscow, Russia

Tal Baz In-Tune Integrated Developmental Therapies, Somerville, MA, United States

Courtney Bitting Imagine Academy for Autism, New York, NY, United States; New York State Association for Behavior Analysis Membership, New York, NY, United States; Association of Professional Behavior Analysts Membership, United States

Damián Borda Faculty of Psychology, Pontifical Catholic University, Buenos Aires, Argentina; Child and Adolescents Psychiatric Hospital "Dra.Carolina Tobar García", Buenos Aires, Argentina

Kirsten Byrnes Audrey Hepburn Children's House, Hackensack University Medical Center, Hackensack, NJ, United States; Psychiatry and Behavioral Health, Hackensack Meridian School of Medicine, Nutley, NJ, United States

Ru Ying Cai Aspect Research Centre for Autism Practice, Autism Spectrum Australia, Melbourne, Vic, Australia; Faculty of Medicine, Nursing and Health Sciences, School of Psychological Sciences, Monash University, Melbourne, Vic, Australia

Pericles Cheng Department of Computer Science and Engineering, School of Sciences, European University Cyprus, Nicosia, Cyprus

Gerard Costa Center for Autism and Early Childhood Mental Health, College of Education and Human Services, Montclair State University, Montclair, NJ, United States

Undurti N. Das UND Life Sciences, Battle Ground, WA, United States; Department of Medicine, BioScience Research Centre, GVP College of Engineering, Visakhapatnam, India

Jonathan Delafield-Butt Laboratory for Innovation in Autism, University of Strathclyde, Glasgow, United Kingdom; School of Education, University of Strathclyde, Glasgow, United Kingdom

Penelope Dunbar Independent Artist and Creative Researcher, Glasgow, United Kingdom

Tibor N. Farkas University of Lincoln, Lincoln, United Kingdom

Gilbert M. Foley NYC Early Childhood Mental Health Training and Technical Assistance Center (TTAC), New York Center for Child Development, New York, NY, United States; Profectum Academy, Profectum Foundation, Mendham, NJ, United States

Stephanny Freeman Department of Psychiatry and Biobehavioral Sciences, University of California, Los Angeles, CA, United States

Sima Gerber Queens College, City University of New York, Queens, NY, United States

Chafica Mansour Gharbieh Education & ABA/VB Consultant, Lebanese International University, Beirut, Lebanon; Autism Learning Institute for Applied Behaviour Analysis "ALI for ABA", Lebanese International University, Beirut, Lebanon; Diagnostic Lebanese Centre for Training, Communication & Behaviour Development, Lebanese International University, Beirut, Lebanon; Education and Development Committee for Arab Network for Autism "ANA", Lebanese International University, Beirut, Lebanon; Lebanese International University "LIU", Lebanese International University, Beirut, Lebanon

Sammy Gharbieh Isabella Biomedical Sciences, University of Greenwich, London, United Kingdom; Nutritional Medicine, Surrey University, London, United Kingdom; Bachelor of Medicine and Bachelor of Surgery, Kings College, London, United Kingdom; Nutrition Consultant for ALI for ABA, London, United Kingdom

Michael D. Hannon Department of Counseling, Montclair State University, Montclair, NJ, United States

Alexandra Harrison Department of Psychiatry, Harvard Medical School, Boston Psychoanalytic Society and Institute, United States; Boston Psychoanalytic Society and Institute, Boston, MA, United States; Psychiatry, HMS, Boston, MA, United States; UMB IPMHPGCC, Boston, MA, United States; SCC Cambridge, United States

Michelle Jaehning Department of Psychiatry, Jersey Shore University Medical Center (affiliated with Hackensack Meridian School of Medicine), Neptune, NJ, United States

Barbara Kalmanson KidsAttuned.org, Fielding Graduate University, Santa Barbara, CA, United States

Niko Kargas University of Lincoln, Lincoln, United Kingdom

Irina Koshkina Medical center for the improvement of the immune, nervous and hormonal systems, Moscow, Russia

I. Liberman Western Galilee Academic College & Galilee Research Institute, Acre, Israel

Carla Vale Lucas Psychological Service, University of Madeira, Funchal, Portugal

Ramiro Pérez Martín Faculty of Psychology, Pontifical Catholic University, Buenos Aires, Argentina; Argentine Psychiatrists Association Board Member, Argentina

John Mendy University of Lincoln, Lincoln, United Kingdom

Kaitlin Mulcahy Center for Autism and Early Childhood Mental Health, Montclair State University, Montclair, NJ, United States

Robert A. Naseef Alternative Choices, Philadelphia, PA, United States

Natalia Neophytou Faculty of Health Science, Centre for Exercise Science and Sports Medicine, University of the Witwatersrand, Johannesburg, South Africa

Filipa Oliveira Psychological Service, University of Madeira, Funchal, Portugal

Daniel Orlievsky Faculty of Psychology, Pontifical Catholic University, Buenos Aires, Argentina; Andrés Bello University, Santiago de Chile, Chile; Universitarie Institute of the Italian Hospital, Buenos Aires, Argentina

Marina A. Ovchinnikova Department of Sports Medicine and Medical Rehabilitation, Institute of Clinical Medicine, I.M. Sechenov First Moscow State Medical University (Sechenov University), Moscow, Russia

Neophytos L. Papaneophytou Psychotherapist, Magic Always Happens, Inc., NJ, United States

Tanya Paparella Department of Psychiatry and Biobehavioral Sciences, University of California, Los Angeles, CA, United States

T. Papatheodorou Norland College, Bath, United Kingdom

Alexander Poletaev Medical Research Center Immunculus, Moscow, Russia; Clinical and Research Center of Children Psycho-Neurology, Moscow, Russia

Stacy Sue Rosello Profectum Academy, Mendham, NJ, United States; Occupational Therapy, University of Pittsburgh, Pittsburgh, PA, United States; Occupational Therapy, Texas Women's University, Houston, TX, United States; Embrace the Child, Ltd., Pittsburgh, PA, United States

Olga G. Safonicheva Department of Sports Medicine and Medical Rehabilitation, Institute of Clinical Medicine, I.M. Sechenov First Moscow State Medical University (Sechenov University), Moscow, Russia

Ruby Moye Salazar Smith College, Northhampton, MA, United States; Karen Horney Institute, New York, NY, United States; Pennsylvania Lifespan Services, Dalton, PA, United States; Profectum Academy, Mendham, NJ, United States

Stephen Seligman Clinical Professor of Psychiatry, University of California, San Francisco, United States; Training and Supervising Analyst, San Francisco Center for Psychoanalysis, CA, United States

Patricia Sermabeikian Bergen Evaluation and Counseling Associates, Fair Lawn, NJ, United States

Luísa Soares Faculty of Arts and Humanities, University of Madeira, Funchal, Portugal; Larsys - ITI–Interactive Technologies Institute, Funchal, Portugal

Ramon Solhkhah Department of Psychiatry and Behavioral Health, Hackensack Meridian School of Medicine, Nutley, NJ, United States; Department of Psychiatry, Jersey Shore University Medical Center, Neptune, NJ, United States

Aditi Subramaniam Massachusetts Society for the Prevention of Cruelty to Children, Boston, MA, United States

Check J. Tan

Gil Tippy Dirty Hands Developmental Alliance, Sonoma, CA, United States

Colwyn Trevarthen School of Philosophy, Psychology and Language Sciences, The University of Edinburgh, Edinburgh, United Kingdom

Ed Tronick University of Massachusetts Boston, Developmental Brain Sciences Program, Department of Newborn Medicine, Harvard Medical School, Boston, MA, United States; Psychology CDU UMB, Boston, MA, United States

Mirko Uljarević Faculty of Medicine, Dentistry and Health Sciences, Melbourne School of Psychological Sciences, University of Melbourne, Melbourne, Vic, Australia

Alisa Vig Simaney Kesher Clinic, Petah Tikva, Israel

Serena Wieder Profectum Foundation, Mendham, NJ, United States

Foreword

Autism spectrum disorder (ASD) is a multifaceted and heterogeneous neurodevelopmental condition, frequently coexisting with a wide range of diverse mental health disorders. The ASD construct developed considerably in the last few decades, with its formal inclusion, as such, in the classification systems only materializing in 2013 with the *Diagnostic and Statistical Manual of Mental Disorders*, 5th Edition (DSM-5). Our understanding of its phenomenological, biological, genetic, and environmental underpinnings and their complex interactions has been rapidly evolving, providing new leads for intervention. It is generally accepted that the core symptoms of ASD, namely, deficits in communication, reciprocal social interaction, and restricted and repetitive behaviors and interests, are not amenable to treatment. However, several interventions have been found to reduce the impact of symptoms, improve daily functioning, support cognition, and promote socialization, thus maximizing the potential of children, young people, and adults with this condition. In addition, improved characterization and treatment of comorbidities, sometimes hard to diagnose but usually effectively treatable, has resulted in a less burdensome course and better overall prognosis.

Unsurprisingly, a large part of the interventions for ASD is delivered through families, support structures, educational establishments, and workplaces. Multiagency collaborations are frequently forged to holistically target individual needs, monitor intervention plans, review benefits and adverse reactions, and optimize professional input. All possible means have been employed in that goal: from communication and parenting modifications to the use of the state-of-the-art technology, from medication treatments to contact with animals, from dietary interventions to art therapies. Although not all approaches have been found to be equally effective, this area of ASD interventions is constantly developing at the same time with becoming increasingly intricate.

In this context the current book by Papaneophytou and colleagues is a welcome addition to the growing body of publications aiming to improve the understanding of ASD and, most importantly, the lives of individuals with this condition and their families. This work is a result of extensive direct experience within this fascinating field from different perspectives, and its constellation results in a holistic, multidimensional, and all-inclusive whole. The chapters of the book explore a wide range of aspects that clinicians who work with individuals having ASD and related neurodevelopmental needs will frequently come across. It will most certainly offer them invaluable insights that will inform their approach and clinical practice and enhance their skills and sense of competence. The book would also be of interest to affected individuals and families and help them identify leads to explore further in their journey. As in their previous publications, the vision of the authors to make a difference through embracing all the needs of individuals and families affected by ASD shines through.

Dr. Marinos Kyriakopoulos, PhD, FRCPsych
Consultant Child and Adolescent Psychiatrist, National and Specialist Inpatient Children's Unit (Acorn Lodge), South London and Maudsley NHS Foundation Trust; Joint Training Programme Director, The Maudsley Scheme in Child and Adolescent Psychiatry; Visiting Senior Lecturer, Department of Child and Adolescent Psychiatry, Institute of Psychiatry, Psychology and Neuroscience, King's College London, United Kingdom

Introduction

Neophytos L. Papaneophytou

Autism is being diagnosed in far more people nowadays compared to what was being considered as *Autistic* 10, 20, or 30 years ago. Families are perplexed as to the reasons why their child is on the spectrum and societies are struggling to understand the reason(s) behind the staggering numbers—particularly in the Western world. Despite the *global* incidence of autism (1 in 65 children being on the spectrum) in some areas in New Jersey, USA research indicates 1 in 30 children are autistic. Culturally, societies appear to have moved beyond the initial effort to "fix" people who are autistic and have accepted the fact that some are simply unique in *their* ways—different from the rest.

Many autistic people thrive, many excel, and many may be less able to be/come successful due to the barriers in mentalizing, actualizing, and dealing with the rest of the society. Even today, Autistic People face prejudice and discrimination in societies and suffer from inadequate means for therapy, education, rehabilitation, or validation. Some "autistic behaviors" may appear to be a threat to the unfamiliar person and as such, people may withdraw and not engage with people who are on the Autism Spectrum.

Just like with our previous publication, *Autism 360°*, reinforcing the multidisciplinary approach to Autism, *Emerging Programs for Autism Spectrum Disorder* offers a spherical approach to Autism with well-rounded scientific discussions based on research and best practices available at present. The (commonly stressful) discovery journey from diagnosis to evaluation, therapy, treatment, education, and a life full of "ebbs and flows" need not condone feelings of defeat, loss, oversight, frustration, or omission. A parent, a sibling, an autistic person, and a family have many ways to work together to overcome the "disability" or abilities of one being autistic. From the evidence and solutions presented in this book, it is clear that solutions are at hand for all those *dealing* with autism

Taking steps to improve quality of life, scaffold the person(s), and engage with the family of the autistic person is expected to enhance the educational, therapeutic, and other environments and lead to hope, positivity, and an increased enjoyment of life. Be it the use of robotics, media psychology, psychotherapy, stress reduction, medication management, improved ways of engaging with the legal system, or simply relating with the *other(s)* are some of the available resources, and the variability of best practices is right on target. The journey is one of transformation and the panacea may reside in each of our hearts and minds. We wish that all embrace Autistic people just like we do with any other friend(s) and family member(s), colleague(s), or neighbor(s), and we look up to their daily achievements, struggles, successes, and introjections. We invite everyone to walk a mile in one's shoes instead of waiting for the other shoe to drop, and we remain faithful to our way of moving forward via Actions not words!

Stress experience and life for parents of autistic individuals: four case studies in focus

1

Neophytos L. Papaneophytou
Psychotherapist, Magic Always Happens, Inc., NJ, United States

Introduction

Loving your family member with autism is easy; having the right mechanisms and capacity to cope with the daily life stressors may not be as easy. According to the American Psychiatric Association (2020), autism spectrum disorder (ASD) is considered a "complex neurodevelopmental disorder characterized by persistent alterations in communication and social interaction and by the presence of stereotyped patterns of behavior, activities, and interests" (p. 1). Poletaev et al. (2014), Personal Communication (2016) look at autism from an epigenetic perspective stating:

> *Autism should be considered as a group of phenotypic (epigenetic) multisystem diseases emerging in utero, the typical characteristic of which are not only neurological disorders but also pathological changes in the stomach, small and large intestines; children with autism are often found with changes in the lungs, pelvic organs, kidneys, adrenals, and other organs.*
>
> *Personal Communication (2016)*

According to the Center for Disease Control (CDC), in the United States, it is estimated that 1 in 59 children have a diagnosis of ASD. Based on CDC reports, in 2020, 1 in 54 eight-year-old children in the United States is *on the spectrum*. Nonetheless, as CDC's Autism and Developmental Disabilities Monitoring Network indicates, significant variations were noted in the percentage of the *prevalence* of autism among different US states:

> *The percentage of children identified with ASD ranged widely across geographic areas from a low of 1 in 76 or 1.3% in Colorado to a high of 1 in 32 or 3.1% in areas of New Jersey (p. 9).*

According to Hill, Berthoz, and Frith (2004), who examined the cognitive processing of people with a diagnosis of ASD, such individuals "are significantly more impaired in their emotion processing" (p. 229). At the same time, they experience more depressive symptoms than other neurotypical individuals and the same goes

Emerging Programs for Autism Spectrum Disorder. DOI: https://doi.org/10.1016/B978-0-323-85031-5.00005-0

for their parents. Freeman and Paparella (2019) explain that the efforts to change the behavior of children diagnosed with ASD have shifted from trying to find the "cure" toward the trend of viewing autism as a "positive identity that doesn't need a cure but rather a neurological condition that represents an equal and valid pathway to adult success" (p. 198). As such the authors offer insight based on cited research explaining the recent efforts to focus on concerns relevant to the diagnosis of autism. Specifically, as it regards "specialized socialization interventions, for example, studies target developing social skills at school ... teach imitation skills ... develop joint attention ... teach play ... recognize emotions and mental states ... address social communication ... and teach social problem solving" (p. 198). Tethering between this new and the older "understanding" of offering help including therapy based on best practices may also involve stress management, skill development, and time management.

In the book *Autism 360°*, Undurti, Papaneophytou, and El-Kour (2019) discuss the overall needs of people diagnosed with ASD, as well as those of their families, suggesting a holistic "360° approach" in all aspects of treatment, development, and facets of life. More specifically, Papaneophytou (as cited in Undurti et al., 2019) addresses the issue of providing allies to the parents who may still be mourning the loss of their fantasy about their child's life and goals. Realizing their child's diagnosis, Undurti et al. suggest, may increase parents' levels of anger and guilt, making the road to acceptance even harder. The "unfairness" that living with ASD entails may delay or exasperate issues such as diagnosis, education, treatment, and overall health—physical and mental. Stress undoubtedly is elevated in any such conditions, particularly if neither formal nor informal methods of support are adequate to answer parents' questions, dilemmas, and/or to address their agony for the future with respect to their child's life.

Drawing from research on infants, Provenzi and Tronick (2020) discuss issues pertinent to trauma, the "power of disconnection" and "reparation" (p. 1). They define reparation as the "human ability to co-regulate emotions and to resolve interactive mismatches and separations by reciprocally engaging in attuned interactive exchanges capable of expanding our capacities for resilience" (p. 1). This also holds true for our relationships with our autistic family members, colleagues, friends, partners, husbands and wives, etc. To the extent where such relationships may be characterized as "messy," the above authors explain that "messiness of social relationships matter" (p. 2). Though the expectation may be that when interacting socially, humans engage in synchronous and fine-tuned exchanges with a complete emotional connection, Provenzi and Tronick define such an expectation as naïve. Instead they explain that:

> *We do not engage with each other the way Ginger Rogers and Fred Astaire dance. Rather, we are apprentice dancers. We move around in our shoes with no memory of the future and a partial perception of the present moment. In other words, we do our dance by improvising and by moving our steps based on our present feelings, emotions, cognitions, and reciprocal attempts of attunement (p. 2).*

In the case of "autism," we may find ourselves dancing with two shoes, one shoe, or no shoes, while waiting for the other shoe to drop in a moment's notice so-to-speak! Just like in cases of free-floating anxiety—another name for a capitulating disorder of our times—generalized anxiety disorder (GAD)—when dealing with autistic family members who have more severe impairment across all areas of functioning, anxiety may be raised (sometimes through the roof).

Why the stress and what does it mean for the parent and the family?

A literature review reveals that much research has been conducted with *mothers* in mind, for the most part. Fathers, however, play an equally significant role in the family structure and their function as equal supporters need not be neglected. Tools and techniques utilized as buffers to stress may allow for an improved quality of life; a less stressful life is of concern to most of us. Quality of life may increase or conversely be impaired by both what is *real*, as well as by what one may *perceive* to be real. Hence, personal and other resources (both formal and informal) available in one's community may allow for interventions leading to the improvement of a parent's mental health status, among other. Do parents experience stress in similar ways around the globe? The theme of having more stress among parents of children who have a diagnosis of ASD seems prevalent regardless of where the family resides.

In as early as 1991, Dumas, Wolf, Fisman, and Culligan stated the effects of parental stress due to caring for a child on the autism spectrum. Thus, "parents of children with autism and behavior disorders experienced statistically and clinically higher levels of parenting stress ... Mothers of children with autism and behavior disorders experienced statistically and clinically higher levels of dysphoria" (p. 97). One may wonder if factors having to do with one's internal universe are relevant in this discussion. Does the way we feel and think about our *own self*, make a difference in the levels of stress we experience?

The answer is yes. Kuhn and Carter (2006) examined maternal self-efficacy and associated parenting cognitions among mothers of children with autism and concluded that parental self-efficacy appears to be associated with well-being, agency, and feelings of guilt among mothers of children with autism. Parent- and family-based interventions designed to support parental well-being and focusing on parenting cognitions may enhance parenting self-efficacy. Does *agency* and a sense of coherence affect the way one responds to stress? Evidently, based on research, it does.

Mak, Ho, and Law (2007) investigated issues pertinent to "a sense of coherence, parental attitudes and parenting stress for caregiving parents of children with autism" (pp. 166–167) in a sample of 157 mothers stemming from community centers in Hong Kong. The authors suggested that both the mother's confidence and her acceptance of the child were important variables. Furthermore, Mak et al. explained that mothers with a stronger sense of coherence experienced less stress, even if their children exhibited more severe ASD symptomatology. Experiencing a coherent environment seems to be a common element in parental stress around the world. Would a parent's state of mind or feeling state affect their experience with their child who has a diagnosis of ASD? A parent's ability to express emotion and share their own feeling states is an important factor.

Alexithymia is a personality trait in which there is marked impairment in one's awareness, processing, and expression of emotional states. Szatmari et al. (2008) studied alexithymia in parents of children with ASD. The authors hypothesized that "(a) parents of children with ASD will demonstrate higher impairment in their emotion processing when compared to controls, and (b) high impairment in emotion processing in parents will be associated with severity of symptoms in children with ASD" (p. 1859). In presenting their evidence regarding the Broader Autism Phenotype (BAP), they explained that when compared to parents of neurotypical children, parents of children with ASD scored higher on the Toronto Alexithymia Scale (TAS-20). Importantly, "children of fathers with *high alexithymia* score higher on repetitive behavior symptoms compared to children of fathers with *low alexithymia*" (p. 1859). A parent's ability to express their own emotional world notwithstanding, do issues of *dependency* affect the levels of stress in a parent and does stress have a lesser effect on parents of neurotypical children?

Dabrowska and Pisula (2010) demonstrated that parents of neurotypical children experienced lower stress levels when compared to parents of children with ASD. Issues such as *dependency* and *limits* when it comes to family opportunities were also discussed. Specifically, mothers of autistic preschool children maintained higher levels of stress when compared to their husbands. According to the authors above, "emotion-oriented coping" could be the predictor for stress in these parents. Phetrasuwan and Shandor-Miles (2009) explained that mothers who experienced compounded parenting stress presented with increased depressive symptoms and thus their well-being suffered. If parents are experiencing additional stress, do they present with any relevant physiological responses consistent with their stress levels?

Foody, James, and Leader (2015) examined parenting stress, salivary biomarkers, and ambulatory blood pressure in parents of children with an ASD. The authors articulated that higher levels of stress in parents of autistic children may manifest in increased problems with the parent's health. The authors focused on "parenting responsibility, distress, anxiety, depression, cortisol, alpha-amylase, and cardiovascular activity between 19 mother–father dyads of children with ASD" (p. 1084). The results indicate that "mothers reported higher parenting responsibility, distress, anxiety, and depression than fathers, while fathers had higher blood pressure and heart rate variability" (p. 1084). Can issues such as the lack of grandparent involvement in the child's life and societal prejudice have a negative impact on the parent's health?

Magalhães and Pereira (2017) discussed various issues of concern and support (or its lack thereof) in regard to elevated levels of stress in mothers of children diagnosed with ASD in Portugal. Issues such as the level of grandparent involvement with the child with ASD and the availability of formal or informal sources of information are of cardinal nature in this discussion. Decreased involvement with parenting groups, family friends, or socializing in general stem from parental fear of potential (or real) judgment or prejudice upon them "sharing intimate information" (p. 247). Hence, the mothers' voluntary "protective option" (p. 247) is understood as justified to some extent. Their level of avoidance does not, however, stop them from seeking friends and looking up information regarding ASD online—though as research illustrates, at a lesser degree than they do with formal support. As the authors explained, mothers need formal guidance and support during the *early stages* of their child's development. Often mothers felt that doctors would postpone or not value their own concerns over their child's development, which may be a phenomenon parents are faced with in more than one culture and country. What happens if in addition to societal issues the parent is also faced with the child's own behavioral and emotional problems? Parents can still cope—we would hope.

Miranda, Mira, Berenguer, Rosello, and Baixauli (2019) investigated stress levels in mothers of children diagnosed with ASD who had no intellectual disability. Their goal was to understand factors that mediate behavioral problems, rendering enhanced coping strategies. What their study ($N = 52$) revealed was that the stress level experienced by a parent was "positively correlated with the children's ASD symptoms and behavioral problems" (p. 464). Alas, as the severity of the child's "behavioral problems" and "ASD symptoms" increased so did the mother's stress level. According to Miranda et al., the more the mothers had "engagement coping and social functional support" (p. 464) the less stress they reportedly experienced. The importance of the study lies on the seemingly simple guidance offered by the authors. Stress *can* be alleviated if the mothers learn to "buffer the impact of stress" (p. 464) via the application of various behavioral strategies on the one hand and an enhanced "engagement orientation" (p. 464) on the other.

What are the reasons parents of people with ASD experience increased stress, one may ask?

Autism is a pervasive, lifetime condition that impairs daily life activities, impedes language development, and renders what some may describe as inept social skills. Parents need to develop adequate parenting skills in order to offer the best they can to their child. Autism sets child-rearing issues on top of the rest of the daily stressors that parents experience. As Miranda et al. (2019) explained citing older research, parents who have children on the autism spectrum experience more stress than the parents of children who have a neurotypical development. After all, in 77% of the cases they studied, such stress levels reached clinical significance. Parents of children with other diagnoses such as Down syndrome or attention deficit hyperactivity disorder, are said to experience less stress than parents of children on the autism spectrum. Might the above affect one's self-confidence and ability to cope as a *good enough* parent? Tehee, Honan, and Hevey (2009) emphasized the fact that "decreasing parental stress could have positive implications for child behavior management" (p. 42). The authors go on to explain that "behavioral programs for children with severe presentation to be more effective when parental stress had been dealt with prior to intervention" (p. 42).

How does the child's symptomatology affect the psychosynthesis of her or his parents?

Salazar (as cited in Undurti et al., 2019) explained the importance of parenting as in order to reach optimal development, infants and children need to receive "sensitive and responsive caregiving" (p. 219). Hence, a parent needs to be attuned to the child's needs since birth, at which time *transactional* conversations are initiated. The success of this process depends on the ability of both parents and their child to communicate their needs clearly to their responding parent. Salazar explains that in cases where the child has an ASD *attunement*, "the sharing of affective states" (p. 220) between the child and parent becomes challenging. Difficulties in what she described as "coorientation" may be detrimental in the child's "integrated development" that involves "motor, cognitive, social, emotional, and communication skills" (p. 220).

Magalhães and Pereira (2017) explained that parents may experience reduced feelings of parenting competence due to the "decreased reciprocity" (p. 241) and the behaviors characterized by a lesser emotional involvement exhibited by the child. Additionally, the "relationship between parents and the siblings of children with ASD may be further compromised and neglected by the immense time and care that the child with ASD requires. Siblings feel neglected, alone and concerned about the future of the child with ASD" (pp. 241–242). In general, the family appears to adopt a more *rigid* mode of adaptation that may lead to the family's isolation, reduced engagement with the family circles, and decreased participation in recreational activities. The above may simply reveal a shaped behavior of the family to shield their child from an unfriendly—if not hostile—society. The family as a unit appears to not function at optimal levels and their quality of life suffers as a result.

Are we not a dynamic family system?

As Papaneophytou et al. (2019) explained, *agape*—the ultimate kind of love—allows both the person diagnosed with ASD and her/his parents (and siblings/family) to heal. As he proposed, all aspects surrounding the family—via the 360° approachto autism—need to be based on and stem from love for our fellow human being. This includes "therapy, education, research, technology, design, development, behavior, daily living and the way we treat each other" (p. xxxi). Crisis and adaptation are factors affecting the entire family as a dynamic system. Being able to adjust is imperative in enjoying a good quality of life.

Models such as the double ABCX model (McCubbin & Patterson, 1983) indicating levels of *adjustment* and *adaptation* describe how *facilitation* by social support and coping enable the family to adapt to a crisis. As such, it appears that certain interrelated so-called risk factors may affect parental stress. These risk factors include the characteristics of the person with ASD, any social support the family may have at its disposal and family members' coping strategies. Since just like with autism, there is a range of behaviors exhibited by people on the spectrum, stress levels of parents may be differentially impacted.

Salazar (2019) reminds us that if:

> *Day-to-day life is more limited, more insular, and less varied, then the child with ASD becomes more rigid, more patterned, and more inflexible. Parents may unwittingly allow repetitive, isolated, and solitary play in an effort to prevent behavioral outbursts (dysregulation). They may encourage an overfocus on preferred, academic interests (the alphabet of colors) in a misguided effort to promote cognitive skills. Or, they may not realize the importance of reciprocal interactions by others such as family members and outside of caregiving. In such situations, both the child and the family need guidance to support the development of flexible social, communication, behavioral, and interpersonal skills so that the child's experiences can be more fully integrated into the world of people and things (pp. 221–222).*

The frequency of behavioral issues and their symptom severity are discussed by Miranda et al. (2019) as factors pertinent to the cognitive sphere. Though such developmental issues are of course characteristic of the specific child, they do act as stressors for the respective parent in question. Other studies have examined the role of personal, as well as social resources, vis-à-vis parenting stress levels and coping.

In their longitudinal study of how resources available to parents affect their levels of stress, Zaidman-Zait et al. (2017) examined the stress level of mothers (younger children with ASD; $N = 283$). According to the authors, results indicate that in instances where mothers applied the social support available to them at high levels and they utilized "active engaged strategies" (p. 155), their levels of stress decreased. The child's behavioral issues and the level at which she or he externalized those, decreased family functionality, and the mother's disengaged strategies of coping were variables indicating higher parental stress.

The perceived level parental attachment is also important in this discussion on stress. Goodman and Glenwick (2012) examined attachment and how its perception in parents of autistic children correlates. In this study, the researchers examined how parents of young children (aged 2–10 years old) with a diagnosis of ASD perceived their child's attachment to them. Their sample of 76 mothers and 30 fathers led them to conclude that "perceptions of child-to-parent attachment were related to other aspects of parenting for fathers more than mothers" (p. 1453).

In their study, Reed, Howse, Ho, and Osborne (2017) explored the severity of ASD in conjunction with the mother's perceived ability to set limits to their child's behavioral issues and their own stress levels ($N = 93$). In this study, the mothers filled out two questionnaires to assess their child's level of functioning in accordance to ASD symptoms (Social Communication Questionnaire) and areas pertinent to their child's behaviors (Strength and Difficulties Questionnaire). In addition, the mothers filled out the Questionnaire of Resources and Stress to assess their own experiences of stress. As Reed et al. explained, "higher parenting stress negatively related to judgements about other's limit-setting skills ... stress negatively impacts a wide range of judgements and implies that caution may be required when interpreting the results of studies in which parenting skills are assessed by self-report" (p. 952).

Does the IQ affect stress levels?

One may think that perhaps—for whatever reason—a higher IQ in individuals on the autism spectrum may lead to less stress for their family and yet, nothing could be further from the truth. According to research discussed by Miranda et al. (2019) "parents of children with high-functioning autism report significantly higher levels of stress and lower levels of adaptive coping and resources than parents of children with typical development. They also describe negative experiences and lower quality of life" (p. 465). Da Paz and Wallender (2017) state that the "IQ level appears to be associated with parenting stress" (p. 2) specifically what is referred to as *manipulative IQ*. Who would have thought that people diagnosed with ASD can—just like the rest of *us*—exhibit manipulative behaviors?

The effect of stress on parents

We are interested in understanding and resolving any issues that may elevate a parent's stress level in association with the increased susceptibility to experience symptoms of depression and anxiety of parents of children on the autism spectrum. It is not unusual for a parent to have excess amounts of guilt and anger that may in turn be detrimental to both their physical, as well as to their psychological, well-being. Difficulties with a child's unpredictable behaviors, hurdles met throughout the diagnosis process, limited understanding of "autism" and impaired social relationships due to poor acceptance all compound to increase the potentially deleterious impact on one's family. Rejection by the extended family and society in general, or the perception of that rejection thereof, paired with unmet needs and the worries regarding the child's future, may deplete a family member's internal core strengths leading them to marasmus, or enable other unpleasant psychosomatic conditions. Can stress levels be predicted based on the behavior exhibited by the child?

Da Paz and Wallender (2017) highlighted the relationship between behaviors resulting from a person's ASD diagnosis as having the "capacity to predict parental stress" (p. 2). Specifically, the authors explain that the more severe the features of autism are in a child the more the mother of that child may experience stress and/or other psychopathological symptoms. As discussed by Da Paz and Wallander, a child's "self-isolated/ritualistic and repetitive behaviors are associated with poorer parent outcomes and with the mother's anxiety and depression" (p. 2). The link between the stress level experienced by a parent and the emotional and behavioral problems (EBPs) experienced or exhibited by children with ASD is discussed, particularly in an environment where there may be comorbid disorders diagnosed (i.e., ADHD). "Early autism" and the associated lack of skills and other deficits "such as a lack of joint attention, social responsiveness, or communication skills" (p. 2) become more evident around the age of 6 years old. At that time, parents may need more support. As Da Paz and Wallander explain, "the lack of perceived change in the child's problems is one of the factors that may justify, at least partly, the absence of changes in the levels of parenting stress, thus indicating the importance of intervention" (p. 2). To the above, social sigma may be more intense as the child with ASD gets older.

Yorke et al. (2018) explain that the more children exhibit EBPs, the more their parents experience psychological distress. The challenges put forth by children with ASD may reflect well beyond mood disorders and the above authors suggest additional research to investigate the effect of such behaviors and *psychosis*. In either case, research portrays a picture whereby the more the parental stress, the less their ability to exhibit good parenting behaviors. Thus stress has a compromising effect on parents' abilities to be, or to remain "good enough," parents.

Parental distress can be predicted to a significant degree according to Da Paz and Wallender (2017). As the child's problems of emotional and behavioral nature increase, the stress experienced by the parents also increases. Conversely, according to the Da Paz and Wallander, "stress related to a dysfunctional parent–child relationship is associated with daily living, communicational skills, and cognitive abilities" (p. 2). Does how well a family adapt to the variables discussed above make a difference regarding their stress levels experienced?

Da Paz and Wallender (2017) discuss the "Double ABCX Model" which is the way a family adapts its view would place it within the range of "maladaptation" and "bonadaptation." Bonadaptation exists in families where there is a "minimal discrepancy between the demands and the family's capabilities, in order to achieve a balance in family functioning" (p. 3). In explaining the use and function of the Double ABCX Model the above authors state the variables it explores:

> *A (the crisis-precipitating event/stressor); B (the family's crisis-meeting resources); C (the definition the family makes of the event), and X, (the crisis). Thus, the model explains the factors associated with families' adjustment to chronic stressors, including life tensions prior to or following the stressful event, the outcome of family processes in response to the stressor (in terms of resources and the definition of the event), and finally factors that are part of the family's attempt to adapt to the crisis, such as coping skills and social support (p. 3).*

Obviously, both the availability and use of "coping strategies" by a family would render different results regarding the stress levels experienced. That, in turn, would "dictate" their quality of life and enjoyment of it herewith.

In explaining the difference between the two main coping strategies people employ, Da Paz and Wallender (2017) articulated:

> *Two blocks of coping strategies have been emphasized: problem-focused coping strategies, which aim to solve the problem or do something to actively change one's perception of a stressor (e.g., engagement and positive reframing), and emotion-focused coping strategies, which aim to reduce or manage the feelings of distress (e.g., escape-avoidance, denial, and distraction) (p. 3).*

Hence, adopting a positive, problem focused strategy will be bound to render less stress and an increased quality of life; maternal stress decreases as coping strategies that help increase, as the authors explained. As such, "for both fathers and mothers, the severity of the disorder and the behavioral problems have a direct and positive effect on stress, with the sense of coherence and active avoidance coping strategies playing a mediator role in both cases" (p. 3).

On a "physiological level" and as Keil et al. (2010) explain, there is evidence indicating that there is a connection between parental autoimmune diseases and ASD in children. Based on the research conducted in Sweden and from analyzing studies that took place in Denmark, the authors explain that mothers of children on the spectrum have a higher risk for diabetes mellitus, ulcerative colitis, and psoriasis. Both fathers and mothers have increased risk of developing rheumatoid arthritis. Conversely, they concluded that children of parents who did have autoimmune disorders had a 50% chance to become autistic by the age of 10 years old. The authors had various hypotheses for this observation they made.

Before we delve into looking directly into the specific details shared by parents in each of the case studies discussed below it is worth looking at some of the elements people who live with people on the autism spectrum are familiar with, or troubled by, in most cases. Are there interventions that may defer, mitigate, or prevent mental health issues in parents of children with ASD?

Interventions leading to improved mental health for parents of children with ASD

Tehee et al. (2009) clarified that ASD renders issues pertinent to "the most complex network of family stressors" (p. 34) and the authors cited research conducted in the 1980s regarding coping strategies vis-à-vis resources available to parents. In order to decrease the vulnerability of parents and their potential levels of stress they must be provided with social support enabling them to meet their "emotional, practical and informational needs" (p. 34). Specifically, Tehee et al. (2009) articulated that:

> *The link between support and information demonstrates that providing parents with information may improve their access to support services, hence improving their ability to cope and effectively reduce stress levels ... parents' needs and concerns may be subject to change as their children enter different stages of development ... services should be user-led and parents' appraisals of the efficacy and availability of resources when planning for service provision should be taken into account. Information and support services should be coordinated in order to ease families through changes in their child's development and tailor services accordingly (p. 42).*

As such, according to the above authors, providing effective ways to assist parents with children on the spectrum is imperative. All elements affecting one's stress and mental health need be investigated. Many parents utilize mindfulness techniques to cope with stress. Does mindfulness work one may ask? Beer, Ward, and Moar (2013) investigated the relationship between mindfulness, parenting, and affective distress in parents of children with ASD. The authors asserted that higher levels of mindful parenting were related to lower levels of depressive symptoms and stress. Conner and White (2014) discussed ways by which mothers of children with ASD have the capacity to protect themselves against the deleterious effects of stress. Hence, the authors proposed that mindfulness-based interventions were ideal in such cases. Does one's personality and level of *hardiness* play a protective role, one may ask?

Weiss et al. (2013) investigated family hardiness, social support, and self-efficacy in mothers of individuals with ASD. The authors proposed that the variables mentioned above are important in how a mother experiences both life stressors and her child. The results of the study indicate that accumulated stressors and parental distress may be understood within the schema of the mother's comprehension of hardiness, which in turn is dependent upon variables such as the availability of social support and the mother's self-efficacy. Hence, Weiss et al. proposed that targeted interventions are needed to enhance parents' hardiness and allow them to deal with compounded impact of long-term stress. Foody et al. (2015) suggested that "parents of children with ASD may benefit from routine health screening (particularly adrenal and cardiovascular function) and referral for stress reduction interventions or supports" (p. 1084). Stress is also associated with self-efficacy. Kuhn and Carter (2006) proposed that the self-efficacy levels of parents played a role in their ability to modulate their own levels of stress. Therefore the authors suggested that "parent-and family-based interventions designed to support parental well-being and focusing on parenting cognitions may enhance parenting self-efficacy" (p. 564).

Da Paz and Wallender (2017) stated that "treatment produced medium to large effect sizes with improvements in parenting stress and general health, and reductions in depressions and anxiety" (p. 1). Interventions that appeared promising included: "stress management, relaxation techniques, expressive writing, mindfulness-based stress reduction, and acceptance and commitment therapy" (p. 1). As Da Paz and Wallander explained, there is a relationship between the "difficult child" and parental stress levels. De Paz and Wallander cite research in support of the fact that *temperament* and other "learned patterns of defiance, non-compliance, and demanding behavior" (p. 2) impact parental stress levels. The behaviors of the child allow parents to "identify family stress as being directly related to behavioral factors of the child, such as hyperactivity, demandingness, and disturbed mood" (p. 2).

The guidelines offered under the American Psychiatric Association (2020) has specific advice for parents of children with ASD, which includes: "learn as much as possible about autism spectrum disorder; provide consistent structure and routine; connect with other parents of children with autism; seek professional help for specific concern and take time for yourself and other family members" (p. 1).

Having a child with autism affects the whole family. It can be stressful, time-consuming, and expensive. Paying attention to the physical and emotional health of the whole family is important. Many national and local advocacy organizations provide information, resources, and support to individuals with ASD and their families. However, could it be that the most important tool when dealing with people with ASD lays with their *very own parents* and *families*? Tippy (as cited in Undurti et al., 2019) explains that though parents need to hear the advice provided by experts, they ought not follow that advice blindly. Alas, Tippy offered suggestions on the kinds of things parents *need* to *want* for their child as: "happiness, respect, meaningful work, independence, love, freedom, - to think, - to do, - to not do, - to make mistakes" (p. 178). It appears that the factor of *love* is a repeated one in the cards of people who for years have worked with and researched ASD and the families impacted by it.

Are there benefits in having early intervention and if so, what?

Magalhães and Pereira (2017) discussed research that focuses on what effects and benefits may be rendered by the adoption of an Early Intervention strategy and family support. Evidently, not all professionals pay attention to the concerns the family may present. Instead, the focus seems to be just on the child and her/his ASD symptoms. Hence, the authors propose that professionals need to ask, identify, and handle parental concerns, as well as offer solutions as to how the parent will be supported. An evaluation of those means of parental support need also take place because Early Intervention may be able to alleviate parental stress pertinent to the child's potential impairments in the areas of lack of eye contact, limited or no speech, behaviors viewed as unusual, low frustration tolerance, and repetitive interest.

The inclusion of children and their families in social activities, education, and recreational activities has the potential to enhance everyone's quality of life. To address this, it is imperative that local authorities show an added responsibility in support of people with ASD and their families. Freeman and Paparella (2019) stipulate "play, joint attention, eye contact and peer interaction" (p. 201) as areas to be included in the social engagement skills proposed. Evidently, the "most effective techniques are those which take into account child characteristics" (p. 201). Teachers, nurses, therapists, pediatricians, psychologists, and social workers are but a few professionals that have a significant role to play in addressing the different areas of functioning impacted by ASD. In working closely with governmental ministries (i.e., Ministry of Labor, Health, and Education), it is imperative that an effort be made in order to not only identify the number of children with ASD during the early stages of development, but to provide the much needed support to them and their families diachronically. Freeman and Paparella insist that though addressing behavioral challenges may be important "social skills and adaptive training lag well behind ... In the absence of a call for change, generally poor outcomes will continue to be reported for adaptive skills of all children, adolescents, and adults with ASD" (p. 208).

Stakeholders need a common paradigm of sorts for plans to be initiated and for goals to be met. Starting with the evaluation process, then the individualized education plan, and through offering appropriate social support—specific to the person/community—resources can be deployed with prudence. The three ministries mentioned above can offer formal, internal support and collaborate with various committees that may be in place to protect children and youngsters—all the while allowing for a smooth transition to all educational settings via a constant collaboration with teachers, parents, and other involved parties.

Salazar (2019) offers specific suggestions on what it is therapists may be able to help the families with following an ASD diagnosis:

1. to build their understanding of the road ahead;
2. to help them understand their child's unique neurobiopsychosocial needs (and their own);
3. to assess their capacities and strengths;
4. to strengthen their confidence and commitment; and
5. to build their engagement, reciprocity, problem solving, and symbolic capacities (pp. 224–225).

As Salazar explained, a good therapist—and we would add that new health insurance trends have almost turned the parents into self-directed therapists—needs to encourage, coach effectively, ignite genuine curiosity, reflect on experiences, and discuss daily life, goals, and issues. Nowadays, best practices call for at least 25 hours per week of intervention and treatment focusing on social skills, basic communication, and play that is appropriate for the child's developmental age.

Wieder (as cited in Undurti et al., 2019), cofounder of the Developmental, Individual-difference, and Relationship model (DIR model) for treating autism, discussed the importance of relationships and the importance of "parent-mediated intervention" (p. 236). Wieder explains that "developmental science is shifting away from behavioral reductionism to a relational developmental perspective with its emphasis on mutually influencing components of dynamic change" (p. 236). The positive effects of parent-mediated intervention are relationship based with long-term effects particularly when it pertains to social interactions in preschool age children.

In discussion of the role of play in the DIR Model, Foley (as cited in in Undurti et al., 2019) explains how children on the autism spectrum have difficulty in play in that they prefer solitary play and often fixate on the sensorimotor level. Hence, if prompted and scaffolded, these children may be able to engage in symbolic play similar to neurotypical children. Foley suggested play as part of "the treatment armamentarium for working with young children with ASD" (p. 382).

Early relationships are also important in the application of the Mifne Approach to the ASD intervention, discussed by Alonim et al. (as cited in Undurti et al., 2019). According to the authors, The Mifne Approach is:

> *A method developed to help the infant discover the sense of self and the pleasure of human contact . . . the development of the self in fact occur during the first year of life within the context of the mother-child relationship. Yet, development of the self in fact is one of the core impairments in the phenomenon of autism (2013). The goal of the treatment is to enable the growth of self-confidence, trust, and to stimulate the infant's motivation to engage in social interaction (p. 281).*

Alonim, Lieberman, Tayar, Scheingesicht, and Braude (2019) explained that this intervention utilizes specifically designed play for infants on the spectrum or the "prodrome" of it; this play is called Reciprocal Play Therapy (RPT). RPT "consists of three components, which may occur in parallel, i.e., 'attractive play,' 'sensory play,' and 'cognitive play'" (p. 281). Through filmed sessions, the authors articulate, this approach offers feedback to participating parents who apply and internalize "therapeutic insights and behaviors in their daily life" (p. 283).

As we discussed above emotional and behavioral challenges need to be targeted along with a skillset which includes academic, social, interpersonal, and communication skills. Provided such variables are processed in and out of "therapy," the quality of life ought to improve not just for the individual with an ASD diagnosis but for the entire family as a dynamic system.

Case studies

Content proposed to the parents of ASD children as food for thought

In our attempt to offer specific, experiential, life content regarding each of the people interviewed here, based both on research and shared clinical experience, we led the parents to some critical thinking around various daily life concerns. Personal communication was conducted by Alexandra Harrison, MD, assistant professor psychiatry at Harvard University on March 13, 2020. Based on our previous work, research, and publications, as well as in line with the works of our think tank, the concerns we anticipated would be universally applied. We feel such *universal concerns* would reflect heavily on families around the globe independent of their country of residence (i.e., autism diagnosis). Hence, we asked parents from various countries to complete our brief, narrative questionnaire (see Appendix A) and shed light on their daily life and stress levels. Parents from Cyprus, Egypt, India, Israel, Russia, and the United States contributed feedback as to their levels of stress, triggers, coping, etc.

Specifically, given each person's individual and clinical data shared, we wanted to explore concerns ranging from the parents' own intuition and medical evaluation process leading to their child's ASD diagnosis, to nutrition and self-reliance, among other experiences, vis-à-vis the parents' of stress (see Appendix A).

Case study 1

The parent reporting is the 59-year-old mother of a 29-year-old male who was initially diagnosed with "atypical autism" at the age of 3 years old. The pseudonym "Amyr" will be used, which means "prince" in Arabic. As per the mother's report, Amyr is also diagnosed with "epilepsy, communication disorder, sensory processing disorder, and intellectual disability." The family's native tongue is Arabic, and English is their second language. Amyr resides at home with his mother who takes care of him along with the help of "a live-in house-keeper/nanny." The mother reports that Amyr suffers from high blood pressure and has knee problems.

Amyr is described as "non-verbal and uses gestures (Makaton signs) and a mobile application" to communicate. According to his mother, Amyr receives occupational therapy twice a week, as well as speech language therapy twice a week. The "rest of the time he has Life Skills sessions and works in a sheltered workshop in carpentry." Amyr's parents are "divorced and his father lives outside of the country." Amyr has a younger sister who is married and lives with her husband and children. Amyr has his own room in his mother's house and can take care of his self-care needs (i.e., bathroom, getting dressed, showered, eating, etc.) "with minimum verbal prompt."

The first section of the questionnaire dealt with "parental concerns—concerns about yourself." The responses of the mother to this section are as follows:

Asked about her concerns and intuition regarding the medical and other evaluation process leading to Amyr's ASD diagnosis, the mother explains:

> *My son has an uncle whom I now realize is on the spectrum but had never been diagnosed. If the family were open on why he is different, we would have had an earlier diagnosis and intervention. ASD was treated like intellectual disabilities back in the 90's, but I started a Disability Persons Organization (DPO) with other mothers and got a program in 1999 specialized in autism to use with our children.*

Asked about concerns over any financial and/or economic survival issues the mother stated:

> *As a single parent, I went through most of my inheritance and savings to maintain medical and education services for my children. I had to marry my daughter off all by myself as the father has been out of our life since the divorce, 20 years now. My concern is about my son having his needs covered by the governmental allowance, which actually would not cover his support services' expenses for half a week, not a month. I will soon reach my retirement and my income will be cut almost to half. So, I will start looking for consultation jobs to make up the difference.*

Asked about concerns regarding requirements for information needed, wanted, or demanded of her family through times by agencies, schools, doctors, etc., the mother explained:

> *I wrote up a "guide for my child's guardians" to lead them as to his needs and how to reach for them.*

Asked about socializing and her own needs for recreation and connection regarding herself and her spouse she explained that "our marriage was affected because of the time spent caring for my son." With regard to the needs for socializing between her and Amyr, the mother stated: "My son has no friends and even in big family gatherings he just sits around the cousins, and they do not initiate more than a 'hello' with him."

Regarding Amyr's sister, the mother states:

> *My daughter was affected by all the time that had to go to her brother's care, but I used to make it up with my quality time for us both together. Like half an hour before she sleeps, so that I catch up on what her day was like. Also, when my son started joining sleep over camps with his own teachers, this allowed more quality time with my daughter. It did make a difference in our relationship.*

The mother was asked regarding any unmet needs she may have had to which she responded: "I need some *me* time without feeling guilty about it." Asked about her own stress levels and/or any related side effects the mother stated:

> *Stress level is always high as my son is low functioning and has no sense of danger. He is also epileptic, and I am always on guard as to when he might get a fit.*

Regarding psychotherapy available to her the mother stated: "I went to psychotherapy (CBT) for two years and it helped me a lot."

Asked about spousal/relationship issues due to ASD in the family, the mother articulated that: "The issue led to the divorce as the father was not very accepting of the son, not of the time I spent with him for care or seeking services."

Asked about any formal techniques employed to reduce stress the mother exclaimed: "I used to do some pottery and painting, but I have no time now for it. At present, I use prayer and meditation to reduce stress."

As far as concerns regarding social, political, legal, or other issues affecting her family the mother said: "COVID-19 and the current social distancing is affecting our life routine."

Regarding any support systems available to her, the mother explained: "My family is my support system. I also have teachers who escort my son for social outings, overnight camps, but these are paid for."

The second section of the questionnaire dealt with parental concerns about their child.

Asked about concerns over the availability and quality of services and resources for her child, this mother reported: "Services are good but costly to maintain." Regarding Amyr's health and any restrictions to her son's imposed by the physical environment, this mother stated: "His epilepsy and keeping it under control. Also, poor sleep and how he drains us all."

As far as concerns over Amyr's speech, movement, processing, self-care, and overall presentation, the mother shared that:

> *His communication is limited, and he does not seem to be bothered to try anything, even the mobile application is hardly used by him unless his teachers insist. His self-care is not bad but his dependence on verbal prompt need to be stopped.*

Regarding Amyr's education, the mother stated that: "He is 29, so this is not applicable." Asked about her concerns as far as Amyr's independent living, the mother shared that:

> *In our country, all children stay at home till they get married. So, my concern is his independent life skills not independent living. He will always live with the family, and when I pass away, he would live with his sister's family.*

Responses to questions regarding concerns about Amyr having friends, finding a life partner, and his self-esteem were qualified as "not applicable" by Amyr's mother. Regarding employment or employability, vocational training, Amyr's mother stated: "He works under supervision in a sheltered workshop and gets no pay in the end because we have to pay the Job Coach who escorts him all the time."

Asked about concerns regarding Amyr's anger and the way he externalizes his anger, this mother explained: "Not applicable. My son is fairly tempered."

Regarding Amyr's eating habits, needs involving nutrition/diet and preferences, the mother articulated:

> *He is on a gluten-free, casein-free diet, so often he cannot join the family lunches as most of the food will be off his list. We easily find alternatives.*

When it comes to concerns over techniques regarding Amyr's stress reduction employed by her family, the mother explained that "taking long walks helps a lot." Regarding any other concerns over Amyr's unmet life needs the mother stated that "His sexual life is limited." The mother did not elaborate on the open-ended questions regarding her child and her family; no more comments were offered.

Case study 2

The parent reporting is the 66-year-old father of a 30-year-old male who was diagnosed with "Autistic Spectrum Disease" at the age of 7 years old; let us call this autistic male Francois. The family's mother tongue is French. The father states that Francois resides at home with his parents who are physically healthy. Francois's parents are his primary caregivers. Francois has a "37-year-old sister who is married and has two children." Francois, according to his father, is not verbal; however, he "communicates using sign language" and "facilitated communication on the computer." He has his own room and he can take care of his own daily living needs "with some help."

Regarding Francois's therapy regimen, the father's response addressed the issue by stating that he "is on a gluten-free diet since a couple of months; he has other nutritional restrictions." Francois's father denied having any concerns over issues pertinent to his son's initial evaluation process and diagnosis of ASD. He also denied having any concerns over financial, informational, or medical records needed through time. The father responded "yes" to concerns pertinent to his own need to socialize, recreation, and connection, but he did not provide further elaboration. He acknowledged he had concerns regarding both himself and his wife socializing with Francois but did not elaborate further.

Francois's father agreed that he had unmet needs himself and that he experienced stress. Despite this, the father indicated that no psychotherapy was available to him. He denied any spousal problems due to ASD in the family. He denied having concerns over stress reduction techniques and his own ability to handle stress, however he did not elaborate any further. He did not discuss any concerns over the social, political, or legal environments affecting his family. Though he did not state which support systems they had at their disposal, he denied having any issues concerning this question and stated "no concerns" over religion or other philosophical systems, or whether any such systems were perceived to be support systems to him, or to his family.

The second part of the questionnaires dealt with parental concerns about their child.

Asked about the type and quality of services and resources available, including their functionality and purpose to Francois and to his family, the father explained:

> *French society is so far unable to provide "advanced" innovative services. Francois is just spending three days a week, half a day in a Center for child with different troubles. They have different activities that he likes very much.*

Though he stated "yes, for sure" to the question about having concerns over Francois's health, he did not elaborate any further. Regarding his concerns about his son's speech, movement, processing, self-care, and overall presentation Francois' father articulated: "Yes, overall, but we are progressing (except for speech, but we understand each other quite well!)."

Asked about concerns over Francois's education, the father explained: "Francois has got a very good education with his mother at home (mathematics, history, literature, chemistry, and physics)." Though his response to the question regarding Francois's independent living ability was affirmative, he did not elaborate beyond the simple "yes, sure." Asked about his concerns over the issue of Francois having friends or not he stated "Yes, he has no friends, but he is OK with his sister, her husband and their friends, as well as with our friends."

His response to the question regarding concerns over Francois finding a life partner or getting married was brief: "Sure, but no hopes for this." Regarding concerns about Francois's self-esteem, his father stated: "Yes and no." Regarding concerns over vocational rehabilitation, employment, training, etc., he stated: "Yes, he could somehow work, but I do not see reasons to hope, at least in France."

Francois's father denied his son had any anger related issues and had no concerns over that issue. Regarding his son's eating habits and concerns over Francois's nutrition habits and preferences, he explained: "Not a big concern. Francois eats well, with some restrictions, but big appetite." Though he stated "yes and no" to the question about having concerns over Francois's ability to employ stress reduction techniques, he did not elaborate any further.

Asked about his son's and his family's unmet needs, Francois' father stated: "Need more opportunities for socialization" and explained that concerns over the family were the "same as for Francois."

Case study 3

The parent reporting is the 31-year-old mother of a 7-year-old boy diagnosed with "ADHD and autism" at 2 years of age. The mother denied any physical health comorbidity and explained the child is healthy and lives at home with both his parents who take care of him. We will use the pseudonym Hercules for this autistic boy.

Hercules's mother stated her son has no siblings, does not have his own room, and he is unable to take care of his own basic needs. Asked regarding any concerns regarding the evaluation process that led to Hercules' diagnosis, she simply stated "following doctor's prescription" but did not offer any additional feedback. Hercules's mom denied having any concerns over financial issues.

Regarding concerns over information needed through the years by Hercules's schools, doctors, agencies, etc., she simply stated: "His activities during school time." Asked about her concerns over her own needs for recreation and connection with her husband, she responded by saying "as such nothing." Hercules's mother denied having any unmet needs of her own and asked regarding concerns over her own stress levels she articulated: "Sometimes overthinking about the future." She denied having any concerns regarding psychotherapy available to her, and stated that "it sometimes happens" when asked about having any concerns over spousal issues due to ASD in the family.

Hercules's mother denied having concerns over formal stress reduction techniques and stated "nothing as such"—it is unclear what she meant by that statement. In a similar fashion, she denied any concerns over her own ways of handling stress and utilizing coping mechanisms. Hercules's mother denied having concerns over the social, political, legal, or other environment affecting her family.

Regarding her actual or potential support systems, Hercules's mother explained that she "always try to help him in doing things." She denied having any concerns about their religion as a support system. When it came to parental concerns over their child, more specifically about the type and quality of services and resources available to Hercules, she explained that "we always try to give him the best." Asked about concerns over Hercules's health and any restrictive environments, she stated: "He cannot adjust in new places." Regarding concerns over Hercules's speech, movement, processing, self-care, and processing, she explained: "Yes, delay in speech is major concern."

Asked about her concerns over Hercules's education she responded by saying: "Not actually, as he is autistic, but yes, sometimes." With regard to concerns over Hercules's potential for independent living she explained: "Yes, a lot. One of the major concerns." She denied having concerns over Hercules having friends, without indicating if he did or did not have any friends. Asked about concerns regarding Hercules finding a life partner or getting married she stated: "I don't know." She did not address the question regarding Hercules's self-esteem and offered a "check mark" at the question concerning Hercules's future employment and vocational rehabilitation.

In regard to concerns over Hercules' potential anger with his mother, father, or others, and the way such anger may be externalized or internalized, his mother stated: "He is attention defeat, so concerned," but did not elaborate any further. She denied having any concerns over Hercules's eating habits and stated "mobile" regarding the question on concerns over Hercules's stress reduction needs. Regarding the open-ended question and her overall concerns for her son, she articulated: "Want him to be self-dependent so that he can lead a normal life."

Case study 4

The parent reporting is the 47-year-old mother of a 14-year-old boy diagnosed with "high functioning autism" at the age of 2½ years old. Let us use the pseudonym Basilis (meaning king, in their native tongue, Greek) for this autistic boy. The mother reports that Basilis lives at home with both of his parent and his 18-year-old-brother. She stated that Basilis has his own room. She reported that Basilis has "some sensory issues" but is otherwise "physically healthy." According to his mother, Basilis is verbal and he currently attends psychotherapy. He actively participates in a Boy Scout troop, which according to his mother "was the most effective." Basilis, his mother explains, "had speech therapy, sensory integration therapies, and special ed at times before." As the mother stated Basilis can take care of his own basic needs.

Asked regarding parental concerns and her own intuition regarding the medical evaluation process leading to Basilis's ASD diagnosis, the mother states: "No concerns there, all smooth." The mother denied any financial concerns. Asked regarding concerns over requirements for information needed by agencies, schools, doctors, etc., the mother stated:

> *School treated him as a Special Needs and hindered his abilities, he was very protected, did not flourish, nobody could see his potential, only saw the special behavioral issues.*

Basilis's mother denied having any concerns over her own, or her husband's needs for recreation and/or socializing. She explained her concerns over her son's inability to "communicate his inner needs easily, he never complains, he is an extreme introvert." When asked about any concerns over any unmet needs of hers, Basilis' mother states: "I wish I could get into his mind."

On the question concerning the mother's own stress levels and any side effects of this stress, Basilis' mother emphatically stated: "My stress levels are not connected to the child!" Asked regarding concerns over psychotherapy being available to her or not, Basilis' mother shared that:

> *Psychotherapy is available. The child has his therapist's number, knows that he can call her any time to talk—he never does. I am concerned about this disinterest to share or discuss anything.*

Basilis's mother denied any concerns emanating from having a person with diagnosis of ASD in the family. Regarding concerns about formal stress reduction techniques by her in order to manage stress she, again, emphatically stated: "N/A as my stress is unrelated to this issue." Asked about her own ways of handling stress and coping mechanisms applied, Basilis's mother offered: "N/A but reading/creative activities help."

Basilis's mother denied having any concerns about the social, political, legal/other environment affecting her family. She also denied having concerns over the actual support systems available to her and/or religion.

Asked regarding parental concerns over Basilis, including the type and quality of services and resources available to her child, as well as to his degree of functionality, Basilis's mother stated: "School is normally working via teleconferencing [and] even the Boy Scouts are having teleconferences." Concerning Basilis's health and any restrictive environments, his mother explained that: "He is too bored for any physical activity and it's hard to convince him to go out a bit." She denied having any concerns about Basilis's speech, movement, processing, self-care, and overall presentation, and she denied any concerns about Basilis's education.

When the question regarding concerns over Basilis's independent living, especially after the parents' passing was posed, the mother exclaimed: "Too early to think about this." Asked regarding concerns about Basilis's having friends or not, this mother stated: "He does not have close friends, but it does not concern him, I am a little concerned."

Basilis's mother stated she is "a little concerned" when asked about him finding a future life partner or wife. She denied having any concerns over Basilis's self-esteem or potential for employability, or for vocational training. Regarding any concerns over Basilis's potential anger she explained: "He has never demonstrated anger."

Asked about concerns over Basilis's eating habits she stated: "They have improved, so none." Regarding concerns over Basilis's techniques used for stress reduction his mother explained: "None, he has been trained" but offered no additional explanation. Though she denied Basilis had any unmet needs, she did offer feedback to the "other concerns" open-ended question:

> *He has become an extreme introvert and is happy spending the day doing assignments, reading, or watching videos about COVID-19, or playing video games. He does not seem to feel the need to interact with anyone, he is closed up in his own world and seems completely content in there. Because he is high functioning, he can take care of himself, as long as we give him food. But he is completely closed "down" and even though, he is being educated in the process, my concern is that he is stuck in a cocoon just when he was ready to get out of it all.*

Conclusion

ASD may at times be, as Ed Tronick, PhD, would call it, *messy* and *ugly*; however, parents can attest to the loving relationship and bonding between them and their autistic children. *Agape* may also include the need for *reparation* among other core elements in social, interpersonal, intrapersonal, and *inter alia* communication. Cognitive skills, trauma, level of education, financial stability, and a positive world view may all be factors weighing in when one discusses levels of stress and parenting. A well-rounded, 360-degree approach to scaffolding and supporting all family members has been suggested by Papaneophytou et al. (2019).

Ruby Salazar's (as cited in Undurti et al., 2019) *sensitive and responsive care-giving* need not only apply to infants but to parents and people on the spectrum as well. Humans respond to warmth and "tender loving care" as others may call this approach. Systems need to adjust their approach to accommodate for children and parents, as well as to the child inside each parent by offering unconditional positive regard, realistic support, and a hands-on approach along the person's lifetime.

The four case studies shared make the dynamic systems we all live in more evident. At the same time they may offer a dramatic picture of the joy, the sorrow, the chaos, the order, the denial, the acceptance, the love, the restricted forms of love, the abandonment, and the commitment many of us experience in a moment or in a lifetime. Humans, despite one's race, nationality, culture, history, creed, orientation, language spoken, educational level, and socioeconomic status, all hurt—or hurt the "other"—in similar ways. We all experience stress in similar ways and we all can benefit from responsive approaches from our schools, doctors, institutions, religious and other support systems, be it through COVID-19 times or thereafter.

We are all, truly, in this together as one. Let us walk a mile in any parent's shoes before we exclaim our judgment or project our critical dark shadow unto the "other." Light reflects more light and a calm positive attunement renders healthier lifestyles for most of us. Mindful parenting and healthy coping styles reduce stress and allow for longer, healthier, and more productive lives.

The *fear of isolation* presented during the COVID-19 era draws parallels with many parent's lives who remain entrenched in a lonely shell, perhaps for decades. One can expand on her/his capacity to become or remain resilient if s/he works on issues pertinent to repairing relationships with others, but perhaps most importantly if one works on repairing one's own self. According to Provenzi and Tronick (2020), "We will be able to overcome the fear of isolation and the consequences of this epidemic by achieving resilience through shared and co-constructed reparation" (p. 7).

Perhaps it is worth reiterating here APA's advice to all parents of autistic people:

1. Learn as much as possible about ASD
2. Provide consistent structure and routine
3. Connect with other parents of children with autism
4. Seek professional help for specific concerns
5. Take time for yourself and other family members (p. 1)

And once again, Salazar's (2019) specific suggestions on what therapists may be able to help the families with following an ASD diagnosis:

1. to build their understanding of the road ahead;
2. to help them understand their child's unique neurobiopsychosocial needs (and their own);
3. to assess their capacities and strengths;
4. to strengthen their confidence and commitment; and
5. to build their engagement, reciprocity, problem solving, and symbolic capacities (pp. 224–225).

Self-care, self-soothing, reaching out to experts and others, supporting each other, and scaffolding oneself all along the way, will enhance one's ability to stay composed, healthy, centered, and able to cope with daily stressors. Call it caring, unconditional positive regard, the *good breast*, love, or *agape*; whatever you call it just open your heart and offer it.

References

Alonim, A., Lieberman, I., Tayar, D., Scheingesicht, G., & Braude, H. (2019). A comparative study of infants and toddlers treated with the Mifne Approach Intervention for autism spectrum disorder. In D. Undurti, N. Papaneophytou, & T. El-Kour (Eds.), *Autism 360°* (pp. 277–300). Elsevier Science, Academic Press.

American Psychiatric Association. (2020). *Practice guidelines for the treatment of psychiatric disorders, autism: Tips for parents*. Retrieved on April 4, 2020, Available from <https://www.psychiatry.org/patients-families/autism/what-is-autism-spectrum-disorder>.

Beer, M., Ward, L., & Moar, K. (2013). The relationship between mindful parenting and distress in parents of children with an autism spectrum disorder. *Mindfulness*, *4*, 102–112. Available from https://doi.org/10.1007/s12671-012-0192-4.

Center for Disease Control. (2020). Community report on autism: Autism and developmental disabilities monitoring (ADDM) network. National center on birth defects and developmental disorders. Retrieved on April 4, 2020, Available from <https://www.cdc.gov/ncbddd/autism/addm-community-report/documents/addm-community-report-2020-h.pdf>.

Conner, C., & White, S. (2014). Stress in mothers of children with autism: Trait mindfulness as a protective factor. *Research in Autism Spectrum Disorders*, *8*(6), 617–624. Available from https://doi.org/10.1016/j.rasd.2014.02.001.

Da Paz, N. S., & Wallender, J. L. (2017). Intervention that target improvements in mental health for parents of children with autism spectrum disorders: A narrative review. *Clinical Psychology Review*, *51*, 1–14. Available from https://10.1016/doi.org.rlib.pace.edu/j.cpr.2016.10.006.

Dabrowska, A., & Pisula, E. (2010). Parenting stress and coping styles in mothers and fathers of pre-school children with autism and down syndrome. *Journal of Intellectual Disability Research*, *54*, 266–280. Available from https://doi.org/10.1111/j.1365-2788.2010.01258.x.

Dumas, J., Wolf, L., Fisman, S., & Culligan, A. (1991). Parenting stress, child behavior problems, and dysphoria in parents of children with autism, down syndrome, behavior disorders, and normal development. *Exceptionality*, *2*(2), 97–110. Available from https://doi-org.rlib.pace.edu/10.1080/09362839109524770.

Foody, C., James, J., & Leader, G. (2015). Parenting stress, salivary biomarkers, and ambulatory blood pressure: A comparison between mothers and fathers of children with autism spectrum disorders. *Journal of Autism and Developmental Disorders*, *45*, 1084–1095. Available from https://doi.org/10.1007/s10803-014-2263-y.

Freeman, S., & Paparella, T. (2019). Treatment in autism spectrum disorder: Areas of unmet need in the United States. In D. Undurti, N. Papaneophytou, & T. El-Kour (Eds.), *Autism 360°* (pp. 193–209). Elsevier Science, Academic Press.

Goodman, S. J., & Glenwick, D. S. (2012). Correlates of attachment perceptions in parents of children with autism spectrum disorders. *Journal of Autism and Developmental Disorders*, *42*, 2056–2066. Available from https://doi.org/10.1007/s10803-012-1453-8.

Hill, E., Berthoz, S., & Frith, U. (2004). Brief report: Cognitive processing of own emotions in individuals with autistic spectrum disorder and in their relatives. *Journal of Autism and Developmental Disorders*, *34*, 229–235. Available from https://doi.org/10.1023/B:JADD.0000022613.41399.14.

Keil, A., Daniels, J. L., Forssen, U., Hultman, C., Cnattingius, S., Söderberg, K. C., … Sparen, P. (2010). Parental autoimmune diseases associated with autism spectrum disorders in offspring. *Epidemiology (Cambridge, Mass.)*, *21*(6), 805–808. Available from https://doi.org/10.1097/EDE.0b013e3181f26e3f.

Kuhn, J. C., & Carter, A. S. (2006). Maternal self-efficacy and associated parenting cognitions among mothers of children with autism. *American Journal of Orthopsychiatry*, *76*, 564–575. Available from https://doi.org/10.1037/0002-9432.76.4.564.

Magalhães, L., & Pereira, A. (2017). Early intervention in autism spectrum disorder: Concerns and support of Portuguese mothers. *Education and Training in Autism and Developmental Disabilities*, *52*(3), 240–251. Available from https://doi.org/10.2307/26420397.

Mak, W., Ho, A., & Law, R. (2007). Sense of coherence, parenting attitudes and stress among mothers of children with autism in Hong Kong. *Journal of Applied Research in Intellectual Disabilities*, *20*, 157–167. Available from https://doi.org/10.1111/j.1468-3148.2006.00315.x.

McCubbin, H., & Patterson, J. (1983). The family stress process: The Double ABCX Model of adjustment and adaption. *Marriage & Family Review*, *6*(1-2), 7–37. Available from https://doi.org/10.1300/J002v06n01_02.

Miranda, A., Mira, A., Berenguer, C., Rosello, B., & Baixauli, I. (2019). Parenting stress in mothers of children with autism without intellectual disability: Mediation of behavioral problems and coping strategies. *Frontiers in Psychology*, *10*, 464. Available from https://doi.org/10.3389/fpsyg.2019.00464.

Papaneophytou, N., Undurti, D., & El-Kour, T. (2019). *Autism 360°*. Elsevier Science, Academic Press.

Phetrasuwan, S., & Shandor-Miles, M. (2009). Parenting stress in mothers of children with autism spectrum disorders. *Journal for Specialists in Pediatric Nursing*, *14*, 157–165. Available from https://doi.org/10.1111/j.1744-6155.2009.00188.x.

Poletaev, A., Poletaeva, A., Pukhalenko, A., Zamaleeva, R., Cherepanova, N., & Frizin, D. (2014). Adaptive maternal immune deviations as a ground for autism spectrum disorders development in children. *Folia Medica*, *56*(2), 73–80. Available from https://doi.org/10.2478/folmed-2014-0011.

Provenzi, L., & Tronick, E. (2020). The power of disconnection during the Covid-19 emergency: From isolation to reparation. *Psychological Trauma: Theory, Research, Practice, and Policy*, *12*(1), 252–254. Available from https://doi-org.rlib.pace.edu/10.1037/tra000061.

Reed, P., Howse, J., Ho, B., & Osborne, L. (2017). Relationship between perceived limit-setting abilities, autism spectrum disorder severity, behaviour problems and parenting stress in mothers of children with autism spectrum disorder. *Autism: The International Journal of Research and Practice*, *21*(8), 952–959. Available from https://doi.org/10.1177/1362361316658775.

Salazar, R. (2019). Full circle autism care includes family relationships and dynamics. In D. Undurti, N. Papaneophytou, & T. El-Kour (Eds.), *Autism 360°* (pp. 219–234). Elsevier Science, Academic Press.

Szatmari, P., Georgiades, S., Duku, E., Zwaigenbaum, L., Goldberg, J., & Bennett, T. (2008). Alexithymia in parents of children with autism spectrum disorder. *Journal of Autism and Developmental Disorders*, *38*(10), 1859–1865. Available from https://doi.org/10.1007/s10803-008-0576-4.

Tehee, E., Honan, R., & Hevey, D. (2009). Factors contributing to stress in parents of individuals with autistic spectrum disorders. *Journal of Applied Research in Intellectual Disabilities*, *22*, 34–42. Available from https://doi.org/10.1111/j.1468-3148.2008.00437.x.

Undurti, D., Papaneophytou, N., & El-Kour, T. (2019). *Autism 360°*. Elsevier Science, Academic Press.

Weiss, J., Robinson, S., Fung, S., Tint, A., Chalmers, P., & Lunsky, Y. (2013). Family hardiness, social support, and self-efficacy in mothers of individuals with autism spectrum disorders. *Research in Autism Spectrum Disorders*, *7*(11), 1310–1317. Available from https://doi.org/10.1016/j.rasd.2013.07.016.

Yorke, I., White, P., Weston, A., Rafla, M., Charman, T., & Simonoff, E. (2018). The association between emotional and behavioral problems in children with autism spectrum disorder and psychological distress in their parents: A systematic review and meta-analysis. *Journal of Autism and Developmental Disorders*, *48*(10), 3393–3415. Available from https://doi.org/10.1007/s10803-018-3605-y.

Zaidman-Zait, A., Mirenda, P., Duku, E., Vaillancourt, T., Smith, I. M., Szatmari, P., ... Thompson, A. (2017). Impact of personal and social resources on parenting stress in mothers of children with autism spectrum disorder. *Autism: The International Journal of Research and Practice*, *21*(2), 155–166. Available from https://doi.org/10.1177/1362361316633033.

Further reading

Provezi, L., Scotto di Minico, G., Giusti, L., Guida, E., & Muller, M. (2018). Disengaging the dyadic dance: Theoretical, methological and outcomes systematic review of mother-infant dyatic processes. *Frontiers in Psychology*, *9*, 1–22. Available from https://doi.org/10.3389/fpsyg.2018.00348.

Rossignol, D. A., & Frye, R. E. (2011). Mitochondrial dysfunction in autism spectrum disorders: A systematic review and meta-analysis. *Molecular Psychiatry*, *17*(3), 290–314. Available from https://doi.org/10.1038/mp.2010.136.

Appendix A

Thank you very much for agreeing to assist us with the publication of our new book/chapter. Our goal is to present the 'stories' and daily life regarding stress levels of parents of children on the spectrum. Please remember this is an *ANONYMOUS* questionnaire and a pseudo name/pseudo-initials only will be used for our publication purposes. All information provided *is* and will *remain* confidential!

Our new book is expected to be published by October 2020. We will keep you informed accordingly.

Kindly provide us with your family/child's information:

Are you the father, or the mother? Your age:
Child's gender:
Child's age now: Age diagnosed:
Diagnoses:

- Are there any comorbid/other diagnoses beyond Autism?

Is she/he residing at home with you? Other?

Who takes care of her/him?
Are they physically healthy?
Are they verbal and/or how do/if they communicate with you/others?
What is their therapy/intervention regimen?
Are the parents together, separated, divorced, other?
Are there any other children/siblings at home, or in your family?
Does the child have her/his own room?
Can he/she take care of his/her own needs (bathroom, get dressed, showered, eat, etc.?)

Below please answer each of the "concerns" listed in a narrative fashion; simply type in the space below each *concern*. Please do not use more words that needed and, in any event, kindly limit each response to below 80–100 words if possible:

1. *Parental concerns—concerns about yourself*:
  a. Concerns about (or simply discuss/explain) your own intuition regarding the medical/ other evaluation process leading to their child's ASD diagnosis:
  b. Concerns about (or simply discuss/explain) any financial and/or economic survival issues:
  c. Concerns about (or simply discuss/explain) requirements for information needed, wanted or demanded of you/family through times by agencies, schools, doctors, etc.:
  d. Concerns about (or simply discuss/explain) socializing and your *own* need for recreation and connection:
    i. For you and your spouse:
    ii. For you and your child:
    iii. For you and other siblings (with or without your spouse):
  e. Concerns about (or simply discuss/explain) any unmet needs of yours:
  f. Concerns about (or simply discuss/explain) your own stress levels (perceived; side effects):
  g. Concerns about (or simply discuss/explain) psychotherapy available or not available to you:
  h. Concerns about (or simply discuss/explain) spousal/relationship issues due to ASD in the family:
  i. Concerns about (or simply discuss/explain) formal techniques employed by you for stress reduction:
  j. Concerns about (or simply discuss/explain) your own ways of handling stress and coping mechanisms applied:
  k. Concerns about (or simply discuss/explain) social, political, legal or other environments affecting your family:
  l. Concerns about (or simply discuss/explain) your actual or potential support systems:
  m. Concerns about (or simply discuss/explain) religion or any other philosophical system [s] you may believe in as support systems:

2. *Parental concerns about your child*:
  a. Concerns about (or simply discuss/explain) the type and quality of services and resources available to your child, as well as to her/his degree of functionality and purpose to your child or to you/parents:
  b. Concerns about (or simply discuss/explain) your child's health and any physical health restrictions or restrictive environments:

c. Concerns about (or simply discuss/explain) your child's speech, movement, processing, self-care and overall presentation:
d. Concerns about (or simply discuss/explain) your child's education:
e. Concerns about (or simply discuss/explain) your child's independent living (especially after the parents' own passing):
f. Concerns about (or simply discuss/explain) your child having friends:
g. Concerns about (or simply discuss/explain) your child finding a life partner (or getting married):
h. Concerns about (or simply discuss/explain) your child's self-esteem:
i. Concerns about (or simply discuss/explain) your child's employment or employability, vocational training/other:
j. Concerns about (or simply discuss/explain) your child's anger with his mother, father and/or siblings and the way that anger is externalized or internalized:
k. Concerns about (or simply discuss/explain) her/his eating habits, needs and nutrition/diet habits and preferences:
l. Concerns about (or simply discuss/explain) techniques employed by your child for stress reduction:
m. Concerns about (or simply discuss/explain) your child's [any] unmet needs:
n. *Open ended*—Other Concerns about:
  i. Your child:
  ii. Your family:

Can bioactive lipids arachidonic and docosahexaenoic acids prevent autism and reduce its severity?

2

Undurti N. Das[1,2]
[1]UND Life Sciences, Battle Ground, WA, United States, [2]Department of Medicine, BioScience Research Centre, GVP College of Engineering, Visakhapatnam, India

Introduction

Autism has both a genetic and an environmental basis. Several factors concerned with inflammation, synapse formation, nerve transmission, and information processing may play a significant role in the pathobiology of autism. The concentrations and actions of brain-derived neurotrophic factor (BDNF), bioactive lipids arachidonic (AA), eicosapentaenoic (EPA), and docosahexaenoic acids (DHA) and their products and neurotransmitters dopamine, serotonin, acetylcholine, GABA (gamma-aminobutyric acid), and catecholamines and cytokines are altered in autism that may account for some of its clinical features and underlying pathobiology. Previously, I proposed that maternal infections may trigger inflammatory events that may adversely affect intrauterine growth of the fetus. This may lead to changes in gene expression profile and proteomics leading to dysfunction of the neuronal function(s) and alterations in the levels of various neurotransmitters accompanied by perturbations in the metabolism of polyunsaturated fatty acids (PUFAs) that ultimately result in the development of autism. PUFAs and their metabolites play a significant role in the synthesis and actions of various neurotransmitters, and participate in synapse formation and information processing in the brain. PUFAs and their metabolites can modulate the production of BDNF and influence gut microbiota and their metabolism.

Some of the factors that play a significant role in the pathophysiology of autism include both internal and external factors. Internal factors include inflammatory conditions that the mother may have at the time of pregnancy, gut microbiota of the mother, and bacterial metabolites.

Factors that influence the development of autism

Several studies revealed that maternal obesity is possibly a factor that can increase the risk of autism in children (Connolly et al., 2016). There appears to be a parallel increase in the incidence of obesity in young women and autism. Obesity is considered as a low-grade systemic inflammatory condition with elevated plasma interleukin-6

Emerging Programs for Autism Spectrum Disorder. DOI: https://doi.org/10.1016/B978-0-323-85031-5.00020-7

(IL-6), tumor necrosis factor-α (TNF-α) concentrations. Obesity is also associated with changes in gut microbiota, alterations in the hypothalamic neurotransmitters, insulin resistance, and dysregulated production of adipokines (Das, 2001, 2002a, 2010). If it is true that there is indeed a correlation between maternal obesity and autism in their progeny, it is expected that autism may also be showing similar abnormalities in gut microbiota, plasma cytokines, and hypothalamic neurotransmitters. Subjects with autism are known to have gastrointestinal problems and dysbiosis of gut microbiota (Bresnahan et al., 2015; Mayer, Tillisch, & Gupta, 2015; Parracho, Bingham, Gibson, & McCartney, 2005). The apparent crosstalk between the gut and the brain (termed as gut–brain axis) may perhaps explain how gut microbiota influence the development and function of brain (Cryan & Dinan, 2012; Mayer et al., 2015). It is likely that gut microbiota produces small-molecular-weight fatty acids called short-chain fatty acids (SCFAs), acetate, butyrate, and palmitate that can reach the brain via vagal fibers and influence brain growth and development. Thus gut microbiota may have a role in the pathobiology of autism. Previously, we showed that subjects with type 2 diabetes mellitus that is common in those with obesity have decreased circulating levels of BDNF. BDNF levels are also low in the brain of those with type 2 DM. In an extension of these studies we showed that BDNF levels revert to normal when diabetes mellitus is prevented by pretreatment with arachidonic acid (AA) and its antiinflammatory metabolite lipoxin A4 (LXA4) (Bathina, Srinivas, & Das, 2017; Naveen, Naidu, & Das, 2017a, 2017b). Furthermore, insulin is essential for brain growth and development. Thus those with obesity and type 2 diabetes mellitus may have abnormalities in brain growth and development due to altered levels of insulin (in the form of insulin resistance), BDNF, and increased concentrations of proinflammatory cytokines and altered gut microbiota (Araki, Yamamoto, Dobashi, Asayama, & Kusuhara, 2014; Das, 2002b, 2010).

Insulin, bioactive lipids, BDNF, and neurotransmitters in autism

Insulin is known to enhance acetylcholine (Ach) levels and Ach, in turn, regulates the production of several other hypothalamic neurotransmitters. It is noteworthy that Ach is a potent antiinflammatory molecule that can suppress the production of IL-6 and TNF-α (Borovikova et al., 2000). Ach stimulates LXA4 production (Serhan, de la Rosa, & Jouvene, 2018). Gut microbiota can regulate serotonin production in the gut by enterochromaffin cells (Reigstad et al., 2015). In addition, human brain is rich in AA and DHA. DHA is also the precursor of potent antiinflammatory molecules—resolvins, protectins, and maresins. One purpose of the presence of large amounts of AA and DHA in the brain is to produce appropriate amounts of LXA4, resolvins, protectins, and maresins as and when needed to prevent inflammatory events and enhance resolution of inflammation and restore homeostasis in the brain. Thus AA, DHA, LXA4, resolvins, protectins, and maresins are not only needed to regulate brain growth and development and synapse formation but also to protect brain from various endogenous ad exogenous inflammatory stimuli. Furthermore, these bioactive lipids are also regulators of the production and action of various neurotransmitters, such as BDNF Ach, dopamine, serotonin, and MSH. It is interesting to note that AA and DHA alter cell membrane fluidity and thus influence the expression of various receptors on the neuronal cell membrane including that of insulin. Thus there is a close interaction among brain lipids (AA and DHA), their antiinflammatory metabolites, BDNF, Ach, serotonin, insulin action, and cytokines that ultimately influence the growth and development of brain synapse formation and its strength, neurotransmission, and inflammatory events in the brain. We and others have also reported that AA and DHA can alter the gut microbiota and their function and metabolism (Yu, Jiang et al., 2014; Yu, Zhu et al., 2014). AA and DHA stimulate glucose uptake by neurons and enhance Ach release (Almeida, Cunha, & Ribeiro, 1999; Ximenes da Silva et al., 2002).

Bioactive lipids, cytokines, and autism

This evidence is in tune with the observation that patients with autism have low plasma concentration of AA and DHA and increased amounts of TNF-α and IL-6 and prostaglandin E2 (PGE2, a metabolite formed from AA that has proinflammatory actions), indicating that autism is a low-grade systemic inflammatory condition (Bell et al., 2004; Jory, 2016; Parletta, Niyonsenga, & Duff, 2016). Several other abnormalities (such as PTEN and p53 alterations, dopamine, serotonin) reported in autism can also be linked to altered concentrations of various PUFAs and their metabolites. Maternal high-fat diet induces behavioral alterations in their offspring that can be correlated to alterations in their gut microbiota (Shelly et al., 2016). Based on this evidence, it is suggested that a rational combination of AA and DHA when fed to the pregnant and lactating mothers, newborns, and children is likely to prevent the development of autism and may be useful to manage or reduce the severity of the disease.

PUFAs are essential for brain development and function

It is evident from the preceding discussion that there is a parallel increase in the incidence of obesity, in general, and maternal obesity, in particular, and neurodevelopmental disorders including autism spectrum disorder (ASD) in children. This correlation between obesity and ASD could be explained in part due to the association of obesity with low-grade systemic inflammation (Das, 2001, 2002a, 2010). There is evidence to suggest that ASD is associated with the activation of microglia and astrocytes and severe chronic inflammation both in the periphery and in multiple brain areas that could be related to increased plasma and CSF (cerebrospinal fluid) levels of tumor necrosis factor (TNF)-α, interleukin (IL)-1, IL-6, and interferon-γ (Al-Ayadhi, 2005; Chez, Dowling, Patel, Khanna, & Kominsky, 2007; El-Ansary & Al-Ayadhi, 2012; Vargas, Nascimbene, Krishnan, Zimmerman, & Pardo, 2005; Wei et al., 2011). It was opined that increased levels of proinflammatory cytokines as a result of maternal inflammation (secondary to obesity) may lead to inflammatory events and oxidative stress (due to an increase in free radical generation) during the development of brain that results in abnormalities in neuronal development, synapse formation, and changes in various neurotransmitters that ultimately results in ASD. In addition, animal studies revealed that pups born from obese mothers have decreased concentrations of BDNF that may result in a reduction in neuronal progenitor cell proliferation, atypical synaptic stability, and a reduction in dendrite length and branching (Hatanaka, Kabuta, & Wada, 2017; Tozuka, Wada, & Wada, 2009; Tozuka et al., 2010; Yu, Jiang et al., 2014; Yu, Zhu et al., 2014), all factors generally seen in mouse models of ASD. These results indicate that strategies developed to suppress abnormal inflammatory events (such as increase in the levels of proinflammatory cytokines) and restore BDNF levels to normal and providing appropriate factors needed for brain development, synapse formation, and restore neuropeptides to normal during the development of brain may help in the prevention of ASD. One such important factor that could be provided through diet is polyunsaturated fatty acids (PUFAs) that are essential for brain growth and development, normal synapse formation, and synthesis and action of various neurotransmitters in the brain, including BDNF.

Perinatal factors that influence development of autism

Insults during critical or sensitive periods in early life can have lifetime consequences and are termed *programming*. Early nutrition during the fetal period from the mother during pregnancy and lactation period and early childhood are important environmental programming factors. Thus nutrition during the fetal life and early childhood can have lifetime effects on metabolism, growth, and neurodevelopment, including pathobiology of autism (Lucas, Fewtrell, & Cole, 1999). The period from the third trimester of pregnancy to 5 years postterm are critical to the growth and development of human brain, breastfeeding is a important factor that can prevent in the development of autism. Breastfed children are not only protected from necrotizing enterocolitis, atopy, and childhood infection but also show higher cognitive development and lower blood pressure in adulthood and have lower frequency of obesity both in childhood and adults (Elliott, Kjolhede, Gournis, & Rasmussen, 1997; Kramer, 1981; von Kries, Kolletzko, Sauerwald, & von Mutius, 2000; Wolman, 1984). These beneficial actions of breast milk could be attributed to its higher content of AA and DHA. In addition, breast milk also contains significant amounts of LXA4, resolvins, protectins, and maresins.

Both AA and DHA form an important constituent of cell membrane and are essential for modulating cellular properties of neuronal cells (Auestad et al., 2003; Das, 2003a, 2003b, 2003c; O'connor et al., 2001). Hence, breastfeeding is important for brain health. This is supported by the observation that higher intake of AA/DHAs by the others before and during pregnancy tend to have children with low incidence of autism (Steinman & Mankuta, 2013). Both AA and DHA and their antiinflammatory LXA4, resolvins, protectins, and maresins suppress the production of neurotoxic

TNF-α, IL-1, and IL-6, protect neuronal cells from the cytotoxic actions of these cytokines, and enhance nitric oxide generation and improve memory formation and consolidation (Das, 2003a, 2003b, 2003c). It is likely that AA and DHA enhance glucose uptake by neuronal cells and augment Ach release by neurons. Increased glucose uptake enhances memory by increasing Ach release. Thus there is a crosstalk among glucose uptake, Ach release, and AA/DHA that ultimately results in improved learning ability. AA and DHA selectively modify membrane stability and integrity associated with reductions of GABA and glutamate uptake and of $(Na^+ + K^+)$-ATPase activity (Albrecht et al., 2000; Almeida et al., 1999; Chan, Kerlan, & Fishman, 1983; Hersi, Kitaichi, Srivastava, Gaudreau, & Quirion, 2000; Minami et al., 1997). Thus a close interaction(s) exists among AA/DHA (PUFAs), Ach, dopamine, GABA, glutamate, brain growth and development, and neuronal function that may play a role in the pathobiology of obesity and autism.

AA and DHA are critical for insulin secretion by pancreatic β cells (Itoh et al., 2003), by their action on GPR40, receptors for these fatty acids and expressed in the pancreas. Furthermore, insulin is needed for the activity of desaturases that are needed for the formation of AA and DHA from their dietary precursors linoleic acid (LA) and alpha-linolenic acid (ALA), respectively (Das, 2006a, 2006b).

Both obesity and autism are associated with altered levels of AA and DHA lending support to their (AA/DHA) role in these diseases.

How and why PUFAs are of benefit in ASD?

AA/DHA and their antiinflammatory metabolites lipoxins, resolvins, protectins, and maresins suppress the production of cytokines IL-6 and TNF-α and thus protect both pancreatic beta cells and neuronal cells (Naveen et al., 2017a, 2017b; Naveen, Naidu, & Das, 2018). Since both LXA4 (antiinflammatory in nature) and PGE2 (a proinflammatory molecule) are derived from AA, it implies that under physiological conditions a balance is maintained between these two metabolites of AA. In AA deficiency states, PGE2 synthesis is increased whereas that of LXA4 is decreased. On the other hand, supplementation of AA does not increase PGE2 levels but increases LXA4 (Tateishi, Kakutani, Kawashima, Shibata, & Morita, 2014; Tateishi et al., 2015). These results imply that supplementation of AA suppresses inflammation and thus can prevent autism.

It is noteworthy that high levels of TNF-α (and IL-6) can suppress the formation of AA and DHA from LA and ALA by its suppressive action on desaturases (Mayer et al., 2002), that in turn may lead to decreased formation of LXA4, resolvins, protectins, and maresins due to their respective precursor deficiency. Thus AA/DHA deficiency state triggered by excess TNF-α production can further augment TNF-α production and aggravate inflammation due to the absence of negative feedback control exerted by AA/DHA on TNF-α production. It is important to note that AA regulates TNF receptor expression, neutrophil function, and free radical generation triggered by TNF (Moghaddami et al., 2003). These results suggest a negative and positive feedback regulation between AA/DHA and their metabolites and TNF production and its action.

Conclusions and therapeutic implications

Plasma levels of PUFAs AA and DHA and BDNF are decreased in autism and there is an excess of PGE2, IL-6, and TNF-α and altered oxidative stress (reviewed in Das, 2013a, 2013b). We observed that AA/DHA and LXA4 enhance the levels of BDNF and vice versa. This coupled with the observation that AA/DHA are essential for the growth and development of brain and synaptic transmission and memory

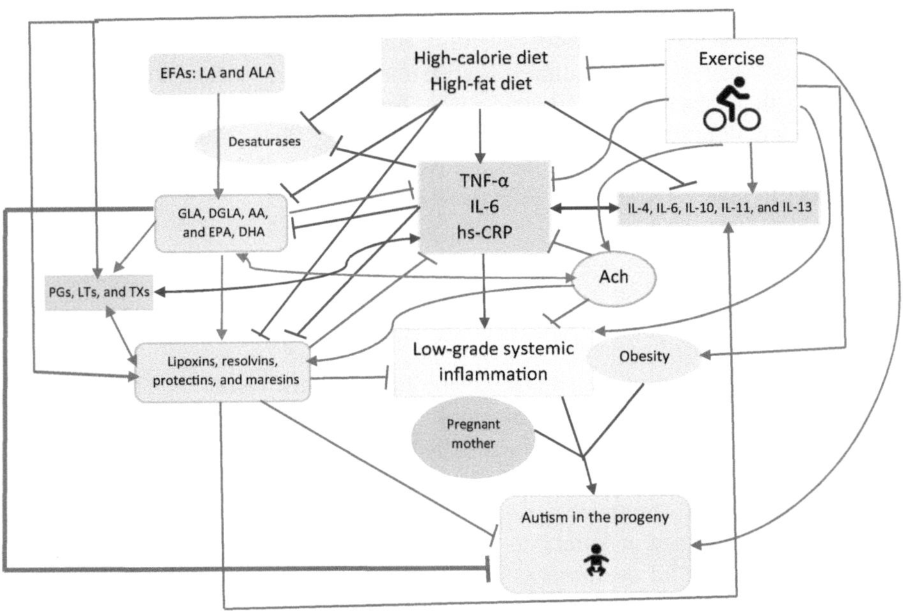

Figure 2.1 Scheme showing relationship bioactive lipids (especially AA and DHA) and autism. Obesity is a low-grade systemic inflammatory condition in which plasma levels of IL-6, TNF-α, and PGE2 are increased. TNF-α inhibits the activities of desaturases that are needed for the conversion of dietary LA and ALA to AA and DHA, the precursors of LXA4, resolvins protectins and maresins. PGE2 is also formed from AA. PGE2 and lipoxins, resolvins, protectins and maresins inhibit IL-6 and TNF-α production. TNF-α produces AA and DHA deficiency that results in decreased formation of LXA4, resolvins protectins and maresins. PGE2 inhibits TNF-α formation. Thus there is both a positive and negative feedback regulation among cytokines, PUFAs, PGE2, lipoxins, resolvins, protectins and maresins. Exercise is antiinflammatory in nature. Exercise increases the formation of LXA4, resolvins, protectins and maresins and enhances vagal tone and Ach formation. Ach has antiinflammatory action by enhancing LXA4 formation. *ALA*, alpha-linolenic acid; *LA*, linoleic acid.

implies that availability of adequate amounts of AA/DHA and other PUFAs during the periods of brain growth and development can prevent autism (Das, 2013a, 2013b). Since AA/DHA are needed for normal synthesis, release, and action of the neurotransmitters dopamine, GABA, Ach, catecholamines, this supports AA/DHA essentiality to prevent autism. Based on this evidence, it is suggested that alterations in the concentrations and activity of neurotransmitters (dopamine, serotonin, catecholamines, and BDNF) and gut microbiota seen in autism could be related to AA/DHA deficiency that could be corrected by AA/DHA supplementation. AA can alter the AKT-mTOR-NO pathway (Gingras et al., 2007), which may explain the role of scaffold proteins SHANK3 in modulating neurotransmitters, growth factor receptors, ion channels, glutaminergic neurons, and AKT-mTORC1 pathways in autism.

Based on all this evidence, it is suggested that AA/DHA supplementation during the periods of growth and development of brain will prevent the development of autism (see Fig. 2.1).

References

Al-Ayadhi, L. Y. (2005). Pro-inflammatory cytokines in autistic children in central Saudi Arabia. *Neurosciences*, *10*, 155–158.

Albrecht, C., von der Kammer, H., Mayhaus, M., Klaudiny, J., Schweizer, M., & Nitsch, R. M. (2000). Muscarinic acetylcholine receptors induce the expression of the immediate early growth regulatory gene Cyr61. *The Journal of Biological Chemistry*, *275*, 28929–28936.

Almeida, T., Cunha, R. A., & Ribeiro, J. A. (1999). Facilitation by arachidonic acid of acetylcholine release from the rat hippocampus. *Brain Research*, *826*, 104–111.

Araki, S., Yamamoto, Y., Dobashi, K., Asayama, K., & Kusuhara, K. (2014). Decreased plasma levels of brain-derived neurotrophic factor and its relationship with obesity and birth weight in obese Japanese children. *Obesity Research and Clinical Practice*, *8*, e63–e69.

Auestad, N., Scott, D. T., Janowsky, J. S., Jacobsen, C., Carroll, R. E., Montalto, M. B., et al. (2003). Visual, cognitive, and language assessments at 39 months: A follow-up study of children fed formulas containing long-chain polyunsaturated fatty acids to 1 year of age. *Pediatrics*, *112*, e177–e183.

Bathina, S., Srinivas, N., & Das, U. N. (2017). Streptozotocin produces oxidative stress, inflammation and decreases BDNF concentrations to induce apoptosis of RIN5F cells and type 2 diabetes mellitus in Wistar rats. *Biochemical and Biophysical Research Communications*, *486*, 406–413.

Bell, J. G., MacKinlay, E. E., Dick, J. R., MacDonald, D. J., Boyle, R. M., & Glen, A. C. A. (2004). Essential fatty acids and phospholipase A2 in autistic spectrum disorders. *Prostaglandins Leukot Essen Fatty Acids*, *71*, 201–204.

Borovikova, L. V., Ivanova, S., Zhang, M., Yang, H., Botchkina, G. I., Watkins, L. R., ... Tracey, K. J. (2000). Vagus nerve stimulation attenuates the systemic inflammatory response to endotoxin. *Nature*, *405*, 458–462.

Bresnahan, M., Hornig, M., Schultz, A. F., Gunnes, N., Hirtz, D., Lie, K. K., et al. (2015). Association of maternal report of infant and toddler gastrointestinal symptoms with autism: evidence from a prospective birth cohort. *JAMA Psychiatry*, *72*, 466–474.

Chan, P. H., Kerlan, R., & Fishman, R. A. (1983). Reductions of gamma-aminobutyric acid and glutamate uptake and $(Na^{+}+K^{+})$-ATPase activity in brain slices and synaptosomes by arachidonic acid. *Journal of Neurochemistry*, *40*, 309–316.
Chez, M. G., Dowling, T., Patel, P. B., Khanna, P., & Kominsky, M. (2007). Elevation of tumor necrosis factor-alpha in cerebrospinal fluid of autistic children. *Pediatric Neurology*, *36*, 361–365.
Connolly, N., Anixt, J., Manning, P., Ping-I Lin, D., Marsolo, K. A., & Bowers, K. (2016). Maternal metabolic risk factors for autism spectrum disorder—An analysis of electronic medical records and linked birth data. *Autism Research*, *9*, 829–837.
Cryan, J. F., & Dinan, T. G. (2012). Mind-altering microorganisms: The impact of the gut microbiota on brain and behaviour. *Nature Reviews Neuroscience*, *13*, 701–712.
Das, U. N. (2001). Is obesity an inflammatory condition? *Nutrition (Burbank, Los Angeles County, Calif.)*, *17*, 953–966.
Das, U. N. (2002a). Obesity, metabolic syndrome X, and inflammation. *Nutrition (Burbank, Los Angeles County, Calif.)*, *18*, 430–432.
Das, U. N. (2002b). Is type 2 diabetes mellitus a disorder of the brain? *Nutrition (Burbank, Los Angeles County, Calif.)*, *18*, 667–672.
Das, U. N. (2003a). Can memory be improved? A discussion on the role of ras, GABA, acetylcholine, NO, insulin, TNF-alpha, and long-chain polyunsaturated fatty acids in memory formation and consolidation. *Brain & Development*, *25*, 251–261.
Das, U. N. (2003b). Long-chain polyunsaturated fatty acids in memory formation and consolidation: Further evidence and discussion. *Nutrition (Burbank, Los Angeles County, Calif.)*, *19*, 988–993.
Das, U. N. (2003c). Long-chain polyunsaturated fatty acids in the growth and development of the brain and memory. *Nutrition (Burbank, Los Angeles County, Calif.)*, *19*, 62–65.
Das, U. N. (2006a). Biological significance of essential fatty acids. *The Journal of the Association of Physicians of India*, *54*, 309–319.
Das, U. N. (2006b). Essential fatty acids: Biochemistry, physiology, and pathology. *Biotechnology Journal*, *1*, 420–439.
Das, U. N. (2010). Obesity: Genes, brain, gut and environment. *Nutrition (Burbank, Los Angeles County, Calif.)*, *26*, 459–473.
Das, U. N. (2013a). Nutritional factors in the pathobiology of autism. *Nutrition (Burbank, Los Angeles County, Calif.)*, *29*, 1066–1069.
Das, U. N. (2013b). Autism as a disorder of deficiency of brain-derived neurotrophic factor and altered metabolism of polyunsaturated fatty acids. *Nutrition (Burbank, Los Angeles County, Calif.)*, *29*, 1175–1185.
El-Ansary, A., & Al-Ayadhi, L. (2012). Neuroinflammation in autism spectrum disorders. *Journal of Neuroinflammation*, *9*, 265.
Elliott, K. G., Kjolhede, C. L., Gournis, E., & Rasmussen, K. M. (1997). Duration of breast feeding associated with obesity during adolescence. *Obesity Research*, *5*, 538–541.
Gingras, A.-A., White, P. J., Chouinard, P. Y., Julien, P., Davis, T. A., Dombrowsk, L., et al. (2007). Long-chain omega-3 fatty acids regulate bovine whole-body protein metabolism by promoting muscle insulin signalling to the Akt–mTOR–S6K1 pathway and insulin sensitivity. *The Journal of Physiology*, *579*(1), 269–284.
Hatanaka, Y., Kabuta, T., & Wada, K. (2017). Disturbance in maternal environment leads to abnormal synaptic instability during neuronal circuitry development. *Frontiers in Neuroscience*, *11*, 35.

Hersi, A. I., Kitaichi, K., Srivastava, L. K., Gaudreau, P., & Quirion, R. (2000). Dopamine D-5 receptor modulates hippocampal acetylcholine release. *Brain Research Molecular Brain Research*, *76*, 336–340.

Itoh, Y., Kawamata, Y., Harada, M., Kobayashi, M., Fujii, R., Fukusumi, S., et al. (2003). Free fatty acids regulate insulin secretion from pancreatic β cells through GPR40. *Nature*, *422*, 173–176.

Jory, J. (2016). Abnormal fatty acids in Canadian children with autism. *Nutrition (Burbank, Los Angeles County, Calif.)*, *32*, 474–477.

Kramer, M. S. (1981). Do breast-feeding and delayed introduction of solid foods protect against subsequent obesity? *The Journal of Pediatrics*, *98*, 883–887.

Lucas, A., Fewtrell, M. S., & Cole, T. J. (1999). Fetal origins of adult disease—The hypothesis-revisited. *BMJ (Clinical Research ed.)*, *319*, 245–249.

Mayer, E. A., Tillisch, K., & Gupta, A. (2015). Gut/brain axis and the microbiota. *The Journal of Clinical Investigation*, *125*, 926–938.

Mayer, K., Schmidt, R., Muhly-Reinholz, M., Bögeholz, T., Gokorsch, S., Grimminger, F., & Seeger, W. (2002). In vitro mimicry of essential fatty acid deficiency in human endothelial cells by TNFα impact of ω-3 versus ω-6 fatty acids. *Journal of Lipid Research*, *43*, 944–951.

Minami, M., Kimura, S., Endo, T., et al. (1997). Dietary docosahexaenoic acid increases cerebral acetylcholine levels and improves passive avoidance performance in stroke-prone spontaneously hypertensive rats. *Pharmacology, Biochemistry, and Behavior*, *58*, 1123–1129.

Moghaddami, N., Costabile, M., Grover, P. K., Jersmann, H. P., Huang, Z. H., Hii, C. S., & Ferrante, A. (2003). Unique effect of arachidonic acid on human neutrophil TNF receptor expression: up-regulation involving protein kinase C, extracellular signal-regulated kinase, and phospholipase A2. *Journal of Immunology*, *171*, 2616–2624.

Naveen, G., Naidu, G., & Das, U. N. (2018). Amelioration of streptozotocin-induced type 2 diabetes mellitus in Wistar rats by arachidonic acid. *Biochemical and Biophysical Research Communications*, *496*, 105–113.

Naveen, K. V. G., Naidu, V. G. M., & Das, U. N. (2017a). Arachidonic acid and lipoxin A4 attenuate alloxan-induced cytotoxicity to RIN5F cells in vitro and type 1 diabetes mellitus in vivo. *Biofactors (Oxford, England)*, *43*, 251–271.

Naveen, K. V. G., Naidu, V. G. M., & Das, U. N. (2017b). Arachidonic acid and lipoxin A4 attenuate streptozotocin-induced cytotoxicity to RIN5F cells in vitro and type 1 and type 2 diabetes mellitus in vivo. *Nutrition (Burbank, Los Angeles County, Calif.)*, *35*, 61–80.

O'connor, D. L., Hall, R., Adamkin, D., Auestad, N., Castillo, M., Connor, W. E., et al. (2001). Growth and development in preterm infants fed long chain polyunsaturated fatty acids: a prospective, randomized controlled trial. *Pediatrics*, *108*, 359–371.

Parletta, N., Niyonsenga, T., & Duff, J. (2016). Omega-3 and omega-6 polyunsaturated fatty acid levels and correlations with symptoms in children with attention deficit hyperactivity disorder, autistic spectrum disorder and typically developing controls. *PLoS One*, *11*, e0156432.

Parracho, H. M., Bingham, M. O., Gibson, G. R., & McCartney, A. L. (2005). Differences between the gut microflora of children with autistic spectrum disorders and that of healthy children. *Journal of Medical Microbiology*, *54*, 987–991.

Reigstad, C. S., Salmonson, C. E., Rainey, J. F., 3rd, et al. (2015). Gut microbes promote colonic serotonin production through an effect of short-chain fatty acids on enterochromaffin cells. *The FASEB Journal*, *29*, 1395–1403.

Serhan, C. N., de la Rosa, X., & Jouvene, C. C. (2018). Cutting edge: Human vagus produces specialized proresolving mediators of inflammation with electrical stimulation reducing proinflammatory eicosanoids. *Journal of Immunology*, *201*, 3161–3165.
Shelly, A., Buffington, S. A., Di Prisco, G. V., Auchtung, T. A., Ajami, N. J., Petrosino, J. F., & Costa-Mattioli, M. (2016). Microbial reconstitution reverses maternal diet-induced social and synaptic deficits in offspring. *Cell*, *165*, 1762–1775.
Steinman, G., & Mankuta, D. (2013). Breastfeeding as a possible deterrent to autism—A clinical perspective. *Medical Hypotheses*, *81*, 999–1001.
Tateishi, N., Kakutani, S., Kawashima, H., Shibata, H., & Morita, I. (2014). Dietary supplementation of arachidonic acid increases arachidonic acid and lipoxin A_4 contents in colon, but does not affect severity or prostaglandin E_2content in murine colitis model. *Lipids in Health and Disease*, *13*, 30.
Tateishi, N., Kaneda, Y., Kakutani, S., Kawashima, H., Shibata, H., & Morita, I. (2015). Dietary supplementation with arachidonic acid increases arachidonic acid content in paw, but does not affect arthritis severity or prostaglandin E_2content in rat adjuvant-induced arthritis model. *Lipids in Health and Disease*, *14*, 3.
Tozuka, Y., Kumon, M., Wada, E., Onodera, M., Mochizuki, H., & Wada, K. (2010). Maternal obesity impairs hippocampal BDNF production and spatial learning performance in young mouse offspring. *Neurochemistry International*, *57*, 235–247.
Tozuka, Y., Wada, E., & Wada, K. (2009). Diet-induced obesity in female mice leads to peroxidized lipid accumulations and impairment of hippocampal neurogenesis during the early life of their offspring. *The FASEB Journal*, *23*, 1920–1934.
Vargas, D. L., Nascimbene, C., Krishnan, C., Zimmerman, A. W., & Pardo, C. A. (2005). Neuroglial activation and neuroinflammation in the brain of patients with autism. *Annals of Neurology*, *57*, 67–81.
von Kries, R., Kolletzko, B., Sauerwald, T., & von Mutius, E. (2000). Does breast-feeding protect against childhood obesity? *Advances in Experimental Medicine and Biology*, *478*, 29–39.
Wei, H., Zou, H., Sheikh, A. M., Malik, M., Dobkin, C., Brown, W. T., et al. (2011). IL-6 is increased in the cerebellum of autistic brain and alters neural cell adhesion, migration and synaptic formation. *Journal of Neuroinflammation*, *8*, 52.
Wolman, P. G. (1984). Feeding practices in infancy and prevalence of obesity in preschool children. *Journal of the American Dietetic Association*, *84*, 436–438.
Ximenes da Silva, A., Lavialle, F., Gendrot, G., Guesnet, P., Alessandri, J. M., & Lavialle, M. (2002). Glucose transport and utilization are altered in the brain of rats deficient in n-3 polyunsaturated fatty acids. *Journal of Neurochemistry*, *81*, 1328–1337.
Yu, H.-N., Zhu, J., Pan, W. S., Shen, S. R., Shan, W.-G., & Das, U. N. (2014). Effects of fish oil with high content of n-3 polyunsaturated fatty acids on mouse gut microbiota. *Archives of Medical Research*, *45*, 195–202.
Yu, M., Jiang, M., Yang, C., Wu, Y., Liu, Y., Cui, Y., et al. (2014). Maternal high fat diet affects Msi/Notch/Hes signaling in neural stem cells of offspring mice. *The Journal of Nutritional Biochemistry*, *25*, 227–231.

Is autism treatable?

3

Irina Koshkina
Medical center for the improvement of the immune, nervous and hormonal systems, Moscow, Russia

"Would you tell me, please, which way I ought to go from here?"—Alice asked.

"That depends a good deal on where you want to get to"—said the Cat.

"I don't much care where"—said Alice.

"Then it doesn't matter which way you go"—said the Cat.

"So long as I get somewhere"—Alice added as an explanation.

"Oh, you're sure to do that, if you only walk long enough"—said the Cat.
Lewis Carroll "Alice's Adventures in Wonderland"

Introduction

Autism is usually considered as a complex disorder of mental and somatic development, which entails a pronounced deficit of social communication, limited interests, difficulty in accepting any "new," and repetitive stereotypical actions. This is in general, but in practice, it turns out that every child with autism differs from other children in their unique features: triggers, the course of the disease, the presence and severity of a particular symptom, etc. Perhaps these differences can help us to answer the question of how to act and how to help every child with autism.

The problem of autism spectrum disorders (ASD) is one of the most urgent in modern neurology, due to the steady growth in the number of children suffering from early childhood autism (Bashina, 1999; Morozov, 2000; Poletaev & Shenderov, 2016; Uvarovskaya & Khairetdinov, 2010). At the same time, while in the year 2000, each quantity of the 10,000 new born children included the quantity

Emerging Programs for Autism Spectrum Disorder. DOI: https://doi.org/10.1016/B978-0-323-85031-5.00024-4

of from 5 to 26 children with autism spectrum disorder, and in the year 2005, one case of ASD occurred already in number of 250–300 new born children, this means that each quantity of from 250 to 300 new born children included one child with ASD. If consider the quantity not from 250 to 300, but only 250 (to divide easily we take number 250 to divide 10,000 by 250), this means that per every 250 new begotten children there occur one child with ASD. If make correlation with the number of 10,000, we will be able to see that in the year 2000 per every 10,000 there were, if take maximum level, 26 children with ASD, and in 2005, there already were found 40 children with ASD (per every 10,000 new born), and in the year 2008, there was found one ASD case already in quantity of 150 (in average) new born children, which means that fact that in the year 2008 per every 10,000 new born children there were found more than 40 children with ASD cases. In accordance with institution, called World Autism Organization, in the year 2008 in average one case of ASD was found within the quantity of 150 children, and this means that over the course of 10 years that the quantity of children with ASD increased very strongly. And in accordance with institution, called American Centre for Disease Control (CDC), the quantity is even bigger (Poletaev & Shenderov, 2016).

To date, there is no clear understanding of the causes and mechanisms of the occurrence of ASD and, as a result, there are no generally accepted tactics and algorithms for treating ASD. In this article, we will consider only two clinical cases of autism from many.

Methods

We analyzed a detailed medical history of each child based on an interview with parents. ELI-Tests immunoassay studies of serum immunoreactivity profiles were performed in both children (Poletaev, 2013a, 2013b). These methods allow us to quantify persistent changes in the synthesis and content of dozens of marker autoantibodies. Obtained results indicate abnormalities typical to the different forms of pathology in the human body and brain (Poletaev & Alieva, 2019; Poletaev, 2013a, 2013b).

Studies of the composition of the general microflora (mainly intestinal) were performed by the Osipov method using gas chromatography of blood and saliva samples and mass-spectrometric detection. This method allows quantification of the content of the main families and genera of bacteria—aerobic and anaerobic, symbiotic, and potentially pathogenic—by their characteristic marker molecules (Osipov, 2010).

Based on anamnesis data, neurological observations, and laboratory data, children were prescribed corrective measures. Correction schemes were selected individually (Koshkina, 2020).

Patient G.M., boy (born 2005)

In accordance with the information that was given to us by the patient's mother, the child was different from his peers since his birth. He did not speak until he reached the age of 3 years. There was stereotypical behavior often, including such perseverations as echolalia, and all this was accompanied with hyperactivity. The child had problems with food consumption (he ate plenty of food containing salt and sugar). He had problems with sleep—he could not sleep alone. Also the patient had problems such as constipation lasting for a period of 3–4 days; dysfunctions of large and small motor skills; lack of interest in peers and games with children; fears (he was afraid of loud sounds, passing cars, new people, new accommodations, sharp smells); aggression; obsession; no interest in the outside world and, accordingly, he did not make any attempts to make contact with the outside world; his position of intelligence was decreased; and from time to time he pronounced memorized phrases from TV shows. The patient was diagnosed with ASD at age of 4 years.

Disturbances in the composition of the intestinal microflora with the predominance of pathogenic species over symbiotic species, and a significantly increased content of *Staphylococcus aureus*, *Streptococcus mutans*, and *Candida* spp. were detected. The boy had abnormalities in the brain's dopamine and serotonin neurons, and also signs of astrocytic gliosis (GFAP) and changes in S100 calcium-binding proteins were noted. With regard to the visceral systems, he had inflammatory changes in the walls of the stomach and large intestine, and changes in insulin receptors (indicating a violation of carbohydrate metabolism) and antigen Spr-06 (indicating violations in the endocrine system). An activation of apoptosis (due to abnormal bacterial and viral activity) was also found.

Our observation and correction of the patient began in September 2014, at the age of 9 years. From September 2014 to May 2015, consultations and medical appointments were undertaken every 1.5–2 months.

Correction of the intestinal microflora was prescribed with the use of probiotics and prebiotics, bacteriophages, antifungal agents of the terbinophin group, and phytopreparations. Homotoxicological drugs, aimed at improving the function of the liver and kidneys, and amino acid complexes were also prescribed. Organotropic drugs were used to restore the function of the adrenal cortex, pituitary epiphysis, and brain cortex. The child's diet consisted of the complete exclusion of sugar and sugar-containing products, and minimization of the consumption of products containing gluten and casein. Measures aimed at activating the lymphatic system (lymphatic drainage massage, trampoline classes) were prescribed. To improve the drainage functions of the kidneys and liver an optimized drinking regime was prescribed and such drinks as berry juice (with cranberries, and lingonberries) and herbal decoctions were recommended.

After a 6-month period of correction, from September 2015, the child began to study in a normal school (learning with a tutor, in a program of inclusion in the classroom with children without neurological disorders). He coped well with the program, socialized, found friends, participated in joint games and field trips. His fine motor skills remained weak, but he coped with the function of writing satisfactorily, wrote dictations, and began training at the school of fine arts. Large motor skills were normalized (he jumped on a skipping rope along with his classmates, and performed all the tasks in physical education classes). He retold the stories he had read. He expressed his thoughts coherently and logically correctly. Periodically, there was an emotional arousal that he could not control himself. His fears significantly decreased. Sleep returned to normal (he started being capable of falling asleep on his own after going to bed in a period of 15–20 minutes). His defecation became regular, daily, and normal consistence. His diet was extended, without selectivity.

His parents were completely satisfied with the results that were achieved, and insisted stopping treatment. The correction measures were discontinued in May 2015. Four years later (in October 2019), there was parental repeat appeal due to the return of symptoms of disorder (uncontrolled excitement, aggression, and unreasonable crying). Learning at school became impossible, since almost everything in his environment and any sensory stimuli (light, sounds, touch) caused strong fears; sleep was disrupted again.

A study was performed to determine the main genera and species of the microbial flora of the child by the method of Osipov (Osipov, 2010). An excess of the following microorganisms were found: *Streptomyces* spp., *Ruminococcus, S. mutans, S. aureus, Eubacterium* spp., *Eggerthella lenta, Clostridium ramosum, Clostridium propionicum, Clostridium difficile, Clostridium coccoides/Blautia coccoides, Prevotella* spp., *Fusobacterium/Haemophylus, Lactobacillus, Corynebacterium* spp., *Clostridium hystolyticum, Bacteroides fragilis, Peptostreptococcus anaerobius 18623, Enterococcus, Kingella* spp., *Porphyromonas, Candida* spp., *Propionibacterium* spp., *Stenotrophomonas maltophilia, Veillonella* spp. Probiotic cultures were prescribed, including Lactobacteria, Bifidobacteria (*Lactobacillus reuteri, Lactobacillus gasseri, Lactobacillus paracasei, Lactobacillus casei, Lactobacillus plantarum, Lactobacillus acidophilus, Lactobacillus brevis, Bifidobacterium bifidum, Bifidobacterium longum, Bifidobacterium breve, Propionibacterium freudenreichii, Lacticaseibacillus rhamnosus, Lactobacillus salivarius, Bifidobacterium animalis subsp. lactis*), and *Propionobacteria shermani*. Functional nutrition based on fermented extracts, vitamins, amino acids, and trace elements was recommended. Inulin, vitamin C, and a fermented blend of turmeric, cranberry, ginger, garlic, black pepper, peppermint, and kelp extracts were also prescribed. Enzyme preparations (amylase, glucoamylase, cellulase, and lipase) were prescribed.

After 2 weeks, the condition stabilized and all pathological behavioral disorders disappeared and the child went back to school. The observation was continued. No problems were noted.

Patient M.V., boy (born 2014)

Threat of placental abruption was presented throughout pregnancy. Hepatitis C was revealed in the mother before pregnancy. Pregnancy was completed by Cesarean section to reduce the risk of child infection, and because the breech presentation of the fetus. At the age of 14 months the child's cognitive skills began to fade, and the parents began to notice abnormalities in behavior and gait (legs were tangled and falls became more frequent). It began soon after the Mantoux reaction was made and after an hours-long flight to Thailand, and severe injury to the right eye socket. At the age of 20 months, paraphymosis was surgically treated under general anesthesia. After that the child ceased to respond when anybody appealed to him by calling his name and he stopped responding to any speech addressed to him. He was doing waving motions with his hands like those were his wings. The patient was diagnosed ASD. Our observation began in December 2016, at the age of 2 years. At the first meeting, the child had a sharp decrease in speech comprehension, did not respond to his name, his large and small motor skills were impaired, his gait was clumsy, and he did not feel well in space. There was no pointing gesture. His tactile sensitivity was abnormally elevated (he didn't allow himself to be touched).

Between December 2016 and December 2018, consultations and appointments were held every 52 months and then every 4 months. During the observation period, we consistently tried to correct such symptoms as reduced intelligence, lack of speech, impaired large and small motor skills, increased tactile and sound sensitivity, and lack of interest in toys and games with peers. Initially the only game that he liked was to pour grits on himself for hours. There was a breach in eating behavior (he ate only nuts, bread, and cookies). There were fears (he was afraid of stairs, steps, playgrounds, etc.).

The child was found to have an increased content of *S. aureus*, *Egertella lenta*, *Candida fungi*, *Aspergillus*, Herpes, CMV and Epstein-Barr viruses. The boy had abnormalities in the brain's dopamine and serotonin neurons, and in addition signs of abnormalities in axons (NF-200), changes in myelin (MBP), changes in GABA–neuron systems, and changes in the endogenous opiate system of the brain. With regard to the visceral systems, he had signs of changes in the kidney, lungs, and liver. An activation of apoptosis (due to abnormal bacterial and viral activity) was also found. Correction measures were carried out in a few stages. In the first stage, the intestinal microflora was corrected, using probiotics, prebiotics, bacteriophages, antifungal agents, and the use of detoxification drugs (homeopathic therapy, naturopathic group). In the second stage, antiviral and immune-correcting therapy was performed. In the third stage, the endocrine system functions (adrenal cortex and thyroid gland) were stimulated, using organotropic drugs. In the final stage, stimulation of the cerebral cortex and cerebellum was performed by use of an individualized diet, using organotropic drugs, amino acids, trace elements, and vitamins of group B.

Two years after the start, an obvious positive dynamic was seen. The child's speech was closer to normal and the volume of vocabulary progressively increased. At the kindergarten matinee, he was the center of attention, danced in the hall, and was the main participant in all competitions and games. He was well engaged in the section of gymnastics and swimming, and fulfilled all the tasks of the coach. He became agile and coordinated in his movements. He easily communicated with other children. There was no socially unacceptable behavior. Before treatment, he was afraid of stairs; of height on the whole, he was afraid of speed and situations in where human is to reach equilibrium not to fall: bicycles, scooters. But after being treated, he stopped being afraid of stairs, speed, height, and he managed to reach equilibrium not to fall, where it was needed—the vivid example of that fact was that he studied riding scooter. In Russia playgrounds, which are situated in large shops, super markets, are called children's towns, the reason for this fact is that that they are similar to little towns. And before treatment the child was afraid of visiting such places, but after being treated, besides he stopped being afraid of such places; moreover, he started being fond of visiting them: play in there, with no problems he came there, was inspecting (studying) such places with curiosity and interest, and easily was leaving such places. Treatment was suspended, due to the achievement of the goal.

Discussion and conclusion

In the two cases described there, children were characterized by similar disturbances in the composition of the intestinal microflora with the predominance of pathogenic bacteria; a significantly increased content of *S. aureus, S. mutans, Candida* spp., and some others were detected.

Both children were found to have abnormalities in the brain's dopamine and serotonin neurons. Both children showed changes indicating the general activation of apoptosis (due to abnormal bacterial and viral activity).

The behavior of both was dominated by increased excitability, there was an increased sound and tactile sensitivity, a decrease in intelligence, and dysfunction of large and small motor skills.

Along with this, each child had their own specific abnormalities. Patient G.M. showed the typical stereotypical behavior, his speech was good but there was episodic echolalia. In laboratory studies, G.M. showed changes in insulin receptors (indicating a violation of carbohydrate metabolism) and Spr-06 (indicating violations in the endocrine system). Signs of astrocytic gliosis (GFAP) were shown along with changes in S100 calcium-binding proteins, which are trophic factors for serotonergic neurons.

The patient M.V. had marked detachment from other persons, fears, and complete lack of speech. His diet was very limited. In laboratory studies, M.V. showed an increased content of cytomegalovirus, changes in axons (NF-200), changes in myelin (MBP), changes in GABA–neuron systems, and changes in the endogenous opiate system. Abnormalities in the immune system, kidney, lungs, and liver were revealed.

Individual differences between patients influenced the choice of correction tactics. In the first case (patient G.M.), the emphasis was placed on the correction of the endocrine and gastrointestinal systems. And in the second case (patient M.V.), the main attention was paid to the correction of the immune system. The patient had indications of immune disturbances: M.V. had some postvaccination complications (this follows from the anamnesis—a "typical" story of his mother about how after the next routine vaccination, typical autistic manifestations began to rapidly increase and progressive loss of speech functions). In addition, his mother had chronic viral hepatitis C during pregnancy, and the child was found to have an excess of cytomegalovirus. Therefore, M.V. also used antidotes (homeopathic and constitutional drugs) that reduce the adverse effects of vaccinations.

The used measures allowed the achievement of positive changes in both children: The patient G.M. normalized cognitive, motor, and mental functions. M.V.'s speech function was successfully restored, his communication skills improved, and he was almost completely socially adapted.

The main conclusion of our work can be formulated as follows: children's autism can be effectively corrected (even difficult cases). In spite of only two examples presented there, we have dealt with nearly 200 autistic children of different ages during the past 5 years. Based on our experience we may conclude that any child with autism can be helped. Most adequate individual correction measures will always give positive results but the degree of severity of the results obtained may differ prominently from child to child.

In general, effective behavior correction of autistic children should include a system of measures aimed, in particular, at correcting microbiocenosis, selecting an adequate diet and correcting the content of vitamins and trace elements.

References

Bashina, V. M. (1999). *Autism in childhood.* Moscow: Medicine Publishing House.

Koshkina, I. A. (2020). A method of treating patients with various types of diseases by improving the immune, nervous and hormonal systems using Koshkina's method. Certificate No. 20-816 on registration of an intellectual property object.

Morozov, S. A. (2000). Special education for autism and autistic personality traits. In N. M. Nazarova (Ed.), *Special pedagogy (textbook).* Moscow: Publishing House The Academy.

Osipov, G. A. (2010). Chromato-mass spectrometric analysis of microorganisms and their communities in clinical samples for infections and dysbiosis. In G. K. Budnikov (Ed.), *Chemical analysis in medical diagnostics* (pp. 293–368). Moscow: Nauka.

Poletaev, A. (2013a). Autoantibodies: serum content or profiles? In A. B. Poletaev (Ed.), *Physiologic autoimmunity and preventive medicine* (pp. 199–207). Sharjah, Oak Park, Bussum: Bentham Science Publishers.

Poletaev, A. (2013b). The main principles of adaptive immune system function: self-recognition, self-interaction, and self-maintenance. In A. B. Poletaev (Ed.), *Physiologic autoimmunity and preventive medicine* (pp. 3–20). Sharjah, Oak Park, Bussum: Bentham Science Publishers, 2013.

Poletaev, A., & Alieva, F. (2019). Markers autoantibodies as indicators of cognitive dysfunction in children and adults. *Archives of Immunology and Allergy*, *2*(2), 42–48, ISSN: 2639-1848.

Poletaev, A. B., & Shenderov, B. A. (2016). Autism: genetics or epigenetics? *ARC Journal of Immunology and Vaccines*, *1*(2), 1–7.

Uvarovskaya, O. Yu., & Khairetdinov, O. Z. (2010). Study of the catamnesis of patients with various forms of childhood autism. In Materials of the 15th congress of psychiatrists of Russia. Moscow.

Classical child autism: can we prevent it?

4

Alexander Poletaev[1,2,†] and Tatyana Batysheva[2]
[1]Medical Research Center Immunculus, Moscow, Russia, [2]Clinical and Research Center of Children Psycho-Neurology, Moscow, Russia

A fairly large number (possibly dozens) of rare monogenic and chromosomal diseases are known in which symptoms of autism are often observed. For example, some children with Down's syndrome (up to 12%), and even more with Martin–Bell syndrome (up to 40%) or Rett syndrome (90%), show typical autistic symptoms. However, children with Martin–Bell syndrome (or Rett syndrome, Down's syndrome, or other genetic disorders) are children with Martin–Bell syndrome (or Rett syndrome, or Down's disease, etc.), and it is not correct to call their diseases "genetic autism."

Classic childhood autism—first described by Grunya Sukhareva (1925) and later by Leo Kanner (1943) and Hans Asperger (1944), (Fitzgerald, 2019)—does not fall under genetic but epigenetic (phenotypic) diseases. The frequency of autism has increased many times over the past half century and is becoming an epidemic, while the frequency of genetic diseases remains stable. (There are no epidemics of genetic diseases.) For debunking pseudoscientific "genetic mythology" in relation to autism, it is important to speak briefly about the genetic polymorphisms (the individual variability of the genome)—about random and for the most part neutral point mutations that occur mainly in noncoding regions of the genome and represent a basic tool of evolutionary variation (Kimura, 1983). The material expression of such mutations is SNP (single nucleotide polymorphisms), including transposition (changing A to G and T to C), transversion (replacement of G to A and C to T), or deletions of single nucleotides (Conrad, Andrews, Carter, Hurles, & Pritchard, 2006). By using genome-wide screening (GWAS), it is possible to detect many variants of a SNP occurring with increased frequency in the genomes of persons suffering from these or other diseases, for example, in children with autism (Anney, Klei, & Pinto, 2012). However, the prognostic significance of these findings will be small since the random SNPs are biologically neutral. Only in a small number of cases, can SNP influence the expression of a macromolecule (enzymes, receptor, or transport proteins). This, in turn, could potentially lead to metabolic changes decreasing a little the general resistance of the body to external influences. The reduction of the overall resistance of the organism to constant environmental pressure will to some extent increase the risk of any disease, from the risk of getting the flu or myocardial

[†] Deceased.

Emerging Programs for Autism Spectrum Disorder. DOI: https://doi.org/10.1016/B978-0-323-85031-5.00023-2

infarction to the increase of the probability of birth of an autistic child. However, a little decrease in the overall resistance can indicate, though rare, an increased predisposition to a specific pathology. The characteristics of the genome may to some extent affect the risk of development of atherosclerosis, diabetes, and gastric ulcer as well as resistance to infectious diseases. For example, when dealing with a leper, 9 out of 10 individuals are resistant to leprosy infection, as determined by their genotype, and only about 10% of contactees are at risk. However, with any structure of the genome in the absence of *Mycobacteria lepra*, no one can get sick. Similarly, no one can get autism without predisposing external influences. From this perspective, it seems important to take a new look at (and to stop taking on faith) exaggerated importance of "genetic predictions."

- *Phenotype cannot be predicted by the genotype (and vice versa).*
- *Epigenetic diseases are phenotypic phenomena.*
- *Classical autism is a phenotypic disease.*
- *Therefore, epigenetic (phenotypic) diseases cannot be predicted from the peculiarities of the individual genome.*

Despite the above, we should not underestimate the role of the genome in the development of autism. The importance of the individual genome is extremely high, and it is from its features that it directly depends on whether a particular disease, including autism, will be formed under potentially dangerous external influences, or whether the body will be resistant to adverse environmental influences.

Autism is formed in the prenatal period of a child's development under the influence of various harmful environmental factors. The harmful factors (technogenic pollutants, other chemical factors, infectious agents, etc.), the pressure of which has increased many times over the past half century, do not act directly on the fetus. They mostly affect the mother's body, causing characteristic changes in it, which, in turn, negatively affect the development of the fetus. Accordingly, the mother's body can be considered as a kind of interface that mediates the influence of the environment on the fetus. In most cases (although not always), the mother's body weakens, shields, and, in part, blocks many harmful influences, thus protecting the forming fetus. And the effectiveness of this protection depends directly on many genetically determined features of the mother's body.

Based on our long-term observations, we assume that autism is formed in the prenatal period (probably in the first half of pregnancy). This also applies to the cases of the so-called "regressive autism": in approximately 25%–30% of cases, the child's parents and their pediatrician note that at first the child's development was almost normal or there were minimal features that did not cause concerns. Later (usually at the age of 1–3 years), a sudden regression occurred, and in a short period of time the child lost previously acquired communication skills, stopped talking, and behavioral stereotypes and other symptoms appeared. Typically, the regression was preceded by an acute infectious disease of the child, intoxication, vaccination, or a stressful event. The question arises: does the phenomenon of regressive autism contradict the ideas about the innate nature of disorders that form at the beginning of pregnancy? In fact, there are no contradictions, and the situation is explained by the fact that in some cases a born child can develop almost normally even having certain disorders formed in the prenatal period. Due to the functioning of many compensatory mechanisms, it may not have any or almost no obvious clinical manifestations until then. In other words, for a long time, the disease is in a latent (hidden) form. However, this situation is unstable, and any additional external event may be the last straw that leads to the failure of compensation and transformation of the disease from a hidden (latent) form to an explicit one with all typical clinical manifestations.

Autism should be considered as a group of phenotypic (epigenetic) multisystem diseases emerging in utero, the typical characteristics of which are not only neurological disorders but also pathological changes in the stomach, small and large intestines; children with autism are often found with changes in the lungs, pelvic organs, kidneys, adrenals, and other organs (Poletaev et al., 2014; Rossignol & Frye, 2012). The multiplicity of somatic disorders is explained by the fact that the formation of autism occurs in the first half of pregnancy and overlaps "critical periods" in the development of different organs. It is not surprising that the death rate from somatic causes in autistic children is 3–10 times or more (depending on the severity of autism) than in "normotypic" children of the same age groups who do not suffer from autism (TreatingAutismPublications. http://www.autismtreatment.org.uk/wp-content/uploads/2014/03/Medical-Comorbidities-in-Autism-May-20131.pdf).

Pesticides, herbicides, abnormal changes in the symbiotic microbiota, excess of heavy metals, chronic deficiency of macro- and micronutrients and vitamins, chronic inflammatory processes, acute infectious diseases, food imbalance, and many other factors and agents can play the role of trigger factors that affect the body of a pregnant woman and can induce the formation of an autistic child (Poletaev & Shenderov, 2016). Note that the factors listed above—seemingly unrelated to each other—are characterized by a common fundamentally important property: all of them are able to induce long-term changes in the state of the immune system of pregnant woman (Poletaev et al., 2014). In turn, the universal response of the immune system to any biologically significant influences (chemical, infectious, toxic) is a persistent change in the production of many antibodies and cytokines that negatively affect the development of the fetus (Poletaev, 2012; Poletaev et al., 2014).

It remains unclear whether the effects of toxins, pollutants, and infectious agents involved in the development of autism are realized through induced changes in the immune system of a pregnant woman, or whether the immune changes are only part of the overall metabolic deviations. This question is fundamentally important because in the first variant of the answer to it many metabolic disorders typical of children with autism spectrum disorder (changes in folate metabolism, glutathione cycle, and many others) should be considered as immunomediated, and correction measures may be limited to targeted immunocorrective measures. And with the second variant of the answer, it will be impossible to perform the correction without a set of additional measures to detoxify the body and normalize violations of certain metabolic cycles.

Depending on many conditions, the mother's environment-induced immune changes may differ, for example, in the antigenic specificity of the induced autoantibodies. This, accordingly, will lead to the formation of different variants of autism in a child (different variants of autism spectrum disorders), differing in characteristic clinical features and, in part, in the affected somatic organs of the fetus. It is clear that different variants of disorders may require differentiated approaches to their neurology and somatic correction. For example, more than 80% of children with autism (as well as most of their mothers) have abnormalities in the opiate system (Poletaev, Poletaeva, & Khmelnitskaya, 2016). This may lead to the deviations not only of pain sensitivity but also of sensory perception in general. The milk protein casein contains several such fragments (casomorphins), and the wheat protein gluten contains several glutorphins. Note that many behavioral deviations in autistic children can be eliminated when removing a certain product from the child's diet (not only milk and gluten) that cause food intolerance reactions (Poletaev, Rizzo, & Batysheva, 2019).

Less than 10% of children with autism have characteristic changes in the system of cholinergic neurons of the anterior basal brain involved in providing cognitive functions (Poletaev et al., 2016, 2019). For the correction of such children, as a rule, prescriptions of nootropic drugs are required. About half of children with autism are characterized by marker signs of axonopathy, disorders of neuromuscular synapses, and myelin sheaths (Poletaev et al., 2016). These children are characterized by motor disorders. It is clear that in such cases special approaches to correction are required, based primarily on specialized training procedures for motor functions.

In most cases, changes in women's bodies that create the risk of fetal development disorders and the birth of a child with autism are formed long before pregnancy. Characteristic immune deviations induced in women before pregnancy (or during pregnancy) can be detected using objective and inexpensive laboratory methods (Poletaev, 2013). It is important to note that in contrast to irreversible genetic disorders changes in the body acquired under the influence of adverse external influences are reversible in most cases. Accordingly, mass-scale screening of women of childbearing age, timely detection of women with abnormal changes and disorders that pose risks to normal fetal development, and their adequate correction —mainly before the planned pregnancy—can dramatically reduce the frequency of birth of children with autism and related disorders and stop the epidemic spread of this pathology.

Conclusion (main provisions)

- The term "autism" refers to a heterogeneous group of systemic pathological changes that are similar in a number of major neuropathological symptoms but affect, in addition to the central nervous system, the organs of the gastrointestinal tract, the pelvic organs of the child, and other somatic organs.
- Autism refers to a kind of pathology of intrauterine development, formed under the influence of very different chemical or infectious agents acting on the body of a pregnant

woman. A significant part of the heterogeneous etiological (trigger) factors of autism realizes its effect through persistent changes in the state of the immune system of a pregnant woman (equifinality of the action of different factors).
- Environmental factors inducing immune changes associated with impaired production of natural autoantibodies and cytokines have multiple negative effects on the developing fetus.
- The severity of violations by the central nervous system and other organs and systems of the fetus and newborn depends on the state of its general resistance to adverse environmental influences and is caused by genetically determined individual resistance and homeostasis features.
- "*The child's health is laid in the mother's womb*" (L.S. Persianinov). This expression is fully applicable to autism and suggests the possibility of preventing this pathology based on mass screening and subsequent targeted correction of the mother's body before the planned pregnancy.
- The most promising biomarkers (informative, reliable, and suitable for mass screening) are some autoantibodies in the blood serum, persistent changes that are the basis of (or accompanies) the formation of autism.
- Analysis of characteristic changes in the content of certain autoantibodies can help reveal women's groups at risk of abnormal fetal development and the birth of autistic children. Also, it can be used to check on the children at risk in the first year of their life and for targeted corrective measures, if necessary.

As a postscriptum

About 400 years ago, Rene Descartes, who was admiring a sophisticated tower clock that could play elaborate theatrical performances, conjectured that the functioning of living beings was not intrinsically different from the work of the wonderful clocks. This idea seemed logical—if a skillful watchmaker was able to make such an amazing clock, what about another Almighty Creator, with his limitless power of creating and combining "wheels and gears" of any shape and size. And he does so to create ants, elephants, and all other flying and jumping, breeding and playing, devouring one another living beings.

Today, however, we tend to disapprove of the Cartesian mechanism. In so doing, we for some reason overlook that in our attempts to explain the principles and mechanisms that underlie the vital activities of living beings from the development of the fetus to the cognitive activity of the brain against the foundation of intermolecular interactions we have not gone far from the classical mechanism of the 17th century. All our accomplishments come down to replacing Descartes' mechanical "levers and gears" with molecular ones, which hardly constitutes a crucial difference. Francis Crick, one of the DNA pioneers, wrote in 1966, "The ultimate aim of the modern movement in biology is in fact to explain all biology in terms of physics and chemistry."

Famous physicist and philosopher Bohm (1969) wrote, "...when physics is moving away from mechanism, biology and psychology are moving closer to it. If this trend continues, it may well be that scientists will be regarding living and intelligent beings as mechanical, while they suppose that inanimate matter is too complex and subtle to fit into the limited categories of mechanism."

Reductionism that is, the same simplifying mechanism but in a modern guise—claims to explain any biological phenomena in terms of interacting molecules. Molecules are components ("bricks") of all living cells, but as such molecules are not alive. Deeper down than the level of the cell, biology stops being a life science. It is the context that creates the meaning; it is meaningless to talk about architecture by discussing single bricks (Zavarzin, 2011). Here lies the fallacy of the universal orientation toward the reductionist ideology in biology and medicine.

Ancient Roman poet Decimus Junius Juvenalis wrote, "*Mens sana in corpore sano*" (a healthy mind in a healthy body). It is not uncommon that individual dietary recommendations coupled with correction of the autistic child's microflora become even more effective for psychoneurological, verbal, and sociocommunicative correction than heavy psychotropic drugs. Thus the views of advocates of the psychosomatic ideology, a semiunderground movement not too long ago, gain new evidence. As well as the ideology of holism as such.

Children's autism is a vivid example of a body-wide systemic pathology of the body that requires a systemic (holistic) approach for its solution and hardly can be explained "in terms of physics and chemistry."

References

Anney, R., Klei, L., Pinto, D., et al. (2012). Individual common variants exert weak effects on the risk for autism spectrum disorders. *Human Molecular Genetic*, *21*, 4781–4792.

Bohm, D. (1969). Some remarks on the notion of order. In C. H. Waddington (Ed.), *Towards a theoretical biology* (Vol. 2, pp. 18–40). Edinburgh: Sketches. Edinburgh Press.

Conrad, D., Andrews, T., Carter, N., Hurles, M., & Pritchard, J. (2006). A high-resolution survey of deletion polymorphism in the human genome. *Nature Genetics*, *38*, 75–81.

Fitzgerald, M. M. (2019). The history of autism in the first half century of the 20th century: New and revised. *Journal of. ReAttach Therapy and Developmental Diversities*, *1*(2), 70–77. Available from https://doi.org/10.26407/2018jrtdd.1.13.

Kimura, M. (1983). *The neutral theory of molecular evolution*. Cambridge: Cambridge University Press, ISBN: 0-521-23109-4, ISBN.

Poletaev, A. (2013). Autoantibodies: Serum content or profiles? In A. B. Poletaev (Ed.), *Physiologic autoimmunity and preventive medicine* (pp. 199–207). Sharjah, Oak Park, Bussum: Bentham Science Publishers.

Poletaev, A., Poletaeva, A., Pukhalenko, A., Zamaleyeva, R., Cherepanova, N., & Frizin, D. (2014). Adaptive maternal immune deviations as a ground for autism spectrum disorders development in the child. *Folia Medica*, *56*(2), 73–80.

Poletaev, A. B. (2012). Maternal immunity, pregnancy, and child's health. In S. Sifakis, & N. Vrachnis (Eds.), *From preconception to postpartum* (pp. 41–57). Rijeka, Croatia: InTech, Open Access Publisher, ISBN: 978-953-51-0353-0, ISBN.

Poletaev, A. B., Poletaeva, A. A., & Khmelnitskaya, A. V. (2016). Changes in the opiate system in autistic children. Possible causes and consequences. *Clinical Pathophysiology*, *22* (1), 48–54.

Poletaev, A. B., Rizzo, K., & Batysheva, T. T. (2019). Food intolerance: Clinical significance and methods of analysis. *Journal of Child and Adolescent Rehabilitation*, *3*(39), 5–10.

Poletaev, A. B., & Shenderov, B. A. (2016). Autism: Genetics or epigenetics? *ARC Journal of ImmunologyVaccines*, *1*(2), 1–7.
Rossignol, D. A., & Frye, R. E. (2012). A review of research trends in physiological abnormalities in autism spectrum disorders: Immune dysregulation, inflammation, oxidative stress, mitochondrial dysfunction, and environmental toxicant exposures. *Molecular Psychiatry*, *17*, 389–3401.
Zavarzin, G. A. (2011). *Kakosphera*. Moscow: Rhutenica.

Further reading

Poletaev, A., & Aliyeva, F. (2019). Markers autoantibodies as indicators of cognitive dysfunction in children and adults. *Archives of Immunology and Allergy*, *2*, 42–48.

Methods to improve imitation in young children with autism: a review

5

Tanya Paparella and Stephanny Freeman
Department of Psychiatry and Biobehavioral Sciences, University of California, Los Angeles, CA, United States

Many studies have linked autism spectrum disorder (ASD) and imitation difficulties (Nadel, 2014; Vivanti & Hamilton, 2014). Children with ASD tend to imitate less frequently and accurately than neurotypical children, and appear to have more difficulties early in development than later on (Williams, Whiten, & Singh, 2004).

In general, for children with ASD, imitating simple one-step actions appears to be easier than sequences of actions (Vivanti & Hamilton, 2014). Studies have also reported greater success for actions on objects in contrast to gestures (Vivanti, Nadig, Ozonoff, & Rogers, 2008) and for actions with a clear goal (Gowen, 2012; Vanvuchelen, Roeyers, & De Weerdt, 2007; Wild, Poliakoff, Jerrison, & Gowen, 2012). Children with autism are more likely to imitate when the object is familiar and the outcome is interesting (Sevlever & Gillis, 2010). Hobson and Lee (1999) also reported that children with autism have difficulty imitating the style in which actions are presented. Overall, the most severe problems with imitation seem to occur for imitation of nonmeaningful gestures and body positions (Gowen, 2012; Vivanti & Hamilton, 2014).

There are several reasons why imitation is a critical developmental skill and should be included as part of a treatment plan for young children with autism. First, research suggests that teaching children with ASD to imitate may contribute to gains in collateral skills that are not directly taught. For children with ASD, better imitation skills appear to be related to improved language (Stone, Ousley, & Littleford, 1997; Thurm, Lord, Lee, & Newschaffer, 2007), play skills (Libby, Powell, Messer, & Jordan, 1997; Stone et al., 1997), and social skills such as joint attention (Rogers, Hepburn, Stackhouse, & Wehner, 2003). Second, the ability to imitate is considered a prerequisite for many other areas of learning, both academic and social (Soorya, Arnstein, Gillis, & Romanczyk, 2003). Further, as children learn to imitate others, their capacity for observational learning also develops, creating a path for more natural learning from watching and modeling others (Bandura, 1977).

Imitation is clearly an important aspect of childhood development, and in previous decades there was a necessary and concerted effort to better understand and specify the nature of imitation difficulties in autism. While autism research on the

Emerging Programs for Autism Spectrum Disorder. DOI: https://doi.org/10.1016/B978-0-323-85031-5.00010-4

construct of imitation extends back over 50 years, the number of studies focusing on imitation instruction for young children with ASD is relatively small. Early autism interventions to teach new behaviors, including successful imitation instruction, was dominated by Applied Behavior Analysis (ABA) (Smith, 2001). In recent years there has been a general shift away from purely behaviorally based treatment for children with ASD toward interventions that are considered to be hybrids of both behavioral and developmental approaches. These have been described as Naturalistic Developmental Behavioral Interventions (NDBIs) (Schreibman et al., 2015). This trend is reflected in this review, with the 10 studies identified offering a mix of treatment approaches that reflect the historical beginnings based in behavioral approaches (ABA), the use of technology to offer video-based and remote treatment [Video Modeling (VM) and telehealth], and six using NDBA approaches over the last 10 years. We limited our search to recent literature to highlight expanding, efficacious, intervention methodologies aimed to improve motor imitation in young children with ASD.

The treatment studies reviewed also investigated different types of imitation. Several measured changes in *spontaneous imitation or mimicry*. This is when a child spontaneously imitates in response to a modeled action. The child spontaneously and unintentionally copies the other person without regard for the function of the act (e.g., unintentionally imitating a sad expression). Other studies targeted *elicited* imitation. This occurs when a child is given an instruction to imitate (i.e., "do as I do"); the imitated act is considered elicited. True *imitation* involves copying both the means and the intention of the action. For example, a child learns how to open a snack container by copying a parent so they can then eat the snack. *Emulation* describes when the child copies the goal of an action, but not the means used to achieve the goal. For example, a teacher puts toy people in a bus one at a time and later a child puts a handful of toy people into the bus (Sevlever & Gillis, 2010; Vivanti & Hamilton, 2014). For the purpose of this review, we use the term "imitation" generally but we also specify the type of imitation investigated in the study outcomes.

Method

Search strategy

Five electronic databases (APA PsycINFO, APA PsycArticles, Melvyl, PubMed, Google Scholar) covering education, medicine, behavior, and psychology were searched in July 2020. The search was restricted to materials published in peer-reviewed journals between January 2010 and July 2020. Keyword search terms were autism, intervention, treatment, teaching, and imitation. This search identified 168 studies for possible inclusion. Removal of duplicates yielded 132 manuscripts. Next, a review of titles and abstracts was conducted with a Level 1 Screening (autism, age, and imitation intervention) excluding 64 articles. The remaining 68 full manuscripts were then subjected to a reference review. No additional studies were identified from the references. The Level 1 Screening (autism, age, and imitation intervention) was then applied to the full 68 manuscripts as, at times, the abstract did not provide enough information for judgment. This yielded 32 manuscripts. The inclusion and exclusion criteria below were then applied to the full text resulting in 10 articles that met all inclusion criteria. In all, there was one randomized controlled design study (RCT), one study with a group experimental design, and eight single subject design articles.

Inclusion and exclusion criteria

A set of inclusion and exclusion criteria was applied to the manuscripts obtained from the search. Included studies:

- Used a quantitative, RCT or group experimental design, or single subject research design.
- Published in the English language.
- Published in a peer-reviewed journal between 2010 and July 2020.
- Included participants between the ages of 1 and 7 years diagnosed with ASD.
- Included at least two participants.
- Examined an intervention for which motor imitation was an outcome. This excluded imitation taught solely for communication purposes, such as gestures to regulate another's behavior or to share attention. It also excluded studies that measured the efficacy of a comprehensive treatment approach.
- Included measurement of imitation as a direct target. Studies were excluded if imitation was measured as a collateral outcome.
- Intervention was person-mediated. Robotic mediated interventions were excluded.

Results

A total of 10 studies were reviewed. Only one was conducted outside of the United States (i.e., Belgium; Warreyn & Roeyers, 2014). The number of participants with autism across studies ranged from 2 to 18. Two studies used intervention methods with an ABA approach, two used VM, one used a Naturalistic Developmental Behavioral Approach (NDBA), four used Reciprocal Imitation Training (RIT) which represents an NDBA approach, and one compared RIT and VM. Interventions were therapist, parent, or sibling delivered, in-person, or via VM or telehealth. There was only one RCT; the majority of studies were single-subject experimental designs and one quasi-experimental pre–post design was included.

Review and discussion of studies

In the 10 identified studies (see Table 5.1 for study characteristics and findings), RIT dominated the methodological choices, including in vivo and telehealth parent-mediated studies, as well as a sibling-mediated study. VM and ABA were other

Table 5.1 Study characteristics and findings.

Authors (year)	Sample size $n =$	*M* Age in months CA (MA)	Methods	Experimental design	Mean/ fidelity	Outcome
Cardon (2012)	4	24–50	Caregiver-mediated VM 3 times a week for 0.6 hr for 12 sessions	MBD by participants	>80%	VM effect on elicited object and gestures imitation
Cardon (2013)	3	34–54	VMIT 3 times a week for 0.5 hr for 4 weeks	MBD by participants	Not reported	VMIT effect for elicited gross motor actions and gestural imitation
Cardon and Wilcox (2011)	6	20–48	RIT VM 3 times a week for 0.5 hr for 5 weeks	MBD by participants	>99% RIT 100% VM	RIT effect on spontaneous object imitation, VM effect on elicited object imitation, VM effect occurred at faster rate
Deshais, et al. (2020)	3	36–84	ABA dose varied by child	MBD by sets of gestures	99%	Possible effect of two therapist concurrent prompting on elicited gestures for children with impaired delayed imitation
Ingersoll (2010)	11 Tx 10 cont	41.4 (21.7) 37.2 (18.6)	RIT 3 times a week for 1 hr for 10 weeks	RCT	90%	RIT effect on spontaneous and elicited object and gesture imitation
Tereshko et al. (2010)	4	48–72	Segmented VM dose varied by child	MBD by participants	Not reported	Segmented VM effect on elicited multiple step sequenced object imitation

Valentino et al. (2018)	2	26–54	ABA 3 times a week, 2–5 times a day, for up to 0.25 hr each session for 30 sessions	adapted alternating treatments design	>98%	Effect of two therapist concurrent prompting on elicited gestures and objects for child with impaired delayed imitation, effect of using a salient stimulus for child with attention difficulty
Wainer and Ingersoll (2015)	5	29–59	Telehealth parent-mediated RIT dose varied by child	MBD by dyads	80% during coaching	RIT effect on spontaneous imitation
Walton and Ingersoll (2012)	4	45–57	Sibling (8–13 years of age)-mediated RIT 2 times a week for 0.25 hr for 10 weeks	MBD by dyads	71%	RIT effect on spontaneous imitation for 3 out of 4 children
Warreyn and Roeyers (2014)	18 Tx 18 cont	68.6 (54) 68.9 (52)	NDBA 2 times a week for 0.5 h for 24 sessions	Pre-test, post-test	Not reported	No significant NDBA effect on spontaneous and elicited total imitation (object, gestural, vocal, symbolic)
Zaghlawan and Ostrosky (2016)	2	48–60	Parent-mediated RIT dose varied by child	MBD by strategies	100%	Modest RIT effect on spontaneous and elicited object and gesture imitation

ABA, Applied behavior analysis; *MBD*, multiple baseline design; *NDBA*, naturalistic developmental behavioral approach; *RCT*, randomized controlled trial; *RIT*, reciprocal imitation training; *VM*, video modeling; *VMIT*, video modeling imitation training (VM with prompts).

approaches used. Of the VM studies, one study compared RIT to VM, one used a mostly behavioral approach to deliver a caregiver-mediated intervention, and one used a behavioral approach to teach multiple step sequenced imitation. The two ABA studies examined the efficacy of using two therapists to provide concurrent prompting.

Reciprocal Imitation Training/Naturalistic Developmental Behavioral Interventions

Historically, interventions to improve imitation skills in children with autism originated in behavioral approaches using operant conditioning protocols with highly systematic adult directed teaching (e.g., Lovaas, Freitas, Nelson, & Whalen, 1967). Despite initial success, concerns arose that imitation actions learned via behavioral methods resulted in little spontaneous imitation outside of the taught, highly structured context (Dawson & Adams, 1984; Ingersoll, 2008).

RIT was developed as a more naturalistic teaching method. It emphasizes the underlying social nature of imitation and aims to improve spontaneous imitation naturalistically through play. The goal of RIT is for the child to imitate the majority of actions of a play partner rather than to accurately produce specific actions in response to a model (Ingersoll & Schreibman, 2006). It is based on dyadic play exchanges in which the therapist imitates the child's actions, establishes a turn-taking routine, and then models new actions for the child to imitate. Prompts are used if the child does not imitate. All spontaneous imitated behaviors are reinforced with natural praise. Intervention strategies include contingent imitation of the child's actions and language, describing the child's actions, and modeling target imitation actions. Thus, with the combination of developmental and behavioral strategies, RIT has the characteristics of a NDBA treatment.

Several studies have shown success using this approach. The most rigorous of these is Ingersoll's (2010) RCT. It is a continuation of her previous single subject multiple-baseline design studies (Ingersoll & Gergans, 2007; Ingersoll, Lewis, & Kroman, 2007; Ingersoll & Schreibman, 2006) that were successful in developing spontaneous and generalized imitation. The 2010 RCT nicely demonstrated that a low-intensity (3 hours per week for 10 weeks) focused intervention improved elicited and spontaneous imitation actions with objects and gestures.

Warreyn and Roeyers (2014) showed modest gains in overall imitation in a study using a customized NDBA approach. Within this NDBA, RIT strategies appeared to contribute largely to the intervention approach but also included were aspects of Pivotal Response Training (PRT), Incidental Teaching, and Responsive Teaching. PRT strategies included teaching in highly motivating activities, following the child's lead, and behavior strategies applied in naturalistic contexts (Koegel & Koegel, 2006). Targeted instructional exercises embedded in typical activities is a strategy used in Incidental Teaching (McGee, Morrier, & Daly, 1999), and reciprocity is a characteristic of Responsive Teaching (Mahoney & Perales, 2003).

While the Ingersoll (2010) study used therapists as interventionists, since then, a few, very small studies (Wainer & Ingersoll, 2015; Walton & Ingersoll, 2012;

Zaghlawan & Ostrosky, 2016) have begun to explore the possibility of siblings or parents delivering intervention. RIT is particularly suited to sibling- or parent-mediated intervention as it can be implemented in natural play settings and during daily routines at home. Results appear to be moderately successful which is notable for a potentially home-based, low-cost, low-intensity intervention. Notwithstanding, each variation in terms of who delivered the therapy encountered unique challenges. For school aged siblings delivering the intervention, difficulties included lower intervention fidelity as new strategies were introduced and inconsistent generalization of strategies to different settings and materials. Also of note, was that the siblings implemented strategies at a lower rate overall than adult therapists. For parent-mediated intervention, barriers to fidelity included competing demands for time and attention in the home and learning style differences. Indeed, Hall, Mastel, Nickel, and Wainer (2019) delayed a planned parent-mediated study in a rural setting to first identify barriers to participation. Barriers included limited time due to child and work needs, personal life events, and family stressors. These are significant and very real concerns contributing to the outcome of an intervention.

Lastly, and especially in light of the current global COVID-19 epidemic, Wainer and Ingersoll's (2015) hybrid telehealth program is of particular interest. They combined asynchronous self-directed internet-based instruction with synchronous remote coaching to teach parents to increase spontaneous imitation in their children with ASD. Although promising, at conclusion they determined that an asynchronous, self-directed program may be sufficient for some, but not all, parents to learn the intervention. Others may require additional support, in the form of remote synchronous coaching and feedback, in order to implement the techniques with fidelity.

Overall, RIT seems to not only increase spontaneous imitation, but also appears to facilitate generalization beyond the teaching context. In addition, teaching imitation skills using RIT has shown collateral gains in play, joint attention, social skills, and language acquisition (Ingersoll, 2010, 2012; Ingersoll & Schreibman, 2006; Warreyn and Roeyers, 2014). RIT also has the potential to be adaptable in situations where traditional therapist/child visits in a clinic setting are challenging.

Video Modeling

VM has also shown to be successful in teaching imitation to children with autism. Using this approach, the child watches a prerecorded video of a person performing an action and is expected to imitate the observed gesture or action with an identical set of objects. Similar to in vivo instruction, the model may be an adult (e.g., teacher or parent), or a child (e.g., sibling, peer model).

The foundation of VM is essentially observational learning. Observing and imitating a model requires that the child remember the observed actions for the duration of the video, and the period of time between the video and the task presentation. This involves attention, retention, and motivation for the child to successfully perform the desired action. Indeed, it seems that VM facilitates all of these necessary elements (Dorwick, 1991). In terms of attention, relevant stimuli are restricted on the video screen, be it for example, a handheld device, computer, or television. The child's attention is focused within a restricted field of vision thus decreasing the likelihood of attending to irrelevant stimuli (e.g., Charlop-Christy, Le, & Freeman, 2000; Corbett & Abdullah, 2005). The consistent repetition of the modeled behavior supports retention, and the opportunity to practice is limitless. Lastly, children with autism are generally drawn to screen content, thus VM as an approach is naturally likely to be motivating (Charlop-Christy et al., 2000; Nikopoulos & Keenan, 2003).

Several studies in the last 10 years have used VM to teach imitation skills to young children on the autism spectrum. These include teaching one- and two-step gestural imitation (Cardon, 2013), caregiver-mediated training to develop imitation of gestures and actions on objects (Cardon, 2012), a comparison of RIT and VM approaches to teach imitation on objects (Cardon & Wilcox, 2011), and multistep segmented object imitation used to teach an eight-step toy construction task (Tereshko, MacDonald, & Ahearn, 2010). The latter was carried out by showing children video clips of increasingly longer segments of a behavioral chain, starting with a one-step action and increasing systematically to the full chain of steps in the task analysis to facilitate imitation of the model.

While these studies are very small, VM appears to be a promising method for teaching imitation of varying types and complexity. Across studies, treatment fidelity was high, children's imitation of the desired actions emerged rapidly, their imitation abilities generalized beyond the teaching context, and maintained beyond the teaching period. Collateral gains in language, play, and social skills were also achieved in two studies (Cardon, 2012, 2013).

In the Cardon and Wilcox (2011) study, which compared RIT and VM, both were effective. Interestingly, however, the children who were taught via VM rapidly increased their imitation skills overall, whereas the children receiving the in vivo RIT intervention demonstrated a steady increase in skill acquisition. Other learning differences are of note and invite questions as to whether some children are less suited to learning via VM. In Cardon (2013), the child who did not make gains in imitation was the youngest (34 months) and most impaired on several standardized measures of developmental function. This is consistent with previous research suggesting that autism severity is related to imitation impairment (Rogers et al., 2003). In Tereshko et al.'s (2010) study, children who performed poorly on delayed match-to-sample ahead of instruction, did not perform well in multistep VM. This suggests that delayed object to picture matching may be a prerequisite to using VM for more advanced imitation. However, given the very small sample sizes in these studies, these observations require further investigation to determine if they truly bear significance on teaching practices.

In sum, VM is an interesting and promising approach. It may be a more motivating approach for children with autism spectrum than in vivo approaches. This could be because it capitalizes on characteristics associated with ASD such as overselectivity, social impairment, and preference for visual stimuli (Corbett & Abdullah, 2005). It can be delivered to children who live in areas where in vivo treatment is sparse, and it is cost effective when compared to in-person treatment. Questions remain about what prerequisite skills are needed for VM to be effective (Lindsay, Moore, Anderson, & Dillenburger, 2013). It has been suggested that children who have stronger imitation skills prior to VM intervention are those who respond more positively to this approach

(Rayner, 2015). Future studies might also explore how differences in response time (i.e., how long to wait before imitation is expected) impact child performance. For example, Zaghlawan and Ostrosky (2016) used 3 seconds with decreased imitation success in comparison to 10 seconds used in other studies (Cardon, 2012; Cardon & Wilcox, 2011; Ingersoll, 2010). However, other confounding factors may have contributed to decreased success. The Zaghlawan and Ostrosky (2016) study was caregiver mediated and also decreased the number of prompts from three (used in Cardon, 2012; Cardon & Wilcox, 2011; Ingersoll, 2010) to two, making it difficult to determine whether the provider, number of prompts provided, or response time could have been the active ingredients contributing to greater success.

Applied Behavior Analysis

Two recent studies found mixed results when revisiting the ABA approach to teach imitation, but they utilized a novel method and examined contributing child characteristics (Deshais, Phillips, Wiskow, Vollmer, & Donaldson, 2020; Valentino, LeBlanc, & Conde, 2018). Taken together, they found that the use of concurrent prompting during gross motor imitation training may be a useful strategy, especially for those who exhibit a particular impairment in delayed imitation. Concurrent prompting involves the use of a second therapist to deliver prompts while positioned behind the participant. This eliminates the delay between the target imitative action being modeled and the response expected by the child. They propose that, although the use of two therapists may require more resources, it may be a necessary avenue toward establishing imitation in some children. If this holds true, additional robust research will be needed to determine which children may benefit from this stepped-up approach.

Discussion

In the last decade, the number of studies examining imitation as a targeted outcome of treatment is surprisingly few. Furthermore, with the exception of two studies (Ingersoll, 2010; Warreyn & Roeyers, 2014), the majority were single-subject experimental designs with six participants or less. The paucity of treatment research is especially notable since imitation is an area of particular impairment in children with ASD, it can be targeted very early in a child's development, and has the potential to impact other areas of learning and social development.

Promising, however, was the finding that RIT appears widely supported as an effective method for developing imitation in young children with autism given the multiple small studies and the RCT. The play-based approach appeals to many professionals who were uncomfortable with the unnatural, contrived instruction of behavioral approaches, and offers a somewhat caregiver-friendly format for parent- or sibling-mediated treatment. The collateral effects on language, play, and aspects of social development such as joint attention, further substantiate the teaching method.

The studies using VM as a treatment approach, though very small, also yielded intriguing results. Although they all demonstrated a positive effect on differing levels of complexity of elicited imitation, most notable was the observation that children appeared to make rapid imitative gains, and also showed collateral gains in language and play. While promising, these preliminary results should be tested in larger scale, more rigorous studies. Similarly, caregiver-mediated treatment via telehealth should be further explored, not only with regard to efficacy, but also with a focus on feasibility. The ability to provide potentially low-cost, low-intensity treatment to children and families in remote or underserved areas is clearly a benefit. However, factors such as computer and internet access, computer literacy, and competing personal or family demands could impede feasibility and outcomes.

Examining further aspects of these intervention approaches in more detail, several noteworthy observations emerged, particularly with regard to child characteristics. Children with ASD can differ significantly in their abilities, ranging from children who are minimally verbal to fluent speakers, from children with comorbid intellectual impairment to children with above average intellectual ability, from children who seek social interaction with peers to those who isolate themselves. With such a wide range of individual differences, of relevance to treatment efficacy then, is the question of fit or how well a treatment approach matches the developmental characteristics of an individual child. Ingersoll (2010) found that the number of spontaneous play actions at RIT pretreatment was associated with amount of improvement in imitation skills. This finding suggests that an initial interest in objects or a greater play repertoire may be predictive of skill acquisition during RIT. In regards to VM, Tereshko et al. (2010) found that children who were unable to perform delayed matching tasks (object to picture) pretreatment, were also not able to imitate an eight-step video model. Further, Cardon (2013) found that the youngest child who was also most impaired made the least gains. Interestingly, the two ABA studies (Deshais, et al., 2020; Valentino et al., 2018) attempted to address how to better support children with weaker skills. They found that using two therapists to provide concurrent prompting for elicited imitation may help children with impaired delayed imitation.

Addressing the method or "how" of interventions is one aspect of intervention research. Another critical aspect is the content or "what" is taught. In this regard, several observations are of note. First, most but not all of the studies, chose to teach meaningful actions on objects. This is consistent with previous research that has shown that children with ASD imitate better when tasks involve objects and when actions are meaningful, and indicates a trend away from teaching children to imitate actions out of context which characterized the early behavioral teaching approaches (e.g., Lovaas et al., 1967). Teaching goal-oriented actions on objects is clearly evident in RIT where the context of the intervention is in meaningful play. Similarly, comprehensive NDBA treatment approaches, such as The Early Start Denver Model (Rogers & Dawson, 2010) teach imitation in the framework of joint activity routines, where the adult models actions that are meaningful in the context of the play activity.

Finally, the studies were very mixed in terms of their methodological rigor and ecological validity. While most reported high fidelity, two studies did not report on a fidelity measure. Some reported on maintenance of imitation skills beyond the treatment phase, others included measures of generalization. Of the studies that did measure imitation maintenance, follow-up evaluation tended toward proximal timelines (e.g., 3 weeks post treatment) rather than longer-term (e.g., 1 year) distal follow-up measures which would better represent sustained skill acquisition and ecological validity. Multiple studies did not include measures of collateral gains in other areas of development. These are all important considerations in designing an informative treatment study and should be included in future research.

The reviewed studies add a strong emerging knowledge base to the research literature on treatments directly targeting imitation in young children with autism. Practitioners can make a more informed decision on imitation targets and approach; however, there continue to be many unanswered questions regarding treatment efficacy and utility. Further research is needed to identify essential components or active ingredients of imitation interventions. Clarification is also needed on which specific types of treatments or strategies seem more suitable for certain children or parents. Finally, especially given the current pandemic and low-resourced environments, a concerted effort should be made to further explore how to effectively deliver video-based or telehealth treatments.

Identifying and targeting pivotal skills such as imitation is important when designing comprehensive effective treatments for children with ASD as they likely increase the probability of overall positive outcomes. This review of the literature helps determine the most current, effective, generalizable, and flexible intervention methodology to target the critical skills of imitation as essential to learning. Hopefully, this knowledge will contribute not only to successful, but also to efficient treatment delivery, as measured by improvements in imitation skills and collateral effects in other areas of development.

References

Bandura, A. (1977). *Social learning theory*. New Jersey: Prentice-Hall.

Cardon, T. (2013). Video modeling imitation training to support gestural imitation acquisition in young children with autism spectrum disorder. *Speech, Language and Hearing*, *16*, 227–238. Available from https://doi.org/10.1179/2050572813Y.0000000018.

Cardon, T. A. (2012). Teaching caregivers to implement video modeling imitation training via iPad for their children with autism. *Research in Autism Spectrum Disorders*, *6*, 1389–1400. Available from https://doi.org/10.1016/j.rasd.2012.06.002.

Cardon, T. A., & Wilcox, M. J. (2011). Promoting imitation in young children with autism: A comparison of reciprocal imitation training and video modeling. *Journal of Autism and Developmental Disorders*, *41*, 654–666. Available from https://doi.org/10.1007/s10803-010-1086-8.

Charlop-Christy, M. H., Le, L., & Freeman, K. (2000). A comparison of video modeling with in vivo modeling for teaching children with autism. *Journal of Autism and Developmental Disorders*, *30*, 537–552. Available from https://doi.org/10.1023/A:1005635326276.

Corbett, B. A., & Abdullah, M. (2005). Video modeling: Why does it work for children with autism? *Journal of Early and Intensive Behavior Intervention*, *2*, 2–8. Available from http://doi.org/10.1037/h0100294.

Dawson, G., & Adams, A. (1984). Imitation and social responsiveness in autistic children. *Journal of Abnormal Child Psychology*, *12*, 209–225. Available from https://doi.org/10.1007/BF00910664.

Deshais, M. A., Phillips, C. L., Wiskow, K. M., Vollmer, T. R., & Donaldson, J. M. (2020). A comparison of imitation training using concurrent versus delayed prompting. *Behavior Analysis: Research and Practice*, *20*, 132–147. Available from https://doi.org/10.1037/bar0000174.

Dorwick, P. W. (1991). *Practical guide to using video in behavioral sciences*. New York: John Wiley & Sons, Inc.

Gowen, E. (2012). Imitation in autism: Why action kinematics matter. *Frontiers in Integrative Neuroscience*, *6*, 117. Available from https://doi.org/10.3389/fnint.2012.00117.

Hall, T. A., Mastel, S., Nickel, R., & Wainer, A. (2019). Parents training parents: Lessons learned from a study of reciprocal imitation training in young children with autism spectrum disorder. *Autism: The International Journal of Research and Practice*, *23*, 1601–1606. Available from https://doi.org/10.1177/1362361318815643.

Hobson, R. P., & Lee, A. (1999). Imitation and identification in autism. *The Journal of Child Psychology and Psychiatry and Allied Disciplines*, *40*, 649–659. Available from https://doi.org/10.1111/1469-7610.00481.

Ingersoll, B. (2008). The social role of imitation in autism: Implications for the treatment of imitation deficits. *Infants & Young Children*, *21*, 107–119. Available from https://doi.org/10.1097/01.IYC.0000314482.24087.14.

Ingersoll, B. (2010). Brief report: Pilot randomized controlled trial of reciprocal imitation training for teaching elicited and spontaneous imitation to children with autism. *Journal of Autism and Developmental Disorders*, *40*, 1154–1160. Available from https://doi.org/10.1007/s10803-010-0966-2.

Ingersoll, B. (2012). Brief report: Effect of a focused imitation intervention on social functioning in children with autism. *Journal of Autism and Developmental Disabilities*, *42*, 1768–1773. Available from https://doi.org/10.1007/s10803-011-1423-6.

Ingersoll, B., & Gergans, S. (2007). The effect of a parent implemented imitation intervention on spontaneous imitation skills in young children with autism. *Research in Developmental Disabilities*, *28*, 163–175. Available from https://doi.org/10.1016/j.ridd.2006.02.004.

Ingersoll, B., Lewis, E., & Kroman, E. (2007). Teaching the imitation and spontaneous use of descriptive gestures in young children with autism using a naturalistic behavioral intervention. *Journal of Autism and Developmental Disorders*, *37*, 1446–1456. Available from https://doi.org/10.1007/s10803-006-0221-z.

Ingersoll, B., & Schreibman, L. (2006). Teaching reciprocal imitation skills to young children with autism using a naturalistic behavioral approach: effects on language, pretend play, and joint attention. *Journal of Autism and Developmental Disorders*, *36*, 487–505. Available from https://doi.org/10.1007/s10803-006-0089-y.

Koegel, R. L., & Koegel, L. K. (2006). *Pivotal response treatments for autism*. Baltimore, MD: Paul H. Brookes.

Libby, S., Powell, S., Messer, D., & Jordan, R. (1997). Imitation of pretend play acts by children with autism and Down syndrome. *Journal of Autism and Developmental Disorders*, *27*, 365–383. Available from https://doi.org/10.1023/A:1025801304279.

Lindsay, C. J., Moore, D. W., Anderson, A., & Dillenburger, K. (2013). The role of imitation in video-based interventions for children with autism. *Developmental Neurorehabilitation, 16*, 283–289. Available from https://doi.org/10.3109/17518423.2012.758185.

Lovaas, O. I., Freitas, L., Nelson, K., & Whalen, C. (1967). The establishment of imitation and its use for the development of complex behavior in schizophrenic children. *Behaviour Research and Therapy, 5*, 171–181. Available from https://doi.org/10.1016/0005-7967(67)90032-0.

Mahoney, G., & Perales, F. (2003). Using relationship-focused intervention to enhance the social-emotional functioning of young children with autism spectrum disorders. *Topics in Early Childhood Special Education, 23*, 77–89. Available from https://doi.org/10.1177/02711214030230020301.

McGee, G. G., Morrier, M. J., & Daly, T. (1999). An incidental teaching approach to early intervention for toddlers with autism. *Journal of the Association for Persons With Severe Handicaps, 24*, 133–146. Available from https://doi.org/10.2511/rpsd.24.3.133.

Nadel, J. (2014). *How imitation boosts development: In infancy and autism spectrum disorder*. Oxford: Oxford University Press.

Nikopoulos, C. K., & Keenan, M. (2003). Promoting social initiation in children with autism using video modeling. *Behavioral Interventions, 18*, 87–108. Available from https://doi.org/10.1002/bin.129.

Rayner, C. (2015). Video-based intervention for children with autism: Towards improved assessment of pre-requisite imitation skills. *Developmental Neurorehabilitation, 18*, 113–121. Available from https://doi.org/10.3109/17518423.2014.890959.

Rogers, S. J., & Dawson, G. (2010). *Early start denver model for young children with autism: Promoting language, learning and engagement*. New York: Guildford Press.

Rogers, S. J., Hepburn, S. L., Stackhouse, T., & Wehner, E. (2003). Imitation performance in toddlers with autism and those with other developmental disorders. *Journal of Child Psychology and Psychiatry, 44*, 763–781. Available from https://doi.org/10.1111/1469-7610.00162.

Schreibman, L., Dawson, G., Stahmer, A. C., Landa, R., Rogers, S. J., McGee, G. G., ... Halladay, A. (2015). Naturalistic developmental behavioral interventions: Empirically validated treatments for autism spectrum disorder. *Journal of Autism and Developmental Disorders, 45*, 2411–2428. Available from https://doi.org/10.1007/s10803-015-2407-8.

Sevlever, M., & Gillis, J. M. (2010). An examination of the state of imitation research in children with autism: Issues of definition and methodology. *Research in Developmental Disabilities, 31*, 976–984. Available from https://doi.org/10.1007/s10803-015-2596-1.

Smith, T. (2001). Discrete trial training in the treatment of autism. *Focus on Autism and Other Developmental Disabilities, 16*, 86–92. Available from https://doi.org/10.1177/108835760101600204.

Soorya, L. V., Arnstein, L. M., Gillis, J., & Romanczyk, R. G. (2003). An overview of imitation skills in autism: Implications for practice. *The Behavior Analyst Today, 4*, 114–123. Available from http://doi.org/10.1037/h0100108.

Stone, W., Ousley, O., & Littleford, C. (1997). Motor imitation in young children with autism: What's the object? *Journal of Abnormal Child Psychology, 25*, 475–485. Available from https://doi.org/10.1023/a:1022685731726.

Tereshko, L., MacDonald, R., & Ahearn, W. H. (2010). Strategies for teaching children with autism to imitate response chains using video modeling. *Research in Autism Spectrum Disorders, 4*, 479–489. Available from https://doi.org/10.1016/j.rasd.2009.11.005.

Thurm, A., Lord, C., Lee, L., & Newschaffer, C. (2007). Predictors of language acquisition in preschool children with autism spectrum disorders. *Journal of Autism and Developmental Disorders, 37*, 1721–1734. Available from https://doi.org/10.1007/s10803-006-0300-1.

Valentino, A. L., LeBlanc, L. A., & Conde, K. A. (2018). Validation of a skills assessment to match interventions to teach motor imitation to children with autism. *Learning and Motivation, 62*, 67–76. Available from https://doi.org/10.1016/j.lmot.2017.02.005.

Vanvuchelen, M., Roeyers, H., & De Weerdt, W. (2007). Nature of motor imitation problems in school-aged boys with autism: A motor or a cognitive problem? *Autism: the International Journal of Research and Practice, 11*, 225–240. Available from https://doi.org/10.1177/1362361307076846.

Vivanti, G., & Hamilton, A. (2014). Imitation in autism spectrum disorders. In F. R. Volkmar, S. J. Rogers, P. Rhea, & K. A. Pelphery (Eds.), *Handbook of autism and pervasive developmental disorders* (4th Edition, pp. 278–301). New Jersey: Wiley & Sons.

Vivanti, G., Nadig, A., Ozonoff, S., & Rogers, S. (2008). What do children with autism attend to during imitation tasks? *Journal of Experimental Child Psychology, 101*(3), 186–205. Available from https://doi.org/10.1016/j.jecp.2008.04.008.

Wainer, A. L., & Ingersoll, B. (2015). Increasing access to an ASD imitation intervention via a telehealth parent training program. *Journal of Autism and Developmental Disorders, 45*, 3877–3890. Available from https://doi.org/10.1007/s10803-014-2186-7.

Walton, K. M., & Ingersoll, B. (2012). Evaluation of a sibling-mediated imitation intervention for young children with autism. *Journal of Positive Behavior Interventions, 14*, 241–253. Available from https://doi.org/10.1177/1098300712437044.

Warreyn, P., & Roeyers, H. (2014). See what I see, do as I do: Promoting joint attention and imitation in preschoolers with autism spectrum disorder. *Autism: the International Journal of Research and Practice, 18*, 658–671. Available from https://doi.org/10.1177/1362361313493834.

Wild, K. S., Poliakoff, E., Jerrison, A., & Gowen, E. (2012). Goal-directed and goal-less imitation in autism spectrum disorder. *Journal of Autism and Developmental Disorders, 42*, 1739–1749. Available from https://doi.org/10.1007/s10803-011-1417-4.

Williams, J. H. G., Whiten, A., & Singh, T. (2004). A systematic review of action imitation in autistic spectrum disorder. *Journal of Autism and Developmental Disorders, 34*, 285–299. Available from https://doi.org/10.1023/b:jadd.0000029551.56735.3a.

Zaghlawan, H. Y., & Ostrosky, M. M. (2016). A parent-implemented intervention to improve imitation skills by children with autism: A pilot study. *Early Childhood Education Journal, 44*, 671–680. Available from https://doi.org/10.1007/s10643-015-0753-y.

Disruption to embodiment in autism, and its repair

6

Jonathan Delafield-Butt[1,2], *Penelope Dunbar*[3] *and Colwyn Trevarthen*[4]
[1]Laboratory for Innovation in Autism, University of Strathclyde, Glasgow, United Kingdom, [2]School of Education, University of Strathclyde, Glasgow, United Kingdom, [3]Independent Artist and Creative Researcher, Glasgow, United Kingdom, [4]School of Philosophy, Psychology and Language Sciences, The University of Edinburgh, Edinburgh, United Kingdom

Introduction

In the human mind, consciousness of "the self as agent" (Macmurray, 1957) is not a singular, homogenous phenomenon, but is a layered set of systems integrated by a hierarchy of phylogenetic principles of brain growth and animated activity that give rise to sympathetic actions and reactions that connect "persons in relation" (Macmurray, 1961). Comparative neuroscientist of emotions, Jaak Panksepp (Panksepp, 1998a; Panksepp & Biven, 2012) identified three levels of neural processing in mammals, each generating an awareness of the Self made in relation to internal and external environments, and mediating between the two. His view advanced by detailed comparative neuroanatomy with penetrating observation of affective expressions and responses common to rodents and primates gave psychology improved description and richer evolutionary understanding of the basic notion of a "triune" brain of MacLean (1990)—the idea that evolution of vertebrate ecology in social groups toward the human cultural intelligence incorporated three distinct, but interconnected levels of processing. First of the *reptilian brain stem*, then the *paleomammalian midbrain limbic system*, and finally the complex neomammalian powers for acquiring adaptive experience recorded in what is known as *the neocortex of the forebrain*.

What a human person experiences in healthy activity of the body and brain with awareness as a singular coherent conscious Self (Sherrington, 1906) is the result of efficient composition of action in the layers of neurobiological processing working in synchrony (Buzsáki, 2006). Regulations of energy in internal embodied well-being of an integrated person is maintained by an affective system linked to the autonomic visceral organs (Panksepp, 1991, 1992), and this is coupled with all voluntary and imaginative neuromotor control of the skeletomuscular system of the body in purposeful movement (Bernstein, 1967). This "inner life" from which all arts, mathematics, and philosophies grow (Langer, 1942; Lashley, 1951) is both graceful or *aesthetic* in its efficiency (Turner, 1991), and gracious or *moral* in intersubjective social cooperation (Trevarthen, 2015).

Emerging Programs for Autism Spectrum Disorder. DOI: https://doi.org/10.1016/B978-0-323-85031-5.00018-9

Efficient communication between all the elements of the intentional and self-conscious nervous system in one rhythm of time (Buzsáki, 2006) is critical. The animal brain evolved as an integrative organ to bring the experiences and activities of all parts of the body into one composite awareness. In human beings the fingers, hands, elbows, and feet move the body in ambient and focal awareness to exploit what the outside world affords for use (Gibson, 1977). Inner vitality coordinates functions of the stomach, liver, and heart, and the information-seeking assertions of neck, head, mouth, and eyes that become powerful media of communication of individual impulses and their effects in social partnerships (Reed, 1996). Every movement acts as a coherent and coordinated whole with its own, singular purpose in transformations of the body made in movement with prospective imagination of the effects (Bernstein, 1967). The innate coherent rhythmic "musical" composition of all willful agency of the individual is elaborated within each body as the common code for shared cultural awareness and understanding (Malloch & Trevarthen, 2009b; Trevarthen, Gratier, & Osborne, 2014).

At the anatomical center of this integrative system of neurons in all vertebrates is the brainstem. At the anterior end of the spinal column it brings together information from the visceral organs on maintenance of inner life, and information from the moving muscles of the skeleton together which sense information about the surrounding world from the distance receptors, the eyes, ears, and nose for sight, sound, and smell. This brainstem "head ganglion" (Coghill, 1929) has access to all of the information from outside and inside the body required for prospective conscious awareness along the intended course of locomotion. Its basic anatomy and neural function is shared across "vertebrates"—all animals with a spine; reptiles, amphibians, birds, and mammals. As the most ancient phylogenetic layer of this neural system, it is the site of rapid integration and evaluation of information across the body and brain, in what Panksepp calls the "Core Self," the first "center of conscious awareness" (Northoff & Panksepp, 2008; Panksepp, 1998b).

Interestingly, and importantly, this Core Self can operate on its own in humans, cats, and rats, without the addition of information from the phylogenetically more recent neocortex—the large, voluminous convoluted brain mass that fills the skull and that most educated people (including cognitive neuroscientists) think of as "the brain" (Merker, 2007; Penfield & Jasper, 1954). In fact, we can be conscious without a cortex, as surgical decortication experiments have shown, and as is proven by children born with rare congenital total loss of neocortex (Shewmon, Holmse, & Byrne, 1999). This simple fact is lost in most contemporary neuropsychology sources, but it is critical to our understanding of autism. The brainstem is the site of coherent integration of information about the world outside in consciousness, and also of the state of the world inside, rich with vital needs of the body, which are afforded opportunity for satisfaction in active appreciation of benefits, and apprehension of dangers, in contacts with the world outside.

Second, above the brainstem sits a complex of pathways and larger nuclei that hold special abilities to store memories and appraise these as benefits or risks of harm. These store and organize past experience so it can be recalled and deployed to help organize action in the present moment, and in the service of future goals. The accumulated memories of the past serve understanding of the consequences of actions in the present, and set goals for a desired and imagined future of purposeful life.

In the third level of organization experiences grow with our expanded cognitive or "knowing" capacities, and with tools of symbolic abstraction that enable defined experiences to be held "off-line" in memories and manipulated in our imagination. This third level of processing occurs across the vast array of brain space we recognize as the cortex. Its unique format presents layers of neurons stacked as vast, broad sheets of integration that can process the rich variety of experiences near-simultaneously. This new element of the brain provides capacities of enhanced perceptual discrimination, memory, abstract reflection, conceptual organization, planning, and evaluation. These "cognitive tools" become the structures that build our human intelligence, knowledge, and technical mastery (Gigliotta, Pezzulo, & Nolfi, 2011; Pezzulo & Castelfranchi, 2009). It is the seat of our postindustrial rational human mind and reflective pragmatic intelligence recorded symbolically in manufactured media.

Our conscious experience in each moment varies and shifts, contingent on changing needs and circumstances. It is a single point in what William James called "the specious present" (James, 1890), a unique moment in time that slips ever forward, its experience structured by the remembered past and anticipated future. We now understand its structure is the product of deep evolutionary layering, adapted for an adventurous animal life that expands our ability to anticipate and prepare for the organic needs of growth, sustenance, and learning especially highly developed in humans. It enables an exceptional capacity to project the imagination into the future, to make plans in the present moment based on a remembered past, for a desired future (Delafield-Butt & Gangopadhyay, 2013; Fig. 6.1).

Jaak Panksepp's three levels of conscious processing demonstrate that what we have traditionally considered "unconscious" is in fact the core of our conscious experience—it is a primary, prereflective consciousness that is evident in, and that structures, everyday actions of the animal. As Solms and Panksepp (2012) put it in their title, "The 'Id' knows more than the 'Ego' admits." We accept this as the hierarchy of human motor intelligence, and how it grows between the intuitive invention of activity in awareness of the body, and the articulate record and interpretation of thinking with semantic codification of foci of interest in gestural and linguistic syntax with affective prosody (Delafield-Butt & Gangopadhyay, 2013; Delafield-Butt & Trevarthen, 2015; Malloch & Trevarthen, 2009a; Trevarthen & Delafield-Butt, 2017).

Autistic experience as a disruption of the primary affective self, and its coherent integration with secondary and tertiary processing

In this chapter we examine lived autistic experience to reveal its nature in light of the vertical organization of mental processing. We build on self-reflection, scholarship, and dialogue between Penelope Dunbar (Pum) and Jonathan Delafield-Butt, made in recorded interviews about Pum's life with autism over a period of five

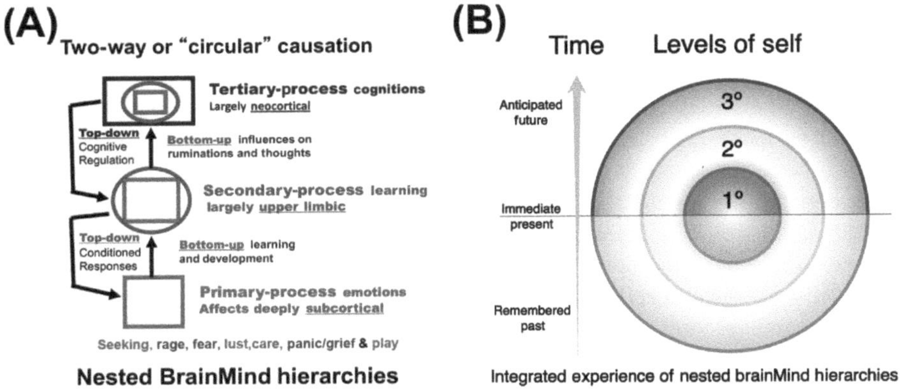

Figure 6.1 Schematics of the nested layers of the self showing (A) their nested organization and (B) their integration and contribution to experience over time. The primary, Core Self is the most phylogenetically ancient and therefore ontogenetically primary self—a site of integration of integrative, evaluative experience and agency. This is brainstem mediated. The secondary self stores with greater precision the memories with greater powers of discrimination for evaluation, but finally the tertiary self is empowered with the cognitive tools built on abstraction from primary experience through its secondary process and considered "offline." Cortically mediated. These layers of processing are reflected in the artwork, "Profile of a collaged mind finding sense and synthesis in the language of movement, fragments and aesthetic coherence." shown in Fig. 6.3.
Source for (A): Reproduced under CC BY 3.0 license from Solms, M., & Panksepp, J. (2012). The "Id" knows more than the "Ego" admits: Neuropsychoanalytic and primal consciousness perspectives on the interface between affective and cognitive neuroscience. *Brain Science*, 2, 147–174.

years, and placed into context of a developing understanding of autism from an embodied, ecological perspective developed earlier between Jonathan Delafield-Butt and Colwyn Trevarthen (Delafield-Butt & Trevarthen, 2017; Trevarthen & Delafield-Butt, 2013a). We have worked to understand the structure of her experience as a person diagnosed with autism spectrum disorder (ASD) from a phenomenological, lived perspective and have set this within new theoretical understanding of autism as a disorder or distortion of a particular kind of embodiment of human agency, distinguishing the regulation of purposes by levels of feeling in body movement, affective appraisals and arousal, and their communication (Trevarthen, 2014). Therefore, the experiences and conclusions drawn from these are relevant for this one particular autistic individual, and we can guarantee their accuracy as reported.

However, autism is not a simple variation of normal motivation and intelligence. It is recognized as a very varied state of personality and in each case manifests its spectrum of conditions idiosyncratically (Gillberg, 1992; Hobson, 1993; Hobson & Hobson, 2011).[1] Therefore, although not all of our findings from Pum's account will

[1] As the autistic community points out, "if you've met one person with autism, you've met *one* person with autism."

generalize or fit as one correct description of the condition, we do emphasize the manifestations in it of general truths applicable to all human beings concerning feeling, arousal, the nested organization of conscious experience, and the effects of these manifest in the embodiment and learning of intentional action. The basic facts of motivation for human life are common to individuals with their different characters and experiences, and a typical disruption of these within autism may be identified.

A brainstem sensorimotor disruption in autism

Our account of autism emphasizes a disruption to efficient primary processing of sensory-motor information, and the self-related affective processing that mediates arousal regulation and coherence of motivation within Panksepp's Core Self (Fig. 6.1; Delafield-Butt & Trevarthen, 2017; Delafield-Butt, Trevarthen, Rowe, & Gillberg, 2019; Trevarthen & Delafield-Butt, 2013a). In this paper, we extend this account of a disturbance of self-regulating vitality to include a specific disruption in the coherence of consciousness vertically, between its three levels of processing. This weakening of coherence appears to start within the primary, brainstem processing that integrates the Core Self, affecting first its internal coherence, and subsequently its elaboration through participation in processes of the higher levels. Weak central coherence of primary consciousness, originating in disruption to brainstem integration, affects the whole psychological system rich with affectivity and the spirit of vitality and awareness. It is not limited to particular higher-order cognitive and perceptual domains of the traditional theory (Happé, 1997, 1999, 2003; Happé & Booth, 2008; Happé & Frith, 2006). Instead, we draw out aspects of conscious experience below tertiary perceptual and cognitive processing to show a more fundamental global "weakening" of conscious coherence that involves affects, arousal, and the center of gravity of one's conscious awareness.

Our account recognizes and appreciates the fundamental contribution to conscious thought, feeling, and awareness the brainstem complex provides, not only in terms of organizing information, but in terms of organizing one's *subjective awareness*. And although the brainstem may be anatomical subcortical, its function is ontogenetically supracortical, giving patterns and structure to cortical development and processing in organization of bodily activity (Merker, 2005, 2013), and the generation of subcortical rhythms that pattern cortical cohesion (Buzsáki, 2006).

An *intrapersonal* coherence between levels of processing appears disrupted, which prevents the development of the innate function of the Core Self in regulating affective states, and that disrupts efficient agency and *interpersonal* communication recognized in formal clinical autistic symptomology.

Autistic challenges of a disconnected and incoherent Core Self

In Pum's experience, she felt a distressing disjunction between her rational, reflective self and her inability to manage her affective states of arousal. Her core affective and integrative corporeal self was disconnected and muted. Her reflective Tertiary Self became obsessively aware of her social expectations, and its demands for her to perform in a socially conformed manner. This logic produced a "false" rationale because it excluded personal feeling and motive, but it dominated her thinking and reflection and came to control her conscious experience and behavior. It was an inflexible, literal appropriation that accepted what she was taught and led to a rational rule-governed understanding of social requirements and engagement in them. Yet, this rational self-control of her behavior neglected her more fundamental needs for self-knowledge and self-satisfaction as an individual animal with impulses and feelings, which were denied to her. Instead, compliance to learnt social scripts were supported at the cost of her emotional well-being. Later, her ability to regulate states of arousal and anxiety were paralyzed by a disconnection and in many respects were completely unaware of what we have come to identify as the feelings and needs of her Core Self. Further, this habitual disassociation into a performed script damaged her ability to manage her basic functioning, and manifested in, for example, eating and sleeping disorders and entrenched mental health problems in her early adult life.

The language of the Core Self is nonverbal, affective, and aneotic (Vandekerckhove & Panksepp, 2009). In childhood learning Pum was instructed how to understand and use social verbal language. And she worked hard to learn speech, reading, and writing through copying particular demonstrations of these, and with obsessive attention to detail of politeness and needs of others. This led to an unintegrated sense of self, which was eventually expressed in mental health symptoms of chronic anorexia and depression. It was only many years later in adult life, after ongoing therapy and some decades of self-reflection and analysis that she came to understand that she had developed a disjunction between what we now know as her Core Self—her core affective, perceptual, and embodied Self—and her more artificial, rational, and reflective Tertiary Self. The logical language of words were not expressive of her true intuitive self-as-agent with its idiosyncratic autism profile, accepting it, and therefore did not communicate what she really wished to do and share.

Meaning, coherence, and the challenge of incoherence

We are a social species that demands meaningful social interaction, even in autism (Jaswal & Akhtar, 2018). Social isolation is a painful experience and can be associated with feelings of shame on both sides (Trevarthen, 2005), it disconnects the *interpersonal* world from a system evolved to share in it (Gallagher, 2014). Similarly, disconnection within oneself can be painful. In Pum's autism, centers of conscious experience evolved to work integratively as a whole were disconnected from each other, an *intrapersonal* disconnection. Failure of a coherent, integrated experience of behaviors and interactions left each less meaningful, and created distress and challenging behaviors as a consequence. Left unattended to in childhood, this lack of depth of meaning created despair and anxiety that became the standard in her adolescence and early adulthood.

On the surface, she had adjusted her social relationships to appear acceptably "normal", but she struggled in private with an array of distressing and challenging behaviors hidden from view. Internal incoherence and neglect of more primitive, subsurface feelings and desires led to significant mental health issues, especially apparent at peak life events, such as the transitions of puberty and to adulthood, and in the event of life's challenges affecting love, loss, desire, and change of "home". Her Core Self that worked to integrate somatic physiology, including satiation in feeding, digesting, sexual awareness, affectionate engagement, and satisfaction, and sleep/wake regulation, was disengaged from her public behavior.

In childhood, Pum learned language rationally, "outside" of her body. She became more and more disconnected from the life of the body and its needs for self-regulation as the years went by. And, by copying sounds, which then became learnt codes for behavior that were socially appropriate, she could present herself as appropriate, but these were personally meaningless to her.

Johnson and Lakoff teach us how "being in the body" grows into language (Lakoff & Johnson, 1980, 1999), a feature missed or reduced in Pum's development. In typical ontogenesis, one develops movement first, and feelings expressed in movement generate the inspiration for expressive language (Delafield-Butt & Trevarthen, 2013, 2015; Iverson, 2010). It is only once this affective experience of being has found its primary, intuitive, and embodied language can it be developed into an expression of reaching out and sharing what is internal with those who are physically external. Only once this is achieved can the meaningful shared communicative verbal language of words be placed on top, and the possibility of authentic communication established.

Lessons in language development offer a particularly useful illustration of how a supportive parent, therapist, or teacher can encourage healthy curiosity and enjoyment of animated learning. The expressive language of the emotions and body come first in development, on which the language of words bears depth of meaning, and purpose. "It is by natural signs chiefly that we give force and energy to language; and the less language has of them, it is the less expressive and persuasive" (Reid, 1764, pp. 106–107).

Implications for self-improvement and therapeutic support of autistic disturbance to the Core Self

If our account of the disruption to the coherence of core experience of self and its communication with higher level processing is correct, then focusing therapeutic intervention on overt behaviors and conventional speech production may miss the mark, overshooting a coherent integration of feelings and impulses of the affective Core Self. Ontogenetically one must work to develop and substantiate the primary levels of processing first, before extending to more advanced forms such as social regulation, speech production, and verbal communication. One must first build an intimate an affective "languaging" of the self (Halliday, 1975, 1978).

The Core Self is principally embodied, enactive, and nonverbal. Stories of language-like understanding can be first formed on a nonverbal sensory and motor level, as artful visual imagery or musical auditory patterns (Malloch, 1999; Malloch, & Trevarthen, 2009a, 2009b), and within the level of the physiological regulation of the communicator's body and its inner life, as in "polyvagal theory" of the emotional nervous system and expressive forms of movement for communication (Porges, 2001). For therapy, deploying creativity and playful movement in an asocial, structured environment paying particular attention to detail and consistency of the routine to support the patient's growth within the condition of autism, rather than setting a priority on teaching technical performance and social rules where one may unwittingly be led to prioritize performance rather than intuitive knowing what is intended and felt, may be more effective in engaging, or facilitating, the whole, integrated self of the individual with autism.

We have found strong physical activity can also be therapeutic, such as in sports, dance, or equine therapy (Ford, 2013; Koch, 2016; Koch, Mehl, Sobanski, Sieber, & Fuchs, 2015; May et al., 2019; Rinehart, Jeste, & Wilson, 2018), or in shared movement-regulating programs, such as that based on the agency-guiding education theory of Geoffrey Waldon (Posner, 2016; Solomon, Holland, & Middleton, 2012). In the activity of "doing," the sensory and motor system embeds, supports and physically yolks experience to the active sensory-affective self. Further, creative process and movements can become tools when they are built into established daily and weekly structured routines that are organized and predictable.

We caution that the individual with autism may need special support to access and maintain these routines adequately. A low arousal, structured, and predictable lifestyle can support overall well-being and regulation. Without support for routines, feelings and self-agency may be inaccessible, blocked by executive function difficulties in planning, preparation, and organization.

First, for growth and learning, one must be confidently centered within oneself. The human organism must come to terms with the innate complexity of its own movements, expressions, and desires, and able to experience these as self-expression of "Me", before one can differentiate him or herself from the actions of another.

> *In the course of emotional development of the individual a stage is reached at which the individual can be said to have become a unit.... At this stage the child can say "here I am." What is inside me is me and what is outside me is not me. The words inside and outside here refer simultaneously to the psyche and to the soma... A satisfactory psychosomatic partnership.*
>
> *Winnicott (2001/1971, pp. 130–131)*

The center is first and foremost our embodied Core Self, the brainstem-mediated ontogenetically primary agent who perceives, feels, and anoetically evaluates without conscious definition, acting without the "superior" reflective consciousness mediated by our cortical cognitive systems (Vandekerckhove & Panksepp, 2011). One must first "get into the body" with the felt life of willful movements (Lakoff & Johnson, 1980, 1999).

Getting into a routine

However, we must appreciate that activities of integrated movement may not be physically or psychologically available or accessible to a person with ASD. There is an anxiety specific to autism provoked by the beginning of any new act (Robledo, Donnellan, & Strandt-Conroy, 2012), and it takes time for the individual to feel safe and allow arousal levels to settle. Accessing movement for personal or social aims can overexcite uncertainty, "Am I going to be able to move my body?" This can be debilitating, and prevent willful transition into the activity. However, with external support for practice of a daily and weekly routine, the impulse to act can recover with feelings of safety, and the body can begin to associate the beginning of that structured routine with a sense of confidence in knowledge of the future activity.

How emotional arousal can be understood, and managed

When a child's or an adult's autism's needs are not met, their levels of arousal increase, and they may appreciate even a sensitive invitation as disorientating. The individual requires an adapted calm responsive treatment, which offers containment and a neutrality that accepts and attempts to moderate their reactions of distress (Douglas, 2007; Fig. 6.2).

At first, the companion, supporter, or therapist may work alongside the individual. This may help to foster oblique communication by removing face-to-face interaction which can be experienced as overwhelming and confrontational for the individual with autism. Imitating and helping to organize the routine of their actions, acting as a coach or guide to help regulation of their movement and to confirm a sense of coherent agency. A therapist who is patient, committed, and observant of patterns of action may act with aesthetic and compassionate feelings that recognize the unique autistic needs of the individual in the present moment.

The practitioner's actions need to be predictable and consistent for the person with autism to feel accepted, safe, and their needs appreciated. Then they can begin to become aware of what those needs are, safe in the knowledge that the other is able to foster trust and lower arousal. From this foundation in mutual regulation of self-awareness and trust, the more creative organic platform of communication for the self through structured, repetitive activity can be developed. This way autonomy can be promoted, and eventually secured. Communication from within the Primary Self leads to a growing potential to meaningfully communicate with another person as a more authentic, confident, and true Self.

Co-opting compulsions for repetitive behaviors, and transforming them into productive, creative, self-sustaining action for personal growth

Self-expression is built and shared in efforts of sport and art, but their aesthetic and moral power in shared vitality can be devalued and often overlooked in

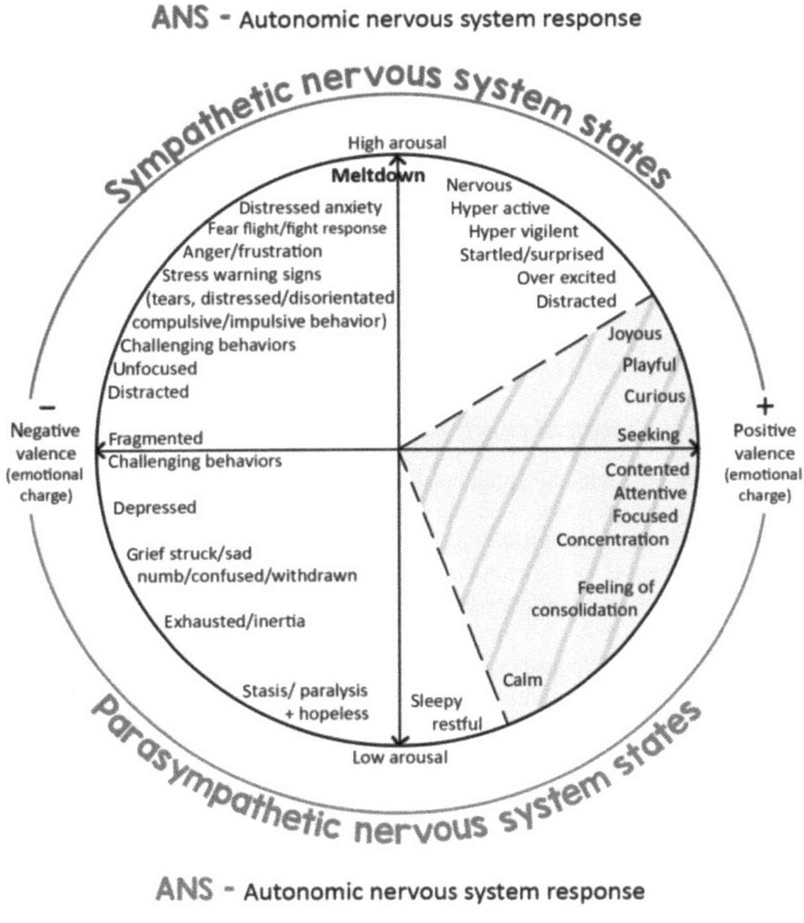

Figure 6.2 Pum's states of subjective, internal regulation of affects and arousal by body activity, their personal expression and interpersonal sharing in movement. The green area indicates the optimum, ideal levels of arousal for practicing structured and creative routines in kinetic expression, and to facilitate "self-to-self" communication across levels (cf. Fig. 6.1). The left-hand side of the chart shows negative valence states, feelings that are detrimental to individual functioning and well-being and that incur further stress. The right-hand side of the chart shows more positively valenced feelings. The higher regions of arousal on this side can still result in an unpleasant and detrimental response. States of happiness and surprise are especially triggering, and stressfully disorientating. Being overexcited makes Pum dissociate and become overstimulated, which often results in an inevitable shift to meltdowns and anxiety, leading to disorientation, confusion and a grief-stricken state.

Psychology, even as music has been by Stephen Pinker, follower of Noam Chomsky's theory of the rational formality of language (Chomsky, 1957), on "the language instinct" (Pinker, 1994).

With the information obtained by detailed analysis of the talents of infants for sharing stories of life in movement (Trevarthen, 2003; Trevarthen & Delafield-Butt, 2013b, 2015), we see these activities and the routines that lead into them as fundamentally important for personal well-being, growth, and mental health of every human being. From before birth, as a foetus alive and responding to feelings with the mother's person, each individual adapts the vital compulsion for rhythms of repetitive action (Stern, 2000, 2010), and coopts this to serve useful purpose in special ways of living in the objective and social worlds. Their cooption affords gains in self-control, self-satisfaction, and learning with a shift in mental processing that is felt, from the start, as a cohesive and integrative embodied experience, a story of human life to be shared (Bruner, 2003).

In infants with autism, their cooption into habits of shared social value is disrupted (St. Claire, Danon-Boileau, & Trevarthen, 2007; Trevarthen & Daniel, 2005). Repetitive movement without a plan or narrative that gives a clear beginning, middle, and end to the project (Trevarthen, Aitken, Nagy, Delafield-Butt, & Vandekerckhove, 2006) can produce compulsive repetition of behaviors. Some stereotypies of gesture, such as hand flapping, can be self-confirming, allowing one to hold a presence of mind for useful benefit in self-regulation (Caldwell, 2000, p. 14–16). Others can be detrimental, such as excessive consumption of water or food, or teeth grinding. When overdone, their beneficial effect is lost to a detrimental, sometimes damaging form of loss of control, such as in compulsive eating, biting, or extensive habits that cause damage to the body. In Pum's experience, the self-affirming quality of repetitive action contains within it a valuable resource to be harnessed.

With care to bring into life a structured routine that has a clear narrative purpose, with a meaningful beginning, middle, and end, security in predictable rhythms of action can be recovered. However, without this structure and routine the autistic individual may lose that coherence of purpose, not know what one is doing or what to do, and it can be very difficult to step over into the activity or the movement, particularly the transition from a mental, imagined into physical, active state. This particular emotional autistic sensitivity can be supported through movement and the creative process set within a regular routine.

Pum has revealed the power of two routines that coopt her autistic need for repetition and regularity, together with her need for body movement, to allow her to feel alive in her body, and in her mind. These two activities are swimming and collage, different in degrees of physical exertion, but similar in their adoption of repetition and routine for beneficial gains, and unique in their particular transformation of states of mind that is of special interest to our developing thesis on the Primary Self.

Pum's swimming routine was developed over ten years of practice. It serves as a self-generated intervention to manage her autism and its associated depressive mood disorder. Its physical exercise benefits regulation of appetite, sleep, hygiene, but also creative imagination. Second, she has always deployed art for cathartic expression, particularly painting. From her creative, artistic research grew a collage praxis. Collage satisfied a need for an expansive, yet concrete visual language.

It further helped her to explore her autism, her sensory sensitivities, disruption to her embodied being, and difficulties managing her lived experiences.

We explore the details of each, in turn. Each is predicated on sensorimotor repetition, sensorimotor loops (cf. Daniel, 2019; Trevarthen, Daniel, & Trevarthen, 2017). Each practice is a routine that involves ritualized regularity of the tasks before, during, and after it, for example in the days of the week, time of day, and pattern of preparation, practice, and conclusion. Each is itself a regular, repetitive routine, but its sensory-motor nature does something peculiar for Pum's state of mind, improving her clarity, reducing her autistic anxiety, and enabling a cohesion in her sense of Self that bridges between her rational Tertiary Self and her Core Self. Both give integration through movement (Fig. 6.3).

Swimming as creative therapy

The cycles of body movement in swimming are repetitive and predictable over a series of timescales. They are carried out in a specially constructed swimming pool environment which stays constant, improving the regularity of the experience. Each length of the pool is the same as the next or the last, and each lap repeats a loop of the same action architecture. Thus the repetitive nesting of voluntary neuromotor actions creates and sustains a regularity of acting, one that is generated and controlled by the individual's own wish, and will, to swim.

Swimming creates a sensation of a moving and floating Self made by making sinuous movements of the whole body pushing against the water by cyclic strokes of legs and arms, coordinated to follow a particular course with more or less vigor. It requires exercise of repetitive sensorimotor loops guided by bilateral actions with unique kinetic and proprioceptive properties. The body is suspended with a feeling of weightlessness and sufficient buoyancy to hold it at the surface in any posture, but able to dive by pushing downwards. With any movement the water provides a tactile feedback over the body's surfaces, and muscular–skeletal feedback is felt internally by proprioceptive stimulation from actions slowed by the resistive forces of the water.

Regular, repetitive sensory-motor loops of arm, leg, head, and body posture in synchrony are paced and forced with direction in space and time to produce fluid movement of the whole body through the water. Separate actions are serially organized and coordinated to work in step with their kinetics slowed by the fluid mass in which they float. A front-crawl cycle of arm moves to push the body forward is made with adjustments of posture and head to afford breathing in time with the successive strokes of left and right arms in alternation, and the two legs kick in contrapuntal, antiphase synchrony. Thus simple actions of the limbs are serially organized and coordinated in time with breathing. Each cycle of limb actions conforms with the cycle of a whole-body pattern marked by breathing, which resets the cycle. A fixed project of these repeated actions moves the body to the other end of the pool where a different set of coordinated movements turns the person around to face the opposite direction, and the exercise repeats.

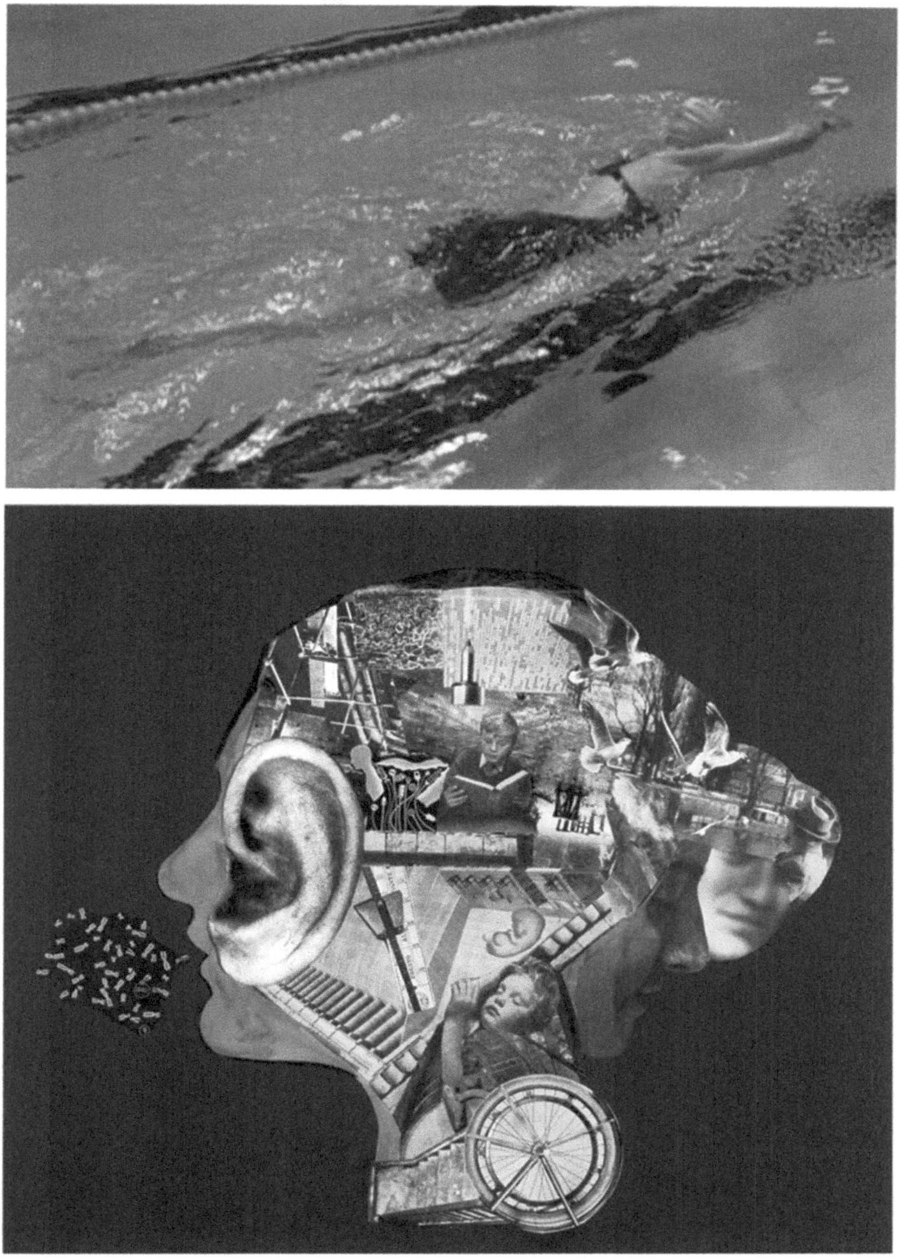

Figure 6.3 Above: Pum enjoying moving her body through the supportive medium of water which offers routines of sensorimotor integration and progress in movement. **Below**: An original collage artwork by Pum that explores and expresses visually a growing understanding of the neurobiological basis of autism spectrum disorder. The foetus represents the Core Self, and the collage spatially positions images in correspondence to the brain locations of various structures to represent those functions. See Appendix 1 for a full key to the component parts.

Using buoyancy of the body held with the liquid mass of water, swimming is regulated by kinetic proprioception of the body surface by a unique tactile feedback of counterbalancing muscular forces sensed simultaneously. With strong patterns of simultaneous feedback from trunk and all four limbs it can be particularly somatically integrative. It sets swimming aside as a unique exercise of all-body monitoring by sensory feedback. This appreciation of intentional action, coupling all modalities of sensory feedback, may have especially positive benefits for individuals with autism, helping them sense in fully-coherent self-control. It generates a physiological and psychological experience of unification: "I am, I become, I act embodied. My body is felt as mine." This relates back to Winnicott's understanding that, from the beginning of individual life, knowing your body as yours is primary, and essential for learning an understanding that your body is separate and distinct from any other person's body. Swimming builds up individual and relational awareness and creates a safe exploration in rhythms of movement for the experience of Self, to appreciate it is intact and truly inhabited with an ambitious will to live.

What are the special beneficial effects of swimming for a person with autism?

As with all repetitive, patterned activity, the exercise of swimming frees the conscious mind to reanimate a deeper, more primary physical awareness. The conscious attention required to perform a skilled routine is significantly reduced, which allows the sensuous part of the mind to become affectively engaged with the body, finding somatic satisfaction in the expression of movement. This can be felt as cathartic.

Generated and integrated within the brainstem at the level of Panksepp's "Core Self," the underlying sensory-motor activity generates a rhythmic regularity and integration of experience at this primary level of integrative processing. The contrapuntal, bilateral repetitive movements together with haptic sensation of the whole-body to resistive forces of liquid flowing across it confirm a strong sensory-motor integration in active experience beneficial for peaceful and pleasurable integration of mind.

Signals from rhythmic brainstem sensory-motor integration, in concert with the rhythms of action generation and sensory responses, are repeated through all their nested cycles in synchrony. The foundational rhythms of body movements, generated and integrated in the brainstem, pattern and structure the more speculative rhythms of neural activity in the cerebral cortices (Buzsáki, 2006). There, our abstract, "off-line" intuitive, anoetic processes and reflections are aroused and coordinated by patterning of interneuronal activity excited from below (Pezzulo & Castelfranchi, 2009; Vandekerckhove & Panksepp, 2011). From this knowledge we advance the hypothesis that increased strength of the brainstem integrative signal excited for swimming generates a coherence of conscious experience by its regular repetition with the improved vigor of simultaneous, all-body sensory and motor signals.

The physical exertion of swimming certainly brings deep physiological benefits. The heart pumps faster, circulating more blood, oxygen, and energy not only to the muscles, but also to the brain, enhancing mental function. There is increased awareness of this link between exercise and thought, with particular attention in the literature to walking. It is a common understanding that walking or swimming or other forms of exercise enable thoughts and especially creative or "divergent" thinking (Keinänen, 2016). Walking has long been associated with facilitating creativity in intellectual pursuits (Keinänen, 2016), from the Socratic peripatetic school (Peripatetic = walking about) advanced by Aristotle and others (Athamatten, 2012), to Nietzsche who claimed in typical overzealous fashion, "Only those thoughts that come by walking have any value" (Nietzsche, 2007, p. 9). Indeed, Henry David Thoreau commented, "Methinks that the moment my legs begin to move, my thoughts begin to flow" (Thoreau & Blaisdell, 2011). Exercise of repetitive body movement can liberate thought.

In the case of Pum's lived experience, the act of mixed purposeful programs of action and their repetitions affords an intense feeling of integration in coherence of mind and body that is not otherwise felt, and that produces within it a sense of calm and affective equilibrium.[2]

Swimming and walking, and indeed any complex well-conceived pattern of behavior, depends on regular cycles of action in an involuntary autonomic system, which assures the supply of oxygen and energy required for the rhythms of exercise. Done well, the body's physiological homeostasis can be maintained for many tens of minutes with the benefit of a constant, regular repetition of action and its felt sensory effects. Pum has developed her swimming practice of biweekly swims of 50 lengths, with regular periods of rest between sustained swimming to stretch the body. Stretches generate further skeletal muscular feedback and give her a growing sense of her body as hers in that moment. The movements and stretches performed together confirm ownership and self-control of her actions.

Collage as creative therapy

Pum is a practiced collage artist. Her practice developed from a need to explore, express, and interrelate ideas and concepts from her own personal research and scholarly work. She has found collage-making exceptionally beneficial, cathartic, and calming. Collage as a medium allows her mind to shift into a fluid multimetaphorical state similar in dynamic complexity to her use of the water in swimming exercise, but with differences of composition and significance.

Like swimming, collage is a repetitive activity that allows discovery of new forms of experience and thought, and that flows with the activity to allow opportunity for the accessibility of affective and reflective self-awareness. It involves intention for regular cycles of repetitive sensorimotor activity—sorting of the paper, selection of images, cutting of fragments—all actions that demand integrated action across the body, stabilizing posture and maintaining coherence of attention and coordinated action.

[2] Interestingly, this stands in contrast to the lateral thinking released for enhancement of the creative imagination in people without autism, and suggests that while some common mechanism is at work, its effects differ in their quality between autistic and nonautistic experience.

Done easily with rehearsed skill, these simple activities can allow the mind to freely associate, playing off the images and their associations in the safety of a known environment that remains peacefully constant and unobtrusive.

Small, elementary micromovements make large shifts of symbolic content with very little effort and only subtle movements of the muscles. A shift of the paper can juxtapose foreground and background in a new way to give rise to a significantly larger cognitive and perceptual shift in the created world. This aesthetic incidental control of the pictorial world can be very strengthening, reassuring, and rewarding. Again, a sense of agency is confirmed. Moreover, while each repetitive micromovement is focused on detail, controlled shifts of attention strive to piece together the detailed parts into a new whole. This strategy of creation exploits her autistic preference for applying detailed focal attention while at the same time allowing a return placement of the selected part into the whole again. Perspectival shifts from part to whole, back to part again, and so on to give the aesthetic feel of the growing picture, and this can enhance a sense of integration and coherence for the autistic artist in their practice. The aesthetic affective resonance of the work of art allows for and reinforces the maker's experience of affective, embodied self-awareness.

As with her swimming, Pum has found collage-making to be a calming activity that allows an integration of the whole self from across the vertical levels of mental processing, allowing thought of the experience to flow from its perceptual elements to recollections of their embodied resonances on combination.

The simple logical efforts, of sticking together a complex picture composition and swimming down a pool are constituted in the pursuit of repetitive sensorimotor action. In collage, this is the selection of print material, the cutting out, and the handling of discreet components. The amount of physical exertion for picture-making is significantly less than for any athletic task, and correspondingly the degree of perceptual and cognitive reflection can be considerably greater, feeding off the images and patterns that transform the elements of the collage in their creative exploration to make their meaning coherent.

This requires a regular to-and-fro shift from internal-to-external percept, a movement from creative interior intuition to concrete external symbols. It enables a stitching together of conscious processing with thoughts and feelings that lie below conscious awareness. This process of composing an integrated picture can be cathartic, easing her internal tension which arises out of an autistic confusion of fragmented parts and contexts.

Collage affords Pum the discovery of a new synthesis of mind, allowing her autistic brain to get into the detail and to feel how each part shape the others, allowing comprehension and a new, literal appreciation of the attractiveness of the message as a coherent whole. By shifting focus across the details in collage-making, the whole visual composition is held and articulated, complete with thoughts and feelings communicated through the silent and still language of imagery. Pum feels this benefit, a satisfaction in the work of interpretation.

Collage is hugely strengthening for Pum, because she has to capture its sense not in words, but in images of tangible static imagery made in scraps of concrete detail. It lets her autistic mind to do what it likes to do, focus on the detail, and lets the autistic brain do what it likes to do, get stuck in and focused in on the activity or project. Then, when one is locked into that activity of repetitive sensorimotor process, the creative process kicks in. Something new happens: a new, integrative state of consciousness. And that new something enables growth of her creative self, enables Self-relating, and an integration of her sensory-affective experience made coherent and meaningful in her exploratory, expressive body movement. It opens new, higher states of reflective self-consciousness. This is incalculably beneficial, its insights translated for healthier everyday living.

The other important feature of collage is that it captures one's interest in the little fiddly movements some individuals with ASD are compelled to repeat, normally with little product or enjoyment to be shared. However, by embedding this repetitive behavior in a structured routine, a creative opportunity is encouraged. Thus, if a supportive and sensitive practitioner can foster one's engagement with concrete materials, one can help the individual with autism access an evolving creative dimension. When acting in an asocial setting, and left alone, the individual collage-maker necessarily communicates with him- or herself, through the aesthetic, signs, and symbols of their work. Thus, when Pum is making a collage, she is engaged in Self-related processing. She is "dialoguing" with different aspects of her Self free from social responsibility or performative requirements. She is solely engaged in communicating to and with her Self. She likens this process to a private form of waking dream, in which she can slowly discover herself.

In Pum's experience, good collage comes from three to four hours of continuous practice. It is in such sustained activity that she begins to synthesize thoughts, feelings, and ideas working below the level of conscious reflection to solve problems, and that is when she begins to feel an intuitive, integrated, and coherent sense of self. It gives her new, inner strength that enables her to survive and cope with the relentless performative demands of her autism disorder and the everyday, practical activities that support her physical, mental, and emotional well-being. This deeply restorative creative behavior has allowed her to understand her need to withdraw from the conventional social world, whilst supporting her growth within her private creative work and research.

Collage is embodied self-reflexivity in changing sensorimotor movements. Movements of the pieces of collage generate feedback that is satisfying, or not. And through appraisals and self-reflection, something new and rewarding can be established. As the repetition of these movements proceed, Pum discovers a transition in her consciousness from its usual state of tense, fragmented, unfocused attention, to one of more relaxed coherence of perception, action, and reflection. This transitioned state allows an appreciation of experiences immediately at hand to include both internal and external awareness. New to this experience is a feeling of integrated coherence, with mind and body working synchronously together in balanced harmony, not felt passively during the flux of daily experience or under the demands of rules and routines in a spontaneously changing external or internal environment. Autism presents disorder in the normal experience of self-conscious purposeful and valued habits of a life alone and in relationships. It can be helped by giving it clarity and strength by changing personal and social demands for action, and social interaction.

Sensitive care for the primary self of a companion with autism: supportive structures for routines of practice

From consideration of the principles of brain control of purposeful muscular activity of the human body in awareness of its environments, objective and social, with appreciation of the efforts and emotions involved, we have outlined a theory of autism, its development and how its problems may be alleviated by relational and sympathetic therapy that adapts the urge for repetitive behavior into constructive routines (Trevarthen & Delafield-Butt, 2013b). The foundation of our approach is in the phylogenetic record of vertebrate brain systems that direct and evaluate movements with many senses for feedback of biomechanical effects between the body and the environment, as well as within the body between its inner vital organs, media for sustaining nutritive well-being, and harmonization of activity in its skeletomuscular system to maintain health and growth of the integrated whole Self (Bosco et al., 2019; Dadalko & Travers, 2018; Delafield-Butt & Trevarthen, 2017).

A focus for therapeutic intervention can be to improve intrapersonal coherence and self-awareness of the different levels of processing, especially the difference between the rational, reflective analytic consciousness (Fig. 6.1; tertiary kind) and a more ontogenetically primitive and core affective and embodied self (Fig. 6.1; primary kind) that is able to integrate the rational thoughts from "above" with the feelings and desires of the present moment, made real in active bodily expression. Strengthening this self-regulation can lead to gains in cooperative awareness if the emotional processes of inner, intrapersonal sympathetic relating are enriched (Delafield-Butt et al., 2019; Delafield-Butt, Zeedyk, Harder, Vaever, & Caldwell, 2020).

It is for this reason that we caution against behavioral therapies such as those based on Adaptive Behavioral Analysis that focus on the performative aspects of communication and action, but that do not work to help the individual to find the particular form of expression that carries their inner feeling. Performative methods train the intellect to control and rule the body in service of socially acceptable norms of shape or form. And while this may yield some benefit for the family and community by creating an apparently adapted individual with socially normalized behaviors, that individual may very likely remain internally stressed deeper in the body, because performative communication can remain disconnected from personal motives, and remain meaningless or empty.

In such a case, the autistic individual can be left stranded, disconnected, and unable to relate to oneself let alone to another. This aloneness can be disorientating and the meaninglessness stressful. It can be explained as a dissonance between the primary self and the social expectations learned by the secondary and tertiary levels of processing, incurring an internal, chronic distress and further cutting off and entrenching dissociation with primary affective experience.

The organization of autism and its phenomena described in this paper give information for individuals with autism, and for parents and professionals who offer care and support for them. We offer simple, practical advice on securing coherent, productive and pleasurable Self-awareness with motive impulses to enrich experience and give value to habits and knowledge. This is not about appropriate behavior or reciprocal communication of facts in shared meaning for social use of conventional tools or media, which is an enterprise that can arouse self-judging anxiety or shame. It is about finding internal coherence in one's sense of self, and making the best of one's autistic impulses and particular needs.

Establishing a routine for safe practice

Pum's account of her active use of swimming and collage for building strength in her ability to self-relate confirms that such creative activity can be helpful not only as therapeutic for autistic anxiety, but for opening new possibilities for thoughtful reflection, personal development, and creative expression that can allow for an integration of the Self, and only later for one's personal experience to be communicated, and shared in safe and sustaining relations. Both activities were conducted alone, in quiet isolation, exploiting familiar environments and set within routines of daily and weekly patterns. A supportive context can be generated by caring others with practical prompts, such as "in ten minutes we will be stopping," or by showing an object that signals "coming to the end" of an activity. These simple steps encourage security in knowing what is to come. By learning what a movement of the body is and how its activity draws to completion clarifies how the feeling is embodied, and lived.

Change and transitions between states of being can cause the individual with autism significant discomfort. Performing simple rituals of preparation and travel to the swimming pool, or setting out the items to start a college, can itself be anxiety-provoking. Without support, the individual may find this anxiety too difficult to overcome alone. By understanding the individual's autism's needs for clear, transparent expectations with explicit prompts, a caring supporter can facilitate management of the individual's growing anxieties about the change-to-come. This can be done simply through rehearsal and help with planning the details and preparing for the routine.

Each step is important: preparing the swimming costume and towel, packing the bag, wearing the right clothes for the outside, leaving the house, and traveling to the pool. Familiarity with this routine is paramount to reducing anxiety, and maintaining consistency in the patterns is extremely helpful. Keeping to a regular time of day and day of the week is very helpful. Once at the pool, regular use of the same changing room, shower, and swimming lane all help to present a degree of constant, regular familiarity in the routine. This will lead to a building up of an affirmative experience where anxiety levels become reduced over the weeks, months, and years. This will promote a growing sense of self-control, self-confidence, and self-empowerment.

It is worth noting that no matter how simple or complex the task to hand, the carer who is observant and responsive to expectations and past experiences, and respectful of reassuring routines, will assist the individual to become more confident and secure. It may be important to help an individual with autism to identify their needs so they may learn how to communicate them, and find how to manage them for themselves, and become better resourced in self-regulation of vitality. The autistic child needs this support to feel the story of each simple routine, so they can practice it again by themselves. From Pum's experience, the ideal help for the child with autism to surpass developmental hurdles is at their own pace, encouraging known routines and actions that already work, however simple they may be.

Supporting an integration of the self, for self-awareness and self-empowerment

The experience of feelings and motives for action and interaction of the Core Self can be very different from that of the higher-order, Conceptually-Oriented Self. This higher-order Self is developed socially with others, and is therefore structured and organized by conventional social expectations, including instructions. It is shaped by outside social environments. Altogether these external influences on the priorities and values of the Tertiary Self may dissociate it from the feelings, desires, and wishes of the Core Self, which may become trapped and unexpressed.

This can lead to "difficult," "disruptive," or "challenging" behaviors. But it can be damaging for an individual to be defined as such, and it neglects the role and responsibility of social expectation and caregiver support when these behaviors result from a mismatch between these social expectations and tolerances, and lack of "connection" an individual's needs and modes of feeling, thinking, and being. This is why we advise support for them to become more happily self-aware, ready and able to ask for help and therefore to manage their autism better, in friendship.

The Core Self is nonverbal, expressive in the language of body movement, gesture, and intonation of the voice. It may be that to emphasize verbal language acquisition in some children—"to get them to talk"—may miss the fact that they don't speak because they are not ready for that level of abstract, verbal narrative and sense-making, and must rely on intuitive nonverbal elements of self-expression. As in typical development, there needs to develop first a "languaging" of the self in actions of the body (Halliday, 1975). In the sensory-motor realm of psychological functioning, the motor life embeds and supports the awareness of the senses, physically yolking them to the sensory, giving structure to and learning of self-consciousness from sensory perceptions.

All behavior is communication

Parents as custodians of mental and emotional life can often be overly concerned with what their child "can't do", overlooking what their child "can do". We say it is fundamentally important for the child and adult with autism to find their own language on their own bodily level, in extraverted and introverted activity. Throwing a ball and catching, jumping on a trampoline, or moving to music gives that child an experience of their body. And at the same time its activity in action is creating life experiences at a cognitive and sensory level, creating new neural pathways. Just by doing something in a structure or project, with or without a caregiver. Thus the best caregiver support is attentive and observant to the opening, to where the child is going to be able to channel communication with their self and body.

Key conclusions, how individual vitality, with emotional appreciation of experience from acting, grows in brain and body of a person with ASD, and how it may benefit from sensitive care

This paper has examined the evidence for a nested hierarchy of human conscious experience that exists at all stages of development of body and brain, and the special nature of autism disorder that disrupts the efficient integration in neural centers of the primary Core Self, and the development of coherence in communication of neural and motor effects reaching between levels to enrich the consciousness of the top level. We identified the need in each person, child or adult, for *intrapersonal communication* to be supported and strengthened as the Self-in-Relations of an intimate and structured social life. This is fundamental learning for self-care and self-development.

By analysis of Pum's personal experience and collaboration with her perspective and insights of her experience of autism, we consider the benefits from two energetic and demanding sensorimotor activities, swimming and collage, which she knows to be beneficial for the integrative access between higher and core levels of her Self, and that she believes can be made beneficial for individuals with autism.

We confirm that genuine *interpersonal* communication in parental care or professional therapy can bring benefit only once the autistic individual is in touch with his or her Core Self, and can source meaningful engagement with others from this place of assertion to move with emotional appraisal. We identify means that caring persons can deploy to help the person with autism become more complete, embodied, and coherent, and to help them express their individuality ready to share an integral meaning in life's movements and what they discover.

Acknowledgment

We thank Ruth Mutch for her kind assistance with Fig. 6.2.

References

Athamatten, E. (2012). Philosophy begins with wander. *Nomadic Sojourns Journal*, *2*, 13–21.

Bernstein, N. A. (1967). *The co-ordination and regulation of movements*. Oxford: Pergamon Press.

Bosco, P., Giuliano, A., Delafield-Butt, J., Muratori, F., Calderoni, S., & Retico, A. (2019). Brainstem enlargement in preschool children with autism: Results from an intermethod agreement study of segmentation algorithms. *Human Brain Mapping*, *40*(1), 7–19. Available from https://doi.org/10.1002/hbm.24351.

Bruner, J. S. (2003). *Making stories: Law, literature, and life*. New York: Farrar, Strauss, & Giroux.

Buzsáki, G. (2006). *Rhythms of the brain*. Oxford: Oxford University Press.

Caldwell, P. (2000). *You Don't Know What It's Like* (pp. 14–16). Brighton: Pavilion Publishing.
Chomsky, N. (1957). *Syntactic structures*. The Hague/Paris: Mouton.
Coghill, G. E. (1929). *Anatomy and the problem of behaviour*. Cambridge: Cambridge University Press.
Dadalko, O. I., & Travers, B. G. (2018). Evidence for brainstem contributions to autism spectrum disorders. *Frontiers in Integrative Neuroscience*, *12*(47).
Daniel, S. (2019). Loops and jazz gaps: Engaging the feedforward qualities of communicative musicality in play therapy with children with autism. *The Arts in Psychotherapy*, *65*, 101595.
Delafield-Butt, J., & Trevarthen, C. (2017). On the brainstem origin of autism: Disruption to movements of the primary self. In E. Torres, & C. Whyatt (Eds.), *Autism: The movement sensing perspective*. Taylor & Francis CRC Press.
Delafield-Butt, J., Trevarthen, C., Rowe, P., & Gillberg, C. (2019). Being misunderstood in autism: The role of motor disruption in expressive communication, implications for satisfying social relations. *Behavioral and Brain Sciences*, *42*, e86.
Delafield-Butt, J. T., & Gangopadhyay, N. (2013). Sensorimotor intentionality: The origins of intentionality in prospective agent action. *Developmental Review*, *33*(4), 399–425.
Delafield-Butt, J. T., & Trevarthen, C. (2013). Theories of the development of human communication. In P. Cobley, & P. Schultz (Eds.), *Theories and models of communication* (pp. 199–222). Berlin/Boston: De Gruyter Mouton.
Delafield-Butt, J. T., & Trevarthen, C. (2015). The ontogenesis of narrative: From moving to meaning. *Frontiers in Psychology*, *6*, 01157.
Delafield-Butt, J. T., Zeedyk, M. S., Harder, S., Vaever, M. S., & Caldwell, P. (2020). Making meaning together: Embodied narratives in a case of severe autism. *Psychopathology*, *53*(2), 60–73.
Douglas, H. (2007). *Containment and reciprocity: Integrating psychoanalytic theory and child development research for work with children*. London & New York: Routledge.
Ford, C. (2013). Dancing with horses: Combining dance/movement therapy and equine facilitated psychotherapy. *American Journal of Dance Therapy*, *35*(2), 93–117.
Gallagher, S. (2014). The cruel and unusual phenomenology of solitary confinement. *Frontiers in Psychology*, *5*(585).
Gibson, J. J. (1977). The theory of affordances. In R. Shaw, & J. Bransford (Eds.), *Perceiving, acting, and knowing*. Hillsdale, NJ: Erlbaum.
Gigliotta, O., Pezzulo, G., & Nolfi, S. (2011). Evolution of a predictive internal model in an embodied and situated agent. *Theory in Biosciences*, *130*(4), 259–276. Available from https://doi.org/10.1007/s12064-011-0128-x.
Gillberg, C. L. (1992). The Emanuel Miller Memorial Lecture 1991. Autism and autistic-like conditions: Subclasses among disorders of empathy. *Journal of Child Psychology and Psychiatry, and Allied Disciplines*, *33*(5), 813–842.
Halliday, M. A. K. (1975). *Learning how to mean: Explorations in the development of language*. London: Edward Arnold.
Halliday, M. A. K. (1978). *Language as social semiotic: The social interpretation of language and meaning*. London: Edward Arnold.
Hallmayer, J., Cleveland, S., Torres, A., et al. (2011). Genetic heritability and shared environmental factors among twin pairs with autism. *Archives of General Psychiatry*, *68*(11), 1095–1102.
Happé, F. (1999). Autism: Cognitive deficit or cognitive style? *Trends in Cognitive Sciences*, *3*(6), 216–222.

Happé, F. (2003). Theory of mind and the self. *Annals of the New York Academy of Sciences, 1001*, 134–144.

Happé, F., & Frith, U. (2006). The weak coherence account: Detail-focused cognitive style in autism spectrum disorders. *Journal of Autism and Developmental Disorders, 36*(1), 5–25.

Happé, F. G. E. (1997). Central coherence and theory of mind in autism: Reading homographs in context. *British Journal of Developmental Psychology, 15*(1), 1–12.

Happé, F. G. E., & Booth, R. D. L. (2008). The power of the positive: Revisiting weak coherence in autism spectrum disorders. *Quarterly Journal of Experimental Psychology, 61* (1), 50–63.

Hobson, P., & Hobson, J. (2011). *Joint attention or joint engagement? Insights from autism. Joint attention: New developments in psychology, philosophy of mind, and social neuroscience* (pp. 115–135). Cambridge, MA: MIT Press.

Hobson, R. P. (1993). *Autism and the development of mind*. Hillsdale, NJ: Lawrence Erlbaum Associates.

Iverson, J. M. (2010). Developing language in a developing body: The relationship between motor development and language development. *Journal of Child Language, 37*, 229–261.

James, W. (1890). *The principles of psychology*. New York: Dover.

Jaswal, V. K., & Akhtar, N. (2018). Being vs. appearing socially uninterested: Challenging assumptions about social motivation in autism. *Behavioral and Brain Sciences*, 1–84.

Keinänen, M. (2016). Taking your mind for a walk: A qualitative investigation of walking and thinking among nine Norwegian academics. *Higher Education, 71*(4), 593–605.

Koch, S. (2016). Body image in autism: An exploratory study on the effect of dance movement therapy. *Autism Open Access, 6*.

Koch, S. C., Mehl, L., Sobanski, E., Sieber, M., & Fuchs, T. (2015). Fixing the mirrors: A feasibility study of the effects of dance movement therapy on young adults with autism spectrum disorder. *Autism: The International Journal of Research and Practice, 19*(3), 338–350.

Lakoff, G., & Johnson, M. (1980). *Metaphores we live by*. Chicago, IL: Chicago University Press.

Lakoff, G., & Johnson, M. (1999). *Philosophy in the flesh: The embodied mind and its challenge to western thought*. Basic Books.

Langer, S. K. (1942). *Philosophy in a new key: A study in the symbolism of reason, rite, and art*. Cambridge, MA: Harvard University Press.

Lashley, K. S. (1951). The problem of serial order in behavior. In L. A. Jeffress (Ed.), *Cerebral mechanisms in behavior* (pp. 112–136). New York: Wiley.

MacLean, P. D. (1990). *The triune brain in evolution: Role in paleocerebral functions*. New York: Plenum Press.

Macmurray, J. (1957). *The self as agent*. London: Faber and Faber.

Macmurray, J. (1961). *Persons in relation: The form of the personal* (Vol. II). London: Faber and Faber.

Malloch, S. (1999). Mother and infants and communicative musicality. In I. Deliège (Ed.), *Rhythms, musical narrative, and the origins of human communication. Musicae scientiae, special issue, 1999–2000* (pp. 29–57). Liège, Belgium: European Society for the Cognitive Sciences of Music.

Malloch, S., & Trevarthen, C. (2009a). Musicality: Communicating the vitality and interests of life. In S. Malloch, & C. Trevarthen (Eds.), *Communicative musicality: Exploring the basis of human companionship* (pp. 1–12). Oxford: Oxford University Press.

Malloch, S., & Trevarthen, C. (Eds.), (2009b). *Communicative musicality: Exploring the basis of human companionship*. Oxford: Oxford University Press.
May, T., Chan, E. S., Lindor, E., McGinley, J., Skouteris, H., Austin, D., et al. (2019). Physical, cognitive, psychological and social effects of dance in children with disabilities: Systematic review and meta-analysis. *Disability and Rehabilitation*, 1–14.
Merker, B. (2005). The liabilities of mobility: A selection pressure for the transition to consciousness in animal evolution. *Consciousness and Cognition*, *14*, 89–114.
Merker, B. (2007). Consciousness without a cerebral cortex: A challenge for neuroscience and medicine. *Behavioral and Brain Sciences*, *30*, 63–134.
Merker, B. (2013). The efference cascade, consciousness, and its self: Naturalizing the first person pivot of action control. *Front Psychol*, *4*, 501.
Nietzsche, F. W. (2007). *Twilight of the idols with the antichrist and Ecce Homo*. Wordsworth Editions.
Northoff, G., & Panksepp, J. (2008). The trans-species concept of self and the subcortical-cortical midline system. *Trends in Cognitive Sciences*, *12*, 259–264.
Panksepp, J. (1991). Affective neuroscience: A conceptual framework for the neurobiological study of emotions. In K. T. Strongman (Ed.), *International review of studies on emotion*. New York: Wiley & Sons.
Panksepp, J. (1992). A critical role for "affective neuroscience" in resolving what is basic about basic emotions. *Psychological Review*, *99*(3), 554–560.
Panksepp, J. (1998a). *Affective neuroscience: The foundations of human and animal emotions*. New York: Oxford University Press.
Panksepp, J. (1998b). The periconscious substrates of consciousness: Affective states and the evolutionary origins of the SELF. *Journal of Consciousness Studies*, *5*(5–6), 5–6.
Panksepp, J., & Biven, L. (2012). *The archaeology of mind: Neuroevolutionary origins of human emotions*. New York: Norton.
Penfield, W., & Jasper, H. H. (1954). *Epilepsy and the functional anatomy of the human brain*. London: Little, Brown, and Co.
Pezzulo, G., & Castelfranchi, C. (2009). Thinking as the control of imagination: A conceptual framework for goal-directed systems. *Psychological Research*, *73*, 559–577.
Pinker, S. (1994). *The language instict*. London and New York: Penguin Books.
Porges, S. W. (2001). The polyvagal theory: Phylogenetic substrates of a social nervous system. *International Journal of Psychophysiology: Official Journal of the International Organization of Psychophysiology*, *42*(2), 123–146.
Posner, D. S. (2016). Review of W. Solomon, C. Holland, M. J. Middleton: Autism and understanding: The Waldon approach to child development. *Journal of Autism and Developmental Disorders*, *46*, 1498–1499.
Rajendran, G., & Mitchell, P. (2007). Cognitive theories of autism. *Developmental Review*, *27*(2), 224–260.
Reed, E. (1996). *Encountering the world: Towards an ecological psychology*. New York: Oxford University Press.
Reid, T. (1764). *An inquiry into the human mind on the principles of common sense*. Edinburgh: A. Kinkaid & J. Bell.
Rinehart, N. J., Jeste, S., & Wilson, R. B. (2018). Organized physical activity programs: Improving motor and non-motor symptoms in neurodevelopmental disorders. *Developmental Medicine and Child Neurology*, *60*(9), 856–857.
Robledo, J., Donnellan, A. M., & Strandt-Conroy, K. (2012). An exploration of sensory and movement differences from the perspective of individuals with autism. *Frontiers in Integrative Neuroscience*, *6*, 107.

Sandin, S., Lichtenstein, P., Kuja-Halkola, R., Larsson, H., Hultman, C. M., & Reichenberg, A. (2014). The familial risk of autism. *JAMA: The Journal of the American Medical Association, 311*(17), 1770–1777.
Sherrington, C. (1906). *The integrative action of the nervous system*. New Haven, CT: Yale University Press.
Shewmon, D. A., Holmse, D. A., & Byrne, P. A. (1999). Consciousness in congenitally decorticate children: Developmental vegetative state as self-fulfilling prophecy. *Developmental Medicine and Child Neurology, 41*, 364–374.
Solms, M., & Panksepp, J. (2012). The "Id" knows more than the "Ego" admits: Neuropsychoanalytic and primal consciousness perspectives on the interface between affective and cognitive neuroscience. *Brain Science, 2*, 147–174.
Solomon, W., Holland, C., & Middleton, M. J. (2012). *Autism and Understanding: The Waldon Approach to Child Development*. London: Sage.
St. Claire, C., Danon-Boileau, L., & Trevarthen, C. (2007). Signs of autism in infancy: Sensitivity for rhythms of expression in communication. In S. Acquarone (Ed.), *Signs of autism in infants: Recognition and early intervention* (pp. 21–45). London: Karnac Books.
Stern, D. N. (2000). *The interpersonal world of the infant: A view from psychoanalysis and development psychology* (2nd ed.). New York: Basic Books.
Stern, D. N. (2010). *Forms of vitality*. Oxford: Oxford University Press.
Thoreau, H. D., & Blaisdell, B. (2011). *Thoreau: A book of quotations*. New York: Dover Publications Inc.
Trevarthen, C. (2003). Memory as motor activity: The brain making time, going places and finding objectives in company. *German as: Frühe Kommunikation und autobiographisches Gedächtnis. BIOS: Zeitschrift für Biographieforschung, Oral History und Lebensverlaufsanalysen, 2/2002*, 213–240.
Trevarthen, C. (2005). Stepping away from the mirror: Pride and shame in adventures of companionship. Reflections on the nature and emotional needs of infant intersubjectivity. In C. S. Carter, L. Ahnert, K. E. Grossman, S. B. Hrdy, M. E. Lamb, S. W. Porges, & N. Sachser (Eds.), *Attachment and bonding: A new synthesis. Dahlem workshop report* (92, pp. 55–84). Cambridge, MA: The MIT Press.
Trevarthen, C. (2014). *Educational psychology in Scotland*. Special Issue: Video Interaction Guidance, 15, 10.
Trevarthen, C. (2015). Stories of truth and beauty in the sound of moving. In P. A. Brandt (Ed.), *Sigata: Annals of semiotics*. University of Liège.
Trevarthen, C., Aitken, K. J., Nagy, E., Delafield-Butt, J. T., & Vandekerckhove, M. (2006). Collaborative regulations of vitality in early childhood: Stress in intimate relationships and postnatal psychopathology. In D. Cicchetti, & D. J. Cohen (Eds.), *Developmental psychopathology* (pp. 65–126). New York: John Wiley & Sons.
Trevarthen, C., & Daniel, S. (2005). Disorganized rhythm and synchrony: Early signs of autism and Rett syndrome. *Brain and Development, 27*, S25–S34.
Trevarthen, C., Daniel, S., & Trevarthen, C. (2017). *Rhythms of relating in children's therapies*.
Trevarthen, C., & Delafield-Butt, J. T. (2013a). Autism as a developmental disorder in intentional movement and affective engagement. *Frontiers in Integrative Neuroscience, 7*, 49.
Trevarthen, C., & Delafield-Butt, J. T. (2013b). Biology of shared meaning and language development: Regulating the life of narratives. In M. Legerstee, D. Haley, & M. Bornstein (Eds.), *The infant mind: Origins of the social brain* (pp. 167–199). New York: Guildford Press.
Trevarthen, C., & Delafield-Butt, J. T. (2015). The infant's creative vitality, in projects of self-discovery and shared meaning: How they anticipate school, and make it fruitful. In S. Robson, & S. F. Quinn (Eds.), *International Handbook of Young Children's*

Thinking and Understanding (pp. 3–18). Abingdon, Oxfordshire and New York: Routledge.
Trevarthen, C., & Delafield-Butt, J. T. (2017). Development of consciousness. In B. Hopkins, E. Geangu, & S. Linkenauger (Eds.), *Cambridge encyclopedia of child development* (pp. 821–835). Cambridge: Cambridge University Press.
Trevarthen, C., Gratier, M., & Osborne, N. (2014). The human nature of culture and education. *Wiley Interdisciplinary Reviews: Cognitive Science*, *5*(2), 173–192.
Turner, F. (1991). *Beauty: The value of values*. Charlottesville, VA: University Press of Virginia.
Vandekerckhove, M., & Panksepp, J. (2009). The flow of anoetic to noetic and autonoetic consciousness: A vision of unknowing (anoetic) and knowing (noetic) consciousness in the remembrance of things past and imagined futures. *Consciousness and Cognition*, *18*, 1018–1028.
Vandekerckhove, M., & Panksepp, J. (2011). A neurocognitive theory of higher mental emergence: From anoetic affective experiences to noetic knowledge and autonoetic awareness. *Neuroscience & Biobehavioral Reviews*, *35*(9), 2017–2025.
Winnicott, D. (2001/1971). *Playing and reality*. London: Routledge.
Winnicott, D. W. (1954). Mind and its relation to the psyche-soma. *British Journal of Medical Psychology*, *27*(4), 201–209.
Winnicott, D. W. (1960). Ego distortion in terms of true and false self. In D. W. Winnicott (Ed.), *The maturational processes and the facilitating environment: Studies in the theory of emotional development* (pp. 140–152). London: Karnac Books.
Zeki, S. (1993). *A vision of the brain*. Oxford: Blackwell.
Zeki, S. (1999). *Inner vision*. Oxford: Oxford University Press.

Appendix 1

Profile of a collaged mind finding sense and synthesis in the language of movement, fragment and aesthetic coherence

A collage by Pum

This collage is a composition of parts that speaks of the relationship between autism, sensory-motor processes, spatiotemporal delays, problems with control, tolerance and connection in the infrastructures of the primary, secondary and tertiary processes of brain communication. This thesis presents a new perspective of autism deploying the concept of a fundamental disruption to the ability to interrelate the different brain regions leaving the Core Self sealed off, disconnected, disembodied, and importantly unavailable to self-regulate in accordance with the organisms ever-changing biopsychosocial environmental needs.

The elements of the collage are presented roughly spatially in corresponding regions of the brain, that is, limbic system and amygdala, cerebellum, vestibular apparatus of the inner ear, thalamus, and neocortex.

1. *Giant ear.* This giant ear represents the sensory apparatus of hearing and the vestibular sense of balance. Pum's sensory sensitivity profile includes hypersensitivity to sound;

she can hear her contact lens drop on a carpeted floor. The inner ear is the site of the vestibular sense and it plays an important part in attention regulation, the ability to focus and concentrate. Pum experiences a delayed audio and visual processing disparity that creates out-of-synch information inputs. Pum is also hypersensitive to smell, the ear is positioned over eye and olfactory bulb

2. *Split torso diagram.* This is spatially placed in midbrain area of limbic system housing the amygdala, hypothalamus and thalamus. Sensory-motor, sensory-affective and cognitive perceptions collide and fragment processing. Output and input exchange and interrelate internal subjective experience to the to external world of objects, others and stimulus. The conflict and tension created by the autistic brain's difficulties between managing the incoming and outgoing communications overwhelm and disrupt the body-mind relationship.
3. *Concrete dam barrier built.* The architecture of compliance and withdrawal—it is a protective, maladaptative defense to protect the ungerminated Core Self (Winnicott, 1960).
4. *The wheel.* The wheel represents motion, movement embedded in the revolution of repetition—the cycle of movement from the microcellular level to the macroskeletal muscular level (Delafield-Butt & Gangopadhyay, 2013; Trevarthen & Delafield-Butt, 2013a, 2013b).
5. *Staircase.* The staircase is like the spinal column. It leads down to a landing in the body, the home of the human being's embodied self, a space where psyche and soma work together to generate mindfulness (Winnicott, 1954).
6. *Metronome needle.* The metronomic is a time-keeping device symbolizing temporal displacement of experience between inner processing and the outer world environment (Delafield-Butt & Trevarthen, 2017).
7. *Face facing backwards, looking inwards.* This area of the collage is synthesized into a depiction of memory, innovation and creativity that is generated through processes orchestrated by the cerebellum region of the brain. Pum has an extraordinary strange and vivid long-term memory. The occipital lobe area at the back of the head is where insight is generated through the coupling-up and categorizing of visual perceptual details into grouped concepts (Zeki, 1993, 1999).
8. *Child with book, looking and learning.* This learning, conditioning, behavioral part of the brain responds to the emotional valance of experiences. Unpleasant experiences become charged with negative associations, while for Pum learning, knowledge acquisition, school work was charged with positive experiences of self-control and acceptance and a high regard from other. Thus, social scripts and social coding was copied and tattooed (the computer chip being indented with programming circuitry) into the neocortex, the tertiary level brain processing.
9. *Scaffolding precariously placed in a ridged, fixed disorganized space.* As indicated by the cloud of strange detailed marks, which appears to the right of the scaffolding poles, this is the region of the forebrain responsible for executive function (the ability to think into the future) planning organization. Individuals with autism have problems with executive functioning (Rajendran & Mitchell, 2007).
10. *Expiration the cloud of breath, or speech bubble of chromosomes, the complex strands which hold and fold their genetic mysteries.* Pum believes that the branch of science epigenetics is showing up just how important lifestyle choices (how the interactions with our environment shape our being, and the expressions of our genes) are. Autism etiology is complex, involving both genetic and environmental factors (Hallmayer, Cleveland, & Torres, 2011; Sandin et al., 2014).

By adopting certain activities (movement based and creative-led activities), we would argue that we can perhaps turn down the influence of any autism genetic material, we can enhance the brain's potential by supporting the autism needs, therefore encouraging the development of a more integrated brain, body and environment, one where the autism syndrome is managed through diet, low arousal lifestyle and emphasis of Primary Self communication, in order to foster an individual's ability to better self-regulate and to better tolerate the inevitable changes that come with being human.

Mind, body, space and time: the Neuro-Geometric approach a new roadmap to symbol formation

7

Alisa Vig[1] *and Serena Wieder*[2]
[1]Simaney Kesher Clinic, Petah Tikva, Israel, [2]Profectum Foundation, Mendham, NJ, United States

The Neuro-Geometric approach offers a new roadmap for understanding and supporting the development of symbolism among children, especially those with neurobiological challenges, such as children with autistic spectrum disorders (ASD). It suggests that children's growing capabilities for regulating, processing, and operating in space enable parallel development of their evolving internal world. The developed internal world is characterized by growing processed presymbolic, symbolic, and abstract thinking on the ground of powerful rudimentary internal forces, impulses, and drives. The approach is based on identifying, supporting, and handling vital mechanisms and processes in the external and internal world that support symbol formation (Fig. 7.1).

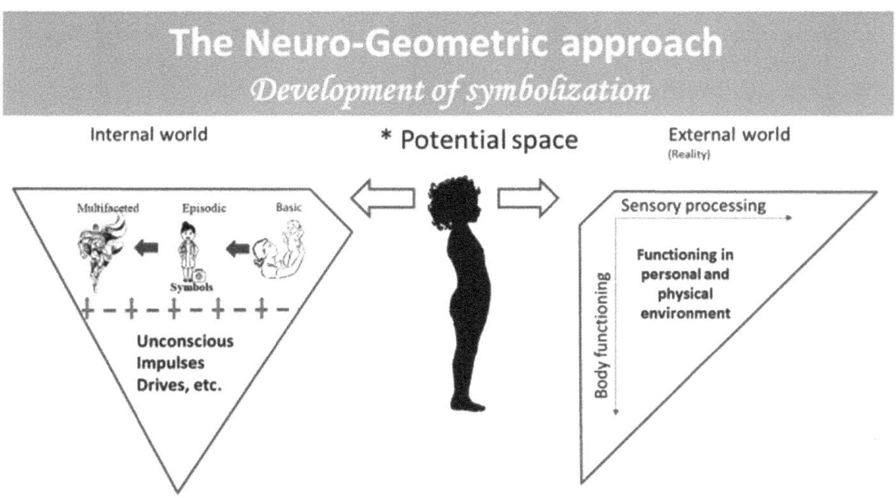

Figure 7.1 Potential space—where experience is transformed into internal symbols that process emotions or meanings.

Emerging Programs for Autism Spectrum Disorder. DOI: https://doi.org/10.1016/B978-0-323-85031-5.00009-8

The Developmental, Individual-Difference, Relationship-based Model (DIR) is the foundation for this approach. It offers a unifying theory and integrated model that promotes fundamental developmental areas of functioning, including attention and regulation, engagement across a wide range of emotions, two-way intentional communication, complex social problem-solving, and symbolic and abstract thinking. It indicates that relationships play a vital role in development through affect-based interactions tailored to the children's unique neurobiological profile. The significance of sensory-motor and visual–spatial processing, even though it is central to all functional emotional capacities including self-developments and the formation of symbolic thinking, has been understated. Visual-spatial processing guides movements through space and sequences involved in the action, thought and relating, coordinating information from other senses, especially auditory (language), and mediating the construction of imagery through interaction and play. The model offers a unifying theory that addresses these developmental components in an integrated framework (Greenspan & Wieder, 2006; Wieder & Wachs, 2012).

This chapter introduces the innovative Neuro-Geometric approach that creates a three-dimensional internal schema connecting existing psychological theories with neurobiological studies. It uses visual–spatial aspects and geometric terminology to support one's understanding of the multifaceted phenomenon of symbolism in simple language and provides opportunities to construct distinct interventions that support development. The following concepts from the field of geometry are briefly described here and will be elaborated in the chapter:

- Points depict realistic, partial, and limited experiences, such as focusing on the color or the object's size. Points have no mental record in the inner world.
- Lines describe the continuous experience of relationships and interactions, especially between children and their primary caregivers. Lines have specific characteristics and are unique in their emotional and physiological hues that generate internal representation in the children's inner world.
- Triangles and polygons express the children's ability to show interest in two or more points, especially people, simultaneously. Since the children can gradually process expanded physical space through vision and movements in a synchronized and integrated manner across time, they can also construct multilayered inner representations of self and others. The role of triangles and polygons are varied and have a significant role in symbol formation, as will be described later.
- Time is another measurement that goes with any of the three preceding dimensions and signifies endurance. It relates to notions such as seconds, moments, future, and past.

This approach's main idea is that children gradually process greater complexity in space, including distance, mobility, and numbers of stimuli, and get involved in their larger environment across time. The children first can focus on points in space. This ability expands to forming lines, and later they perceive triangles and polygons. These evolving capacities enable the children to see the real world in 3D and build a parallel three-dimensional internal map. These abilities also help them sense depth in themselves, others, and the world around them. Three milestones of symbolic development are defined in the chapter to simplify the vast and rich sequence of symbolic development. These milestones include internal representations of basic symbols (1), episodic symbols (2), and multifaceted symbols and abstract thinking (3).

The chapter's first section discusses the importance of play and symbols to one's development. It provides a historical perspective on symbolism by reviewing some of the existing psychological theories, including psychoanalytic ones. Special attention is given to the term "potential space," which Winnicott (1971) coined, since this chapter's scope is the space between the real and psychic worlds. The second section reviews neurobiology studies and traditional psychological approaches, including Freud's (1961) and Klein & Riviere (1964; 1988) theories in the light of updated research. The third part summarizes the DIR model as the Neuro-Geometric scheme's groundwork and the approach itself. The three-dimensional Neuro-Geometric representative map of the outside world is outlined to facilitate effective treatment planning. The approach is presented along with clinical illustrations and its application at home and in educational settings. Unique strategies that are used in this approach are also detailed, including (1) affective container, (2) affective agent, (3) visual–spatial play, and (4) dynamic drawing.

Part I: Background: symbolism, play, and psychological approaches

Symbolism and play

Symbols are representations of ideas, experiences, perceptions, and thoughts that enable separation of perception of the real world and imagination (Greenspan & Wieder, 2006; Wieder & Wachs, 2012). Symbols can be represented in various modalities, including verbal, visual, auditory, movement or sensual, and complexity levels, and it enables agility, complexity, and unlimited expression of emotions and ideas. For example, a stop sign represents a simple universal symbol of "stop" or "no entry." A lion, on the other hand, is a complex symbol. Depending on the lion's body posture, size, or colors, it may represent a theme of nurturance, aggression, or power. Various elements, such as scary background sounds or unpredictable movements, can intensify the symbolic meaning.

Children's ability to create, understand, and use symbols develop in parallel with play and language. For example, children will first use a single word "pacifier" to symbolize their wish and later, a broader expression, "I want a pacifier," or "Give me the pacifier!" The latter conveys expanding ideas of self, actions, or feelings. In the play, a broad emotional range will also gradually develop. Power and control, as well as vulnerability, can be safely explored in symbolic play by taking different roles, such as a lion or prey. Children who act as superheroes will feel omnipotent or feel helpless and powerless playing a mouse.

Symbols and symbolic thinking have a significant impact on children's development in numerous realms, including emotional, communicative, social, and cognitive ones. Children use transitional objects (Winnicott, 1953), usually physical objects incorporated into their daily routine, to provide psychological comfort. These objects remind them of their caregivers' loving and caring behavior when in distress. For example, to overcome anxiety, a child afraid of the dark can use different solutions. At first, the child may hug a beloved teddy bear to which she is attached not to feel alone and comfort herself. Later, with further emotional development and ideas of what might be hidden in the darkness, she will be able to use imaginative objects to overcome the fear itself by setting a "monster trap" or wishing on a "magic wand" to reassure herself and allow her to feel powerful and safe in this situation. Interchangeably, she may verbally (symbol) express her concern (internal world) to her parent and receive a more precise soothing and supportive response to her distress from darkness (reality). The parent who realizes that the child's behavior is a reaction to the darkness, and not, for instance, to hunger or longing, can then soothe the child by singing or hugging her. The language, in this case, starts to serve as a transitional phenomenon.

Many have questioned whether children with developmental challenges, including ASD, can develop symbolic capacities, especially when some might only attend to an object's physical traits such as texture, sound, or smell and not to what it represents. If so, will a child who initially relates only to the shiny color of Superman's cape, or its silky fabric, be able with further development to have it represent the power to rescue those in danger? Similarly, will a child who throws objects when mad later symbolize this expression of aggression or anxiety by playing knights at war? How does sensory-motor play develop into symbolic? Symbolic development will be considered from several theoretical psychological perspectives that contribute to the consolidation of the Neuro-Geometric approach.

Psychoanalytic approaches—the "I" (self)

Psychoanalytic theories have evolved over the years. Originally, the emphasis was put on impulses and uncovering influences from one's history. Symbols in play or behavior were used mainly to learn about one's unconscious. Now psychoanalytic approaches focus more on understanding the symbolization processes based on previous and current relationships and their internalization.

Freud, the founder of psychoanalytic theory, for example, focused on the role of internal forces and impulses, including the need to obtain pleasure and gratification (1961). He describes a little boy that "never cried when his mother left him for a few hours." The child would throw objects or toss a reel with a string tied to it and pull it back, "repeated untiringly." Freud indicates this play symbolized the child's emotional experience and his attempt to obtain control over a situation by casting and retrieving the reel. He explained that rediscovering the reel represented the pleasure and gratification that the child desired in his relationship with his mother, that is, her reappearance (different ideas regarding this description will be discussed later). Klein, from Freud's followers, developed the field of child-psychotherapy, asserted that play represents children's unconscious and internalized relationships. Her object-relations theory broadens the scope from Freud's theory of impulses to a theory that focuses on an internalized relationships, mostly unconscious, that affects one's psychological framework later (Klein, 1988; Klein & Riviere, 1964).

Klein's successors, Bion and Winnicott, related to relationships but gave a central role to the function of the "real mother" (vs internalized mother) in children's mental development. They indicated that symbols represent the internalized experience of children with their caregivers. Winnicott (1968, 1971) describes three important concepts concerning the mother's functioning that allow the development of symbolism among children. First, he emphasizes "holding" as an essential parental function that protects the baby from external intrusion and includes nurturing the baby, considering rhythm, tone of speech, and visual or auditory sensitivity. He emphasizes that holding varies in response to the needs of the baby since each baby has its unique characteristics. The second concept is "a good enough mother." It refers to the mother's ability to respond to the baby's needs in a varied manner that is good enough but not necessarily perfectly matched to the baby's needs to encourage the most optimal growth. The third concept, "potential space," is a metaphoric space that Winnicott coined to refer to the central area between fantasy and reality. It is where reality, such as distress from being alone, is mediated by the mother's attentiveness to the child's emotional needs. Her attentiveness consists of the two previously described concepts, "holding" and "good enough" that enable symbols to develop in the potential space. For example, by softly approaching, hugging, and talking to the baby, offering her a teddy bear, she calms down. The teddy bear gradually serves as the baby's soothing function, symbolizing the real mother when she is not available (Winnicott, 1953).

Bion emphasizes *containment* as a significant parents' mental function that supports symbolism (Symington & Symington, 1996). The baby might experience sensory impressions that are meaningless and unorganized for him, such as voices, odors, or touch (β elements/points). He uses the term "conversion" to describe the action in which the parent reflects the baby her chaotic and disorganized experiences in an organized manner, without having to repel these emotions or to throw them back on the baby. The parents' role is to regulate and contain the distressed of the baby. The parent's success would be affected by her ability to stay calm. In such cases, the parent's response, "I am here, and you will be fine," creates cohesiveness and continuity in the baby's experience. This soothing state enables the experience to be symbolized. The parent's calming words organize the baby's chaotic experience. However, suppose the caregiver cannot bear the distress, and at the same time, experiences powerful emotions such as anger, helplessness, or guilt, she will not be able to serve as a "container" for the baby. Her experience will continue to be chaotic, thus not allowing the creation of a symbolic representation of being contained (Symington & Symington, 1996).

Intersubjective approaches—the "me, you, and us"

Later intersubjective theories evolved, focusing on the role of actual interpersonal relationships in development and not only internal ones. Based on observations of embryos and infants, Stern (1985) described the course of development as a gradual consolidation of the self that emerges from sensory, affective, and interactive everyday life experiences. He described the baby's first experiences in the world as assortments of unrelated sensory experiences, which through the daily interactive exchanges, consolidate to growing "islands" of self. For example, a baby may feel distressed during hunger or because of a wet diaper. A few minutes later, a wave of relief comes from a gratified desire and sensations of dryness and cleanliness. Gradually she identifies the parents as the source of the pleasure and feelings of relief. She can identify the rhythm, soft voice, or type of touch as, "Hey, it's my mother who has made me feel good." In the higher stages of development, children begin to recognize islands of "lack of change in themselves," changes in others, and the separateness between themselves and others. For example, a toddler may cry when she falls, and her parent will share her emotional experience saying, "Oh, you fell, it surprised you, it hurts!". The parent's emotional tone that matches the child's one becomes attached to the "falling" experience. Yet, the toddler will pick up on the slight difference in the pain she hears in her parent's voice, whether softer or more forceful and dramatic, which will help her to symbolize her experience. Later on, she will be able to express her internal world that gradually becomes clearer, organized, and separate from others through language and play (Stern, 1985).

Beebe and Lachmann (1988) also emphasized the importance of mother–infant space for developing self and internal representations created by the partners' interactive patterns. With their unique characteristics, such as rhythm and length, these patterns create expectations by the children and enable them to predict the next piece in the interaction. They can expect what is not currently in their receptive field but exists in the imaginary field. For example, a mother, playing peek-a-boo with her son, creates an expectation that she will see her face just a few seconds after her face is covered. The baby knows that the moment of exposure will come soon. Until this moment arises, the "real mother" is visualized and represented in her mind. They suggest that these patterns create the presymbolic ability. They referred to the potential space that was offered by Winnicott, as it occurs in the space between two individuals—between the mother and the infant, and not only within the baby.

Developmental approaches—the "I, you, the environment and culture"

In parallel to psychoanalytic and intersubjective approaches, developmental theories expand the framework and emphasize the interrelatedness of various individual functionings to the child's growth, the environment, and the culture. Bowlby (1969) emphasizes the biologically preprogrammed evolutionary drive of infants to search for physical proximity. Stimuli of danger get the baby to signal distress and cause the caregiver to approach and protect him. The sense of safety creates the connection and is the internal working model in the attachment process. Later, with the children's physiological and cognitive development, the call for help and support based on the internal representations becomes more dynamic and sophisticated.

Piaget (1962) coined the term "object permanence," describing the child's growing ability to understand that an object exists even if the child does not see it (e.g., the bottle or the mother). He defined the process of cognitive development as related to the children's ability to learn how to operate in the world by mimicking what she sees and create her own schemas. For example, a child will pretend she eats from an empty plate. The increasing complexity of symbols and flexibility of thought is a significant leap in thinking and imagining capacities that release her from relying solely on trial and error behavior.

Erikson (1950) claimed that symbolization grows through conflict resolution between motor development and the children's body-control, personal needs, and social requirements, such as controlling defecation and hygiene education. These conflicts hold different feelings, such as shame, control, and aggression. Children use symbolic play to cope with social demands and express their needs following their growing psychosocial development and understanding of the world. According to Vygotsky, the development of symbolic ability is attributed to social activities and culture, as well as emotional aspects. In return, the symbol's quality allows children to have a new base on which they can learn to function in the real world (Vygotsky, 1929/1994).

The DIR Model drew upon these theories and integrated them into functional, emotional, and developmental capacities that anchor the symbolic process (Greenspan & Wieder, 1997). Wieder emphasizes the three-dimensionality of experience with movement in space and time, both visually, auditorily, and accompanied by sensations. This can be observed, for example, in children "lost in space" who have difficulty knowing where they are or who they are in relation to others, especially if others are moving, but also encounter visual–spatial processing-based challenges that derail back and forth communication, and executive functioning. These children may also have difficulty using symbolic processes being bound to concrete images that impede the flexibility of imagination and fantasy (Wieder & Wachs, 2012).

In summary, the overview of various approaches from the end of the 19th century to the present gives an expanding scope on play, internal representation, and symbolism. Symbolic development occurs, in part, due to the need for a sense of safety that children experience using pretense. Psychoanalytic, intersubjective, and developmental theories emphasized the child's sense of safety in their interpersonal relationships or the world surrounding them. Suitable challenges may support symbolism if a sense of safety is maintained, while unmatched ones may negatively affect symbolization.

Part II: A dialogue between neuropsychological research, psychological theories, and autism

Neuropsychological research and theories

People's ability to interact effectively with others and objects in the world stems from neurobiological sensory systems like the visual, auditory, tactile, balance, and interoception, where sensations are conveyed to the brain for processing and executing (Ayres, 1972). Research supports the link between neurobiology, qualitative relationships, and psychological functioning. For example, studies show that wide-open and broad body postures that involve, for example, the balance and interoception systems, which express strength and dominance, increase testosterone and self-confidence levels. In comparison, closed and low positions increase levels of cortisol and anxiety. Others show that difficulties in the postural balance system increase anxiety and lower self-esteem (Bart et al., 2009; Carney, Cuddy, & Yap, 2010; Shefer, Gordon, Avraham, & Mintz, 2015).

Synchrony and parental mentalizing are concepts that relate to the quality of infant–parent relationships. The two concepts that clearly embrace the two partners' neurobiology profile refer to the delicate infant–parent dance of compatibility and combine elements of sensation, movement, and voice in addition to content. For example, when a baby cries, a mother's tone of voice or movements may initially be very soft and empathetic to synchronize with the baby's mental state. A few seconds later, it might change to fit the baby's new emotional state. As a result of this type of interaction, the baby has a sense of being understood. Researchers found a link between a higher level of synchronization and the mother's mentalizing ability to reduce anxiety, secure attachment, and level of oxytocin. Symbolic functioning of children, as was measured in symbolic play, verbal IQ, and the children's use of internal state words, was associated with a higher level of synchronization (Feldman, 2007; Feldman & Greenbaum, 1997; Shai & Belsky, 2016). However, the DSM 5 manual (American Psychiatric Association, 2013) mentions difficulties in processing sensory input as one criterion for diagnosing ASD. Other studies also specify that communication difficulties may arise from challenging integrating auditory, somatosensory information, sensory-motor sequencing, and processing difficulties, resulting in ASD and atypical behaviors (Mueller & Tronic, 2019; Russo et al., 2010; Trevarthen & Delafield-Butt, 2013).

It is interesting to see that research that links neurobiology and mental states echoes various psychological literature voices. For example, Freud's psychosexual theory highlights that impulses' energy is defined in the body's organs. He also claimed that "ego is first and foremost physical." According to Freud (1961), the ego is consolidating from inner and external sensations but declared the need to continue investigating internal sensations' perceptions. These statements may stem from his background as a neurologist. Nearly 90 years later, Torres (2012) studied the feedback received from body movements in the brain. She found that the feedback is more randomized and less accurate in children with ASD. She concluded that people with autism might have body awareness problems; feeling where their body is in space and their ability to control movements and postures are poor. Considering Freud's theory, in conjunction with Torres' research, one might assume that children with ASD may have challenges forming psychological self, at least, in part, because of neurobiological challenges.

Other psychoanalytic theories also referred to processing issues and sensory flooding as influencing symbolism's formation (Klein, 1988; Ogden, 1989; Stern, 1985; Symington & Symington, 1996). For example, in her later writing, Klein emphasizes the importance of a child's sensory experience, especially touch, body movement, and hearing, to create the parent–child unit, reduce anxiety, and create integrated internal representations. Ogden (1989) also describes the autistic experience as a fragmented sensation and meaning. He shares his personal attempt to experience it by dismantling the sounds of the word "napkin" into "nap" and "kin" and by playfully repetitively pronouncing these sounds. He declared that by referring only to one aspect of the object, in this case, the sounds, the object lost its meaning for him (as an object made of fabric). Reportedly, after the partialization of the experience, it took him some time to integrate the object, the word "napkin," and it's meaning. Here dismantling the world may be gratifying sound play with no interest in the object. Hence, it is agreed that sensual experience, including auditory or visual stimuli, has a significant effect on the creation or distortion of mental representation.

Constraints of traditional psychological theories

Traditional psychological theories are prevalent and have a definite perspective. Yet, they have some significant constraints. First, they do not take into consideration updated neurodevelopmental research. Such research can provide additional lenses to these theories, including, for example, individual differences related to the influence of sensory-motor processing and integration on relationships, play, and emotional development. Integrative thinking may enrich one's clinical understanding and affects interventions. For example, in Freud's description of the reel play (1961), he interpreted the repetitive behavior as a symbolic expression of the child's anxiety about the separation. A wider and comprehensive clinical perspective raises the question of whether this behavior resulted from challenges in integrating auditory and somatosensory information, self-regulation, or motor planning that prevented the child from signaling his distress every time the mother disappeared. Second, though clearly described and referred to in the literature, neurobiological components are not systemized in assessment and treatment. For example, in Winnicott's clinical work with Little (1990), the mind, body, and external environment are considered. That includes treating in a darker room, as well as the touch on her head. Yet, these are reported in a rather anecdotal manner and not in a systemized way. Third, symbolism's roadmap is too often generic and limited. The traditional theoreticians describe a mechanism of basic representations and symbols. For example, there is unity between theories and research that anxiety or emotional and sensory flooding affect relationships and may derail one from developing symbolism and the capacity to deal with distress. Yet, earlier theories are not clear on the formation of advanced symbols and do not clearly understand how children proceed from basic representations to more complex ones.

A clinical vignette will illustrate the importance of integrating psychological and neurodevelopmental knowledge in therapy. A 9-year-old child with ASD, auditory oversensitivity, and processing issues, began to shout in terror during a dyadic session. The psychologist noticed loud indistinct construction noises from the street that she did not notice before, and assumed that the child reacted anxiously to the noise. The terrified child ignored any comments or attempt to reflect the situation in a verbal nor nonverbal manner while in the room. The therapist then invited the mom and the child to the street. At first, the child was still terrified, screamed in terror, and covered his ears with his palms (what Bion referred to as β elements). Apparently, the falling wreckage from the roof created a noise that flooded the child. Outside, the therapist helped him integrate what he heard (the loud noise) with what he saw (wreckage falling) and his emotional response. The psychologist used vocalization ("boom, boom") to echo the falling wreckage, first with a similar rhythm, and soon introduced playfulness in the patterned vocalization. Gradually, the child watched the workers clearing the wreckage. The terrifying feeling was managed by generating coregulative patterns that prepared the child for the "next fall," supported by the therapist's vocalization matching the fall's noise. Gradually, the child's level of anxiety was reduced.

Later, back in the room, the therapist supported the child processing the distress, using a dynamic drawing (as described below), to integrate the child's physical and emotional experience. Through back and forth interactions with the therapist, the child's vocal, visual, and the emotional experience was represented in the drawing to encourage an internal representation of his distress. The drawing enabled the child to externalize his experience, and by seeing it unfold, he could let go of the flooding sensation destroying him. The anxiety and auditory sensitivities in this incident were also linked to his reactions to barking dogs discussed a few weeks earlier in therapy (alpha in Bion's terms), supporting the consolidation of physiological and psychic ego. His experience was intertwined using neurodevelopmental interventions, drawing, vocalization, and rhythm that supported a sense of safety, and traditional emotional techniques, including intersubjective emotional relatedness and curative attachment experience (Stern), conversion (Bion), holding (Winnicott), as well as interpretations (Freud and Klein). Together these interventions reduced his anxiety of the unknown intrusion on his senses, increased his sense of safety, and accessed his cognitive ability to understand, organize, communicate, and symbolize the emotional experience.

Part III: Integrative approaches

The Developmental, Individual Difference, Relationship-based (DIR) model developed by Greenspan and Wieder introduced major paradigm shifts from behavioral reductionism to relational dynamic developmental systems that function simultaneously in the context of the family and environment. Anchored in the 20th century's psychodynamic theories, it integrated the multiple dimensions of human development, identifying essential capacities throughout life. The "D" casts the functions of development into functional, emotional, social, and cognitive capacities that include shared attention, attachment, and engagement, communication, complex social problem solving, and symbolic and abstract thinking. The "I" represents the individual neurobiological differences in the child's neurological, psychological, physiological, sensory, and motor processing, and the ability for sequencing and synchronization, through which experience is understood. The "R" focuses on the vital role relationships play in learning, social–emotional growth, and mental health. Putting parent–child relationships at the core of human needs, DIR embraces the interactions that provide the experience necessary to create a child's sense of self and agency, intentionality and initiative, and emotional well-being in the context of the family's culture and environment. Together DIR provides a unique profile to understand a child's challenges and guides the comprehensive interventions needed for adaptation and emotional and developmental progress. Parents are supported through coaching and reflection. Other caregivers, including teachers and therapists, are trained in the same approach. Therapies are brought in (OT, PT, Speech and Language, creative arts, psychotherapy, etc.) as needed. The focus is always on the developmentally appropriate experiences needed to build higher emotional and intellectual capacities based on each child's profile (Greenspan & Wieder, 1997, 2006; Vig, 2019; Wieder & Wachs, 2012).

More recently, Porges introduced Polyvagal Theory related to the autonomic nervous system and identified the mechanism of neuroception, distinct from conscious perception, that can detect if the environment is safe or dangerous and provides the neurophysiological substrates for adaptive behavior. He links the autonomic nervous system's evolution to affective experience, emotional expression, facial gestures, vocal communication, and contingent social behavior. His theory is relevant to understanding infant–mother interaction when social cues are misread or unavailable and do not regulate prosocial responses, disrupting the relationship's security, also experienced as anxiety, that is, the increased heart rate of the vagus nerve. It clarifies the autonomic nervous system's important contribution to the central nervous system platforms of behavior and development (Porges, 2009).

The Neuro-Geometric approach—basic terminology

The Neuro-Geometric approach extracts the theory and mechanisms identified in the DIR model, including the relation between body, space, time, and mind. It constructs an internal three-dimensional representative map of the outside world for symbolism. It is a bottom-up approach that emphasizes regulation, attention, attachment, communication, and organization as the foundation for higher level presymbolic and symbolic development. The approach uses geometric conceptualizations of dimensions, including *points*, *lines*, *triangles*, *polygons*, and *time*, to represent daily experiences, relationships between individuals, emotions and affect, and the physical environment in simple and coherent language to create a common language between parents, therapists, and educators:

- *Points* describe the chaotic and fragmented first experiences of the infant in the world. The infant's actions stem from an unplanned relationship with the human and nonhuman environment based on what lures her at the same moment and her impulses. They depict realistic, partial, and limited experiences, such as focusing on animals' types or sorting them by their size and color. It can also be observed in the attraction to the sight, texture, or temperature of objects, for example, children enticed by the movement of leaves, hand flapping, and cold or rough surfaces. Points have no mental record in the inner world of the infant. The infant's point of attraction has no depth or volume, and she goes solely after her senses. For example, overwhelming or anxiety-provoking experiences described by Bion, such as β elements, can be translated into the geometric terms "point."

- *A line* describes a connection between a baby or a child and a caregiver, represents a baby–parent continuous and synchronized relationship's experience. The integration of sight, voice, or touch creates lines between self and others. The consolidation of lines in the real world enables the emergence of mental representation in the baby's mind. The baby may expect and search for her mother, even when she disappears from the visual field, as the baby now has her image in her mind.

  Lines' characteristics are varied and include length, space, clarity, endurance, directionality, axes (up–down, side to side, and diagonal), sensory modalities (visual, auditory, tactile, etc.), continuity (flow vs. broken), and mobility of the child, parents, or both parties. For example, a child with sensory-motor vulnerabilities (if she is hypo- or hyperreactive, or unable to locate, turn, or move toward the stimulus) may struggle to form steady interactions. She may benefit from physical interactions that include deep pressure or tickling to regulate her body. Later maybe only a light touch (e.g., high five) or even just funny facial expressions from across the room will be enough to maintain the line steady and for a longer time (modality, axes, endurance). In other cases, children may initiate or maintain lines in a quiet and calm environment. They may find it difficult in a more complex situation. Gradually, they will create a line even when other children are involved or moving around in a mall (mobility, clarity).
- *Triangles and polygons*—As the child develops and increasingly interacts with her parents and the environment, the parent's images are formed and stored in her mind where "out of sight is no longer out of mind." With this constancy, she can shift her attention to exploring other objects or people in her environment that capture her interest. A triangle emerges when the child then turns to her parent (who is image in her mind), shifting her attention back and forth across space and time to share the new experience with the parent. This dynamic process then creates another image in her mind, which is now three-way, or a triangle, having expanded from the line that had just connected the parent and child. Triangles are created between self, another person, and additional points, whether an object or a person, and they represent joint attention. In Fig. 7.2, after forming a line with her mother, the baby can generate a triangle when she shares her enthusiastic interest in the puppet. Polygons are created from four or more additional points, including oneself, and three or more other objects or individuals. For example, the ability to create a playful interaction between three children and a ball. All lines, whether between two points, three (triangles), or four and more (polygons), share similar characteristics, such as size, length, width, and flexible mobility.
- *Time* is an independent phenomenon representing the duration of experience related to perceptual, visual–spatial, and emotional elements in each of the previous dimensions. In early situations, when there are no mental representations, like in the experience of points, the child does not perceive the factor of time. She may continue her activity for a long time without any meaningful change since time has little effect on the occurrence (e.g., spinning wheels). Later, during the formation of lines, representing the expectation that the parent will interact with her, she will gradually notice the meaning of time. She will incorporate what she observes her parents doing day-to-day in her play across time and space. For example, her dad is cooking dinner, and later she pretends to make dinner for her doll. The perception of time develops and affects the child's emotional world and her mind's ability to create meaning and symbols. She can now anticipate upcoming situations and understand her parent saying, "Mommy will come soon!" or "Tomorrow we will go to the dentist." The child evolving sense of time allows her to express past, forthcoming, or imaginary events also in her play.

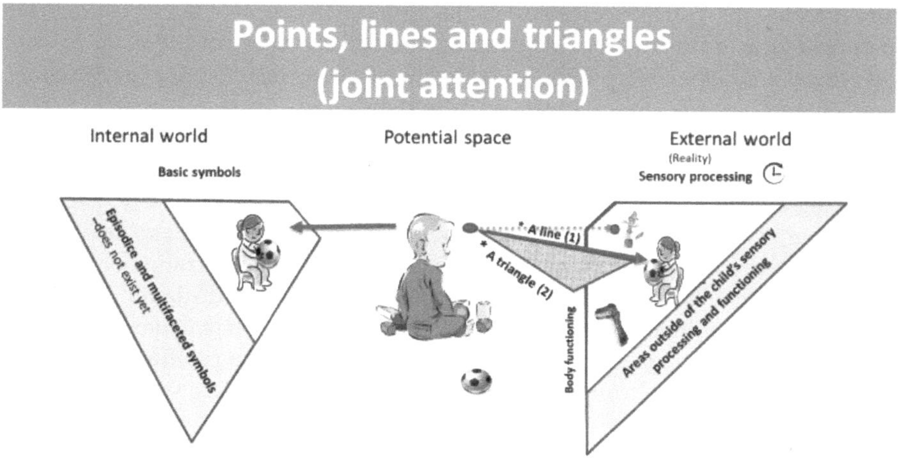

Figure 7.2 *A line* is created by affective interaction that enable the child to built basic internal representation. *A triangle* is consolidated from the growing capacity of the child to connect what he sees (real caregiver and puppet), the imaginary caregiver in his mind, and the ability to get back and share the emotional experience with the "real caregiver".

Symbol formation using the Neuro-Geometric approach and its unique methods

Three symbolic milestones are identified to clarify the vast and rich sequence of development generated from powerful internal forces of energy, including impulses and drives (see Fig. 7.1). These milestones include internal representations of *basic symbols*—children's ability to create mental representations of primary caregivers (1). *Episodic symbols* describe the ability to perceive, process, and use internal representations that include the self and caregivers in emotionally involving simple daily occurrences such as waiting eagerly for food while Mommy is cooking or fearful anticipation of a doctor's visit's office (2). Later, *symbols and abstract thinking* that express complicated feelings, ideas, values, and emotions are constructed due to the child's ability to perceive more complex events along a continuum of time and space (3). Developmentally appropriate methods illustrate how to proceed from points to lines, triangles, and polygons to support symbolic development. These methods include (1) affective container, (2) affective agent, (3) visual–spatial play, and (4) dynamic drawing.

Basic symbols: mom, dad, pacifier, teddy bear, blanky, and others

Babies cross from a physiological womb to a new world of numerous overwhelming sensations, including sights, smells, voices, and motion, which can be defined as *points*. Points are objects or specific aspects of an object or person. The caregiver, now as "a psychological womb" (Foley, 2006), needs to support the baby on this journey into the "real world" by organizing and processing the fragmented stimuli/points the baby experiences in the new environment. Older children with neurobiological difficulties, such as autism, attention deficit disorder, or anxiety, may share a similar disorganized experience as young babies. The imbalance in their sensory system (over, under, or mixed reactivity to sensations) and other neurobiological challenges may drive them to shut down the dynamic and confusing world by focusing on one facet of the object like color, size, scent, or category such as placing toy animals or cars on a line (a point in space). Alternatively, one might move from one point to the next (many unorganized points), not attend or play with one object purposefully. These reactions do not generate internalization or representation of the caregiver or objects in one's mind. The fragmented stimuli exist at this stage only in the perceptual field. Hence, a cry at this phase may express the baby's distress, but not her request for soothing by her mother or the pacifier, who are not mentally registered in her mind with a function of comfort, unless seen.

Gradually, children should be able to self-organize the world more coherently by the feeling of being fully held physically and emotionally. The limited visual space (distance between the mom's arms and face, which allows for the best attentiveness) and the simultaneous soft vocalizations create intimacy and security. They begin to synchronize sight, voice, and movements, such as reaching out to the parent's hair or mouth. The infant evolving active role in the relationship now leads to her ability to distinguish her mother from others based on knowing her looks, voice, touch, and smell. Soon, the mental representation emerging in her mind, even when the parent disappears from her sight for a few seconds, for example, in a pick-a-boo play or when mom prepares her bottle. In these situations, her parent's mental representation will help her stay calm and regulate, knowing that the parent will show up shortly, whether in the play or with the warm bottle. In Fig. 7.2, the child, for example, first attends for a few seconds to each of the three points (puppet, clown, mother), with no preference. Later, with the mother's affective interaction tailored to her needs, a line is formed, enabling her to focus on the mother and have her in her mind, even when looking at the puppet. The process, in which the baby can keep mental representations of the puppet and the mom, and not only in the perceptual field, forms moments of shared attention when the child shares her emotional enthusiasm from the puppet with her "real mother."

Two unique methods are especially useful to achieve basic lines and triangles at this phase of basic symbols. The use of affect, the active ingredient in DIR intervention, is the foundation of these methods and evokes the energy and aliveliness that give meaning to interactions, thoughts, and feelings.

1. *Affective container* is a method in which the parent or therapist facilitates the room's affective tone to increase cohesiveness, regulation, and synchronization in the parent--child interaction. It focuses on the level of the arousal of the interactive partners. The child may be under- or overaroused, self-absorbed, or craving movement. Different affective tools may be used to set the tone of the relationship and hence the environment they are sharing (the container), including playful vocalization and rhythmicity. For example, a therapist may help the mom playing tag to set a more exciting affective tone when she

experiences the child's drowsiness, by saying in an upbeat, playful manner "run, run, run." The affective container facilitates creating a line, that is, the interaction between the two. In another case, the therapist may feel one or two of the partners are too excited and may soften the interaction using a slow and soft tone while facilitating the session. The use of affect can also be useful in an education setting in which the teacher can use this understanding to facilitate a cohesive and learning environment in the classroom by either upregulating or down-regulating the occurrence using interactive affective elements (Vig, 2019).

2. *Affective agent* is a caregiver who tailors his voice, looks, proximity, and movement in relation to the child to coregulate and engage the child in a line. He focuses on the child's attentiveness and the quality of interaction. He uses affect cues tailored to the child's profile to engage her through tone of voice, facial and body gestures, pacing, and rhythm. The caregiver observes the child, determining how to gain her attention and engagement to enhance and optimize their interaction, and fill it with pleasure and comfort. For example, the teacher, who is the affective agent, can encourage a child's curiosity and learning by supporting her attentiveness as will be described later (Vig, 2019).

Clinical example 1: Creation of a line in therapy

A 3-year-old child is wandering around the room. He is touching a swing (point), moving to a shiny bus (point), and touching a small hoop (point). Then he notices his therapist (point). The therapist playfully pulls the hoop that the child holds, accompanying it with a simple vocalization that reflects the intensity of the child's effort to hold it (modalities, affective agent). The child briefly meets her gaze (short line). She continues by playfully swaying back and forth, side to side, up and down, in a "where am I" fashion while both still hold onto the hoop (affective agent, stability—mobility). The child is laughing. The therapist continues to surprise him, slowly swaying in but in unpredictable directions (affective agent, line—mobility, axes). The child can maintain his gaze, now a moving line between them as he finds her. Later, she feels confident enough to abandon the hoop, and she hides behind a chair (line: mobility, distance, space, endurance). He is expecting her smile and looks for her. The therapist intervention supports the formation of an internal representation, emphasizing her presence using affect and movement across time and space that attracted the child.

Clinical example 2: Creation of line and triangles in a classroom

A 10-year-old child in a special-ed classroom was repeatedly playing with pieces of a torn paper. He does not respond to the teacher, who is calling his name (point). The teacher approaches him in a playful manner (line: distance). She touches his arms to alert him. He glances at her and turns back to his pieces of paper (line: break-off). She then initiates playing high-five with him, which he likes (affective agent, line). When she moves back to the whiteboard, the child keeps looking at her (line: motion, distance, space). The author, who has been observing, coaches the teacher to keep the child attentive by reinforcing the "line." She was directed to monitor the "sense of the line," and stay close to him if she feels the "line" is breaking down. A few minutes later, the teacher moved away, and he still was attentive to her. She uses an animated tone now and clear facial expression to attract the other children, afraid to lose their attention (affective container). Another girl answered the teacher's question, the child looked at his classmate, then turned back to the teacher, and added to his classmate's answer (triangle). Now, the child could construct a polygon out of the points, meaning the self, whiteboard, teacher, and the girl. He progresses from being focused on a single point (torn paper) and narrow space to follow the teacher across time and space, which created involvement and a meaningful learning experience.

Episodic symbols: playing family, doctor, policeman, or firefighter

Episodic symbols represent real life experiences that are emotionally engaging for the children. Between ages 2 and3, the toddler is on the move and observing or interacting with others, using all their sensory and motor abilities to understand the environment around them and develop a functional play based on their experiences. For example, a child in this age can watch from the living room a sequence of her mother opening the refrigerator, taking out vegetables and cooking a bowl of soup for her, or getting dressed and going to work. She may later reenact these scenes in her play kitchen, put on her mother's shoes, and walk around with her bag. Her body is now more competent, and she can climb and balance in ways that were unattainable a few months earlier. Episodic symbols describe the ability to perceive, process, and use internal representations of these occurrences.

These new capacities and experiences fuel the expanding emotional world of the child. For example, Sarah was told she has a doctor's visit tomorrow and appears to react with some anxiety, but that afternoon she searches for her doctor kit and finds dolls and teddy bears to examine. When her mother notices this, she comes over and tells playfully to "the doctor" (Sarah) she isn't feeling well. Sarah quickly changes patients and examines her. Unlike months before, when she would try every utensil in the kit, based on past experiences in the "real" doctor office, she takes out the stethoscope and the "shot." Her play reveals her concerns and offers her to master her anxiety, changing passive to active, to manage her anticipation and leads to a reassuring conversation. The play unfolds in a series of scenes that express the child's emotional world, including nurturing, comfort, reassurance, assertion, and power. This wider range of emotions in real life is symbolized in parallel processes in the internal world, as described in Fig. 7.3 (Greenspan & Wieder, 2006; Wieder & Wachs, 2012).

However, when children's sensory experiences or processing capacities are constricted, the symbolic representation will also be limited. Children that overfocus on toys or get distracted while playing may not register what others are doing around them, like others building a castle, or the chef in the kitchen cooking. They may be too absorbed in their obsessions or repetitive play. Pretending to be a doctor may not have meaning to them, or the doctor is someone to be avoided. Their difficulty to play functionally or symbolically may be related to other reasons, beyond poor attention, sensory processing, motor planning, and execution difficulties. It may suggest gaps in shared attention, engagement, and reciprocal interactions and communication. It is important to go down the developmental ladder to strengthen these earlier levels.

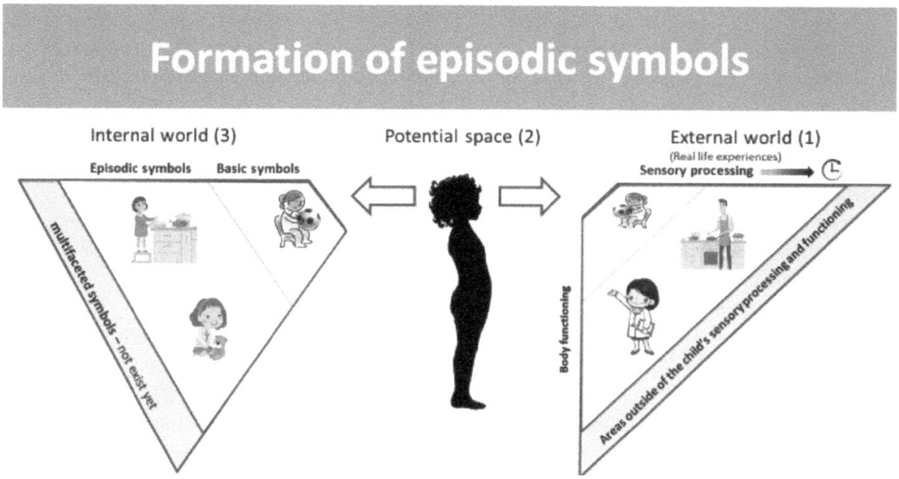

Figure 7.3 The children's ability to process information in expanding across space and time in real-life situations (1). Potential space—their daily experience is processed in play and art (2). Formation of episodic symbols in the internal world (3). This is a spiral process in which the internalize experience (3) also affect the child play (2) actions and choices in his environment (1).

Visual–spatial play is a type of play that encourages sensory-motor play, emphasizing and encouraging the dynamic use of the real space to its full potential. The goals of visual–spatial play first would be to increase mobility, being aware of one's own body and the environment. Later, the goals would expand to being aware of others who are moving in the space and being able to track their movement as well as the child's movement in relation to others and the environment. These include childhood games such as freeze tag, treasure hunts, monkey in the middle, and all sports involving moving through space (Wieder & Wachs, 2012). More advanced visual–spatial symbolic play will facilitate integrating pretend and imaginary play, while considering the physical environment and others. Such play will support symbol formation. The focus is on creatively using the space and building an imaginary world in the room to facilitate the formation of a parallel internal world. One can use different tools including, designating different corners of the room for different activities, inventing a new use for furniture (turning a folding sofa into a pirates' boat), building an obstacle course for an imaginary scene (e.g., a thief running from a cap or creating a cave underneath a chair draped in a blanket). Also, playing in space includes creating roads or pathways to destinations where the king and queen figures reside or are hiding, arranging the stage for their story, and moving soldier figures through space to set an ambush in war.

Case illustration:

A child with regulatory and visual–spatial challenges turned to his mom during a session, pointing to a tiger puppet he desired (triangle). Once he got it, he became overly excited, and his muscle tone tightened. His mother, who held the meaning of the "tiger," playfully invited him to a simple tag game, "You can't catch me!" (affective agent). He looked at the tiger, bringing it closer and further from his eyes as if he was having difficulty with convergence and focusing, not responding to his mom's playful attempts (point, no-line). She touched him to get his attention and reflected his feelings, "You are super, super excited about the tiger!" in a rhythmic voice (affective agent). The child looked at her for a few seconds and turned back to the puppet (broken line). The therapist suggested Mom put on a lion hat, act scared, and run to hide in the "cave" under the table in the corner of the room (visual–spatial play), reversing their expected roles. The therapist encourages the playful upregulating tone in the room (affective container). The playful manner that the mom used and her facial expression (affective agent) caught her child's attention and enabled him to attend to her and engage playfully. He came toward her (line: long, distance, axis) and pretended he was hunting her. He focused on the lion's mane, as well as her eyes, and identified it when he got closer (line: motion). First, he was hesitant and slow but soon became fast and sharp in his movements. He got closer to his mom and pulled back. The symbols in the play, including the tiger and the attack, got deeper in meaning and included content as well as dynamic and more forceful movements and voices. She whispered, "Where should I run?" (symbolic visual–spatial play), relinquishing control to him. He pointed to the chair on the other side of the room. "Oh, to the mountain?" and she ran away (triangle, visual–spatial play). He tries to get her and shouts playfully, "I will hunt you!" (line). The child who first focused on a point (the puppet) and did not know what to do, was later able to use his body playfully in the space to enjoy a richer plot integrating dimensions of time, space, and body, which enabled him to create personal symbols in his mind. The shift occurred when his mother playfully introduced affect in the idea of being hunted, giving her son the upper hand to feel powerful and continue the chase.

Multifaceted symbols and abstract thinking: superheroes, witches, and rulers

Multifaceted symbols and abstract thinking require a sophisticated level of perception and processing of multisensory stimuli, including visual, vestibular, and tactile in wider space and units of time, as well as emotional ones. Children can connect nuances in facial expression, body postures, and intonation in others, and bring multifaceted depth to social interaction and emotional experiences in general. Envy, anger, cruelty, aggression, competitiveness, and death, as well as justice, and altruism, reflect the emotions that build the child's internal world. Perception gradually relies more on the children's inner world. Yet, there is still an important role in this equation for action or sensory experience as feelings are always coupled with sensation. Symbolic play enables children to get more control and understanding of these multifaceted feelings and situations. Witches, dragons, pirates, ghosts, fairies, knights, and superheroes become the main characters in complex themes that process the compounded emotions from the "real world." These symbols reflect the child's emotional developmental level. In this case, discovering powerful aggression and the magical power needed to defeat enemies, find safety, and be victorious. Difficulties in using these frightening and heroic symbols actively in play, and the magical solutions they offer, deprive the children of the opportunity to test reality, reflect on their meaning, and release the anxiety they experience with the realization of aggression that exists in human nature and the world they live in. With further emotional development, they begin to differentiate fantasy and reality, reflect on the meaning of these symbols, and develop abilities to define values and complex emotions such as shame, guilt, jealousy, morality, empathy, etc. Whether or not they are on the autism spectrum, not all children reach this abstract reflective level. These challenges may affect their ability to create causality and become emotionally constricted and anxious (Wieder, 2017).

Dynamic drawing is a special intradisciplinary method that encourages emotional processing, symbol formation, and abstract thinking. The dynamic nature of emotions is embodied in the drawing process to support child development, meaning that the drawing change in parallel to the unfolding dialogue with the child, gradually getting deeper into the emotional world. The method relies on neurobiology research indicating that children with ASD and others may have difficulties sequencing, integrating, and processing auditory and sensory-motor input. The caregiver starts by establishing physical and emotional proximity (space) and emotional involvement (affective agent), drawing external characteristics of the child, such as the color of eyes or hair playfully ("Let's see who I am drawing. Who has a curly hair?"). The purpose is to maintain a line and a triangle (e.g., child, therapist/parent, drawing) during the intervention. Later, observed behavior or facial expression are drawn (e.g., "Wow, I see you are jumping"). In the third phase, the child's inner world is explored in a lively dialogue, and the child's revealed thoughts, feelings, and imagination are represented in the developing drawing. The dynamic drawing includes dyadic coregulated interactions (lines) that help children process and symbolize feelings of joy, fear, anger, anxiety, and themes such as intimacy or reflective thinking. The intervention is tailored to the child's profile, taking into consideration, for example, issues of pace, language, communication, attention span, etc.

As indicated above, emotional and social issues can be processed using this technique, including, for example, splitting, a situation where a child perceives people as either bad or good (mind). In this case, one would follow the child's lead, focusing first on the elements that the child "disapproves of" in her "evil" friend. A drawn black heart, for example, can symbolize this, and later small anecdotes that she does like about her friend will be added to the drawing. Finally, the child will have this drawing that has changed through the process and includes on one piece of paper, the positive and negative feelings and experiences concerning her friend. This visual representation of her psychic world helps the child "carry the moment of symbolization" across time, using two-dimensional space, which can be experienced more comfortably and in a controlled manner. Anxiety is an internal experience, often covering or defending against other feelings that are too difficult to feel or express and can also be processed using dynamic drawing.

A mom trained to use this technique at home describes how she went through with her son when the child lost sight of his parents for a few minutes and got extremely anxious: "Wow! You came out, and suddenly you didn't see either of us?" "Did you get scared?" (history, time). She accompanied this dialogue by drawing the situation and his frightened face and heart, using engaging tone to entice eye-contact and involvement (line, triangle). "Oh, and then you found daddy," and drawing the relief in his facial expression and heart over the previous anxious face (time). The drawing's facial expression and the heart reflected the change in the emotions as the story evolved. Her son was able to show this drawing with relief to his dad later (triangle, time, alfa function/mind). The dynamic drawing was used to coregulate the child, supporting lines and triangles, while reflecting on his anxiety about the separation and the fear she experienced.

In another case, a girl in a social skills group that took place in one of the author's clinic had a hard time processing the multifaceted situation underway in the group and often regressed and reacted in a way that was described by her school psychologist as a "psychotic regression." Analysis of these occasions in the clinic helped the therapist understand that the girl's processing speed is slow. When an occurrence is too fast (time) for her, she presents with regressive behavior, especially around scary emotions (mind), even when she initiates them. In these cases, she might lie down and start to talk like a baby, perhaps a safer experience, as babies are protected. A few tools were used to help her regulate and get a sense of security in the group. For example, in a play sequence where a scary scene of a witch was brought into the story, the therapist paused the acting (space, time) and asked her to direct the scene and show (body) how she wanted the witch to be. She was asked to describe the witch's fingernails' length, the tone of voice (loud or soft), and clothing. In this case, a dynamic drawing was also used to slow down and narrow the space (space, triangles, time). That helped her get back to her play with her peers and the therapist, bringing new ideas, and using different symbolic objects in the room while managing her anxiety (α function/triangles–polygons). Consultation to her school team, focusing on the issue or processing and supporting tools, helped reduce her anxiety levels there as well.

Summary

The Neuro-Geometric approach maps development, interaction, and experiences in geometrical concepts of space, including points, lines, and polygons, to create a common language between therapists, parents, and educators. It provides a new reference system and terminology to the DIR model to promote children's development with special needs and uneven development. The approach proposes that children construct an internal three-dimension representational map that parallels their experience of the outside world and boosts symbolic formation.

The Neuro-Geometric approach brings a unified perspective embracing current neurobiological research and existing psychological and developmental theories to support lacking capacities for development, including symbolization and abstraction defined as the highest DIR functional emotional developmental capacity. It rests on recognizing individual differences and relationships and understanding that neurobiology affects children's functional abilities, emotional experiences, and overall development. The approach integrates knowledge from all disciplines related to development, including speech and language therapy, occupational therapy, and psychology. While not every child with autism reaches the same development level, each possible step up the developmental ladder is important. Other children who experience emotional constrictions would also benefit from this integrated model in treatment.

The Neuro-Geometric approach's wide scope enables the therapists to provide a dynamic and modified container for parents and children. The therapists' ability to integrate their understanding of the child's impulses and fantasies, intersubjective experience, developmental levels, neurobiological differences, and the environmental factors enable the therapist to build a comprehensive treatment program. Those programs are established on understanding the children's challenges and strengths, prioritize and map the resources, and provide integrated and effective interventions. While traditional approaches often focus solely on psychological intervention, including interpretation or transferences and reverie, the Neuro-Geometric approach emphasizes establishing therapeutic relationships that also consider the physical space and experience as a catalyst for an emotional and interactive experience. It supports interwoven interventions, including bottom-up and top-down approaches that vary with the children's experience, encourages intersubjective emotional relatedness-techniques of here and now in everyday life while keeping interactions playful, spontaneous, and authentic. Unique developmentally appropriate methods illustrate how to proceed from points to lines, triangles, and polygons to support development in general, and symbol formation and abstract thinking in particular, including (1) affective container, (2) affective agent, (3) visual–spatial play, and (4) dynamic drawing. The Neuro-Geometric approach can be applied in therapeutic and educational settings, and in-home programs by keeping the natural caregivers of the children involved and informed. It enables therapists to provide tools for parents and educators to support development in daily situations.

To summarize, the approach asserts that one cannot talk about potential space or symbolism without talking about the real world of children, including their interactive world, and their ability to function in their physical spaces, in addition to their emotional world. Any attempt to split these worlds will result in compromised intervention and obstacles in therapy. The Neuro-Geometric approach provides an integrated intradisciplinary knowledge base for all therapists, including those in mental health, speech and language therapists, occupational therapists, and others to effectively and comprehensively treat children with ASD and related disorders.

References

American Psychiatric Association. (2013). *Diagnostic and statistical manual of mental disorders* (5th ed.). Arlington, VA: Author.

Ayres, A. J. (1972). *Sensory integration and learning disorders*. Los Angeles, CA: Western Psychological Services.

Bart, O., Bar-Haim, Y., Weizman, E., Levin, M., Sadeh, A., & Mintz, M. (2009). Balance treatment ameliorates anxiety and increases self-esteem in children with comorbid anxiety and balance disorder. *Research in Developmental Disabilities*, *30*(3), 486–495.

Beebe, B., & Lachmann, F. M. (1988). The contribution of mother-infant mutual influence to the origins of self- and object representations. *Psychoanalytic Psychology*, *5*(4), 305–337.

Bowlby, J. (1969). *Attachment. Attachment and loss: Vol. 1. Loss*. New York: Basic Books.

Carney, D. R., Cuddy, A. J. C., & Yap, A. J. (2010). Power posing. *Psychological Science*, *21*(10), 1363–1368.

Erikson, E. H. (1950). *Childhood and society*. New York: Norton.

Feldman, R. (2007). Parent–infant synchrony and the construction of shared timing; physiological precursors, developmental outcomes, and risk conditions. *Journal of Child Psychology and Psychiatry*, *48*, 329–354.

Feldman, R., & Greenbaum, C. W. (1997). Affect regulation and synchrony in mother-infant play as precursors to the development of symbolic competence. *Infant Mental Health Journal*, *18*, 4–23.

Foley, G. M. (2006). Self and social-emotional development in infancy. In G. M. Foley, & M. G. Hochman (Eds.), Mental health in early intervention: Achieving unity in principles and practice (pp. 139–174). Baltimore, MD: Paul H. Brookes.

Freud, S. (1961). *Beyond the pleasure principle*. New York: Norton, Original work published (1920).

Greenspan, S. I., & Wieder, S. (1997). Developmental patterns and outcomes in infants and children with disorders in relating and communicating: A chart review of 200 cases of children with Autistic Spectrum Diagnoses. *The Journal of Developmental and Learning Disorders*, *1*, 87–141.

Greenspan, S. I., & Wieder, S. (2006). *Engaging autism: Helping children relate, communicate and think with the DIR Floortime approach*. Cambridge, MA: Perseus.

Klein, M. (1988). *Envy and gratitude: And other works 1946–1963*. London: Virago.

Klein, M., & Riviere, J. (1964). *Love, hate and reparation*. W W Norton & Co.

Little, M. I. (1990). *Psychotic anxieties and containment: A personal record of an analysis with Winnicott*. Northvale, NJ: Jason Aronson.

Mueller, I., & Tronic, E. (2019). Sensory processing and meaning making in Autism Spectrum disorder. In U. N. Das, N. Papaneophytou, & T. El-Kour (Eds.), *Autism 360°* (1st ed.). Academic Press. (2019).

Ogden, T. H. (1989). *The primitive edge of experience*. London: J. Aronson.

Piaget, J. (1962). The stages of the intellectual development of the child. *Bulletin of the Menninger Clinic*, *26*(3), 120–128.

Porges, S. W. (2009). Reciprocal influences between body and brain in the perception and expression of affect: A polyvagal perspective. In D. Fosha, D. J. Siegel, & M. F. Solomon (Eds.), The healing power of emotion: Affective neuroscience, development & clinical practice. W. W. Norton & Company, pp. 27–54.

Russo, N., Foxe, J. J., Brandwein, A. B., Altschuler, T., Gomes, H., & Molholm, S. (2010). Multisensory processing in children with autism: High-density electrical mapping of auditory-somatosensory integration. *Autism Research*, *3*(5), 253–267.

Shai, D., & Belsky, J. (2016). Parental embodied mentalizing: How the nonverbal dance between parents and infants predicts children's socio-emotional functioning. *Attachment & Human Development*, *19*(2), 191–219.

Shefer, S., Gordon, C., Avraham, K. B., & Mintz, M. (2015). Balance deficit enhances anxiety, and balance training decreases anxiety in vestibular mutant mice. *Behavioral Brain Research*, *276*, 76–83.

Stern, D. N. (1985). *The interpersonal world of the infant: A view from psychoanalysis and developmental psychology*. New York: Basic Books.

Symington, J., & Symington, N. (1996). *The clinical thinking of Wilfred Bion*. London, pp. 12–13.

Torres, E. B. (2012). Atypical signatures of motor variability found in an individual with ASD. *Neurocase: Case Studies in Neuropsychology, Neuropsychiatry, and Behavioural Neurology*, *1*, 1–16.

Trevarthen, C., & Delafield-Butt, J. T. (2013). Autism as a developmental disorder in intentional movement and affective engagement. *Frontiers in Integrative Neuroscience*, *7*, Article 49.

Vig, A. (2019). A comprehensive approach to inclusion: Theoretical and clinical implications using the developmental, individual differences, relationship-based – DIR® Model. In U. N. Das, N. Papaneophytou, & T. El-Kour (Eds.), *Autism 360°* (1st ed.). Academic Press.

Vygotsky, L. S. (1929/1994). The problem of the cultural development of the child. In R. van der Veer, & J. Valsiner (Eds.), *The Vygotsky reader* (pp. 57–72). Oxford: Blackwell. (Original work published in 1929).

Wieder, S. (2017). The power of symbolic play in emotional development through the DIR lens. *Topics in Language Development*, *37*, 259–281.

Wieder, S., & Wachs, H. (2012). *Visual/spatial portals to thinking, feelings and movement: Advancing competencies and emotional development in children with learning and Autism Spectrum Disorders*. Mendham, NJ: Profectum Foundation.

Winnicott, D. W. (1953). Transitional objects and transitional phenomena – A study of the first not-me possession. *International Journal of Psycho-Analysis*, *34*(2), 89–97.

Winnicott, D. W. (1968). *The child, the family, and the outside world*. Harmondsworth, Middlesex: Penguin Books.

Winnicott, D. W. (1971). *Playing and reality*. New York: Basic Books.

Educational readiness for autism spectrum disorders: the integration of experience and development

8

Serena Wieder
Profectum Foundation, Mendham, NJ, United States

The daunting challenge of educating children on the autism spectrum involves the uniqueness of each child and how to offer education based on strengths and the fundamental capacities necessary for life span functioning. Few would argue that education is essential but there is much confusion about different terms, often used interchangeably, such as learning, training, education, experience, and development. Many questions arise. How does education relate to development? How does education relate to experience? What is the best learning environment for education? What training skills will be offered or knowledge acquired? Is it the diagnosis, or functioning, or individual differences that will drive educational options? The terms may overlap but all aspire to realize each individual's developmental potential in order to achieve outcomes that meet the life span needs of individuals and families. To reach unity for the individual on the autism spectrum, a roadmap is needed where theory and intervention meet and development and education are integrated (Greenspan & Wieder, 1997c).

The Developmental, Individual Difference, Relationship-based (DIR)[1] model introduced major paradigm shifts from behavioral reductionism where "one-size" fits all, to relational dynamic developmental systems that function simultaneously in the context of the family and environment. It integrated the multiple dimensions of human development identifying capacities that are essential for all individuals throughout life and where relationships are central. This chapter will highlight the foundations and principles of development necessary for effective education, the emotional readiness for learning, and the integration of experience into functional emotional capacities. The DIR Model for education goes beyond focusing on specific behaviors, symptoms, or rote learning by examining how children use everyday experiences to carry out emotionally meaningful goals based on their developmental levels. This is accomplished through affect-based interactions with parents, caregivers. teachers, therapists,

[1] DIR is the registered trademark of the Interdisciplinary Council on Developmental and Learning Disorders.

Emerging Programs for Autism Spectrum Disorder. DOI: https://doi.org/10.1016/B978-0-323-85031-5.00028-1

and peers. The focus is on the developmentally appropriate experiences needed to build higher levels of emotional and intellectual capacities based on each child's profile.

The DIR framework and its derivative Functional Capacities for Development (FCD) provide a multidimensional approach to the properties and barriers to education utilizing three interrelated pathways (Wieder & Greenspan, 1993; Wieder & Wachs, 2012). The "D" casts the functions of development into functional, emotional, social, and cognitive capacities (see below). The "I" represents the neurobiological individual differences in the child's neurological, psychological, physiological, sensory, and motor processing through which experience is understood. The "R" focuses on the vital role relationships play in learning, social emotional growth, and mental health. Putting parent–child relationships at the core of human needs, DIR embraces the interactions that provide the experience necessary to create a child's sense of self and agency, intentionality and initiative, and emotional well-being (mental health) in the context of the family's culture and environment.

The evolution of the DIR model

Before discussing the model it is important to describe the origins of DIR theory and practice and the theoretical, clinical, and research support for it serving as an educational model. It offers autism opportunities for ongoing development beyond standard educational parameters. The components of the DIR model have long theoretical, clinical, cognitive, educational, and research traditions reaching back into the last century. Greenspan and Wieder, the codevelopers of this model (1997), cited the various frameworks that influenced their model, including the psychodynamic traditions of Freud, Erikson, Anna Freud, Klein, and Mahler. Others included Spitz, Bowlby, Winnicott, Fraiberg, and Provence, who described the critical impact of disrupted and impoverished environments on attachment and emotional development. Meanwhile, Brazelton, Escalona, Ayres, and Miller identified the individual differences in the infant's capacity to organize experience, adapt, process a range of sensory and motor stimuli, and respond to social interactions (Greenspan & Wieder, 1997c).

This body of theory and research on emotional development evolved separately from the impact of the social world and cognitive development which separated cognitive from emotional processes. For Piaget, affect and cognition were complementary in the human condition, but he rejected the idea that affect can create intelligence, or that intelligence can create emotions, though he did concede the functioning of intelligence depends on the energy affect provides (Piaget, 1962). Vygotsky believed social interaction played a fundamental role in the development of cognition. He proposed that for a student to learn a new concept or skill, it had to be within the student's "zone of proximal development," that is, close to what the child already had developed, was meaningful, and could be performed independently. The impact of affect as a motivating force was only reported later (Vygotsky, 1978). For Feuerstein, cognitive functions were enhanced through mediated learning experience

(MLE) (Feuerstein, Rand, & Rynders, 1988). He focused on the relationship between the mediator and learner and the role of affect in motivating learning, but neither he nor Vygotsky were directly concerned with emotional development and the role of internalized relationships.

Only later did it become apparent that the separation of thinking and feeling distorted understanding of both processes and an integrated perspective was needed (Ratner and Stettner, 1991). Furthermore, individual differences were not yet integrated into either theory or research of early emotional or cognitive development (Greenspan & Wieder, 1997c). Presenting a more experiential and functional view was John Dewey, an educational reformer of the last century and a founder of pragmatic philosophy, who believed education is a process of experience acquired not only with the environment but through interactions within relationships and developmental capacities. He revolutionized the theory of education from transmitting knowledge to the importance of experience and believed educators should teach children how to think by doing, rather than relying on rote memorization (Dewey, 1938). This view was expanded by David Kolb, a psychologist and educational theorist, who not only stressed the importance of concrete experience (hands-on learning), but added reflective observation, abstract conceptualization, and active experimentation in his learning cycle (Kolb & Kolb, 2017). Currently, experiential learning has been adopted by many in education and will be discussed below.

The DIR model integrated the above elements by putting emotions, cognition, and experience together. DIR evolved during a 6-year-long NIMH preventive intervention study of high-risk infants in multiproblem families in the late 1970s and early 1980s. During this study children with autism were identified and Greenspan, Wieder, Nover, and Lieberman (1987) discovered developmental and relationship-based approaches were not yet part of the developmental disability world or autism. They shifted their attention to the treatment of children with autism introducing the critical impact of sensory and motor processing challenges, and were the first to integrate these with emotional and relationship-based approaches from infant mental health. With DIR, they pioneered a dynamic systemized developmental model for comprehensive intervention and parent-mediated treatment of autism and related disorders (Greenspan & Wieder, 1997c, 2006).

Parents have long been insisting on the education of their autistic children since Kanner's description of infantile autism in 1943 (Donvan & Zucker, 2016). Yet, autism did not become a diagnosis in DSM III until 1980, amended or revised five times since then based on advances in developmental science, the latest in 2013 (American Psychiatric Association, 2013). In the United States the passage of IDEA (Individual with Disability Education Act) mandating education for special needs was granted in 1987 (34 CFR). The structured TEACCH educational model developed by Eric Schopler was underway years earlier in a statewide program in North Carolina established in 1972 (Schopler, Mesibov, & Hearsey, 1995). Ivor Lovass published his paper on ABA (Applied Behavioral Analysis) promoting discrete trials to correct the deficits of autism in 1987 (Lovass, 1987). The increasing prevalence of ASD that came with growing awareness and parent-led movements generated multiple methods and theories, and research ballooned seeking better early identification, causes, and treatment effectiveness. In 2001 the National Research Council of the National Academy of Sciences, in a landmark report, *Educating Children with Autism*, called for *autism* had already pioneered all these features (Lord & McGee, 2001).

Twenty years later, Project Aim reported on the most comprehensive metanalysis of 130 studies, representing 6240 participants on the autism spectrum between 0–8 years, in seven interventions (behavioral, developmental, naturalistic developmental behavioral intervention (NDBI), TEACCH, sensory-based, animal-assisted, and technology based). They analyzed 15 outcome categories indexing core and related ASD symptoms and found that *developmental and NDBI interventions had high quality evidence to support children with ASD in achieving a range of developmental outcomes*. Interventions were coded as developmental if they were described as being motivated by *constructivist theories of learning* (a theory of education that believes the learners' comprehension and knowledge is based on their own experiences). Also, if they were *heavily child-led and implemented according to a typical developmental sequence, to facilitate the development of foundational skills that would translate to gains in developmentally downstream domains changing the trajectory for the future*. Evidence suggested that developmental interventions may be *particularly effective for supporting the acquisition of social communication*, a core challenge for young children with ASD. Included were Hanen models, and responsive teaching. Behavioral intervention showed some evidence for effectiveness, but lacked methodological rigor. Other approaches did not have sufficient evidence meeting their criteria (Sandbank et al., 2020).

Once again, scientific reviews like Project Aim, as well as a decade of randomized control trials support DIR's developmental approach. Findings in a DIR-based RCT study by Solomon et al. included significant improvements in parent–child and social interaction, social emotional development, reduced autism scores on ADOS and symptomology, as well as improved parent stress and depression (Solomon, Van Egeren, Mahoney, Quon-Huber, & Zimmerman, 2014). Significant improvements in another DIR-based RCT study found significant improvements in joint attention, enjoyment, social interaction, and reduced symptoms, and while language tests did not show advantages, they were found for social conversations (Casenhiser, Binns, McGill, Morderer, & Shanker, 2014; Casenheiser, Shanker, & Stieben, 2011). In addition, the PACT (Preschool Autism Communication Trials) parent-mediated video aided intervention (Green et al., 2010), and its 6-year follow-up after intervention had ceased, the longest RCT studies in the field, demonstrated the long-term effectiveness of parent-mediated relationship-based approaches (Pickles et al., 2016).

In recent years autism research has turned to the search for biomarkers, neural signatures, and genetic studies which hold promise for the future but are not yet readily translated into intervention. However, preventive intervention studies for at risk siblings of children with autism where 20% are likely to have autism, examining the effects of very early intervention are now available. A few will be mentioned here. A 5-month parent-mediated video-aided intervention (12 sessions between 9 and 14 months) reduced the severity of subsequent prodromal autism symptoms at the 39-month follow-up, as well as producing positive impact on parent–infant interactions

(Green, Wai Wan, Guiraud, & Holsgrove, 2013). Another study of parent-delivered intervention, Promoting First Relationships, for infants at risk for ASD, showed effects on electrophysiological and habituation measures of social attention where the pattern of responses appeared closer to normative response of control low risk groups. This study suggested early parent-mediated intervention (PMI) has the potential to impact brain systems underpinning social attention (Jones, Dawson, Kelly, Estes, & Webb, 2017). The robust findings of Project Aim and these other studies support the fundamental process development and relationships play in education for changing the trajectories for children with autism.

Just what is the developmental, individual difference, relationship-based model?

In this new vision of development and integrated interdisciplinary intervention. milestones do not hold the answers. Instead, DIR integrated the multiple lines of development and individual differences in a model which focuses on emotional experience and interactive relationships. It assumes each child is born with the capacity to organize experience that progresses to higher levels as the child's nervous system matures and the child can engage the world both emotionally and cognitively in more complex ways. Greenspan integrated intellect and emotion through the dual coding of experience, that is, both intellect and affect simultaneously give meaning to experience. Affect is a key feature in DIR as a theory and practice. In the Affect Diathesis Hypothesis, Greenspan (2001) posits that there is a fundamental neurogenic disconnect between affect and experience in the processing of individuals with ASD. It is theorized that the deficit in affect–experience integration compromises symbol attainment, memory, motivation, and the formation of relational ties and interpersonal interaction. Typically, affect captures attention, emotion, and intellect expressed through tone of voice, gestures, pacing, and synchrony in preverbal and verbal communication. Affect is the active ingredient which provides the emotional signaling to alert, engage, convey feelings and meanings, and integrate experience (Greenspan, 2001; Greenspan & Wieder, 2006). For example, when a child studying history imagines the fears of facing a battle for freedom and whether he would have fought, he not only comprehends what happened and why, but also responds emotionally and is reflective, learning about himself and others. Or, the toddler who knows which of his Dad's hands hold the most M&Ms as his Dad entices him and does not have to count them to know which one to pick!

The primary focus of DIR intervention is to enable children to master the full range of emotional and cognitive abilities as they progress through the six functional emotional developmental capacities. These capacities are inextricably related to *affect*, which plays an organizing and integrating function. The six active processes provide purpose and function to experience, from sharing attention and enjoying the security of attachment, to communicating and organizing behavior to solve social problems, to generating symbolic ideas and images that advance cognition, creativity, and empathy. These processes start at birth, develop in the early years, and function simultaneously with subsequently emerging capacities. For example, attention accompanies every intentional act. Each capacity can be assessed at any age for their duration, emotional range and self-regulation based on what is systematically observed in the child's functioning. It is also important to attend to what is not observed and thereby becomes the goals for intervention. For example, reciprocal communication builds upon shared attention and engagement (may work well when fun, but what if scared or angry?). It is needed for complex social problem solving (when you ask to go to the park and are told to get ready) and symbolic play (you insist you do not want to be the "bad" guy because Superman is your favorite).

Individual differences, such as a child born with hyper- or hypoarousal, or sensory sensitivities to touch and sound, may have difficulty organizing affective domains of joy, pleasure, and exploration. They may evidence apathy or disregard attempts to engage and communicate. Attuned and insightful caregivers who reflect on their and their child's experience find ways to engage and interact (Oppenheim & Koren-Karie, 2009). Stress related to health, family change, moves, and other events affect developmental functioning (e.g., regressions during the Covid pandemic). Specific learning difficulties related to cognitive and individual differences also need to be identified (e.g., math difficulties because of visual spatial deficits or dyslexia), as do emotional challenges such as anxiety, depression, obsessional patterns, and poor self-regulation and impulsiveness. It is critical to embrace the complexity of development and meet each child at their level as both over- and underestimating a child present risks impeding progress. This developmental perspective supports lifelong learning and while in ASD development is uneven, or barriers must be overcome, ascension to each level should be pursued at all ages. Not every individual reaches the same level, but each level gained adds meaning and functionality to life at any age. Moreover, every person benefits from relationships throughout life (Greenspan, & Wieder, 2003, 2006). Table 8.1 elaborates on each of the functional emotional development levels.

Experience in the emotional development of self

"It was a great experience!" Or, maybe not! Either way, these words capture the emotions one has encoded in mind, body, and experience and now have personal meaning. They will have context as they associate with a special place or event, and others who were present. Or, one might be alone in that "Aha" moment of discovery and understanding, an exhilarating emotion. Experience is accompanied by sensation and motion in one's body, often felt again when remembered as experience goes beyond words and images. When children learn through experience that meets them at their level and connects to their feelings, it has meaning and is felt inside and out. Experience takes many forms from spontaneous, incidental, or semi-structured, to the systematic acquisition of knowledge and skill when attached to

Table 8.1 Functional emotional developmental levels (FEDL).

The "D"—Developmental Capacities of Emotional and Intellectual Functioning The child's functional emotional developmental levels (FEDL) examine how different lines of development (motor, cognitive, emotional, language, visual spatial, sensory) interact with each other and with caregivers to create capacities to support the development of functional emotional and intellectual capacities in order to be able to carry out emotionally meaningful goals. Each capacity develops early in life and continues to develop as the next capacities evolve and become integrated. 1. Regulation and Shared Attention (between child and caregiver). The capacity for calm, focused, regulated interest in the sights and sounds of the outer world while able to attend and share interests with the caregiver (0–3 months). 2. Forming Attachments and Engaging in Relationships. Child and parents become more engaged as they interact with each other with warmth, trust, and intimacy. They each use their senses to enjoy each other through looks, hugs, songs, and dancing together. Over time the child will need to remain regulated, related, and engaged across the full range of emotions, even when disappointed, scared, angry, or other stresses, and later develops the ability to express these symbolically (1–5 months). 3. Intentional Two-Way Affective Communication. A purposeful, continuous flow of interactions with gestures and reciprocating emotions gets underway. The child begins to act purposefully with expanding awareness of her body and the functions it can perform. With greater motor control and abilities to reach; sit and turn; crawl and creep; and give and take or drop objects, she is better able to communicate her desires and intentionally begins to takes charge of her experience. Her interpersonal world is growing, as is her awareness of her body in space and in relation to others who may also be moving (4–10 months). 4. Complex Social Problem Solving. Having developed the capacity to problem solve using social interactions, the child learns the back and forth rhythm of interactive emotional signaling and begins to use this ability to think about and solve his problems. He can take in the signals or intent of others to see if they want what he wants and finds emotionally meaningful, such as taking Daddy by the hand and pulling him to the door to go outside and play. But he is also beginning to recognize when daddy is busy. All of the child's senses work with his motor system as he interacts with others to solve problems. Difficulties may arise when he becomes aware that things are not as they should be based on the prior experiences recorded in his mind, and he encounters new difficulties he must solve as his experience expands (9 and 18 months). 5. Creating Emotional Ideas. The child begins to represent or symbolize her intentions, feelings, and ideas in imaginative play and/or language, using gestures, words, and symbols. His ideas now have a sequence and a purpose. The first symbols come from experiences in real life that can now be enacted in pretend dramas as the child experiments with different roles and feelings. Emotional themes expand as the child transitions from dependency, to separation, to conflicts and aggression with attending developmental anxieties and symbolic solutions (18–36 months). 6. Emotional Thinking, Logic, and Sense of Reality. At about 3 years, the young child begins to combine ideas to tell a "story" as he develops more logical thinking and a better understanding of self and others, and what is real or not real. His stories use imaginative characters or animal figures who talk and are often magical as he discovers he needs more power to encounter the conflicts in life, but reasoning skills click in to understand sequential bridges and he becomes increasingly logical and realistic.

(Continued)

Table 8.1 (Continued)

Over the next few years, the child's emotional and mental abilities move toward abstract thinking and he develops the ability to distinguish reality from fantasy, self from nonself, one feeling from another; and to make distinctions concerning time and space (3–6 years).
Three additional processes elaborate on the sixth to expand cognitive and emotional range.
7. Multicausal and Comparative Thinking. At this level, the child "deepens the plot" as he can explore multiple motives, give opinions, and compare and contrast ideas. The child can express how she or he would feel "in your shoes" and predicts what you will do based on your "affect cues" such as deception, fairness, and justice. He can also hold two conflicting ideas or emotions in mind at the same time, e.g., I am angry but also love you!
8. Relativistic or Gray-Area Thinking. Here, the child differentiates more of his thoughts, rather than thinking only in "black and white" terms. The lion may pay a price for killing the zebra who kicked him and broke his leg, or being disappointed by a friend does not mean he has to dissolve a friendship. The child now considers different possibilities and contingencies and is aware of different outcomes related to how he would feel under different circumstances.
9. Self-Reflection or Thinking Using an Internal Standard. Now the child has a clearer sense of herself; she can look at and reflect on her performance and feelings. She can question why she is feeling a certain way and contrast this with how she usually feels, or she can compare her current efforts with earlier ones. This kind of reflective mindfulness allows her to make inferences about herself and others and creates new choices and ideas.
The "I" of DIR: Individual Differences in Sensory Modulation, Sensory Processing, Sensory Affective Processing, and Motor Planning and Sequencing
These neurobiologically based individual differences are the result of genetic, prenatal, perinatal, and maturational variations and/or deficits. In DIR careful attention is paid to the body and how it responds to sensation, both supporting or compromising functioning and defines the experience a child with autism has of his body's functioning. A 200 case chart review identified the impact of altered patterns of sensory motor responsiveness on the development of children with ASD before it was officially recognized as a diagnostic feature in DSM 5 (Greenspan & Wieder, 1997b, 1999). Recently, Torres, a neuroscientist, studied the feedback received from body movements in the brain. She found that the feedback is more randomized and less accurate in children with ASD and concluded that people with autism might have problems with body awareness, feeling where their body is in space, and their ability to control movements and postures are poor (Torres, 2012).
These individual differences can be characterized in at least five ways:
1. Sensory modulation, including hypo- and hyperreactivity in each sensory modality, including touch, sound, smell, vision, proprioception, vestibular, interoception, and movement in space.
2. Sensory-based motor disorder (dyspraxia and postural disorder). These include deficits in using the two sides of the body; planning, sequencing, and executing novel movements; experiencing postural insecurity against gravity.
3. Sensory processing in each modality, including auditory processing and language and visual–spatial processing. Processing includes the capacity to register, decode, and comprehend sequences and abstract patterns.

(Continued)

Table 8.1 (Continued)

4. Sensory-affective processing in each modality, e.g., the ability to process and react to affect (emotions), including the capacity to connect "intent" or affect to motor planning and sequencing, language, and symbols. This processing capacity may be especially relevant for ASD (Greenspan & Wieder, 1997c).
5. Motor planning (praxis), including the capacity to sequence actions, behaviors, and symbols, including symbols in the form of thoughts, words, visual images, and spatial concepts.
"R" of DIR: Relationships activate development and anchor mental health
Development is constructed by the relationships in a child's life. It is a dynamic bidirectional process in which parents need to recognize the child's individual differences, provide emotional and physiological coregulation, and facilitate the child's social, emotional, and cognitive capacities, all in real time. Early relationships (attachments) are conceptualized as highly significant influences on the child's development across multiple domains. Research has shown that children on the autism spectrum do enjoy secure attachments and benefit from sensitive and insightful parenting (see things from the child's point of view). Dolev, Oppenheim, Koren-Karie, and Yirmiya (2014) found the emotional quality of relationships assessed by attachment and insightfulness even predicted educational placement in inclusion programs 4.5 and 8.5 years later, more than IQ and interactive competence.
Relationships go beyond the primary attachments to establishing an expanding social network with other adults, teachers, therapists, and peers. All can activate development and learning and are essential in every aspect of education. Developmentally appropriate interactions mobilize the child's intentions and affect enabling the child to broaden his/her range of experience at each level and forge pathways from one functional developmental level to the next. In contrast, interactions that do not accommodate the child's functional developmental level or individual differences can undermine progress. For example, a caregiver who is too stressed or depressed may not be able to engage an infant who is underresponsive and self-absorbed, or be available to a child who is anxious or impulsive. When a child does not have the interactive support of a parent or caregiver, he may not feel sufficiently secure to explore negative emotions symbolically and can result in constrictions of affect, anxiety, rigidities, and obsessions (Greenspan & Wieder, 2006). Both the child's and caregiver's emotions reflect the complexity of their experience and nuanced interactions. Does the relationship tolerate affective range, both trust, security and love, as well as tolerance for negative emotions (anger, jealousy, disappointment, etc.)? Is it able to repair following ruptures. Does the relationship support differentiation and individuation, identifications, and social roles (Wieder & Foley, 2018). Project AIM (see above) highlighted social communication changes the trajectory of autism and parent-mediated intervention show long-term impact (Green et al., 2010). Together, the D, the I, and the R produce a dynamic profile of the child and parent/family at any point in time and help caregivers tailor their interactions to the child's developmental level of comprehension. Within the DIR framework it is possible to understand a child's experience, his relationships, emotional well-being and challenges (mental health), and thinking. Its functional emotional capacities provide the foundation for successful education (Wieder, 2013).

meaning and need. You "get it" and "own it," and it becomes part of your implicit repertoire of what you know and can do, making you the agent of your intent. It allows you to know your feelings and desires, and to develop the sense of who you are. When learning is emotionally based it becomes an internal reinforcement that motivates interaction and spontaneity where emotion and cognition are intertwined (Wieder & Greenspan, 1993).

Experience has its own developmental progression where individuals have an active role. From the start infants initiate signals and read signals, communicating hunger, fussiness, or fatigue with the intent to get caregivers to respond. When they show preferences and pleasure they begin to shape experience, leading to their or caregiver's purposeful actions. The 10-month-old has already selected his favorite foods and toys, as well as parent or sibling, while still in his highchair. Over time the toddler plays a greater role in his experience as she develops movement and language, and moves into problem solving sequences, creates her own ideas discovering what is in the kitchen cabinet as she stacks the cans, or bangs the pots loudly, delighting in her new drum and everyone's attention. At 24 months, the toddler might drag daddy to the door and point at the swing set in the yard. At 3 or 4 years, he might ask to scooter to the park to climb the tall rock wall, now able to *communicate* what he wants and why. He feels *comfortable* in his chosen environment, has stored a feeling of self-*control* in his body, is *confident* he can take on the challenge and expects to be *competent*, no longer having to be coaxed through his fears, pleasing his parent and moreover himself with his new physical and emotional abilities. He might even imagine himself climbing Mt. Everest and reaching the top of the world after hearing his Dad once call from below naming the rock wall Mt. Everest, so proud of his daring son, advancing to symbols capturing this wonderful experience. Henceforth, the rock wall will be Mt. Everest, now an internalized image he can take with him wherever he is and representing skill and triumph. This experience encompasses the first five functional emotional developmental capacities, from self-regulation and shared attention (I), to the emotional confidence both he and his father felt taking on this goal (II), to communicating desire and intent (III), achieving the climb to the top (IV), and creating an experience of skill and triumph on the top of Mt. Everest (V). Individual differences reflected in his ability to carry out this climb with such competence increased his sense of confidence and self-esteem, as well as pleasure with his father who shared his success, further deepening their relationship. The FCDs (Foundational Capacities for Development) amplify the emotional outcomes of this experience which now belong to him and are in his implicit repertoire of who he is and what he can do (Wieder & Wachs, 2012). Not every child on the spectrum, is ready or able to initiate this elaborate sequence and may need to be pursued by our availability and presence (relationship) as we convey we are there for him and appreciate any cue he can organize. Developing a sense of self is a moving target throughout development as the child identifies his goals, engages in social problem-solving in day-to-day encounters in life, and is supported by relationships that applaud his success and also support him through challenges. Children don't choose their bodies and therapies and movement are very important and do make a difference. Every child can climb their own mountain as development is lifelong and has its own timetable.

Emotional and developmental readiness

Development is complex and so is readiness. This section will describe DIR's comprehensive intervention approach that is ideally suited for readiness for all approaches to education, and especially suited for experiential education described below, as from the start it utilizes daily life interactions and play to learn. It is a model that can be prioritized in typical and special educational systems. Every program needs to be tailored to the individual and family needs of the student and adjusted in accordance with progress and/or with transitions to new environments as schools and programs change. Evaluating progress should not wait to decide yearly promotions as teachers and parents are the first to know how well a child is really doing well before then. The primary intervention starts with parent-mediated developmental relationship-based interactions at home (floor time, semistructured problem-solving activities at home, and family guidance). Floor time is a treatment method as well as a philosophy for interaction. It is the term used for those experiences in which you follow your child's lead in areas that are of interest to him, give him pleasure, and build on them in interactive ways that expand his emotional capacities and tolerance, helping him climb the developmental ladder. The window into the child's emotional and intellectual world most easily opens when you enter into *his* orbit at *his* eye level and on *his* terms and can be carried out by parents, teachers, aides, and caregivers. The Profectum Parent Tool Box (PPT) provides a webcast floor time training program.

Educational programs can start with developmental placement (inclusion, special education) and are relationship based where teachers offer a meaningful experiential approach with comprehensive interdisciplinary services as needed (tutoring, speech and language, augmentation, occupational, physical, movement, creative arts therapies, and mental health). There is no rote learning and reinforcement comes from the interactive relationships and the child's inherent pleasure and interest. The DIR-FCD IEP Goal Bank reflects DIR theory and guides consistent and unified intervention goals that can be used in any setting. Parents participate regularly to enjoy their relationship in school where they can also get guidance and help with the family. After school programs include play dates and social activities, various sports and special interest activities, as well as nutrition, mental health, and medical following. This daunting array of interventions requires priorities guided by experienced interdisciplinary professionals who understand the child and family as well as the learning challenges. Parenting stress research has indicated that a parent's healthy response style can be cultivated with intention as the most basic and powerful tool that parents have is an engaged, joyful parent–child relationship, supported by the team's relationship with them to remain hopeful and intensive in treatment and in their relationship with their child. When parents are too stressed, confused by choices or their role, interaction can suffer and hamper progress. As noted above research and clinical practice has shown intervention that works with the family and is parent mediated reduces stress and depression (Solomon et al., 2014).

Experiential learning: the process of learning

Exposure to experience is not enough. Parents may take children to many interesting places but until the experience sparks curiosity and creates need and desire in the child, it is not yet an opportunity to learn. Experiential learning is a process of learning through "hands on experience," reflecting on the results, and applying what is learned. It needs to be used to realize its benefits, whether it is an action solving a problem, tasks of daily living, mastering a skill, responding to someone else's need, or creating an idea to share with a friend. In some cases the child may be curious and even appreciate the goal, but if he does not have the ability to execute the actions, he may appear inattentive or wander off. Even if a child is trained or reinforced to perform an action, he may not understand why and may go through prompted motions without learning or enjoyment. In education, if experience is not meaningful (out of awareness) or relevant to the child, and out of his proximal zone of development, it is unlikely to be initiated, and does not come under the child's intentional control. Some examples follow.

Ari wants to make a fruit salad for his sister's Judy's birthday celebration, healthy foods being the theme of the month in his second grade class. His teacher arranges a trip to a small supermarket nearby and they prepare for the trip. Ari, of course, picks his favorite fruits and copies the names from a fruit chart. The teacher does not correct his spelling at this point. He wants to add picture stickers to his shopping list, but they get stuck on his fingers or fall and get stuck on the floor. He gets very upset but instead of giving him more stickers, the teacher asks what else can he do if he wants a picture of the fruit. Ari looks around, sees the colored pencils he used the other day, and sighs with relief. Not as "pretty," but his own. When asked if these were his sister's favorite fruits, Ari pauses and adds strawberries to the list. Meanwhile he talks about how much fun it is to play with her but also how she can annoy him. With list in hand, he and a friend go to the supermarket with their teacher, each finds the aisle with their favorite things and check off what they found. Their parents sent in envelopes with cash so the children could pay at check out. Back at school they reflect on their trip, how they found the aisles, what was packed, and what had to be weighed or refrigerated, who else was shopping, etc. As they cut the fruit, they noticed which fruits were easy to cut or peel, or squished easily, deciding which they would prefer the next time, agreeing or disagreeing with each other. Finally, the task was done and Ari decided he would decorate cupcakes next time, or just bring a basket of strawberries, as fruit salad was too "messy". Embedded in this experience was not only Kolb's experiential learning cycle, but the focus on Ari's relationship with her sister, taking her perspective, expressing his feelings, struggling through frustration, debating with his classmate, and thinking of what he would do the next time, in this highly interactive hands-on opportunity. Kolb's cycle includes explore (what would be relevant), experience (hands on engagement), connect (prior knowledge and experiences), share (integrate different ideas), and reflect (cement into his brain) (Kolb & Kolb, 2017). The FCD's 5Cs add the emotional experience Ari is having in this process building his self-awareness of how he feels and experiences himself (comfort, able to communicate, in control, confident, competent) (Wieder & Osgood, 2020). These are anchored in the "D," the first five functional emotional developmental capacities. He is regulated and shares attention throughout. He is engaged with his teacher and also reveals a special relationship with his sister that tolerates positive and negative emotions. He communicates his preferences but also shows flexibility choosing a fruit his sister likes. Ari is also very invested solving the problem (in this case his desire) to carry out his goal (he practices skills—reading, copying, pasting—as well as finding the fruit aisle, paying, and finally cutting the fruit), forming a clear opinion about what he would do next time, actually abstracting from this experience! Experiential learning involves meaningful learning that Ari will be able to generalize and gained skills, while he also increased his sense of self and others.

Some worry about frustrating a child or get impatient, take over, or tell the child what to do. This does not help the child as much as experiencing his or her own efforts to figure something out, experimenting, or doing it in her own way. Instead work side-by-side with a child, as in the above example, encouraging the child to develop strategies to solve the problem whether successful or not, staying engaged emotionally and cognitively around failure and frustration as with success. It is emotional understanding of the interaction which opens the door to further learning and this can be conveyed in gestures when language is not forthcoming. Such two-way communication is often the child's first lesson in logic and reality.

Another example of experiential learning takes place in an 8th grade special education school. The topic is conflict between neighboring countries and having to flee. The teacher asked the students to bring in what they would take with them if they had to get ready to flee a war zone as quickly as possible. The next day, the desks were pushed to the side and the students had to find a space to set up on this first night "on the run." Could they carry everything they brought and what would they leave if necessary? Lots of negotiations followed for space, things they forgot to bring, crying siblings, insufficient food and water, crowded tents, the drop in temperature, and how to manage their anxiety. They huddled in the darkened room, asked what would happen if...what if they got separated....would they ever see their homes or relatives again...-what else should they do, and more. As they became refugees that day, the meaning of war, flight, and fear was palpable, not just a newspaper or TV report, or page in their history book, but an experience which would be ever present in their hearts and minds as they witnessed wars, saw the destruction of natural disasters, or met refugees seeking safety trying to restart their lives. Common sense, calculations, flexibility, self-regulation, communication, empathy, and fairness had to prevail to survive, as well as relativistic and reflective thinking, taking them through all the functional emotional levels of development. Although already symbolic and they could read and converse, this experience deepened their comprehension, empathy, and reflection on what it means to flee danger and the uncertainty of the future.

In contrast to the above, it is not always possible to immerse students in real-world experiences and they must be learned in the safety of the classroom or home. Virtual reality (VR) technology is increasingly becoming a tool to bring interactive opportunities to practice social and emotional skills, as well as daily living and communication skills. These programs take into account specific environmental challenges such as sensory overload, visual spatial confusion, and the communication difficulties and anxiety in socially charged situations such as being stopped by a policeman, having someone block or say something mean, knowing who to ask for help. A 2018 review found moderate evidence that VR-based treatments can help children with ASD, though it could not state that VR-based treatments can improve the results of traditional treatments, but encourage further development as they are promising and have advantages for ASD symptomatology (Mesa-Gresa, Gil-Gómez, Lozano-Quilis, & Gil-Gómez, 2018). Pilot studies continue to develop this approach for building joint attention in school settings (Ravindran, Osgood, Sazawal, Solorzano, & Turnacioglu, 2019) and have been used to promote social cognition (Kandalaft, Didehbani, & Krawczyk, 2013).

Symbolic play: the transformation of experience

Climbing the symbolic ladder to represent experience, ideas, emotions, and to distinguish reality from fantasy is crucial in education. Symbolic development begins with signs and gestures to communicate, followed by language and the ability to form mental images of objects that are not in sight. These images and words represent thoughts and emotions and can also be expressed in multiple forms such as creative arts, music, and movement. Symbolic play is the transformation of experience as it goes beyond "the real thing" and has a "hidden curriculum" where all developmental components come together. At first, pretense involves real-life experiences reflected in the functional use of objects and the different roles the child perceives in his direct experience, such as doctors, teachers, mechanics, and farmers. Dependency themes are typical when toddlers imitate feeding their baby dolls, showing affection, and other life events conveying closeness and being cared for. As they transition into the next level, now experiencing the bigger world of preschool, dramas of separation, exploration, and assertiveness such as cars crashing or invading monsters and pirates, they begin to experiment with independence and its inherent dangers and magical powers.

During play affect cues convey meanings and emotions; warm and accepting looks are associated with feelings of trust and safety, but through menacing looks and gestures the child learns about threats and danger. Imaginative play allows the child to create dramas and express ideas and feelings relying on the symbolic images they can now manipulate and control in what Winnicott calls "the space in between" fantasy and reality, their inner and outer "worlds" (Winnicott, 1971). It is how children learn to prepare for later encounters and emotions in the real world within the safety of their relationship where they can express feelings symbolically, including anger and aggression without discharge and fear of retaliation. They learn to negotiate and compromise, able to follow rules but also confident and self-assured, able to reason about cause-and-effect, differentiate fantasy and reality, see shades of gray, take on the perspective of others with empathy, and enjoy a whole range of emotional experience essential for relating to peers and success in school when higher levels of thinking are required in all subjects.

Is play always fun? Sensory, motor, and representational play escort the child into the domains of his mind which he has experienced with pleasure and curiosity as he becomes symbolic but may meet monsters and witches. Fortunately, imaginative play suspends reality and provides access to the "power" of magical thinking to fulfill wishes and defeat enemies. But what if what she imagines is scary, confusing, or invokes anger, jealousy, hatred, or aggression, anxiety may increase and will make reality testing episodic resulting in confusion if not terror. The parent or teacher can provide the support to pause, giving the child the space to think, take perspective, regulate the anxiety, and recognize the "idea" and their feelings. As students learn the underlying motives and meaning of literature, history, bias, and justice, they will be more prepared to identify with what is morally right or not and how emotions drive experience and action. If experiential in approach, abstraction and reflection will generalize. Through symbolic play and reflection children convey feelings and understanding of themselves and how others function and think as they agree and disagree, debate. take on the perspective of others (theory of mind), as they step into various dramas related to their actual lives, literature, or history and employ math, logic, or science as well as emotional thinking to solve problems. Symbolic process allows children to go beyond their own experiences to understanding the larger world, and is essential for educational progress and social communication in work and personal lives (Wieder, 2017).

Thus it is emotional understanding and perspective in interaction that opens the door to further learning. For the toddler or preverbal child this can be conveyed through affective gestures that signal patience and acceptance of the child's experience. Think of the delight in playing peek-a-boo again and again sharing the experience. For the school age child desperate to play on the basketball team but never picked, resenting his clumsiness and poor skills, belonging can come in the form of being score keeper or for another the goalie on the hockey field. Special Olympics works for others. Continuous relationships are especially important as children become more aware of their challenges and often one issue may be masking others.

While autism's processing challenges might alter the expression of feelings or ideas, it does not mean they do not exist or cannot still develop. It is important to remember development can be uneven, compelling us to persist and understand the "telegraphic" communication being sent when gaps in language, response lags, retrieval difficulties, poor comprehension, confused sequencing of thoughts and actions, disorganization, or frustration and anxiety impede coherent communication. These are barriers but emotions are a driving force even when it cannot be communicated directly. Age must be considered developmentally and strategies that work with younger children to gain practical experience can be adapted to other ages. Emotions do not depend on age and affect brings playfulness and pride into every level. The parent/teacher and child climb the symbolic ladder together and the relationship provides the impetus to keep going. Teachers offer this experience through role play, drama, writing, conversations, and debates, as well as individual floor time in class. The level of play is predicted by adult willingness to engage in the child's inner world.

Another feature of ASD is the anxiety and confusion associated with uneven development or rejection and trauma, and their potential to disrupt progress. The sources of anxiety are many, from poor comprehension or frustration communicating ideas and feelings, to the alarm of sudden sensory reactivity, compromised motor systems, or feeling lost in space. For others unpredictability or impulsivity, or the anxiety associated with social expectations at school or work may be overwhelming. At times, even developmental progress can contribute to anxiety, such as when trying to understand what is real or not. The ambiguity and conflict between the magical and the logical (i.e., poor reality testing) leaves many children with ASD overwhelmed with anxiety. They may stay invested in fantasy and learn through the symbolic lives of the characters, like Peter Pan who never wants to grow up and pleads with Wendy to return to Neverland. Or, find solutions which bind them to the familiar, such as numbers, restricted interests or the comfort of obsessive or repetitive behaviors, when next steps are not readily apparent. While bioneurological processes may underlie such responses, they are amenable to interaction and engagement when the adult joins and connects to their experience, patiently, persistently, in rhythm with the child's intent and symbolic solutions. Mindfulness training and therapeutic interventions, individual and group, can be helpful.

Educational or emotional readiness?

Both emotional and educational readiness are a function of developmental readiness and environments that are comfortable and give children some control over their learning, following their lead and interests. Understanding the executive function challenges can help set the stage for greater success, but does not replace the opportunity for the child to understand what is getting in his way and trying to figure something out, experimenting, becoming mindful, and doing it in his own way. It is very important for the parent or teacher to stay mindful of the child's experience, read her cues, and mediate different ways to solve the problem. What matters is encouraging the child to develop strategies to solve the problem, whether successful or not, and staying engaged emotionally and cognitively around failure and frustration as with success as indicated above while progressing. When a student keeps rejecting help or simply shuts down, not uncommon in adolescence, the challenge becomes the teacher's who must understand what the resistance means. Perhaps to the student "help" means, "You are wrong, you don't listen, you are learning disabled, you need to be fixed!" Sometimes, the rejection of help is followed by insisting the student tell you how he feels, creating another barrier for the student who experiences this as an invasion of his privacy and being pushed against the wall. The student and teacher collide with an intensity that cannot be overcome in that moment as the interaction has different meanings for each. Invariably, the student is sent off to the resource room or simply left behind despite all the good intentions, ending in despair. This experience might be coupled with unkind peers or bullying as they navigate the halls, the lunch rooms, and school yards when they are alone and unsupported. This student is far from readiness to learn until he is understood and has a trusting relationship to acknowledge his experience and find solutions together. It is emotional understanding of the barriers to interaction that opens the door to further learning. For the young or preverbal child this can be conveyed through affective gestures and simple words, that signal patience and acceptance of the child's experience. For the adolescent yearning to just be like other kids who resents his "special needs," standing by, listening carefully, and giving them back control over what they want, can restore their confidence and build trust. Some adolescents tell you they already have what they want, e.g., friendships, belonging, independence, often remote realities. How to respond without diminishing the student's self-esteem takes mindfulness, reflection, and a relationship to stay engaged, and matching the student's developmental level that will help reach these goals.

Changing the trajectory for the future

In conclusion, there is no one educational approach or curriculum that meets the needs of all students on the autism spectrum given the wide-ranging heterogeneity of ASD. For some intensive experiential programs are best and others are ready to be fully included. But all students are on a lifelong developmental path, have individual needs, and relationship-based interactions activate their potential for comprehension, learning, and social communication. The DIR model integrated emotions, cognition, and experience and provides a framework for establishing foundations for the future on a typical developmental trajectory and suits all educational models at all stages. It is the emotional basis of learning that keeps the pathway to progress open and relationships are the key to progress.

References

American Psychiatric Association. (2013). *Diagnostic and statistical manual of mental disorders* (5th ed.). Washington, DC: American Psychiatric Association.

Casenheiser, D., Shanker, S., & Stieben, J. (2011). Learning through interaction in children with Autism: Preliminary data from a social communication-based intervention. Autism.

Casenheiser, D., Binns, A., McGill, F., Morderer. O., & Shanker, S. (2014). Measuring and supporting language function for children with autism: Evidence from a randomized control trial of a social-interaction based therapy.

Dewey, J. (1938). *Experience and Education*. New York: Touchstone.

Dolev, S., Oppenheim, D., Koren-Karie, N., & Yirmiya, N. (2014). Early attachment and maternal insightfulness predict educational placement of children with autism. *Research in Autism Spectrum Disorders*, *8*(8), 958–967.

Donvan & Zucker. (2016). *In a different key*. New York: Penguin Random House.

Feuerstein, R., Rand, Y., & Rynders, J. E. (1988). *Don't accept me as I am*. New York: Plenum.

Green, J., Charman, T., McConachie, H., Aldred, C., Slonims, V., Howlin, O., … The PACT Consortium. (2010). *Parent mediated communication-focused treatment in children with autism (PACT): A randomized controlled trial. Lancet*. Published online May 21, 2010.

Green, J., Wai Wan, M., Guiraud, J., Holsgrove, J., et al. (2013). Intervention for infants at risk of developing autism: a case series. *Journal of Autism and Developmental Disorders*, *43*, 2502–2514.

Greenspan, S. (2001). The affect diathesis hypothesis: The role of emotions in the core deficit in autism and the development of intelligence and social skills. *Journal of Developmental Learning Disorders*, *5*, 1–45.

Greenspan, S., & Wieder, S. (1997b). Developmental patterns and outcomes in infants and children with disorders in relating and communicating: A chart review of 200 cases of children with autistic spectrum diagnoses. *Journal of Developmental Learning Disorders*, *1*, 87–141.

Greenspan, S., & Wieder, S. (1997c). *The child with special needs: Encouraging intellectual and emotional growth*. Reading, MA: Perseus Books.

Greenspan, S., & Wieder, S. (1999). A functional developmental approach to autism spectrum disorders. *JASH*, *24*, 147–161.

Greenspan, S., & Wieder, S. (2006). *Engaging autism: The floortime approach to helping children relate, communicate, and think*. Cambridge, MA: DaCapo Press/Perseus Books.

Greenspan, S., Wieder, S., Nover, R., Lieberman, A., et al. (1987). *Infants in multirisk families. Case studies in preventive intervention. National Center for Clinical Infant Programs (1987)*. New York: Clinical infant Reports, International Universities Press.

Jones, E., Dawson, G., Kelly, J., Estes, A., & Webb, S. (2017). Parent-delivered early intervention in infants at risk for ASD: Effectson electrophysiological and habituation measures of social attention. *Autism Research*, *10*(5), 961–972.

Kandalaft, M. R., Didehbani, N., Krawczyk, D. C., et al. (2013). Virtual reality social cognition training for young adults with high-functioning autism. *Journal of Autism and Developmental Disorders*, *43*, 34–44.

Kolb, A., & Kolb, D. (2017). *The experiential educator: Principles and practices of experiential learning*. Hawaii: EBLS Press.

Lord, C., & McGee, J. (Eds.), (2001). *Committee on educational interventions for children with autism. Educating children with autism. Division of Behavioral and Social Sciences and Education, National Research Council*. Washington, DC: National Academy Press.

Lovaas, O. I. (1987). Behavioral treatment and normal educational and intellectual functioning in young autistic children. *Journal of Consulting and Clinical Psychology*, *55*(1), 3–9.

Mesa-Gresa, P., Gil-Gómez, H., Lozano-Quilis, J. A., & Gil-Gómez, J. A. (2018). Effectiveness of virtual reality for children and adolescents with autism spectrum disorder: An evidence-based systematic review. *Sensors*, *18*(8), 2486. (Basel, Switzerland).

Oppenheim., & Koren-Karie. (2009). Parents' insightfulness regarding their children's internal worlds: Assessment, research, and clinical implications. In C. Zeanah (Ed.), *Handbook of infant mental health* (3rd ed., pp. 266–280). New York: Guilford.

Piaget, J. (1962). The stages of the intellectual development of the child. *Bulletin of the Menninger Clinic*, *26*(3), 120–128.

Pickles, A., LeCouteur, A., Leadbitter, K., Salomone, E., et al. (2016). Parent-mediated social communication therapy for young children with autism (PACT): long-term follow-up of a randomised controlled trial. *Lancet*, *388*.

Ratner, H. H., & Stettner, L. J. (1991). Thinking and feeling: putting Humpty Dumpty together again. *Merrill-Palmer Quarterly*, *37*(1), 1–26.

Ravindran, V., Osgood, M., Sazawal, V., Solorzano, R., & Turnacioglu, S. (2019). Virtual reality support for joint attention using the floreo joint attention module: Usability and feasibility pilot study. *JMIR Pediatrics and Parenting*, *2*(2), e14429.

Schopler, E., Mesibov, G.B., & Hearsey, K. (1995). Structured teaching in the TEACCH system. In Schopler, E., Mesibov, G.B. (Eds.), *Learning and Cognition in Autism. Current Issues in Autism*. Boston, MA: Springer.

Solomon, R., Van Egeren, L., Mahoney, G., Quon-Huber, M., & Zimmerman, P. (2014). PLAY project home consultation intervention program for young children with autism spectrum disorders: A randomized controlled trial. *Journal of Developmental & Behavioral Pediatrics*, *35*(8), 475–485.

Sandbank, M., Bottema-Beutel, K., Crowley, S., Cassidy, M., Dunham, K., Feldman, J. I., ... Woynaroski, T. G. (2020). Project AIM: Autism intervention meta-analysis for studies of young children. *Psychological Bulletin*, *146*(1), 1–29.

Torres, E. B. (2012). Atypical signatures of motor variability found in an individual with ASD. *Neurocase: Case Studies in Neuropsychology, Neuropsychiatry, and Behavioural Neurology*, *1*, 1–16.

Vygotsky, L. S. (1978). In M. Cole, et al. (Eds.), *Mind in society: The development of the higher psychological processes*. Massachusetts: Harvard University Press.

Wieder, S., & Foley, G. (2018). The developmental. Individual difference, relationship based model for assessment and intervention (the DIR model), autism spectrum disorders. In E. Hollander, R. Hagerman, & D. Fein (Eds.), *Autism spectrum disorders*. Washington, DC: Amer Psych Pub Inc.

Wieder, S., & Greenspan, S. (1993). Climbing the symbolic ladder in the DIR model through floor time/interactive play. *Journal of Autism*, *7*, 4.

Wieder, S., & Osgood, M. (2020). The role of experience and emotional developmental readiness in education. Zero to Three Conference Online Presentation.

Wieder, S., & Wachs, H. (2012). *Visual spatial portals to thinking, feeling and movement: advancing competencies and emotional development in children with learning and autism spectrum disorders*. Mendham, NJ: Profectum Foundation.

Further reading

DIR-FCD IEP Goal Bank. (2020). Profectum Foundation. Mendham, NJ.

Foley, G. M. (2006). Self and social-emotional development in infancy: A descriptive synthesis. In G. M. Foley, & J. D. Hochman (Eds.), *Mental health in early intervention: Achieving unity of principles and practice* (pp. 139–173). Baltimore, MD: Paul H. Brookes Publishing.

Green, J., Pickles, A., Pasco, G., Bedford, R., Wan, M. W., Elsabbagh, M., ... Johnson, M. (2017). Randomised trial of a parent-mediated intervention for infants at high risk for autism: Longitudinal outcomes to age 3 years. *Journal of Child Psychology and Psychiatry*, *58*, 1330–1340.

Greenspan, S., & Wieder, S. (1997a). An integrated developmental approach to interventions for young children with severe difficulties in relating and communicating. *Zero to Three*, *17*, 5–18.

Greenspan, S. I., & Wieder, S. (2011). Relationship-based early intervention approach to autistic spectrum disorders: The DIR model 1068. In D. G. Amaral, G. Dawson, & D. H. Geschwind (Eds.), *Autism spectrum disorders* (pp. 1068–1080). New York: Oxford University Press.

Wieder, S. (1993). The emotional basis of learning. In B. Spodak (Ed.), *Handbook of research in the education of young children* (pp. 77–87). New York: Macmillan Publishing Company.

Wieder, S. (2012). DIR: Developmental, individual-difference, relationship-based model: A dynamic model for the 21st century. In D. Zager, M. Wehmeyer, & R. Simpson (Eds.),

Research-based principles and practices for educating students with autism (pp. 82–98). New York: Routledge/Taylor & Francis.

Wieder, S. (2013). DIR: Developmental, individual-difference, relationship-based model. In F.R. Volkmar (Ed.), S. Rogers (Section Ed.), *Encyclopedia of autism spectrum disorders*. New York: Springer.

Wieder, S. (2017). The power of symbolic play in emotional development through the DIR lens. *Topics in Language Development, 37*, 259–281.

"Aggression" in young children on the autistic spectrum: the dysregulation–"aggression" hypothesis

9

Gilbert M. Foley[1,2] *and Tal Baz*[3]

[1]NYC Early Childhood Mental Health Training and Technical Assistance Center (TTAC), New York Center for Child Development, New York, NY, United States, [2]Profectum Academy, Profectum Foundation, Mendham, NJ, United States, [3]In-Tune Integrated Developmental Therapies, Somerville, MA, United States

The dysregulation–"aggression" hypothesis: an introduction

Infancy, toddlerhood, and early childhood are periods of rapid growth, transition, and transformation. It is expected that under such dynamic conditions, sensory, emotional, and behavioral lability would be the rule rather than the exception. Patterns and expressions of dysregulation also change over this developmental trajectory. In infancy, dysregulated states are usually associated with distress behaviors, including discomfort crying and other frenzied signaling (with an underlying "intent" to bring a caregiver into proximity), hyperarousal, and difficulty calming. Typically, toddlers are apt to exhibit tantrum-like behavior, which is manifest by breaks in emotional control expressed physically in aggression, anger, body flailing and thrashing, or in oppositional and withholding behaviors. In the preschool years, dysregulation may be expressed by verbal combativeness, overtly directed physical aggression, and noncompliance or withdrawal. It is expected under conditions of stress that children may return to "younger" patterns of regulation and are likely to need support from parents in response to their manifest behavior and needs.

Aggression weaves itself as an expression of dysregulation throughout the early years and reflects a limitation in regulating arousal levels under stress. When examining the expression of "aggression" in young children on the autistic spectrum, especially, the questions as to when aggressive behavior is truly an aggressive act or when it is secondary to dysregulation from other sources and systems, become salient. The hypothetical answers may give clues to prevention, intervention, and practical guidance to parents and other professionals.

In traditional definitions of human aggression, immediate intent to do harm and a belief on the part of the perpetrator, that his/her actions will indeed inflict harm,

Emerging Programs for Autism Spectrum Disorder. DOI: https://doi.org/10.1016/B978-0-323-85031-5.00031-1

are operative constructs. Hostile aggression is formulated as being driven by impulsive, thoughtless anger in response to a provocation but still with the ultimate aim of harming the target (Baron & Richardson, 1994; Berkowitz, 1993; Bushman & Anderson, 2001).

In this paper, the authors are proposing and will argue that in young children on the spectrum, "aggression" is often misattributed and better explained as arising from dysregulation in multiple systems and is more often than not a secondary or overlay behavior that in many cases is without the intent to inflict harm, so central to the standard definitions. Thus the dysregulation—"aggression" hypothesis.

More specifically, the authors are proposing three assumptions to frame this discussion: (1) aggressive behavior is a communicative act; (2) "aggressive" behavior can arise out of faulty appraisal of self/other states and situations predicated on misinformation from compromised neurosensory processing, including movement, neuroception, regulation of arousal, and the perception of affect; and (3) that the contributory components are intertwined in such a way as to make the experience of aggression complex, perplexing, and hard to tease apart, thus the approach to analysis and clinical reasoning needs to be comprehensive and dynamic in nature.

Hidden triggers—latent meanings

The idea then, that "aggression" in young children on the spectrum may be sparked by hidden triggers and bear latent meanings will be explored in this paper. In brief, the hidden triggers to which the authors refer are largely related to sensory-movement, neuroception, regulation of arousal, anxiety, and other affective states, that are often imperceptible to the untrained eye. For example, a child on the spectrum, with hypersensitive tactile reactivity as a specific type of sensory challenge among the expected sensory differences associated with autism spectrum disorder (ASD), may experience an accidental brushing by a peer as danger and threat and respond by lashing out. The hidden trigger in this case is the tactile defensiveness, giving rise to a magnified subjective tactile experience, a misinterpretation of the meaning of event (i.e., aggressive/attack) and a subsequent response predicated on the faulty perception and appraisal. A child playing dodge ball who throws the ball too hard and randomly, may have an underreactive proprioceptive system and receives less than accurate feedback as to the force of his thrust and may not possess the age expected postural control and ability to modulate the velocity of his heaves. Visual—spatial differences may further contribute to what appears to be throwing randomly and "aggressively." Consider the child with compromised pragmatic language skills who doesn't know how to enter a desired play group with verbal felicity and resorts to running and barging-in. If combined with some of the same proprioceptive and visual—spatial challenges discussed above, the barging-in may be very disruptive to peer play, may destroy block constructions or other play products, and possibly hurt other children.

The notion of latent meanings is multifold. That is, the risk for misinterpretations of meaning by the child himself of experiences and intents of parents and peers, as well as misattributions of meaning and intent by caregivers and peers to the behavior of the child are greater for children with ASD than typical children. If these behaviors are not understood more deeply, they will likely be interpreted as intentional acts of disruption and "aggression." Overtime, if the behaviors persist relatively unmodified, the child is likely to be perceived as a "behavior problem" unable to adjust to the routines and prosocial climate of the classroom and at best, be referred for a deeper look or at worst, expelled.

The child himself is at risk of forming latent meanings with regard to himself as rejected, unlovable, incompetent, and defective in some way. Thus these hidden misfortunes, if uninvestigated and untreated, can set in motion a cycle of cumulative adversity resulting in outcomes far greater and more complex than the original difficulties in themselves!

That cycle of cumulative adversity can spiral further to impact the parent–child relationship and resonate across the family system in negative ways. Parents look to the young child's postural, facial, vocal, and behavioral signals to guide their parental ministrations. If those signals are relatively clear and readable and parental responses are successful in engaging and regulating their child, a positive bidirectional feedback loop is formed which promotes mutually satisfying and meaningful patterns of interaction, physical caregiving, and attachment. If those signals are ambiguous or confusing to read and are "out-of-synch," as they can often be with children on the spectrum with specific sensory disorders, patterns of interaction can become strained and dyssynchronous. Singletary (2015) suggests that the child with ASD may experience traumatic anxiety secondary to the inability to use the mother as a source of homeostatic regulation and feel an acute absence of the mother, heightening feelings of isolation and fear.

Further, the child's distorted experience of the sensory world and greater risk for dysregulation and patterns of problem behavior, can leave parents feeling bewildered, frustrated, and helpless in how to successfully parent their child. Conflicts between parents about how to respond and manage the behaviors may arise, creating tension and charged dynamics across the family system precipitating shifts in alliances and faults in the family structure.

Theories of aggression: an overview

Conceptualizations with regard to the origins, functions, and vicissitudes of aggression in human development and behavior provide both a framework for understanding and a source of guidance to its management. S. Freud's (1920/1955) formulations about aggression evolved over a period from 1911 to 1926 during which he reconceptualized aggression from being a derivative of libido to a motivational force equivalent to sexuality in its own right. Posited to be innate and directed at both the external environment and the self, it is a destructive impulse in counterpoint to libido and sometimes analogized to the physiological processes of catabolism and metabolism. Aggression is apt to become absolutely destructive when unmoored or unneutralized by libido. When in the service of the life force, such as in the mastication of food, for example, aggression is instrumental in motivating behavior toward meeting basic needs and is instrumental in taking initiative, being independent, and mastering the environment.

A. Freud (1965) elaborated the developmental infrastructure of ego formation—that agent of personality responsible for reconciling and balancing the drive to gratification with a capacity for drive inhibition—in support of adaptive conformity to the constraints and conditions imposed by the child's environment. In the process of ego formation, aggression serves development, for example, by motivating and empowering the child to leave-the-nest and explore the larger world, an essential ingredient to learning and the formation of a reality orientation. Building on those initial forays into the world, the toddler's drive to environmental mastery and autonomy is in part a derivative of aggression or assertion. A. Freud (1965, p. 180) concluded, "The aggressive strivings, if fused in the normal way with the libidinal ones, are socializing influences rather than the opposite. They provide the initial strength and tenacity with which the infant reaches out for the object world and holds on to it."

Klein (1952) focused almost exclusively on the unfolding of the innate aggressive drive and the adaptative "positions" toward objects the archaic psychic system assumes to protect itself from annihilation by aggression. She suggested that a vital developmental task of the young child is to come-to-terms with the aggressive drive and the anxiety it inflicts by posing an irrational and omnipotent threat to destroy the child and those she/he loves. A growing capacity to perceive and relate to the whole love object and an ability to engage in acts of reparation when aggressive ruptures or fantasies of aggressive annihilation threaten, the child learns that his aggression is neither omnipotent nor unmanageable, and will not permanently destroy himself and those he loves.

Lorenz (1966) within an ethological and evolutionary framework suggested that aggression is a species preserving instinct. From an evolutionary perspective, the capacity to protect oneself and offspring from predators and other threats from environment and forces of nature, was central to survival. Those with the power to fend-off-threats and assert a will-to-survival were more likely to endure and thus the aggressive traits that were adaptive were passed on in the gene pool.

Social learning theory (Bandura, 1965) ascribes aggression to modeling from experiences of observed aggressive behavior of a live model, a symbolic model as in video or books or an instructional model as in a description or explanation. Learning is contingent on attention, encoding, replication, and motivation both social and intrinsic. Cognitive and learning processes are thought to be operative in mediating social behavior.

The frustration–aggression hypothesis (Dollard et al., 1939) suggests that when a goal response is thwarted, stereotyped and aggressive behaviors are likely to ensue. For example, if one's aim is to open the top drawer of a dresser to retrieve a desired article of clothing and the drawer sticks, after numerous failed attempts, frustration mounts and problem solving diminishes into fixed or stereotyped action patterns such as more forcefully pulling at the drawer with escalating aggressive force until it is broken in rage. This construct may have particular salience for children on the spectrum who by virtue of their disorder tend to already be prone to repetitive and stereotyped behaviors and are apt to face recurring frustration when they are unable to translate intentions into successful and satisfying executions.

General Aggression Model (Anderson & Bushman, 2002) is a more complex and multifactorial conceptualization that acknowledges a cascade process. It considers how personal and situational factors influence cognition, feelings, and arousal, which in turn affect appraisal and decision-making that influence aggressive or non-aggressive behavior. Broadly, it is most in line with the hypotheses and clinical reasoning presented here

A closer examination of hidden triggers in young children on the autistic spectrum

The hypothesis that dysregulation in multiple systems may be a decisive source of "aggressive" behavior in young children on the spectrum is not a big leap, given what is known about sensory processing differences and the incidence of dysregulated states in young children on the spectrum. Thus the dysregulation–"aggression" hypothesis.

Children with ASD have greater difficulty with regulation of sensation, affect, and behavior (Foley, 2020). Atypical responsivity to sensory inputs in the form of over- or underreactivity is among the criteria for ASD in DC: 0–5 (Zero to Three, 2016). These challenges can interfere with the moment-to-moment lives of these children, and have been shown to be associated with higher levels of family impairment and parental stress (Ben-Sasson et al., 2013). It is also hypothesized that some of the symptoms of ASD itself may be related to, if not actually secondary, to sensory processing disorder. Significant relationships have been found between sensory processing disorder in children with ASD and restricted and repetitive behaviors (Gabriels et al., 2008). Likewise, severity of atypical patterns of sensory responsiveness in children with ASD has been found to predict to greater social impairment (Hilton et al., 2010). Atypical sensory processing is likely to set off a cascade effect that impairs the temporal processing of social information, in turn, contributing to altered patterns of speech perception (Stevenson et al., 2017). Among the symptoms with which sensory differences may be implicated are an increased risk for difficulties in regulation of sensation, affect, and behavior (Williamson & Anzalone, 2001). (Samson et al., 2014) found that children and adolescents with ASD had significantly more symptoms of emotion dysregulation than typical comparisons including greater evidence of sensory abnormalities. A meta-analysis of 14 studies found a significantly high difference in the presence of sensory modulation disorders in children with ASD compared with typical comparisons (Ben-Sasson et al., 2009). In fact, atypical patterns of sensory processing are among the most pervasive of symptoms of the disorder, impacting up to 87% of individuals with ASD (Lord, 1995). A recent review of the research in the field supports the claim that sensory symptoms play a primary role in the neurobiology of autism and the characteristics that define it. Further, these sensory deficits predict to higher-order weaknesses in cognitive and social capacities and explain a significant part of the variance in social and communication symptoms measured in diagnostic assessments (Robertson & Baron-Cohen, 2017).

Sensing movement

Movement is a powerful medium through which humans' express intentions and volitional acts of will. Further, the body is a mirror of emotional states manifest in nuances of posture, both static positioning, and dynamic configurations. Action and gestures, in a shared social space and as part of an interactive exchange, are among the ways humans communicate vigor and vivacity or the "forms of vitality" (Stern, 2010).

> *Movement is also informed and shaped by a sense of self in relationship to others from the beginning of life in the form of an interdependent, interactive dance. This dance influences the temporal dimensions of the interaction and the partners' interpretation of content. The content of the interaction influences the substance and outcome of the interaction, while the temporal impacts the timing and sequencing of the interaction. It is out of precise timing and rhythms of two motor systems interacting in concert with one another that inter-subjective narratives between infant and caregiver are spawned and "communicative musicality" are generated.*
>
> *Delafield-Butt & Trevarthen (2018, p. 124)*

While movement was previously thought to be the expression of a one-way command from the brain, it is a more complex process involving the dynamic interplay of, and bidirectional communication between, the peripheral and central nervous systems. Further, it is now known that through the process of reafference, which is a movement-dependent signal present when movement is self-initiated, humans differentiate between external stimuli and their own responses to them, perceive the trajectory of their own movement, and orient in space. In turn, sensation produced by movement, particularly in the form of proprioceptive and kinesthetic feedback, is important not only to building but also to continuously monitoring and updating internal sensory and motor maps and models for action control. Thus movement is intimately wedded to sensory feedback in a continuous, dynamic, and bidirectional way (Amos, 2018).

Research suggests that this important sensory feedback loop may be impeded in ASD, possibly by hypotonia, which may hinder the transmission of sensory signals from central structures. A disruption in this sensory feedback system, especially kinesthetic, essential to continuous movement production and control, suggests that the brain is being presented with partial, confusing, selective, and intermittent information. Thus movement and perception are not being integrated in typical ways and are likely to evolve differently with the response output taking the form of novel coping strategies, some of which may be characterized as "autistic behaviors" (Amos, 2018).

In autism, there is evidence of a lack of balance between deliberate motions (signal) and automatic ones (noise).

> *When systems that track the balance between signal and noise are not working reliably, the person may be unable to correctly estimate the path and timing of a stimulus and regulate an efficient and effective response.... Inaccurate estimates of a stimulus that are relayed to the body's motor system can produce challenges to self-synchrony (self-coordination), movements that undershoot or overshoot their target, as well as interruptions in the coordination of movement involved in typical social interactions.... Difficulties in establishing or maintaining self-synchrony inevitably play out as challenges to interactional synchrony (coordination with others).*
>
> *Amos (2018, p. 298)*

Thus, further confounding the sensory-social matrix and "the interdependent and interactive dance."

The cumulative upshot of these sensing movement challenges in ASD are anxiety and distress triggered directly by a compromised capacity to efficiently enact desired intentions through actions of the body and the lack of a robust and efficient motor memory, so that even routine movements that would typically be subsumed as a part of the implicit and automatic motor memory system must be tackled as if novel. Indirectly, anxiety, distress, and frustration are associated with constrictions in the social dance so dependent on movement, timing, sequencing, and self-other-synchrony (Delafield-Butt & Trevarthen, 2018; Torres, 2018).

Experiencing safety vs fight, flight, freeze

The way in which both sensory and motor processing transpires within the central nervous system is thought to reflect autonomic nervous system (ANS) involvement (Lane, 2002). Through decades of research, (Porges, 2009, 2017) illuminated the intricacies of the ANS and expanded our understanding of both its structure and its function. Traditionally the ANS was considered to be comprised of two subsystems: parasympathetic and sympathetic, which were considered to have an antagonistic influence. The (traditional) sympathetic system responds to stress by shifting it towards a defensive position, that is, fight/flight/freeze. The (traditional) parasympathetic system supports health, growth, and restoration, and is responsible for stabilization of autonomic processes which, among other things, protects the heart and enhances oxygenation to the brain. Their primary neural pathways are vagal—stemming from the 10th cranial nerve.

However, according to (Porges, 2009, 2017), the vagus, which connects brainstem areas with structures throughout the body, including the heart, lungs, neck, thorax, and abdomen, has, in mammals, two separate branches: dorsal vagus (old) with pathways that are unmyelinated and reach organs located below the diaphragm, and ventral vagus (new) with pathways that are myelinated and reach organs located above the diaphragm. This branch of the vagus collaborates with four other cranial nerves (V, VII, IX, XI) to construct the social engagement system.

This newer understanding of the ANS emphasizes a phylogenetic ordered hierarchy of subsystems which react to challenges in a *reverse* evolutionary order. The old dorsal vagus reacts to stress by reducing blood flow to brain and muscles, withdrawing, dissociating, and shutting down—freeze. The sympathetic track reacts to stress by increasing blood flow to muscles to mobilize movement/action—fight or flight. The new ventral vagus affords an innovative evolutionary and more adaptive "defense" to stress by activating the social-engagement circuitry, a key feature of which is the act of looking and listening.

> *Since the process of looking at a person constitutes both an act of engagement and projects the bodily state of the observer, the person being "looked at" will feel that the "looker" is welcoming or disinterested.*
>
> *Porges, (2017, p. 48)*

Subtle cues communicate a great deal, conveying messages of understanding, shared feelings, and of the security of safety, when the sender is in the prerequisite calm physiological state. The way one looks at another in synchrony with the prosody of vocalization, not unlike music, composes the melody expressing information about the feeling and physiological state of the speaker.

When the new ventral vagus works well, it mobilizes the social engagement system. It accomplishes this by calming the viscera and inhibiting mobilization, enhancing regulation of striated muscles in face and head, increasing prosody, improved listening, expanding emotional expressivity, and supporting quick/efficient changes in metabolic inputs/outputs from the heart in response to external/internal stresses.

When the new ventral vagus doesn't work well, individuals are less available for symbiotic/reciprocal cueing and social interaction. In these situations, the first line of defense is the sympathetic system. However, sympathetic activation is most efficient when used in short bursts of mobilization which are functionally adaptive in response to real danger, and are correlated with production of adrenaline. When sympathetic activation is called for frequently, for longer periods of time, in an erratic fashion, or when there is an inability to escape or physically defend, the hypothalamic–pituitary–adrenal (HPA) circuitry kicks in and floods the system with cortisol. This state then tilts the system towards the last line of defense which is expressed through immobilization and dissociation—freeze/shutdown. This defense mechanism, as in feigning death, may discourage a predator, but in the face of a host of other threats, can in itself prove life threatening.

Thus "... our nervous system has more than one defense strategy and ... the decision of whether we use a mobilized fight/flight or an immobilization shutdown defense strategy is not a voluntary decision" (Porges, 2017, p. 55). Instead, the decision is made through a prereflective, nonverbal, process of neuroception. Through neuroception, the nervous system detects stress and evaluates risk: safety/danger/life threat. This is a task fundamental and crucial to survival. The safety/threat evaluation process is mediated through cues from the environment, especially auditory. If danger is detected, physiological state automatically shifts to optimize survival. When all is well, this process is out of awareness. When a shift occurs, individuals tend to become aware.

When neuroception functions accurately, it affords a match between the level of threat and the autonomic response. Nevertheless, as was noted above, the capacity to distinguish between safety, danger, and life threat is based on cues, especially auditory and visual cues, so for some individuals, such as those with ASD, this becomes a challenging task, often resulting in mismatch after mismatch throughout their days. Thus in an interaction between two individuals, the same facial configurations of one person engaging another, may trigger a range of outcomes, depending on the physiological state of the target individual. If there is a relative state match between the two individuals, one in which the social engagement system is easily accessible, a reciprocal prosocial interaction is more likely to occur. However, if the target in the communication is in a state of mobilization of fight/flight/freeze, there is a greater risk of an asocial interaction of withdrawal or aggression. This mismatch is apt to be magnified because the mobilized state leads to decreased muscle tone in the face and head, difficulties with gaze, facial expressions, hearing the human voice and speech prosody all of which further confound interactive signaling and cue reading in support of prosocial interaction. In such a dysregulated state, the mobilization circuitry of withdrawal or aggression may be difficult to regulate so as to enable the social engagement system to come back on track (Porges, 2009). The reduced social engagement capacity combined with the dissonance in threat appraisal constitute a breeding ground for anxiety. Enabling the social engagement system and managing the anxiety become key components of regulating "aggression" and important aims of intervention.

The complexity and perplexity of the autistic spectrum

When these factors are taken together, children on the spectrum are significantly more vulnerable to states of dysregulation, which the authors hypothesize, increases the risk for aggressive-like or actual aggressive behavior. Thus the dysregulation–"aggression" hypothesis. For example, consider the following scenario: during circle-time, a child with ASD sits among neurotypical children as the teachers lead the group in morning meeting. One of the teachers, sitting close by the child with ASD, suddenly sneezes. The child with ASD abruptly jumps onto her lap, surveying her face with hypervigilance—sensing danger, most likely by the surprise of the sound. Just a few milliseconds after that, another child, sitting next to him, turns her head to the teacher and politely asks if a tissue is needed. Suspending this moment in time, you would appraise the visual exchange between the teacher and the child asking about the tissue, as one that expresses adaptive pragmatic communication. The child with ASD, on the other hand, is still fixating his gaze on the teacher—his visual system not able to flexibly shift between peripheral and central functioning, his auditory system not primed to process the human voice accurately, and his autonomic system not able to shift out of the danger zone. In this state, he is not capable of swiftly adjusting and assimilating the flow of information unfolding around him, and is thus not perceiving the communicative act of the other child as being initiated and directed toward the teacher rather than toward him. Based on his high-alert state, and the auditory surprise, he shifts his body towards the other child (the source of danger) and shoves her in a way that looks significantly excessive. In reality, the forceful shove is an expression of an overshooting motor system rather than an intentional act of aggression. This cascade of mismatches would, usually, evoke the typical request from adults to "use words," and to "say sorry"—both of which are behaviors only possible to access if the child were functioning with an available social engagement system. The well-intended request to "use words" and "say sorry" are apt to trigger even greater stress and anxiety, possibly precipitating another sympathetic behavior, or, even worse, collapse into the shutdown/dissociation zone.

If, instead, this scenario was reframed, applying the dysregulation–"aggression" hypothesis, and an intervention of coregulation to address the stress/anxiety and to inhibit the mobilization system and enable a return of the social-engagement system, then perceiving oneself in relation to the other would become truly possible. The ultimate therapeutic goal then is redefined as an attempt to increase arousal regulation in the face of stress.

An intervention paradigm in a regulation framework

Regulation of arousal is rooted in the concept of physiological homeostasis (Cannon, 1932) or the self-correcting tendency of the body to maintain a relative constancy or biological equilibrium among a range of functions, even in the face of changing external and internal forces. It is thought to be among the oldest capacities of the human being. Arousal regulation exerts a critical force on levels of alertness, attention, awareness, and consciousness. It influences all developmental domains, all learning and relationship capacities. The concept of homeostasis has been extended by analogy to other systems and functions including the capacity for self-regulation, which for this chapter, is defined as the child's developing capacity to flexibly modulate and grade reactivity to sensation, affect arousal and behavior, appropriate to the demands of the physical and social environment and to recover from dysregulated states. all with relative autonomy, in support of goal-directed actions across a broad range of functions (Carver & Scheier, 2016; Foley, 2017; Murray et al., 2015).

Six main areas of regulation are identified in the literature (Lillas & Turnbull, 2009): (1) a capacity for deep sleep cycling; (2) a capacity for alert processing;

(3) a capacity for connection to visceral cues; (4) a capacity for clarity of states and smooth transitions between states; (5) a capacity for adaptive stress responses; and (6) a capacity for efficient stress recovery. The functioning of each of these capacities is intertwined with all the others, and as a whole, they contribute to adaptive behavior across development.

Babies, however, are not born with mature regulatory capacities fully formed. Instead, they are delicately nurtured in a dynamic relational course—first through external-regulation, then through coregulation, out of which robust self-regulation skills develop, inclusive of the ability to access self-regulatory capacity in times of stress.

External regulation begins in utero and continues to be the main vehicle for regulation throughout the first few months of life when the physical proximity and body of the caregiver affords an emotional climate of safety and serves to organize neurobiological functions. Out of this intimate relationship, an "internal working model" is formed for the lifelong possibility that one person can serve an "external regulatory" function to the physiological systems of another.

Around 2–3 months of age, coregulation comes into the foreground. This style of regulation takes the form of repeated patterns of behavior that assume an almost automatic quality and hold the potential to shape neural pathways. These interactions have common qualities, such as repetitive-rhythmic rounds in multimodal exchanges using gaze, touch, affect cues, body postures, physical handling and caregiving, and markers of arousal and physiological states (Feldman, 2007).

Coregulation unfortunately is where the breakdown often occurs for many children with sensory, motor, and arousal vulnerabilities. This is also the reason for the strong emphasis on providing carefully tailored and attuned coregulation experiences for any child who functions with a vulnerable nervous system, as do children with ASD.

Because sensory and motor processing is so integral to these regulatory capacities, children on the spectrum are especially vulnerable to regulatory irregularities. This predisposes them to behavioral difficulties including those that appear to be aggressive or in fact may be aggressive, in that they have sufficient intent. The regulatory and arousal/state difficulties that contribute to breaks-in-control include (1) faulty appraisal of the safety/threat status of the environment; (2) corresponding mismatched states of mobilization of flight/flight/freeze between the child, environment, and other, as described in neuroception; (3) poor recovery from dysregulated states contributing to prolonged and sometimes escalating states of hyperarousal; (4) ambiguous, muted, or poorly differentiated states of arousal often complicated by organization weaknesses and/or abrupt changes in state, making reading of intent and motivation confusing. This cluster of possible complications requires these children to be afforded more specialized interactive regulatory opportunities.

Within the regulation framework, an intervention paradigm derived from the dysregulation– "aggression" hypothesis and based on clinical trials, focuses on the following: (1) regulation of arousal, sensory and movement capacities; (2) the enabling of the social engagement system; and (3) the management of anxiety, implemented in a relational context. The model of the development of regulatory capacity discussed above, progressing from external-regulation to coregulation to self-regulation, guides the specifics of intervention. This progression is neither linear nor lockstep, either in typical development or in intervention. Furthermore, a therapeutic process which aims to address aggression (or the possibility of it developing) needs to be designed in such a way that it constantly and continuously takes into account the hidden triggers (the intricacies of sensory and motor processing as well as the ongoing neuroceptive surveillance), and the latent meanings (the experience of misappraisal of threat vs safety). These constructs need to be in the foreground of the therapeutic process, not only during moments of aggressive-like behaviors, but also in-between these moments as part of an ongoing stream of interventions which aim to create a clinical climate of safety. Building a climate of safety means taking into account the basic experiences of the nervous system that are associated—prereflectively—with safety. This starts with the therapist assuming a stance of sustained physiological calm, a soothing bodily posture and well managed anxiety, which is easier said than done in a high arousal situation, and where the role of reflective supervision can prove helpful. Slowing down, "avoiding undue haste" and reducing the overall level of stimulation, including levels of light, sound, and motion are critical ingredients in external regulation. In addition to that, rhythm and repetition of theme with subtle variation are extremely powerful tools for calming and reassuring, as they are virtually imprinted in the human nervous system from the rhythm and repetition of mothers' heartbeat and respiration in utero. Nevertheless, the reduction in pace and intensity of the sensorimotor aspects of any given communicative act should not be confused and/or correlated with the flattening of the affect. On the contrary, the essential affect (whether it be happiness, excitement, sadness, or anger) in its crystalized form should be preserved, held, and processed for/with the child. In order for that to happen, the essential affect needs to be processed and communicated in a way that the child can perceive it, experience it, tolerate it, and share it. In order for that to happen, the therapist needs to adjust and align to the child's individual sensory profile.

This is what is referred to as attunement. Attunement and mirroring are at the core of coregulation. They are important constructs borrowed from the infant mental health and psychotherapy literature and practice repertoire that have important implications across disciplines. These constructs are to some extent two sides of the same coin. Attunement is a process by which parents and therapists register, adjust and align their feeling state to that of the child—a feeling with, a shared and particular knowing. Mirroring is the means by which attunement is communicated often by changing the modality from observed action to heard sound, sometimes with words but not infrequently (especially when the affect is negative) with brief rather than continuous expressions of intoned and soothing melodic vocalizations combined with gestures and postural adjustments that convey the affective essence. The aim of this process is not merger or enmeshment with the child, but rather that of two separate beings finding a common note and being known. This acknowledgment and alignment of feeling states communicates to the child an expression of being uniquely understood and pierces the well of isolation. Attunement and mirroring are often the "ports of entry" to establishing the prerequisite state of shared safety and transitioning from the mobilization mode to the engagement mode. The state of safety and engagement promotes trust and deepens the relationship, allowing the child to more fully "use" the other to help regulate and "climb the developmental ladder" to higher order modalities of self-regulation such as symbols, language, and executive functions. As noted, the crafting of carefully tailored and attuned coregulatory experiences for children on the spectrum with "aggressive" behavior is a core component of the intervention model. This involves affording the child incremental opportunities to develop, through experience and practice, in relationship, the rudiments of self-regulation. Given that recovery from dysregulated states is a key element of self-regulation, children must be afforded opportunities to be dysregulated so that they can practice regaining the regulated states with decreasing amounts of coregulation.

In the process of coregulation, interactive mismatches between therapist and child are inevitable. Even in typical development, interactional mismatches are more the norm than the exception, but it is in the capacity to repair that the essence of intimate relationships is to be found. Because of the challenges described above, children on the spectrum are more stretched in learning to repair mismatches. Every child must stay sufficiently regulated in the breech to enable a repair and this is a vulnerable gap for children on the spectrum. In addition, the child must learn to tolerate the loss of attention and gratification, important antecedents in early coping. In typical development, the dyad learns to coregulate and self-correct, cocreating the bridge to repair and reunion. In the therapeutic context, attention must be payed to timing, often waiting and watching and allowing for more time than might feel comfortable to enact a repair, thus the need to manage one's own anxiety. Important features of the intervention include: heightening cues, using gestures and supporting the child's regulation and arousal in the mismatch gap to enable the engagement system to stay "in gear."

In the therapeutic moment of aggressive-like behavior, the therapist uses the dynamics of proximity and distance to provide a safe "holding environment" for the child. This requires careful monitoring of the child's affect, posture, movement, and state of mobilization (flight/fight/freeze) cues in order to intuit how close is close enough so as to nurture feelings of safety and security without inducing intrusion panic. The signaling of shared feelings, intent, and physiological state can be communicated through covarying intonation and prosody of vocal attunement and the intensity of the mutual gaze. The regulation of states of high arousal is optimized when the intensity of affect is synchronized between therapist and child within lags of split seconds and the intensity of mutual gaze is titrated and attuned to the child's sensory system, tolerance, and level of arousal.

Eye gaze is a compelling, almost magnetic form of connectedness that focuses, organizes, and sustains us. Erikson (1982, p. 40) suggests the "developing eye-to-eye relationship is a "dialogue" as essential for psychic development and, indeed, survival of the whole human being as is the mouth-to-breast one for its sustenance.... The playful, and yet planful, dialogue that negotiates the first interpersonal encounters, the lights of the eyes, the features of the face and the sound of the name, become essential ingredients of a first recognition of, and by, the primal other. . .. Where such contact is established, the human being will thereafter always look for somebody to look up to and all through life will feel confirmed by "uplifting" encounters." The therapeutic aim is to create "uplifting encounters" of which eye gaze is a compelling ingredient and a potent force for breaking fixed action patterns such as aggressive-like behavior and shifting the focus of attention to intense engagement rather than diffuse flailing and enactment. However, with children on the spectrum, eye gaze must be used judiciously and gently as in a rhythmic dance with encounters, partings, and reunions as in a pas de deux or it can be misappraised as a form of aggression in and of itself. Knowing that children on the spectrum tend to visually focus on the periphery when looking at the face, eye gaze must sometimes begin at that point of contact, from the periphery, rather than frontally (Klin et al., 2003). In fact, the child may actually be making eye contact in a position that appears to be one of gaze aversion.

Differentiating self-other boundaries and sensory-affective states are features of intervention that aim to demarcate, distinguish, and consolidate behaviors and feelings. In states of high arousal and mobilization of fight or flight, feelings, behaviors and targets of "aggression" are apt to become undifferentiated, diffuse, and indiscriminate. There is a tendency to "sympathetic" escalation, that if not bounded and quietened can precipitate psychic as well as behavioral chaos. With children on the spectrum, body boundary formation may be compromised in part by tactile sensitivities, poor self-coordination, and compromised motor planning and accuracy, which render these children less discriminating when in the throw of strong feelings. The target of "aggression," for example, may be perceived at the level of part-object rather than as a whole person, so the child may only distinguish striking an arm or kicking a leg or throwing indiscriminately at a vague form, possibly compounded by visual–spatial difficulties. Feeling states may become difficult for the child, as well as adults, to discriminate, such as the blurring of excitation and aggression. When the child is engaged in a "sympathetic" act the aim is to differentiate and address both the underling affect that may be at play as well as the seemingly "aggressive" act itself.

Demarcating boundaries by using your body; containing the child playfully with equipment or corralling or physically holding, if that can be tolerated; using vocal cues-"ah-aH-AH"; creating visual markers to define spatial areas are differentiating techniques that may be helpful. Tactile and "heavy work" activities can heighten body boundary awareness. Distinguishing children from one another by saying and gesturing, maybe touching, if it can be tolerated, "John, Martha; Martha, John," and mirror feedback may give added visual information in support self-other differentiation.

As children progress toward the capacity for self-regulation, which begins with the ability to mobilize acts upon request (Do) and inhibit actions upon demand (Don't) (Kopp, 1982), and as they move up the developmental ladder toward greater capacities to symbolize, play imaginatively and use language, strategies drawn from psychodynamic play therapy are integrated into the intervention repertoire. The aim is to support the child's developing capacity to flexibly modulate and grade reactivity to sensation, affect arousal and behavior appropriate to the demands of the physical and social environment, and to recover from dysregulated states, all with relative autonomy, in support of goal-directed actions across a broad range of functions (Carver & Scheier, 2016; Foley, 2017; Murray et al., 2015).

Reviewing the array of concepts and techniques from psychodynamic play therapy that may be applicable is beyond the scope of this chapter, but several that have been found to be clinically useful will be addressed. Essential and basic is a strong working alliance built on sensitive, responsive, reliable and benevolent emotional availability. First, the capacity to play symbolically is in itself not only thought to be self-curative but also supportive of the development of self-regulation. Play can be thought of as an "in-between stage, falling between enactment and putting into words as a precondition for controlling thoughts" (Sandler et al., 1980, p. 121). Symbols themselves, whether they be in the form of objects that stand for something else and hold emotional meaning, gestures, images, or words all serve to mediate between a felt need and a behavior. The adult, for example, in a traffic jam who uses running self-talk about what he/she feels and might want to do, but does not, binds the rage impulses in fantasy and words rather than enacting them in behavior. So, symbolic processes, serve as a kind of shock absorber or buffer by containing unruly impulses such as aggression. Likewise, the angry child who throws the doll instead of pushing a child, binds the aggression in a play object that may stand for the actual human object of his anger.

This phenomenon is related to displacement, in which impulses are discharged by shifting them from one object to another. Although considered a defense mechanism, displacement can be used as a conscious strategy to help children learn to shift their impulse discharge from an inappropriate object to a more appropriate one—"You can't bite John but you can bite the pillow."

For this strategy to work, however, a child must be able to comprehend and process the language, stay relatively regulated, inhibit, shift attention, and so forth—all self-regulatory capacities. With a child in high arousal, this is not likely to happen so automatically, even if the child possesses these skills in the regulated state. This strategy must be considered in the context of the sensory-affective-regulatory strategies and of course the qualities of the therapeutic relationship, as discussed previously. To start, displacement often requires using gestures, your body, sensory regulatory interventions, and being with the child at the right place and time with the appropriate substitute objects at hand and introducing them virtually surreptitiously in the moment. Not always so easy! Over time, and when rehearsed in the regulated state, conscious and instrumental use of displacement may become increasingly internalized and more automatic for the child. Ultimately, the aim is for impulse enactment to be subsumed not only in play and objects, but in language. Anna Freud said, "My father once remarked on the philosopher who said that the man who first hurled a word of abuse at his enemy instead of a weapon was the founder of civilization. That is really what analysts are aiming to do in getting patients to verbalize" (Sandler et al., 1980, p. 122).

A particular kind of play that can be especially helpful in working through aggressive feelings is destruction–repair play. In such play, the child creates, destroys, reconstructs, and recreates again, such as building with blocks or clay, knocking down the structure or squashing the clay form and then rebuilding or remolding, sometimes over and over. Aggression, for all children, is a powerful force to be reckoned with. In fantasy children may imagine their aggression has magical power and consequences far beyond reality—power to destroy them, those they love, and the even the world. Children are not infrequently afraid of their own aggressive impulses. Destruction–repair play is one way they can experiment with the reality limits of their aggression, discovering that its power and consequences are neither omnipotent nor irreparably damaging.

Aggression and other intense feeling states must be met without putting the child in fear of retaliation, harsh rebuke, or an in-kind response on the part of the therapist. By the therapist "containing" the strong affects without excessive response and "metabolizing" them for the child, the message is sent that these big feelings will neither destroy you, nor me, nor scare me away, but that they can be managed and understood. The child may learn from this balanced response on the part of the therapist that the aggression will not inflict irreparable harm to the therapist and frees the child from exercising a rigidly constricting inhibition to protect the therapist, allowing the child instead to "use" the therapist in a more trusting, open, and corrective way. The aggressive acts may be reflected or interpreted depending on the child's level of language comprehension, (e.g., when you were angry, your body moved so fast and all about and with such strength that you knocked down Mary's fort and even hit her). It is often more effective to wait until the "iron is cool" and the child is regulated, as in the high-aroused state, a reflection or interpretation may not be able to be heard or processed and could even exacerbate the negative feeling state—regulate, relate with affect attunement, and then reflect and reason.

Limit setting to protect the child and others, may sometimes be necessary. When in a regulated state, the incident in question may be revisited with the child, if able to process at the verbal level, and limits explored in the event of a future incident of strong feelings and unruly behavior. If the child is able, her/his involvement in formulating the nature of the limits can be a helpful exploration in the service of managing anxiety, exercising self-control over thoughts and behaviors and internalizing self-discipline. Anna Freud suggested that the place between absolute freedom and absolute control is sublimation—an adaptive process through which unruly impulses are transformed and invested in constructive and helpful behaviors and endeavors. Implementing these mental health principles and strategies may call for Occupational Therapist (OT) and play therapist to work collaterally, cotreat and/or have ongoing consultation.

Revisiting the power of play as a self-regulatory promoting activity in itself, the qualities of play that are mutative include; (1) practice in intentionally shifting between internal states of fantasy and imagination and external physical/descriptive reality; (2) play as regulatory practice; (3) play as novelty and investigation; and (4) play as roles and rules (Foley, 2017). The very nature of imaginative play has regulatory implications in that it requires the child to intentionally shift between states of consciousness, imposing internally focused fantasy and imagination over physical/descriptive reality. Much of self-regulation relies on the ability to volitionally shift between varying states of arousal, consciousness, attention, and internal and external reality. These capacities are rehearsed as an intrinsic part of symbolic play.

Play affords children near limitless opportunities to rehearse "shifting gears," grading and modulating an array of functions—range of vocal volume, action and activity level, speed, attention, position, starting and stopping, and so forth—in response to the demands of imagination and peers in a naturalistic, self-initiated way without the need for an imposed task. Further, play is also an arena for practicing sympathetic nervous system modulation through coregulation.

> *Play requires an ability to mobilize with the sympathetic nervous system and then to down-regulate the sympathetic excitation with face-to-face social interaction and the social engagement system . . . play is an efficient neural exercise using social interactions to "co-regulate" physiological and behavioral state.*
>
> *Porges, (2017, p. 80)*

Play is a spontaneous experience and the unexpected is apt to happen—a ball rolls under a piece of furniture; a lid can't be removed; a playmate doesn't cooperate. These novel experiences may demand changes in action and revision of play theme, sometimes requiring investigation into the novel event and engaging problem-solving efforts, both physical and social, that result in exercising nimbleness and adaptability, modulation and variation in a range of functions, including frustration tolerance. As the sociodramatic strand of play evolves, the story line frequently involves the assignment and adherence to roles and rules. These experiments with social conformity include practice with inhibition, impulse control, and compliance with the rules of social order and discourse, all dimensions of higher order self-regulation.

In this chapter, the authors have argued that "aggression" in young children on the autistic spectrum may, in many cases, not meet the criteria of intentionality-to-do-harm and belief that their acts will indeed inflict harm. This suggests that care must be taken in attributing motives and meaning to these acts. Closer to impulsive or reactive "aggression," the authors posit that (1) states of dysregulation of sensation and movement; (2) faulty neuroception and nervous system response to misappraised threat with mobilization of fight/flight/freeze, (3) poorly modulated states of arousal; and (4) consequent affective states of anxiety, toxic stress, and frustration are the major precipitants of what may appear to be "aggression" in young children on the spectrum. Thus the authors propose the dysregulation–"aggression" hypothesis to better explain many aggressive-like behaviors in young children on the autistic spectrum.

An intervention paradigm derived from the dysregulation–"aggression hypothesis," based on clinical trials and a collaboration between a treating occupational therapist and psychologist has been outlined. The model integrates sensory-movement intervention and arousal regulation; the enabling of the social engagement system and the management of anxiety and negative affective states, implemented in a relational context, with relevant concepts and practices from psychodynamic play therapy. Informed by the Developmental Individual difference Relationship-based (DIR) model, (Greenspan & Wieder, 2006; Wieder & Foley, 2018) the intervention approach outlined here, could be considered an elaboration and deepening of the "I," relational in its overall approach; it embraces the "R" with the aim of advancing development, the "D."

References

Amos, P. (2018). Seeing movement: Implications of the movement sensing perspective for parents. In E. Torres, & C. P. Wyhatt (Eds.), *Autism: The movement sensing perspective* (p. 295). Frontiers in Neuroscience.

Anderson, C. A., & Bushman, B. J. (2002). Human aggression. *Annual Review of Psychology*, *53*, 27–53.

Bandura, A. (1965). Influence of models' reinforcement contingencies on the acquisition of responses. *Journal of Personality and Social Psychology*, *1*(6), 589–595. Available from https://doi.org/10.1037/h0022070.

Baron, R. A., & Richardson, D. R. (1994). *Human aggression* (2nd ed.). Plenum.

Ben-Sasson, A., Hen, L., Fluss, R., Cermak, S. A., Engel-Yeger, B., & Gal, E. (2009). A meta-analysis of sensory modulation symptoms in individuals with autism spectrum disorders. *Journal of Autism and Developmental Disorders*, *39*, 1–11. Available from https://doi.org/10.1007/s10803-008-0593-3.

Ben-Sasson, A., Soto, T. W., Pedraza-Martinez, F., & Carter, A. S. (2013). Early sensory overresponsivity in toddlers with autism spectrum disorder as a predictor of family impairment and parenting stress. *Journal of Child Psychology and Psychiatry*, *54*(8), 846–853. Available from https://doi.org/10.1111/jcpp.12035.

Berkowitz, L. (1993). *Aggression: Its causes consequences and control*. McGraw-Hill Book Company.

Bushman, B. J., & Anderson, C. A. (2001). Is it time to pull the plug on hostile versus Instrumental aggression dichotomy? *Psychological Review*, *108*(1), 273–279.

Cannon, W. B. (1932). *The wisdom of the body*. New York: Norton.

Carver, C. S., & Scheier, M. F. (2016). Self-regulation of action and affect. In K. D. Vohs, & R. F. Baumeister (Eds.), *Handbook of self-regulation: Research, theory and applications* (pp. 3–23). New York: Guilford Press.

Delafield-Butt, J., & Trevarthen, C. (2018). On the brain stem origin of autism: Disruption to movement of the primary self. In E. Torres, & C. P. Wyhatt (Eds.), *Autism the movement sensing perspective* (pp. 119–139). Frontiers in Neuroscience.

Dollard, J., Miller, N. E., Doob, L. W., Mowrer, O. H., & Sears, R. R. (1939). *Frustration and aggression*. Yale University Press. Available from https://doi.org/10.1037/10022-000.

Erikson, E. (1982). *The life cycle completed: A review*. W.W. Norton & Company.

Feldman, R. (2007). Parent-infant synchrony: Biological foundations and developmental outcomes. *Current Directions in Psychological Science*, *16*(6), 340–345.

Foley, G. M. (2017). Play as regulation: Promoting self-regulation through play. *Topics in Language Disorders*, *57*(3), 241–258.

Foley, G. M. (2020). Adjusting the lens on the spectrum through a developmental, individual-difference, relationship-based model: A developmental, parent mediated, play-based intervention. In U. Das, N. Papaneophytou, & T. El-Kour (Eds.), *Autism 360* (pp. 367–386). Elsevier.

Freud, S. (1955). *Beyond the pleasure principle* (J. Strachey, Ed & trans., The Standard Edition, Vol. 18). Hogarth Press. (Original work published 1920).

Freud, A. (1965). *Normality and pathology in childhood.* International Universities Press.

Gabriels, R. L., Agnew, J. A., Miller, L. J., Gralla, J., Pan, Z., Goldson, E., ... Hooks, E. (2008). Is there a relationship between restricted, repetitive, stereotyped behaviors and interests and abnormal sensory response in children with autism spectrum disorders? *Research in Autism Spectrum Disorders, 2*, 660–670.

Greenspan, S., & Wieder, S. (2006). *Engaging autism: Using the floortime approach to help children relate, communicate and think.* DaCapo Press/Persius Books.

Hilton, C. L., Harper, J. D., Kucker, R. L., Lang, A. R., Abbacchi, A. M., Todorov, A., & LaVesser, P. D. (2010). Sensory responsiveness as a predictor of social severity with high functioning autism spectrum disorders. *Journal of Autism and Developmental Disorders, 40*, 937–945. Available from https://doi.org/10.1007/s10803-010-0944-8.

Klein, M. (1952). Some theoretical conclusions regarding the emotional life of the infant. In M. Klein, P. Heimann, S. Isaacs, & J. Reviere (Eds.), *Developments in psychoanalysis* (pp. 198–236). Hogarth Press.

Klin, A., Volkmar, F., & Charwaska, K. (2003). Automatic attention cueing through eye movement in 2-year-old children. *Child Development, 74*(4), 1108–1122. Available from https://doi.org/10.1111/1467-8624.00595.

Kopp, C. B. (1982). Antecedents of self-regulation: A developmental perspective. *Developmental Psychology, 18*(2), 199–214.

Lane, S. (2002). Structure and function of the sensory systems. In A. C. Bundy, S. L. Lane, & E. A. Murray (Eds.), *Sensory integration: Theory and practice* (pp. 35–68). F. A. Davis Company.

Lillas, C., & Turnbull, J. (2009). *Infant/child mental health, early intervention and relationship-based therapies: A neurorelational framework for interdisciplinary practice.* W. W. Norton & Company, Inc.

Lord, C. (1995). Follow-up of two-year-olds referred for possible autism. *Journal of Child Psychology and Psychiatry, 36*, 1365–1382.

Lorenz, C. (1966). *On aggression.* Harcourt, Brace & World. (Original work published 1963).

Murray, D. W., Rosanbalm, K., Christopoulos, C., & Hamoudi, A. (2015). *Self- regulation and toxic stress: Foundations for understanding self-regulation from an applied developmental perspective.* Washington, DC: Office of Planning, Research and Evaluation, Administration for Children's and Families, U.S. Department of Health and Human Services, OPRE Report #2015-21.

Porges, S. (2009). The polyvagal theory: New insights into adaptive reactions of the autonomic nervous system. *Cleveland Clinic Journal of Medicine, 76*(Suppl 2), 586–590.

Porges, S. (2017). *The pocket guide to the polyvagal theory: The transformative power of feeling safe.* W.W. Norton & Company.

Robertson, C. E., & Baron-Cohen, S. (2017). Sensory perception in autism. *Nature Reviews, Neuroscience, 18*(11), 671–684. Available from https://doi.org/10.1038/nrn.2017.112.

Samson, C. S., Phillips, J. M., Parker, H. J., Shah, B., Gross, J. J., & Hardan, A. (2014). Emotion dysregulation and the core features of autism spectrum disorder. *Journal of Autism and Developmental Disorders, 44*(7), 1766–1772.

Sandler, J., Kennedy, H., & Tyson, R. L. (1980). *The technique of child psychoanalysis: Discussions with Anna Freud.* Harvard University Press.

Singletary, W. M. (2015). An integrative model of autism spectrum disorder: ASD as a neurobiological disorder of experienced environmental deprivation, early life stress and allostatic overload. *Neuropsychoanalysis*, *7*(2), 1–101. Available from https://doi.org/10.1080/15294145.2015.1092.

Stern, D. (2010). *Forms of vitality*. Oxford University Press.

Stevenson, R. A., Segers, M., Ncube, B. L., Black, K. R., Bebko, J. M., Ferber, S., & Barense, M. D. (2017). The cascading influence of multisensory processing on speech perception in autism. *Autism: The International Journal of Research and Practice*, 1–16. Available from https://doi.org/10.1077/1362361317704413.

Torres, E. (2018). Inherent noise hidden in nervous systems' rhythms leads to new strategies for detections and treatments of core motor sensing traits in ASD. In E. Torres, & C. P. Wyhatt (Eds.), *Autism the movement sensing perspective* (pp. 197–210). Frontiers in Neuroscience.

Wieder, S., & Foley, G. M. (2018). The DIR (developmental, individual difference, relationship-based) model: A parent-mediated approach to interdisciplinary assessment and comprehensive intervention. In E. Hollander, R. Hagerman, & D. Fein (Eds.), *Autism spectrum disorders* (pp. 231–251). American Psychiatric Association Publishing.

Williamson, G. G., & Anzalone, M. (2001). *Sensory integration and self-regulation in infants and toddlers: Helping very young children interact with their environment*. Zero to Three Press.

Zero to Three. (2016). *DC:0–5 diagnostic classification of mental health and developmental disorders of infancy and early childhood*. Zero to Three.

Good autism education is just good education

10

Gil Tippy
Dirty Hands Developmental Alliance, Sonoma, CA, United States

Good autism education is just good education. The problem is, we as a society have forgotten what good education is. One of the reasons this chapter is necessary is that we have modeled autism education on the very worst of general education paradigms. In this time, during and after the coronavirus pandemic, when we have seen how badly our educational systems fail when they move to purely "academic" practices, we should be even more aware of what education really should be. Instead of purely transmitting the facts and figures of a culture, education must be the process of opening a student's eyes to the possibility that they have within them the ability to figure out how the world might be different than it is right now in front of them. Education needs to allow students to look within, and realize that their inner faculties are all that they need in order to take this challenge before them and move it in the direction that they pick as a final destination. Anything other than that as an overarching goal is pointless in this age of an antediluvian deluge of facts and information. So, good education is education that supports the student's growth and development in the direction of the student's greatest expression of their innate talents and potential. Any education that is not supporting development in the direction of the student's greatest expression of their innate talents and potential is not good education.

I cannot tell you how many parents came to me for the first half of our sequestering during this pandemic and told me about all the wonderful resources to be found on the internet. You can't blame them, they were suddenly alone at home with their children, they had no idea what they should be doing with them, and "experts" in their designated fields dangled the world's greatest expertise in a number of subjects before their eyes. Everyone wanted to expose their child to the greatest proponents of hundreds of subjects, academic and otherwise. What could be wrong with that? All of a sudden, parents saw a glimmer of hope. The teachers whom they had been paying could be replaced, through the magic of the Internet, with the world's greatest at their particular discipline. Their children, whom they love dearly, would actually be getting the very best information in the world, whereas before they were only getting whatever their particular teacher was able to teach them. Surely, in this particular way, what was about to happen at home was going to be even better than anything that ever happened at school. Their children were actually lucky. Sure, it was very difficult to have their child at home, but at least they would learn from the best.

Emerging Programs for Autism Spectrum Disorder. DOI: https://doi.org/10.1016/B978-0-323-85031-5.00022-0

The truth is, they were right in a particular way. Their students were extremely lucky. But they were not lucky because these parents had the ability to access the greatest geniuses; they were lucky because they were in the presence of their loving parents, of their loving extended family, of the people who knew them best. Learning from the greatest practitioner of something does not guarantee you good instruction. In fact, what you might learn from that person is unlikely to be of much use to you. The simple how-tos of anything are really not as useful as pondering and muddling through trying to figure out how to do something. So, even though people were thrilled at the beginning of the physical isolation during the pandemic to find out the web had miraculous resources, it did not take them long to see that pure access to information is just about the least useful kind of education.

There is a time and a place for this kind of education. At the beginning of any subject you need to know the signposts and symbols, the "givens," of the topic. That, I think, is what kindergarten is intended to do, in the United States anyways. You enter a kindergarten, and you are told where to sit, and that it matters where you sit. You are told that the person at the front of the room is the teacher, and that she is a big deal! You had better listen to what she has to say! She may seem nice, but she's actually a task master! Her rule is total, and she is divinely inspired!

You also learned that the order in which things go matters. First you do this, then you do this, then you do this. You were taught the building blocks of the language: the letters, the sounds. You learned the fanciful squiggles that are meant to represent the numbers that are meant to represent something about quantity. And you learned the rules of the society.

For instance, you learned that you should be nice to people, even if they take your favorite crayon. You learned that hitting is forbidden in the society, as are biting and scratching. You learned to keep your clothes on, and to put them on again when you come out of the bathroom. In short, in addition to learning the facts of academics, you learned the rules of decorum as they are expressed in your society. Once you enter a kindergarten, you can never go back. Your feet are irreversibly on the track of "education."

When you move to first grade, things begin to heat up. You learn even more of the facts, at a more accelerated rate. The same thing is true of second grade, by the end of which you are expected to be able to read and do simple math. But then comes third grade, and things begin to change if you are getting a useful education. In third grade your actual education, of the kind we said was good education at the start of the chapter, begins to happen in earnest.

In third grade things get much more ambiguous. The simple task of memorizing, which served you so well in kindergarten, first grade, and second grade, is no longer sufficient. The teacher begins to introduce the possibility that there could be more than one answer to a problem. They begin to introduce the idea that you might have something in your head, that no one else may have, which might be a viable way to solve the problem in front of you. Simply knowing the facts of the case didn't answer the problem for you. The facts, the letters, numbers, and details that you learned were only useful to you if you could work some kind of internal magic on them. Useful to you only if you could apply the power of your mind to imagine how things could be different if they were not as they were in front of you in that moment. So, if your education had only focused on memorization and routinization, when you got to third grade you would be in big trouble!

The third-grade curriculum changes dramatically in good schools. The first three grades, kindergarten, first, and second, are about learning the academic facts. Third grade is about taking those facts and making something out of them. The first three grades are going to the grocery store to buy ingredients, but third grade is about taking those ingredients and creating dinner. It really doesn't matter how good you are at walking up and down the grocery aisles if you cannot imagine the transformation you have to make on the food you have bought in order to make a delicious meal. Ingredients are not dinner, and the simple acquisition of facts is not education. Or, to be more honest about it, the simple acquisition of facts is not the kind of education that would be of any use to a fully functioning person in an adult society. And yet, this is the kind of education that we offer to persons with developmental challenges.

What I am considering "good" schools or "good" classes for neurotypical kids, are much more the exception than they are the rule. In the vast majority of schools, we here in the United States stay focused on the acquisition of facts much more than is useful. We direct curriculum from the state education office, so that all the fourth graders in a given state are learning the exact same thing on the exact same day. Creative, brilliant teachers, who entered education because they wanted to light the fire of learning in other people, are frustrated and saddened because they can't be creative and innovative in the way that they would like to. When curricula are directed from education offices on the state level, they tend to focus on things which can be tested because they have to have a way to prove that "education" is happening. A test is the easiest way to prove this, supposedly. The easiest things to test are the facts around any subject. So, instead of pursuing the deeper human meaning of the age of exploration, for example, students instead get tested on the dates and the facts. Even in this age, where we would like the students to consider how European aggression in this country impacted the already existing native peoples, when it comes time for testing, we go for the facts. They may now be more enlightened facts, by our standards of the moment, but to do easy standardized testing, we fall back on facts.

This system has created a culture amongst our school children where they cram all the facts they can into their heads on the night before they're tested, dump them onto the examination paper on the day that they are tested, and then forever forget them. The facts are not of any particular use to them, because they are moving on in their classes to another giant set of facts, which they will cram into their memories the day before the test, dump on the paper on the day of the test, and then forget forever. Students call this "cram and dump" or "binge and purge." This cycle goes on *ad nauseam*, and the students who are the very best at this we call the valedictorians of the classes. These students go to our very best universities, where they continue the process, and if they are really good at it, they graduate with advanced degrees. To use medical students as an example, what really matters to them in terms of advancing in their careers is class rank and grade average. The way that one does well in these two areas is by memorizing the facts and regurgitating them. Unfortunately, this leads us to the crisis of medical doctors who cannot diagnose, and medical systems which no longer expect them to diagnose.

It isn't just medical doctors who are in this situation. For every medical doctor who has to follow the treatment recommendations of their health system and its algorithms, and prescribe tests whenever they can be justified for the patient based on their symptoms, there is an auto mechanic doing the exact same thing. They may have gone to the best auto repair school in the world, but when they get out, they read the code that the computer spits out at them when they plug into the automobile's diagnostic system, and then they replace the modules that seem to be implicated, whether they are faulty or not. The age when a doctor could look at you, talk to you, listen to you, and diagnose you, and the age when your mechanic could put their ear to the hood of your car and figure out what simple fix would solve your problem, is over. And the reason this age is over is the reason why our schools habitually fail our students in general, and our students who arrive with special challenges, particularly. If your educational paradigm is based on the idea that you should only teach what is easily tested, students will never rise above the level where they can simply recall facts. They will be stuck in the world of the immediate now, and will always see challenges as insurmountable obstacles. They will not be able to problem-solve, and will be dependent upon prompting, and unvarying decision trees, to navigate their lives.

Good classroom education is education that allows you to imagine that you could look at the problem and cause a change to happen which would lead you in the direction of solving the problem in front of you. It would allow you to imagine the world as different than it is directly in front of you. If it were a very simple problem, for instance, how to divide ten beads into two equal parts, in other words divide them in half, then all you would have to do is a fairly simple "transformation" on the pile. A good education would allow you to do that. You would be able to imagine what you could do to that pile of 10 beads which would result in two equal piles. That's really all there is to all of education. You have to be able to imagine that you could look at the situation and be able to apply something from within your mind that would cause a useful transformation on the problem in front of you. A one-step transformation, like the one in the example above, is the building block. From that simple transformation, you can build all of learning. So, whether you were trying to do simple addition and subtraction, or you were trying to calculate all of the various equations you would have to calculate to send a human being on a rocket to the moon, it is all the same thing. If you can imagine what direction you need to go, and you believe that you have within you the ability to modify what's in front of you in a way that will be useful to move in the direction of your final goal, then you have all of education. That is very rarely what is going on in schools for ostensibly neurotypical children, and it is even rarer in schools for students who have developmental challenges. Perhaps the name of this chapter could have been, "bad education for autism is simply bad education."

I am an American, and have never lived anywhere but the United States, but I teach all over the world, and that experience leads me to believe that autism education in much of the world looks like autism education in the United States. If you live in a part of the world where you are providing the kind of education that I'm talking about as being good autism education, then I would love to hear from you, and hear what it is you are doing nationally. But my experience generally brings me into contact with people who are extremely frustrated with the education that has been provided either for them, or for their loved ones. After years of working in the autism field I think that I have been able to narrow down what goes wrong in general in autism education here in the United States. It is not intended to be an indictment of anyone, or any particular methodology of autism education, it is fully intended to be an indictment of almost every methodology in autism education! I intend to lay-out how all methodologies can fail, and hopefully, how all methodologies could conceivably succeed.

Human beings develop. They develop in more or less predictable ways. By observing human beings as they develop, either individually or in large hoards, theorists over time have proposed theories about human development. Most developmental models think of developmental steps, or milestones, or capacities that growing children achieve or realize on their way toward "typical" human development. Most of these models think of these steps as building upon each other, with a solid foundation in earlier developmental steps being necessary for solid and enduring existence at later developmental steps. As a clinical psychologist, and as a professional teacher, I have been exposed to many developmental models, and I think I have a general idea of some of their common elements.

When they are born, human children are not very well organized. Their small skulls and small brains are not yet fully developed. Nobody sleeps in the house of the zero to 3-month-old. They are simply too disorganized. But slowly, with the support of their loving caregiver or caregivers, they begin to calm, their brains make important neuronal connections, they harness their caregivers' frontal lobes, and they become available and engaged. Once they're available and engaged, they begin to interact. They acknowledge that their caregivers have asked them something or shown them something. They smile in response to smiles, and they show an interest in sharing their interest. Before too long, they begin to use words, and they begin to try to get their needs met. They are able to do this with skill, interacting with their caregivers in simple, but very effective ways. They ask for things, and they receive them.

This developmental capacity, where a child is able to get simple needs met, asking for and acknowledging things, verbally, gesturally, or with sounds, is the developmental capacity where I encounter most of the students who have come to me over the years, regardless of their chronological age. They are in general very good at responding to questions, although they may sometimes pretend that they do not hear the questions. They are often very good at doing things that are requested of them. They are motivated by getting their needs met, and can make themselves clear to their caregivers around issues of food and things which particularly interest them. If they have been in school, they can often point to things and name them, using their good memories. They often have been taught to speak through being reinforced for speech production, so they have a cadence and a speech volume that neurotypical people do not recognize as typical. They can sign their names, but they do it by attacking letters in ways that neurotypical people might not. In general, they reside at the developmental capacity where they can get their simple needs met, where they can answer simple questions, and where they can use their good memories to negotiate the academic curriculum. In short, even the most verbal, even the oldest students I generally encounter permanently reside at, or below, the level of someone entering the typical United States Third Grade.

There are two essential parts of education: the givens, and creative problem solving. Part one only makes sense if you intend to teach the second part. The second part can't be applied without the facts of the first part. The second part is universal to every aspect of human existence. The first part is content specific, but very easily learned. The first part is accomplished by use of the powerful human memory. The second part is accomplished by the application of the human mind, after the mastery of a particular developmental milestone or capacity. Part one is incredibly easy to teach, involving only simply displaying the facts. The second is very difficult to teach, involving getting students to reach into their own powerful minds. But, once the second part is learned, and trusted, the first part becomes short and quick. If education put the second part securely as the focus, students would be free to learn anything. Unfortunately, most education focuses on the first part, for many reasons, and only occasionally waves at the second part in passing. When you only teach the first part, the memory-based part, the facts and the givens, it is only what I call, "As If" education or "The Education Show." Autism education, almost universally, focuses on the first part and entirely ignores the second. Much of education for people with developmental challenges is "The Education Show."

Sometimes, educators think they are teaching creative problem solving by asking students to give their opinions about a topic. Giving your opinion is not necessarily the same as thinking through a problem. Really, often your opinion does not matter. So, textbooks that offer questions at the bottom of the chapter usually present them as fact-based in questions one through ten, and then put one or two "creative" extra-credit questions at the bottom. Usually, the "creative" questions ask a student for an opinion like, "What do you think of the founding fathers at the Constitutional Convention?" Your opinion is nice, but it's not problem-solving. A real question leading to problem-solving might be, "What other ways might the founders have solved the conflict around counting enslaved people in the Constitution, other than the 3/5 solution?" Or, "Look today at a problem related to race, and trace its origins to the Constitution's 3/5 solution." That would require conceptualizing the problem. "How did we get here from the 3/5 beginning?" It would require being able to take a first logical step in the correct direction. Then, it would require you to work by logical steps back to the Constitutional Convention. Just asking for an opinion is pandering to the audience. It is telling students how prime they are. It is a failure, because instead of telling them they are special, they need to be taught how they might solve a problem. They need to be creative problem-solvers.

The pandemic has made some things about education crystal clear to me. After more than 40 years in education, the pandemic drove home, in a way that was no longer intellectual for me, the primacy of the childcare function of school. Families suddenly faced with the challenge of managing jobs and their children at home faced economic disaster. Even though I had struggled while my son lived with me alone, getting him to and from school, connecting with his education while holding a full-time job 45 minutes away from his school, I was still unprepared for just how important childcare is in today's society.

We all have survival needs. There are two basic levels of survival. The first is moment-to-moment survival. The, "I need a breath," or "I need shelter" level. This level is the immediacy of biological survival. Organisms will focus on these first, have to focus on these first. So, with the pandemic, families had to figure out how to survive in the moment. They had to put food on the table. It was then that the childcare aspects of school came into sharp focus. Finally, I saw the light, because of the thing I was dreading most in the world. The coronavirus allowed me a way to understand something I had never understood and constantly questioned. "Why do people choose harmful, ineffective interventions, and keep their children in rotten schools where they make no progress?" The answer, at least partially, is that they need the beloved children to be safe and cared for, while they have to focus on making money to pay for food and shelter. So, if you have a safe place where your child can go, and they return reasonably safe and sound at the end of the day, that can be good enough. Only if you already have that, are you free to begin to consider whether the school is giving your child a useful education for their continued growth. People will stick with schools that they suspect are not meeting long-term goals out of their fear that they may not find another school that is better, and that to remove their child from a school that has already enrolled them is too great a risk. In defense of parents everywhere, very often, they are right! It is much more likely that to remove a child from an available placement in a school puts the child at risk of a less suitable school placement, or no school placement at all.

I am going to outline some risks that every person, at every level of education has to be constantly vigilant against. I do not wish to imply that any particular school or methodology is bad. I only wish to point out where the temptation to not provide effective, developmentally appropriate education lies. Any teacher could protect themselves, and so could every school.

Every educational system, at every level, is subject to a certain kind of bias, even if they have lofty mission statements about growth and development and helping students face the future with freedom. But schools, like individuals, have to meet their basic survival needs. For their survival, educational systems need to run smoothly, be stable, and most importantly, meet the needs of the teachers and the administrators. If the survival needs of the classroom staff, and of the school, are not being met, then the lofty goals of the mission statement will not be addressed.

On the classroom level, teachers work hard to make their classrooms into environments conducive to sound education. They want safety, order, and a smooth workflow. Special education classrooms are very difficult places to manage effectively, so when a teacher gets a flow going, they want to keep up the momentum. But, schools make it almost impossible for this kind of flow and continuity to exist, despite the best efforts of the most inspired and inspiring teachers.

Let's imagine a special education classroom where there are typically eight kids. When this class was started there were four students who are easy to manage: low energy, or not particularly mobile or verbal. Then, let's imagine there were two kids who were verbal and mobile, but also funny and endearing. They required a lot of attention and energy and teaching! Let's imagine that the final two students were more difficult to manage in the context of a classroom with eight students. Maybe they were bigger than the other students, and had difficulties with communicating, so were unpredictable. Sometimes, they were physically aggressive. These two students were the most difficult students to educate in this classroom configuration.

The teacher found this configuration of students very difficult to educate given her resources. These two unpredictable, sometimes physically aggressive students made the classroom feel dangerous, or at least not under the teacher's control. The teacher felt the pressing need to protect the four quiet students, who shrank away quietly to the corners. The teacher paid attention to the two verbal, personable students, because it was gratifying, and also, because these two students were very good at advocating for attention. Very quickly, the two physically aggressive, unpredictable students were identified as the problem.

If the school and the teacher are not constantly vigilant, certain subtle changes begin to take place. No good-hearted, dedicated special education teacher makes these changes consciously, certainly not out of malice. But a teacher has to think about day-to-day survival for her students and her staff, so things begin to shift. The classroom looks for more support for their work with the two students identified as problems. They try to get the specialty teachers to take them out of the class, so that they can use their available in-class resources for the education of the other students, which they sometimes cannot address because of the need to be attentive to the unpredictable students. Calls for extra occupational therapy, physical therapy, speech and language therapy, gym time, and counseling time go out. Soon, the teacher appeals to the administration, saying that the class is unteachable with the two difficult students. Eventually, the two unpredictable students are moved from the classroom to another more intensive classroom with a higher level of support. If no such classroom is available within the school, then the two students move to another education setting that is more restrictive. That leaves the first class with six students, who feel much more teachable, and the classroom feels safer. It no longer feels like every day is a struggle for survival, for the staff, and maybe even for the remaining students.

But now there are two vacancies in the classroom. Who should fill them? The teacher who has worked so long and hard to finally have a teachable, safe class, for the staff, and for the more vulnerable students does not want two unpredictable or aggressive students added, so she advocates specifically for students who are like her current students. This process goes on for a long while, new students, ejection of challenging students, retention of manageable students. Finally, the teacher ends up with a class of eight manageable students, with the cohort of some who need little attention, and make few demands, and some who are verbal, funny, and endearing, who make the class fun to teach. When this stasis is reached, after a very long time, years even, that is when the real education crisis happens.

These classrooms, like all systems, spectacularly resist change. As any systems theorist will tell you, systems are not just inertial, resisting movement, they actively attempt to get back to the state they were in when they were comfortable. So, classrooms that feel manageable fight to keep that feeling. The biggest threat to that is the subtraction, and the following addition, of students.

The alleged goal of education is to help students to grow and develop. A way to measure this in special education settings might be to keep track of how many students are being promoted to less restrictive educational settings. Eventually, the goal for students is to move to a regular education setting with no accommodations. But every time a student gets promoted, a classroom crisis of the kind I have been discussing happens. The teacher does not want to give up the student who has made so much progress, in whom the teacher and staff have invested so much blood, sweat, and tears, who is so gratifying, and now, so easily fits into a manageable classroom. The teachers and staff know that the replacement is not going to be as easy and gratifying, and that the classroom may become very difficult to manage again. A card player throws away bad cards, and draws new ones, hoping for better cards. They never throw away good cards and draw what are most likely worse cards that will hurt their hands.

I don't believe teachers and other staff retain students who should move to less restrictive settings for the conscious goal of hurting their progress. And I don't believe they constantly hold back student progress to make students not appropriate for the next less restrictive level of education, consciously. But I do believe that teachers are human, and that they will make sure that their survival needs are met, and only then can they rise to the lofty goal of education.

I don't think special education stand-alone schools or classrooms are the only places that need to be vigilant for this kind of unconscious creep. I think public schools go through the same process as it relates to students with increased educational needs. Once they have identified the students who are causing problems, danger, or are consuming a lot of administrative time, or producing low test scores, then the process of moving these students to alternate settings begins.

If the school has to report test scores in the aggregate, and has test scores somehow tied to funding, or tied to even being allowed to continue to be autonomous, you can be sure those kids who are getting low test scores will be moved out. If a child is an administrative problem, or considered dangerous, the child will be expelled, continuing the "path to prison" curriculum. This "path to prison," or "school to prison pipeline" has been much written about, so I do not want to more than acknowledge it here. The process I am describing is one part of this much written about phenomenon. Students stay who make the school easy to run, and who make the school look statistically good, until they age out of special education at 21 or 22 years old. But if the school is a private school, particularly a special education private school, most particularly a for-profit private, special education school, the problem is greatly compounded.

I do not believe that any school or person enters the field of special education with less than pure intent. I only want to point out where schools and individuals need to be most vigilant. The pressures at all times, but particularly in these times of economic challenge, are tremendous. Private special education schools need a certain number of students to remain solvent. Their primary budget line is salary, so they need to pay as few educators as possible to teach as many students as possible. Clearly, this equation implies that the most manageable students are retained, and the students deemed too expensive in teacher time, or administrative time (especially administrative time!) be somehow removed. That, as pernicious as it is, is not the problem I want to address. The most insidious problem is that there is tremendous pressure not to move kids to less restrictive settings, and to not provide education that helps students to develop in order that they not move to less restrictive settings. Educational curricula are created for compliance and management in settings like these, not for student growth. Student growth makes no financial sense. It is my belief that this is one of the main reasons why, in the field of autism education, almost all of the curriculum that is written is based in compliance and prompting. Once you have a student at the level in his development where he will listen to what the teacher says, sit quietly, and respond to simple prompt driven tasks, essentially, you have the perfect student, if you are only interested in the financial life of your school. If you are a private, ungraded school, you keep a student at virtually the same level until the state and federal government stops paying for their education at 21 or 22.

There is at least a tacit acknowledgment of this situation that can be found in the way the laws are written for special education in the United States. At the age of 14, students in special education are supposed to begin what is optimistically called "transition planning." What this essentially means is that students have to begin to have a plan about where they are going at the end of their free and appropriate public education. What happens at this stage in many programs is that people change their prompt-based compliance education into a prompt-based compliance education. The only difference is that the new prompts are about how to do your laundry, and how do use public transportation. They cease to be about addition, subtraction, how to write your name, and how to sit in a seat in a classroom.

These prompt-based, growth-inhibiting curricula are in favor because schools need to function, with some degree of safety, and with a great deal of economy. Our children need somewhere to go where they can be kept safe, and somehow we have been deceived into believing that the only way this can be done is to control them, on the theory that otherwise they are entirely unmanageable. But control and compliance is nowhere to be found in our definition of good education. So how can we know if the school is merely struggling for its own survival, or if it is attempting to hold the space, support the student, and promote the kind of human growth and understanding that we all believe are the true goals of education?

When I entered the world of starting private schools, I was full of hubris, and thought I knew what any school I helped to start would eventually look like. I thought that the school would start with a balance of students who make quick developmental progress in a good developmental, not behavioral, program, and students who would make very slow but steady progress in a good developmental, not behavioral, program. I believed that eventually all of the quick-developers would be moved to less restrictive environments, that the slower-developers would continue at the school, and eventually the school would be filled with the slower-developers, because as quick-developers moved out, slower-developers would take more time, and so would fill all the available slots. I thought this was the fate of every new private special-education school. I do see what I imagined would happen in some of the very best schools I consult to around the world, but that is not what I typically see happening. What I much more often see happening is that if the school has a student, and the student is not particularly problematic, the student stays forever. If the student could make quick developmental progress, the school will do what it can to find ways to make sure that the student doesn't meet criteria for other programs. If the student could be making steady developmental progress, but slowly, the school will keep them, if they can get the student to the point where they are not dangerous, or resource intensive. By resource intensive I mean someone who requires a great deal of expensive therapies or administrative attention. So, I see students retained, or slowed down in their growth because they are not expensive in time, energy, or money to teach, and because the school feels it can operate comfortably with them in the student body.

There are ways to remedy some of the long-term, institutionalized abuses within the system. Schools and postsecondary treatment programs could be reporting certain statistics that would make it easier for perspective consumers to understand what they are going to get when they enroll a loved one in a program. First, there are programmatic statistics that relate to the general make-up of the population, then there are statistics related to the movement of the students through the system, and most importantly programs need to demonstrate that they are presenting a program that actually leads to all students making developmental progress in the direction of their greatness. In other words, schools need to demonstrate that they are providing what we have all agreed upon as a good education.

I think every adult who is making decisions for a child should be able to ask for a certain kind of data from every school they are ever considering for their child with developmental challenges. First, they should be able to access, right on the school or treatment program's website, simple demographic information. This should include information about Socioeconomic Status (SES) of the students in the program, diversity of program in terms of race, and gender diversity. These statistics are required by some large school boards, and by state departments of education, but they are generally not made easily available to prospective consumers. Since the schools already have to compile these data for regulatory entities, they should be readily available, and schools should display them proudly, as evidence of their commitment to education without prejudice.

When considering a program it should be easy to access a simple set of statistics that answer the question, "What is the average length of stay of students in your program, reported in number of years?" The reason I refer to this as a set of statistics is because these data need to be reported in three ways: mean, median, and mode. Any of these could be deceptive alone, but together they are the "givens" which you could use to understand what might be happening in an educational program. Mean, which is derived by adding all the lengths of stay together and dividing by the number of students, is greatly affected by students being removed quickly from the program. For instance, a program could be operating like the program I described above, dismissing challenging students quickly, and hanging on to students who make no problems but also make little developmental progress. Let's imagine a program that is operating like this. If they only reported the mean, it could look like their students stay a reasonable time and get discharged. What actually would be happening however, is that there are a number of students who get discharged immediately, and a number who stay until they age out of the school, with little or no developmental progress. So, in this case, mean is not a measure that tells you all you want to know.

If you add median to the way of describing the average, which is simply the number that falls in the center of the reported numbers, then you get a little more information. In the above example, you may get one of the long-term student's length of stay, or, if there are more students who are ejected quickly, you may get one of the short stays student's length of stay. This number alone does not tell you much, but if you add it to the information about the mean, you can begin to have some understanding of what the program is like. Add in the third way of averaging, and you can tell quite a lot.

Mode is the number that appears most in a data set. In the above school, the mode will be the length of stay that happens the most frequently. If it is one of the low numbers, then you can guess that the average way that the program functions is to exmit students early in their tenure at the school. If it is one of the high numbers, you can guess that they keep students for a long period of time. If you add mode to median and mean, you would have a good idea of how a school treats admissions and exmissions.

Let me give you an example. Let's say a school's mean length of stay is 7.6 years. You might think that this is a school that supports students in their growth, and then exmits them when they have moved developmentally to a point where their appropriate setting is less restrictive. If their median is 17 years, you might then understand the school completely differently. This must be a school with many short-term students, who bring the mean down dramatically. If you then find that the mode is also 17 years you would know that here is a school that tends to hang on to kids for a long time if it can, and who exmits a fairly large number of kids very quickly. They might be behaving in the way I described above.

This is already more data than you would most likely get from most schools, but it is obviously not enough. I propose that you should ask the following question: "How many of the students in your special education program leave the program, at your prompting, to go to less restrictive levels of support, in a different program, not run by you?" In order for this statistic to be on a website, there would have to be a governmental agency auditing it for compliance and for accuracy. Many schools could not honestly answer this question without revealing that their program actually exists for the benefit of the school, and not for the growth of the students. If you find a program that can readily and proudly report this statistic, and it shows that students regularly leave the program before they age out, discharged to a less restrictive environment because of their developmental progress, you should trust that they have the goals of good education at the core of their program.

A school dedicated to appropriate, effective, respectful developmental support will be able to point proudly to their students who have moved up developmentally and been exmitted to less restrictive environment. They will be able to demonstrate, empirically, how the students in their programs are making developmental progress, using valid, reliable measures. If their length of stay is high, they should be able to explain how any given student continues to make developmental progress, and should be able to graph that development. They should be able to show you curricula focused on the support, and development of creative thinking, not just the transmission of facts. They should be able to demonstrate that students do not stop at the level of compliance and the ability to get simple needs met. They should be able to demonstrate that they support students as they grow into the creative problem solvers they were meant to be, so that they can move into society in the freest possible way of their choosing.

Good autism education is just good education, and bad autism education is predicated on the very worst of neurotypical education. There are examples of great schools and other institutions offering effective, appropriate, respectful developmental education to students, but they are rare and valuable. It is possible to avoid the seductive traps set by profitability and the desire for comfort on the part of individuals and systems, but it takes vigilance and oversight. Educators enter the field with a sincere desire to help people, but are thwarted in a thousand ways by the educational industrial complex and profiteers. The goal of this chapter is to alert consumers, as well as educators, to some of the ways to find those schools that deliver what we all want: good education for all students. Nothing less is acceptable.

Treatment of eating disorders of infants diagnosed with autism applying the Mifne method: a clinical case study

11

H.A. Alonim[1,2], *T. Papatheodorou*[3] *and I. Liberman*[4]
[1]The Mifne Center, Treatment, Research, Training, Rosh Pinna, Israel, [2]School of Social Science, Bar Ilan University, Ramat Gan, Israel, [3]Norland College, Bath, United Kingdom, [4]Western Galilee Academic College & Galilee Research Institute, Acre, Israel

Preamble

The following letter was received by the Mifne Center from the mother of an infant displaying eating disorders and diagnosed with suspected autism.

> Dear Mifne
>
> My name is... (name removed). I am 30 years old and my husband... (name removed) is 31. We have twin daughters and the baby Tanya (pseudonym), aged 10 months.
>
> We are contacting you regarding Tanya, and enclose a 45-minute videotape which we made of Tanya. She has a behavioral disorder and an eating disorder. The clinic for eating disorders wants to make us an appointment, and after that another checkup with a Developmental Neurologist. She was 5 months old when we began to realize something was wrong, when she started turning her head from side to side. So we don't know whether Tanya is autistic or not, but in our hearts, we are afraid so. The things bothering us about Tanya are as follows:
>
> 1. Her abnormal head movements (we have been told this might be because of excess fluids, or maybe she does it for self-stimulation). This could be stopped by attracting her attention.
>
> 2. Her heavy breathing and fixing her look in one direction (we have been told that she does it for self-stimulation) and that this could be stopped by attracting her attention.

Emerging Programs for Autism Spectrum Disorder. DOI: https://doi.org/10.1016/B978-0-323-85031-5.00002-5

3. When she is awake, she refuses the bottle. We would feed her by squeezing the nipple of the bottle and squirting milk into her mouth, and this is how she drinks till today.

4. Lately, she moves her eyes upwards or sideways and stares, and when we touch her or interrupt her, she stops it.

Tanya is taken care of by her grandmother during our working hours. We are applying to you for a second opinion, and to help Tanya as long as she is small and it is still possible to make changes according to the principles of your treatment. We cannot sit back and do nothing during these next 3 to 4 months, waiting for an appointment for another test.

Looking forward to hearing from you.

After Tanya's initial assessment by the Mifne clinical team, Tanya and her family were admitted to the Mifne Center. Tanya's case study will be discussed in this paper, in the context of extant literature about ASD and eating disorders, to illustrate the application of the Mifne method and demonstrate its impact on Tanya and the family.

Introduction

The autism spectrum disorder ASD is a neurodevelopmental condition consisting of a wide range of impairments on communication, social, and behavioral aspects (APA, 2013). Children with ASD often show significant sensory processing dysfunction, demonstrated in their social emotional regulation and diverse patterns of interaction; their strong aversion to sensory stimuli resulting in behaviors and coping mechanisms such as isolation and retreat, or repetitive sensory stereotypical behaviors (Mueller & Tronick, 2020). Most of the children also display characteristics of eating disorders, appearing as sensory and behavioral disturbances, and nutrition difficulties are common from the early stages of life of children with ASD (Alonim, 1999, 2010; APA, 2013; Schwarz, 2003). A range of such behaviors have been noticed in Tanya, as outlined in the mother's letter.

Though there are as yet no clear biological markers for ASD, brain and genetic science studies provide strong evidence that there is a transaction between genetic predisposition and environmental factors, which influence the early brain development, when dynamic and significant growth of neurons takes place, creating a web of cells that control sensory–emotional–cognitive regulation (Courchesne et al., 2011; Yirmiya & Charman, 2010). Nutrition is increasingly linked with ASD, included among environmental assaults (such as air pollution and toxins, drugs, medical condition, and medication) and it is being investigated in terms of etiology of ASD and its impact on nutrient sufficiency of infants with ASD displaying eating difficulties and disorders.

Eating disorders, nutrition, and feeding in ASD

Most infants, diagnosed with ASD, display feeding problems and signs of eating disorders from early stages in their life (Alonim, 1999, 2010; Wing, 1987). They also have significantly more medical problems that interfere with food intake such as food allergies and present gastrointestinal problems (Mason-Brothers et al., 1993). Feeding problems range in severity from subclinical levels (such as picky eating, food selectivity, and undereating) to clinical extremes (such as chronic food refusal) that can lead to severe medical conditions (Budd & Chugh, 1998).

It is argued that most of the eating problems in children with ASD may be due to sensory and motor impairment and learned behavior (Schwarz, 2003). Children with autism often manifest sensory hypersensitivity and poor motor control, which may lead them to restrict the textures of food eaten (Ahearn, 2001; Prontnicki, 1995; Williams, Dalrymple, & Neal, 2000). Children with severe motor impairment and almost all children with severe speech problems also experience some degree of difficulty in feeding (Sullivan et al., 2000). Infants, who later develop eating problems, often present feeding difficulties or even reject food while being breastfed. Difficulties include abnormal sucking reflex, rejection of breast feeding, refusal to eat, and difficulty in swallowing. Many children are also afraid of the food disappearing when they swallow it. This is a sense that cannot be contained and may cause feelings of guilt and anxiety that may spread to other areas of functioning (Alonim, 1999; Alonim et al., 2007).

Environmental factors such as lack of exposure to developmentally appropriate food and age-appropriate social exchanges, limited opportunities to model appropriate mealtimes, and/or mismanagement of feeding problems might maintain and/or reinforce further eating disorders and make it difficult for a child to maintain a nutritionally adequate diet (Babbitt et al., 1994; Cornish, 1998; Raiten & Massaro, 1986; Whitely, Rodgers, & Shattock, 2000; Williams et al., 2000). Certain behaviors that occur during mealtimes (e.g., crying, screaming, agitated behavior, aggressive and disruptive behavior) can interfere with food consumption further (Ahearn, 2001; Luiselli, 1989). Furthermore, families with restrictive diets may reinforce and maintain negative feeding patterns (Cumine, Leach, & Stevenson, 2000).

The impact of ASD on family

Feeding problems or refusal to eat intensify parental concerns and worries regarding undernutrition, dehydration, health problems, and even hospitalization. As a result, eating becomes a battle ground with parents giving in, allowing their child to eat preferred food, in preferred ways and places, as is evident in Tanya's case. This however reinforces further such eating habits (Alonim, 2010). The pressure and tension created impact on the child, influence their siblings, and bring about disequilibrium in family life.

During the first weeks of life, in which the baby regulates himself physically and emotionally, the mother–baby interaction reveals intricate sensitivities that have significance for the baby's reflective perception. The mother's emotional availability provides a matrix for the growth of the baby, as she picks up the signals that the baby transmits, and these constitute the basis for communication. However, an overanxious mother is not emotionally available to react constructively to the baby's signals. Her anxiety may transmit a message of threat, against which the baby has to construct defense mechanisms. In such a situation, there is a lack of synchronization (Alonim, 2013; Trevarthen, 2007).

The lack of synchronization, when escalated, forms a sort of a vicious circle: the baby does not respond to the mother's (or any family member's) attempts for interaction which, in turn, being interpreted as rejection and/or failure, may accentuate their emotional state, leading to responses that may be perceived by the baby as a threat. These early interactions and experiences, however, are critical in brain development and formation, especially during the first 2 years of life (Bauman, 1999).

This situation accentuates further parents' anxiety, as it evident in the letter written by Tanya's mother. It increases fear and confusion that is often compound by a sense of guilt, failure, and shame (Alonim, 2010). Parents of children with autism have to cope with additional pressures like deficiency in emotional and social mutuality, lack of verbal or social feedback (Salazar, 2020). In the course of the years, many of these families undergo a significant rise in depression and anxiety and the increased difficulties they experience impact on the quality of life of a family and ability to cope with the situation (Minuchin, 1978; Friedrich & Friedrich, 1981; Raiten & Massaro, 1986; Luiselli, 1989; Mason-Brothers et al., 1993; Prontnicki, 1995; Schwarz, 2003; Massie, 2007; Siman-Tov, 2009; Pierce et al., 2011; Mueller & Tronick, 2020; Salazar, 2020), a situation clearly evident in Tanya's case.

Thus addressing the psychological needs and functioning of the family, especially in the early stages of diagnosis of autism, becomes crucial and equally as important the treatment of autism. Historically, treatment methods took an atomistic approach, focusing on behavior management, but a paradigm shift is underway from working with the child to working with the family as a unit seeking equilibrium at all levels of relationships within the family (Salazar, 2020).

The Mifne method

The Mifne method is derived from Bowlby's (1969) attachment theory and Minuchin's (1978) family systems theory, and it is based on the principles of the biopsychosocial model (Engel, 1980). The basic underlying concept of the therapeutic model is the view that the family is an organic unit. No matter what the etiology is, ASD affects the whole family. Therefore the Mifne method identifies the infant, the parents, and, in a broader sense, the nuclear family, as the focal point for treatment. The program addresses the particular needs of the infant, diagnosed with autism, and each member of the family. The therapeutic environment attempts to encourage gradual evolution of the infant and each family member, toward individual and mutual growth. A unique aspect of the Mifne method is its application to the treatment of eating disorders of infants.

The Mifne method's underlying assumption is that learning, development, and socialization are functions of contact in early infancy (Winnicott, 1965). An infant with autism has a different understanding of his environment, which might pick up only part of the information around him and cause him to develop an unclear perception of his world (Alonim et al., 2007). An unclear situation is very frightening for a baby, especially if he is very sensitive. Most of the infants with autism are oversensitive, and carry fears (Alonim, 2013).

The Mifne method is a residential program with a duration of 3 weeks. Each family at the Mifne Center has an individual therapy program. It consists of two major components: (1) the infant treatment through reciprocal play therapy (RPT); and (2) the family therapy, briefly outlined below.

Infant treatment through reciprocal play therapy

The aim of the RPT, developed at Mifne, is to reinforce the infant's innate abilities, and their self-confidence, by means of enjoying and experiencing interactive play within a containing and supportive environment. It enables the infant to discover the sense of the self and the pleasure of human contact. RPT takes place in the therapy room, where the infant spends 8 hours daily with therapists, who alternate during the day, and the parents. RPT consists of attractive play, sensory play, emotional play, and cognitive play.

Family therapy

The work with parents is aimed at enabling them to broaden their ability to achieve an insight into themselves, to understand their own behavior as an outcome of the way they perceive themselves as individuals, and of their role as parents. In working with parents, the Mifne approach uses a variety of techniques; clinical meetings, individual and joint couple meetings, family sessions, feedback, and team consultation with the parents. Each parent is given the opportunity to reach insights into how they and their baby affect one another and to gain an insight into the attachment relationship between mother and infant, father and infant, mother and father, and the structure of the family as a whole.

The program addresses the particular needs of each family member and is designed to match their infant's developmental stage. Family therapy aims to give the family the opportunity to reflect upon themselves and their special infant, to get a better understanding of his and their needs and to be able to consider each step of their infant's treatment.

Monitoring and evaluation of the Mifne program

The treatment program is systematically monitored and evaluated through:

1. An initial assessment of the infant's level of attachment, level of eye contact, level of eating habits. The infant's functioning is rated at four levels: low, mild, moderate, and high.
2. The therapist's clinical reports, where the therapists record their observations at the end of each therapy session with the infant.
3. The Daily Evaluation Scale of Observation, which is completed by each therapist at the end of their session with the infant, to rate their functioning, on a scale 0–10, across four developmental areas, that is, engagement, play, communication, and functioning.
4. The summative Daily Evaluation Scale of Observation which is completed at the end of each day by the therapists by reviewing their clinical reports, the video recordings of RPT and their individual completion of Daily Evaluation Scale of Observation. The summative Daily Evaluation Scale of Observation are analyzed to evaluate the progress made at the end of first, second, and third week of treatment.
5. Parents self-assessment before and on completion of the Mifne treatment program across five dimensions: parents' interrelationship, parental confidence, parental overprotection, parental stress, and parental crisis.
6. Records of weekly meetings of the therapists with parents, when they review the infant's and their own progress.

(For further details about the Mifne program, see Alonim, Lieberman, Tayar, Scheigesicht, & Braude, 2020.)

With parental consent the RPT treatment is recorded, as it happens, and data is collected to evaluate the progress made by the child.

Tanya's treatment at Mifne Center

In this section, we discuss Tanya's and her family's therapy process and its impact on both Tanya and the family. We start by outlining the initial parental concerns about Tanya's development and eating, the assessment of Tanya's, and parental and family functioning. We then discuss the findings from qualitative and quantitative measures and their impact on Tanya and the family.

Parents' concerns about Tanya's development before treatment

In the letter sent to Mifne by Tanya's mother, the parents were concerned about their daughter's complicated development, but mainly about her refusal to eat. In a further interview with the parents, it was revealed that Tanya did not feel hunger and was unaware of the tastes and textures of different foodstuffs. Tanya used to be fed while she was asleep. After she had fallen asleep in their arms, her parents would feed her formula from a bottle, so she was not aware she was eating. The mother never let Tanya cry, because she could not bear it. She said she could not cope with the child feeling miserable. Prior to being admitted to the Mifne Center,

Tanya was referred to a Children's Developmental Unit in the Hospital, where she received a diagnosis of *Suspected Autism.*

Assessment of Tanya's development and functioning

The Mifne clinical team assessed Tanya's functioning by analyzing the home video recordings across three criteria, that is, (1) level of attachment, (2) level of eye contact, and (3) level of eating habits. These criteria were assessed at four levels: low, mild, moderate, and high. Tanya's functioning was assessed at low level across all three criteria. The assessment showed that, although Tanya was 12 months old, she was functioning like a 4–5-month-old baby. She avoided eye contact, her body was rigid and tense, and her fists were clenched. She did not react to tickling and did not smile; her face was screwed up unhappily. She did not like to be held or hugged by her parents or anyone else and recoiled from the touch of soft objects (such as furry animals, velvet or woolly material). She usually became very tense and stiff when picked up and held. She expressed her willingness or unwillingness by crying or whimpering. She would throw out her arms in a pushing or rejecting motion, when she did not want something. She expressed her lack of satisfaction or tiredness by turning over or lying on her back. Tanya displayed various repetitive behaviors, including moving her limbs, rolling her eyes in circle movements, or her head from side to side. She mostly uttered sounds of crying and shouting. She showed she wanted to eat by falling asleep in her mother's arms to be fed while she slept.

Assessment of parental and family functioning

On arrival at Mifne Center, the parents met with two senior psychologists for an assessment of their relationship and family functioning. The meetings consisted of a three-part process. Initially the parents provided a free report on their situation, then responded to a series of questions raised by the psychologists, and finally they provided a self-assessment of their situation across five categories, that is, (1) parents' interrelationships, (2) parents' confidence, (3) parents' overprotection, (4) parents' stress, and (5) parents' crisis. The self-assessment was made at four levels of functioning, namely, low, moderate, mild, and low. The assessment revealed a family in crisis. Parental confidence was low and parental overprotection high, parental stress and parental crisis were at moderate level, while parental interrelationships were assessed at mild level.

Both parents are gentle and sensitive people. The father is an introverted, "down to earth," concrete and practical person, while the mother is the dominant figure and the leader in the family. The mother is strict with their daughters, who are afraid of her reactions; the father is easier and more flexible with them. This is often a cause of conflict between the couple. For both parents, unresolved issues from childhood unconsciously impacted on their coping mechanism. As a coping mechanism, the father resorted into withdrawing and keeping busy with video games. Neither of the parents went out much. Both of them convey a sense of closeness on the one hand, and yet loneliness on the other. The couple instantly realized that this was an opportunity to treat the entire family situation, apart from the treatment of Tanya, and they were open and ready for this.

Family therapy at Mifne Center

Tanya's treatment through reciprocal play therapy

Tanya's treatment started with RPT in the treatment room. The treatment room is quiet and relaxed space, free of external high sensory stimulation. During the treatment, there were many opportunities for intimacy by means of massage, play, and body contact. At the beginning of treatment, an agreement was made with Tanya's parents that she would no longer be fed in her sleep. Food would only be provided during her waking hours only.

Tanya's treatment and progress as recorded in the therapists' daily clinical reports

The therapist's clinical reports provide a picture of the treatment process and Tanya's gradual progress, during and on completion of the treatment program, across various behaviors of the ASD. These are briefly discussed below.

Eating: habits and amount of food—In the initial days, Tanya was offered her bottle of formula when she was awake. She refused to eat or rejected it, accompanied by retching. After 4 days, one of the therapists sat her on her lap and placed a small amount of the familiar pudding mixed with nonfruit flavoring on her lips. The food was put into Tanya's mouth only when she opened it and showed willingness to eat. Tanya gradually began to eat from the therapist's finger. Her menu was gradually enlarged to include blended vegetables, and soft porridge. At the same time, Tanya was placed on a chair with her head on the same level as that of the therapist. The aim of this process was to increase Tanya's awareness of eating. Tanya began to take food from a spoon. She looked from the spoon to the therapist's eyes, and the eye contact was intense and showed an awareness of the feeling of hunger. During the course of treatment, there was an improvement in Tanya's ability to bite, chew, and swallow. A few days before the end of treatment, she began to touch the mashed food. She showed an interest in the cookie she was given, held it in her hand and after playing with it for a while, tasted it.

Eye contact, facial and emotional expressions—As Tanya's confidence and her sense of security with the therapists grew, her eye contact with them gradually increased, too. In meetings with the parents, the mother reported a significant increase in Tanya's eye contact with her, when playing together.

Acceptance and reaction to people and objects—A week after their arrival at the Mifne Center, Tanya held out her arms for her parents to pick her up. When her father picked her up and held her close to him, hugging her, she gradually stayed in this position for quite a long time, feeling more comfortable and relaxed. During the first days, Tanya recoiled from the touch of soft objects. In spite of this, these objects were offered to her from time to time. She gradually became interested in them; she became curious about simple objects and interested to try out what was offered to her. She started to develop preferences for different types of games by examining them.

Curiosity, concentration, initiative in play—During treatment, Tanya was put down on her stomach on the floor of the playroom and was gradually exposed to various toys such as balls, boxes, bottles, soft toys, bells and rattles, and to tactile material such as rustling paper, sand, water and soap, and body lotion. At first, Tanya lay on her stomach, looked at the toys with interest, paid attention to the sounds made, followed the objects with her eyes, made sounds, and gurgled. Tanya gradually began to move toward the toy that interested her. As treatment continued, Tanya discovered the possibilities offered by play. She showed the ability to understand a game. For example, when a therapist put rings on a tower one after another, Tanya lifted them off. After a few days Tanya started to display initiative. She pulled interesting objects towards herself and also tried to reach them on her own, pulling herself on her tummy. During the third week she mostly initiated interactions with the therapist by reaching out to her.

Vocal sounds and speech sounds—During the first week Tanya mostly uttered sounds of crying and shouting. During the second week a change set in; she uttered more frequently sounds of joy. During the third week Tanya began not only to express joy, but also to utter vowel sounds as well as a few syllables.

Repetitive behavior—During the first week Tanya displayed various repetitive behaviors, including moving her limbs, and eyes from side to side. In the second week, she only displayed one repetitive pattern: playing with her fingers. During the third week she did so rarely and no other repetitive behaviors were observed.

Physical contact and detachment—During treatment, the therapists would massage and stroke her face and other parts of her body either gently or roughly. As contact became established and Tanya felt more secure with the therapists, she increasingly enjoyed the physical touch and she expanded the variety of expressions for intimacy and body contact. After 10 days, the therapist taught Tanya how to turn into a sitting position. When Tanya began to sit up, she enjoyed this new situation; she had a better and wider view of her surroundings, which affected the way she played. She let the therapists pick her up in their arms and move around with her in the room, dancing and jumping. Following her increasing confidence in the therapists, she began to enjoy being rocked and swayed. As Tanya's skills and functioning increased her level of detachment gradually decreased.

Tanya's progress—findings from the summative daily evaluation scale of observation

Tanya's progress reported in the therapists' clinical reports is further supported by descriptive analysis of data, collected through the *Daily Evaluation Scale of Observation* over the 3 weeks of treatment, 22 days in total. Table 11.1 shows that, at the completion of the treatment, there was improvement across a range of

Table 11.1 Means, standard deviations, and overall progress of treatment for selected variables (N:22 days).

	First week		Second week		Third week[a]		Progress[b]
	Mean	SD	Mean	SD	Mean	SD	
Acceptance	0.71	0.76	2.86	0.90	5.38	0.74	6.0
Detachment	6.00	0.58	4.86	0.38	3.25	0.71	−4.0
Physical contact	1.29	0.49	3.00	0.82	5.38	0.74	5.0
Eye contact	0.71	0.76	2.29	0.49	3.63	0.52	4.0
Sounds	2.43	0.53	5.57	0.53	6.00	0.00	3.0
Initiative	0.29	0.49	2.00	0.00	3.50	0.53	4.0
Eating: habits	0.93	0.67	2.50	0.50	4.06	0.42	4.0
Eating: amount	1.14	0.90	3.14	0.70	5.38	0.52	4.0
Repetitive behavior	0.93	0.67	2.43	0.45	4.06	0.42	−4.5

[a]Calculated on the basis of the average on all the days of treatment beyond the second week.
[b]The value noted, either a positive or a negative, indicates the difference between the average score on the first and the last day of treatment.

symptoms of ASD. Attachment underwent the greatest change, followed by physical contact, reduced repetitive behaviors, and reduced detachment. Eating (habits and amount and food consumed), eye contact, and initiative also showed progress at similar rate. The least improvement was recorded on sound production. The progress observed across these behaviors is visually represented in Fig. 11.1. It can be seen that there is steep and consistent decrease of detachment and repetitive behaviors as other behaviors improve, during the 3 weeks of treatment.

Nonparametric statistical analysis, Spearman Rho, revealed strong ($r > 0.90$) and significant correlations between a range of symptoms of the ASD. In relation to eating (habits and amounts of food consumed), there is a positive correlation with eye contact, initiative, and physical contact and a strong inverse correlations ($r > 0.90$) of eating habits and eating amount with repetitive patterns ($r = -0.941$, and $r = -0.903$, respectively) and detachment ($r = -0.982$, and $r = -0.946$, respectively). The correlation is lower but still strong between eating habits and speech sounds ($r = 0.830$). Whilst the correlation of these variables does not denote cause and effect, the triangulation of qualitative (Table 11.2) and quantitative (Table 11.1) findings are indicative of the impact of treating eating disorders on the improvement of other symptoms of ASD.

Family therapy

Family therapy started by addressing the key challenges and needs faced by each member of the family. The focus of the family therapy for the mother was to address her guilt and fear about Tanya. When Tanya refused to eat, the mother felt guilty because she thought that she failed her daughter. The therapy sessions intended to help the mother to differentiate between Tanya's desire to eat and her

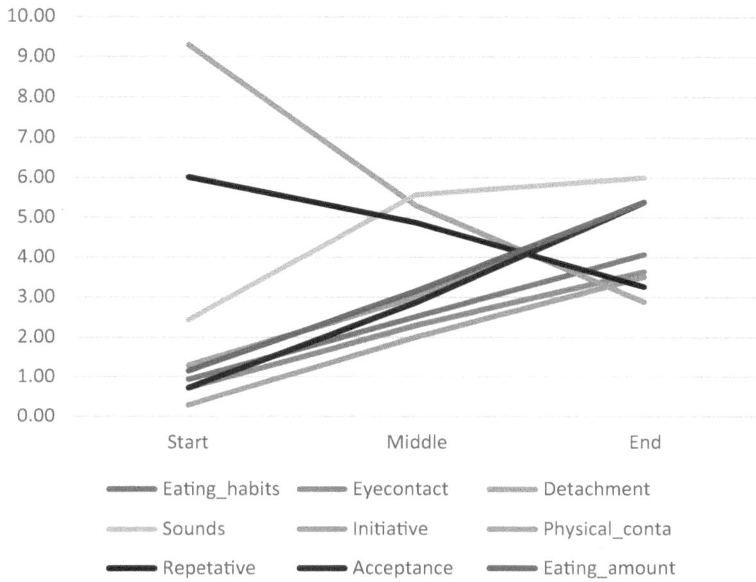

Figure 11.1 Visual representation of the progress made at the end of the first, second, and third week of treatment (22 days).

own sense of success or failure. The feedback sessions of the psychologists with the father dealt mostly with his passivity in the spousal relationship and how he could support his wife not only by expressing how he felt towards her, but in actual fact. The husband was aware of his wife's feelings of guilt and expressed empathy and support for her, saying "We are both in the same boat and we'll overcome this together." However, he was also aware that his wife was a strong and determined person and he took a passive stance in their relationship. The parents had the chance to communicate with each of the older daughters individually to understand their needs and talk about their relationships with them, an emotional aspect of which had previously been lacking.

Family progress during and on completion of family treatment

From the psychologists' reports and parents' own feedback during weekly meetings, it was evident that as family therapy progressed, the parents' couplehood improved. The mother became much gentler, more flexible, and begun to see and treat her husband as a partner. The father became more engaged with his family and got out of his withdrawing and isolating activities. With the flexibility they adopted as a result of the therapy, both parents were capable of continuing to stimulate Tanya's development. The mother underwent a process of learning how to get closer to her daughter, to enjoy being with her daughter, and was able to stay with her longer. She learnt to hug Tanya and not only when she cried. She also learnt that crying

Table 11.2 Spearman correlations matrix between variables and eating habits (n of session = 22).

	Eating habits	Eating amount	Eye contact	Sounds	Initiative	Physical contact	Repetitive	Detachment
Eating_amount	0.996**							
Eye contact	0.967**	0.960**						
Sounds	0.837**	0.841**	0.820**					
Initiative	0.962**	0.962**	0.949**	0.838**				
Physical contact	0.975**	0.970**	0.967**	0.858**	0.970**			
Repetitive	−0.955**	−0.949**	−0.974**	−0.813**	−0.958**	−0.954**		
Detachment	−0.989**	−0.981**	−0.978**	−0.865**	−0.958**	−0.977**	0.960**	
Acceptance	0.976**	0.971**	0.981**	0.855**	0.964**	0.984**	−0.964**	−0.988**

**$P < .001$.

Table 11.3 Parental and family function before and after treatment at Mifne Center.

Parental/family functioning	Beginning of treatment	End of treatment
Parents' overprotection	*H*	*Mo*
Parents' relationship	*Mo*	*H*
Parents' confidence	*L*	*Mo*
Parents' stress	*Mo*	*L*
Parents' crisis	*Mo*	*L*

Rating: *L*, low; *M*, mild; *Mo*, moderate; *H*, high.

does not necessarily express unhappiness, and that Tanya is able to cope with crying. She started increasingly to provide Tanya with challenges.

The father experienced a real connection with Tanya for the first time. In the past, he felt that Tanya ignored him and he was afraid of her. He thought she did not understand and so he never spoke to her. In the wake of many hours of treatment and their staying together for many hours in a family atmosphere, he began to get to know her better. He started to initiate contact with her and became very excited when she let him hug and kiss her. He became very gentle and kind to her. He said that Tanya was beginning to feel more secure and more open with him. The way he became closer to Tanya and also in the end succeeded in feeding her gently, gave them both a great deal of confidence.

The final parental self-assessment of the progress made during therapy showed that parental overprotection was reduced from a high to moderate level, while parental level of stress and crisis were also reduced from moderate to low levels. Parental confidence increased from low to moderate level and their relationship improved from moderate to high level (Table 11.3).

Family follow-up by the Mifne clinical team

Initial follow-up communication of the Mifne clinical team and the parents revealed that Tanya was doing well, and the girls played a lot with her. However, the parents were in conflict regarding the setting of limits. There seemed to be tension between them, as the mother gave in to Tanya. She was afraid of losing the contact she had made with her daughter. She had gone from extreme strictness to giving in too easily.

Further communication confirmed that parental conflicts about their interaction with Tanya reduced. The parents were amazed at Tanya's abilities and her progress. They highlighted that "she stays on her feet for a minute; has high-level eye contact; when visitors come in, she looks at them, holding out her arms and she crawls to the door to see who is coming. All is well where eating is concerned; she eats everything we offer her." The father had chosen to stay at home with his daughter for a few months and helped her make progress. By the age of 18 months, Tanya was able to close the developmental gap between herself and her peer group.

Conclusion

Infants' relationships with the world are mediated via their mouths (Winnicott, 1965). In the initial months of life, representing the neurophysiological regulation stage, feeding is a central factor in the infant's ability to regulate himself. A lack of regulation lies indeed at the root of ASD pathology (Courchesne et al., 2011; Yirmiya & Charman, 2010). Contact and communication are integral components of the regulation process. Owing to the primal instinct of the need to eat and the elements of communication it involves, basic anxieties are channeled into this need, which may spread to other areas of functioning (Alonim et al., 2007).

Tanya's assessment by the clinical team at Mifne Center concurred with the diagnosis of suspected autism, conducted at the Children's Developmental Unit in the Hospital. Tanya displayed a wide range of behaviors at social, emotional, and communication developmental areas, including severe eating disorders. The latter were linked with sensory difficulties and associated with eating habits reinforced by parental concerns of inadequate food intake.

According to the findings of this case study, obtained via the qualitative and quantitative instruments, the more Tanya became willing to eat, the more interest she displayed in her surroundings, increasing her level of attachment. Both qualitative and quantitative measures have shown that, at the end of the treatment, there was improvement across developmental areas to varying degrees. From the descriptive statistics, the greatest improvement was revealed in increasing acceptance of people and physical touch and at the same time reducing detachment and repetitive behaviors. Further, parametric statics revealed strong correlation of eating disorders (habits and amount of food) across various symptoms of the ASD. Whilst correlation between variables does not indicate cause and effect, the fact that the treatment focused on Tanya's eating disorders and on the basis of triangulation of qualitative and quantitative data, it is reasonable to argue that (1) as eating improved, a parallel improvement was observed in other symptoms of ASD; (2) family therapy was equally important; as the findings at the conclusion of the treatment and posttreatment reports have shown, shared parental understanding and responsibilities, and family cohesion brought about long-term changes in the family dynamics and functioning that strengthened Tanya's capabilities.

Consistent with previous research (Alonim, 2004; Alonim et al., 2020; Massie, 2007; Pierce et al., 2011), this case study has demonstrated that treatment at the early stages of life is crucial in improving an infant's functioning in other related developmental areas, while a family oriented and focused treatment minimizes stresses that ensures long-term improvement. In the wake of the support provided by the findings of this study, we may say that there is an association between the breakthrough in the infant's eating patterns and her ability to respond to her caregivers, to develop contact and social communication in a less stressful environment, stresses that ensures long-term improvement.

References

Ahearn, W. H. (2001). *Help! My son eats only macaroni and cheese: Dealing with feeding problems in children with autism. Making a difference: Behavioural intervention for autism* (pp. 51–73). Austin, TX: PRO-ED, Inc.

Alonim, A. (2010). *Investigation of family therapy and treatment of children's eating disorders employed by Mifne intervention program for young children with autism* (Ph.D. thesis). Chelmsford: Anglia Ruskin University.

Alonim, A., Lieberman, I., Tayar, D., Scheigesicht, G., & Braude, H. D. (2020). A comparative spectrum infants and toddlers treated with The Mifne Approach intervention for Autism Disorder. In U. Das, N. Papaneophytou, & T. El-Kour (Eds.), *Autism 360°*. London: Elsevier.

Alonim, A. H. (1999). *Eating disorders in autism.* A paper presented at a conference at Bar Ilan University, Tel-Aviv (Hebrew).

Alonim, A. H. (2004). The Mifne method. *Journal of Child & Adolescence Mental Health, 16*(1), 39–43.

Alonim, A. H., In Acquarone, S., Crespin, G., Danon-Boileau, L., Maestro, S., Massie, H., ... Trevarthen, C. (2007). *Signs of autism in infants. Infants at risk – Early signs of autism* (pp. 118–138). London: Karnac Books.

Alonim, H. A. (2013). Commentary on "The protest of a 6-month-old girl: Is this a prodrome of autism?". *Journal of Infant, Child and Adolescent Psychotherapy, 12*(3), 156–163.

APA. (2013). *Diagnostic and statistical manual of mental disorders* (5th ed.). Arlington, VA: Author.

Babbitt, R. L., Hoch, T. A., Coe, D. A., Cataldo, M. F., Kelly, K. J., Stackhouse, C., & Perman, J. A. (1994). Behavioral assessment and treatment of pediatric feeding disorders. *Developmental and Behavioral Pediatric, 15*(4), 278–291.

Bauman, M. (1999). Autism: Clinical features and neurobiological observations. In H. Tager-Flusberg (Ed.), *Neurodevelopmental disorders* (pp. 383–399). Cambridge, MA: MIT Press.

Bowlby, J. (1969). Attachment and loss*: Vol. 1.* Attachment. London: Hogarth Press and Institute of Psycho-Analysis.

Budd, K. S., & Chugh, C. S. (1998). Common feeding problems in young children. *Advances in Clinical Child Psychology, 20*, 183–212.

Cornish, E. A. (1998). Balanced approach towards healthy eating in autism. *Journal of Human Nutrition and Dietetics, 11*(6), 501–509.

Courchesne, E., Mouton, P. R., Calhoun, M. E., Semendeferi, K., Ahrens-Barbeau, C., Hallet, M. J., ... Pierce, K. (2011). Neuron number and size in prefrontal cortex of children with autism. *Journal of the American Medical Association, 306*(18), 2001–2010.

Cumine, V., Leach, j, & Stevenson, G. (2000). *Autism in the early years.* London: David Fulton.

Engel, G. L. (1980). The clinical application of the biopsychosocial model. *American Journal of Psychiatry, 137*(5), 535–544.

Friedrich, W. N., & Friedrich, W. L. (1981). Psychosocial assets of parents of handicapped and nonhandicapped children. *American Journal of Mental Deficiency, 85*, 551–553.

Luiselli, J. K. (1989). Behavioural assessment and treatment of paediatric feeding disorders in developmental disabilities. *Progress in Behaviour Modification, 24*, 91–131.

Mason-Brothers, A., Ritvo, E. R., Freeman, B. J., Jorde, L. B., Pingree, C. C., McMahon, W. M., ... Mo, A. (1993). The UCLA-University of Utah epidemiological survey of autism: Recurrent infections. *Journal of European Child & Adolescent Psychiatry*, *2*(2), 79–90.

Massie, H. (2007). The prodromal phase of autism and outcome of early treatment. In S. Acquarone (Ed.), *Signs of autism in infants: Recognition and early intervention* (pp. 1–17). London: Karnac.

Minuchin, S. (1978). *Families and family therapy*. Cambridge, MA: Harvard University Press.

Mueller, I., & Tronick, E. (2020). Sensory processing and meaning making in autism spectrum disorder. In U. Das, N. Papaneophytou, & T. El-Kour (Eds.), *Autism 360°*. London: Elsevier.

Pierce, K., Weinfeld, M., Desmond, J., Hazin, R., Bjork, R., & Gallagher, N. (2011). Detecting, studying, and treating autism early: The one-year well-baby check-up approach. *Journal of Pediatrics*, *159*(3), 458–465, e6.

Prontnicki, J. (1995). Presentation: Symptomatology and etiology of dysphagia. In S. Rosenthal, J. J. Sheppard, & M. Lotze (Eds.), *Dysphagia and the child with developmental disabilities: Medical, clinical, and family interventions* (pp. 1–14). San Diego, CA: Singular Publishing Group.

Raiten, D. J., & Massaro, T. (1986). Perspectives on the nutritional ecology of autistic children. *Journal of Autism and Developmental Disorders*, *16*(2), 133–143.

Salazar, R. M. (2020). Full circle autism care includes family relationships and dynamics. In U. Das, N. Papaneophytou, & T. El-Kour (Eds.), *Autism 360°*. London: Elsevier.

Schwarz, S. M. (2003). Feeding disorders in children with developmental disabilities. *Infants and Young Children*, *16*, 317–330.

Siman-Tov, A. (2009). *Construction and validation of a model for variables related to the adjustment among parents of a child with autism* (Ph.D. thesis). Israel: Bar-Ilan University.

Sullivan, P. B., Lambert, B., Rose, M., Ford-Adams, M., Johnson, A., & Griffiths, P. (2000). Prevalence and severity of feeding and nutritional problems in children with neurological impairment: Oxford Feeding Study. *Developmental Medicine and Child Neurology*, *42*, 674–680.

Trevarthen, C. (2007). Signs of autism in infancy: Sensitivity for rhythms of expression in communication. In S. Acquarone (Ed.), *Recognition and early intervention* (pp. 21–45). London: Karnac Books.

Whitely, P., Rodgers, J., & Shattock, P. (2000). Commentary: Feeding patterns in autism. *Autism: The International Journal of Research and Practice*, *4*(2), 207–211.

Williams, P. G., Dalrymple, N., & Neal, J. (2000). Eating habits of children with autism. *Pediatric Nursing*, *26*(3), 259–264.

Wing, L. (1987). Feeding problems in autism. *Communication*, *21*, 7–9.

Winnicott, D. W. (1965). *The maturational process and the facilitating environment*. London: Hogarth.

Yirmiya, N., & Charman, T. (2010). The prodrome of autism: Early behavioral and biological signs, regression, peri- and post-natal development and genetics. *The Journal of Child Psychology and Psychiatry*, *51*(4), 432–458.

Applied behavior analysis and verbal behavior interventions in children with autism spectrum disorder and associated learning difficulties

12

Chafica Mansour Gharbieh[1,2,3,4,5] *and Sammy Gharbieh Isabella*[6,7,8,9]
[1]Education & ABA/VB Consultant, Lebanese International University, Beirut, Lebanon, [2]Autism Learning Institute for Applied Behaviour Analysis "ALI for ABA", Lebanese International University, Beirut, Lebanon, [3]Diagnostic Lebanese Centre for Training, Communication & Behaviour Development, Lebanese International University, Beirut, Lebanon, [4]Education and Development Committee for Arab Network for Autism "ANA", Lebanese International University, Beirut, Lebanon, [5]Lebanese International University "LIU", Lebanese International University, Beirut, Lebanon, [6]Biomedical Sciences, University of Greenwich, London, United Kingdom, [7]Nutritional Medicine, Surrey University, London, United Kingdom, [8]Bachelor of Medicine and Bachelor of Surgery, Kings College, London, United Kingdom, [9]Nutrition Consultant for ALI for ABA, London, United Kingdom

Introduction

Autism Spectrum Disorder (ASD) is a development disability defined by deficits in social interaction and communication and the presence of restricted, repetitive patterns of behavior, interests, or activities that may persist throughout life (American Psychiatric Association, 2013). Autism exists with any level of intelligence, but many individuals with autism suffer also from learning disability (O'Brien & Pearson, 2004). With medical therapies mainly being supportive in nature, behavioral interventions are currently the mainstay of ASD and associated learning difficulties management. Behavioral interventions encapsulate three distinct but relatable fields: philosophy of the science (i.e., behaviorism), basic experimental research (i.e., experimental analysis of behavior), and applied research (i.e., applied behavior analysis) (Dillenburger & Keenan, 2009). In particular, the Applied Behavior Analysis and Verbal Behavior (ABA/VB) approach has largely been adopted to induce behavior change and is now one of the most widely used interventions for ASD (Dillenburger & Keenan, 2009).

ABA is based on the principles of "operant conditioning," which aims to foster "positive" behaviors and prevent "negative" behaviors (Cooper, Heron, & Heward, 2007).

Emerging Programs for Autism Spectrum Disorder. DOI: https://doi.org/10.1016/B978-0-323-85031-5.00032-3

This is achieved by applying specific phenomena such as functional behavior assessment and reinforcement strategies (Foxx, 2008). The "function" of a behavior is the desirable outcome that a behavior produces, which then causes the behavior to persist (Foxx, 2008; Hanley, Iwata, & McCord, 2003). Reinforcement strategies then involve providing the desired rewards following a positive behavior, to increase the likelihood that the behavior will occur again (Foxx, 2008). Rewards are also provided when the targeted behavior is not displayed within a predetermined period of time, a strategy known as "differential" reinforcement (Tassé, Havercamp, & Lecavalier, 2002). Correspondingly, the concept of "extinction" involves withholding the reinforcer if the negative behavior occurs (Tassé et al., 2002). Combined, these efforts can generate significant changes in behavior which, overall, appear to be valuable in ASD.

Despite findings that long-term ABA interventions lead to positive effects in multiple domains of behavior (Reichow & Wolery, 2009), there is still debate about the ideal intensity of the program, with some studies suggesting that 40 hours a week are needed in order to achieve the best outcomes (Mohammad Zaheri, Koegel, Rezaee, & Rafiee, 2014). Eldevik, Hastings, and Hughes (2009) indicated that a high treatment intensity was the only variable that independently predicted IQ and adaptive gains. These findings are important, as the success of such interventions must be feasible, accessible, and cost-efficient for families and carers of children affected. Therefore the aims of this study were threefold: (1) to evaluate the use of the ABA/VB approach as a comprehensive means of managing core and associated ASD features; (2) to assess the long-term efficacy of such an approach; and (3) to evaluate levels of parental stress throughout the intervention.

Methods

Participants

Participants were referred to the center, at the Autism Learning Institute for Applied Behavior Analysis (ALI for ABA) in Ain Anoub, Lebanon. Each participant had a verified diagnosis of ASD based on the criteria of the Diagnostic and Statistical Manual Fifth Edition (DSM 5) from a licensed professional prior to referral. The study enrolled 10 children, aged 4–7 years.

- Every child accepted by the center would already have a diagnosis of autism. As part of ALI for ABA teaching system, every child has an Individual Education Plan (IEP), which links with the national curriculum. Each child's teaching program involves breaking down tasks into learnable elements and teaching them until mastery is achieved.
- The child is constantly rewarded for desired behaviors with systematic use of positive reinforcement, praise, and positive pairing techniques.
- Each element of the teaching process is continuously charted and assessed. This enables staff to identify strengths and weaknesses and to help the child progress in a positive and targeted direction.

There were two classes at the ALI for ABA Center, five children in each class, which made up the sample for this study. Each class has two teachers and one assistant. All 10 children have the diagnosis of autism. The following is a brief summary of the children:

Ali A: Ali A was a 6-year-old boy (at intake) diagnosed with autism with a moderate level of disability, Ali has two brothers, and they are typically developing children. Ali's parents are both educated with Baccalaureate. There is a history of mental retardation and speech delay in Ali's family. As for his behavior, he engages in self-stimulatory behaviors such as flapping hands, and flickering fingers. He is aggressive towards himself and others. As for his medical history, Ali did not suffer any of the childhood illnesses. He was not breastfed. As for his diet, he has an excess of sugar, artificial sweeteners, dairy meat, and wheat products. As for his language, Ali is a nonverbal child (uses few sounds and few meaningful words), he requests his needs by crying or sometimes by pulling hands and leading adults to the desired items. His language skills were characterized as being severely delayed. As for his development history, he walked at the age of 14 months. Ali is toilet trained. Ali had received psychomotor and speech therapy since the age of 3.

Ali G: Ali G was a 5-year-old boy (at intake) diagnosed with autism with a moderate level of disability. Ali has two siblings, and they are typically developing children. Ali's parents are both educated with Baccalaureate. There is no history of mental retardation or speech delay in Ali's family. As for his behavior, he engages in self-stimulatory behaviors such as mouthing objects, throwing objects on the floor in repetitive manners, flapping hands, and flickering fingers. As for his medical history, Ali did not suffer any of the childhood illnesses. He was not breastfed. As for his diet, he has an excess of sugar, artificial sweeteners, dairy crisps, chocolate, and wheat products. As for his language, Ali is a nonverbal child (uses few sounds), he requests his needs by crying or sometimes by pulling hands and leading adults to the desired items. His language skills were characterized as being severely delayed. As for his development history, he walked at the age of 15 months. Ali is not toilet trained. Ali had received psychomotor and speech therapy since the age of 4.

Ayoub: Ayoub was a 4-year-old boy (at intake) diagnosed with autism with a moderate level of disability, Ayoub has one sibling, his brother is a year younger than him, and he is a typically developing child. Ayoub's parents are both educated with a university degree. There is history of Attention Deficit Hyperactive Disorder (ADHD) and speech delay in Ayoub's family. As for his behavior, Ayoub engaged in self-stimulatory behaviors such as mouthing, spinning, and swirling objects. As for his medical history, Ayoub did not suffer any of the childhood illnesses. As for his health, Ayoub was breastfed for only couple of months. As for his diet, he is a picky eater with very limited diet consisting of biscuits, crisps, bread, and carbohydrate. As for his language, Ayoub is a nonverbal child who sometimes uses a person's hand to request something he can see. He requests his needs by crying. His language skills were characterized as being severely delayed. As for his development history, Ayoub walked at the age of 16 months and he had some fine and gross motor difficulties. Ayoub is not toilet trained. Ayoub had received psychomotor and speech therapy since the age of 2.

Hadi: Hadi was a 5-year-old boy (at intake) diagnosed with autism with a moderate level of disability, Hadi has a twin brother who also has autism, Hadi's parents are both educated with Baccalaureate. There is a history of mental retardation and speech delay in Hadi's family. As for his behavior, Hadi engages in self-stimulatory behaviors such as flapping hands, and gazing. As for his medical history, Hadi did not suffer any of the childhood illnesses. Hadi was breastfed for few months. As for his diet, he has an excess of sugar, artificial sweeteners, dairy and wheat products. As for his language, Hadi is a verbal child (uses two words sentences). His language skills were characterized as being moderately delayed. As for his development history, Hadi walked at the age of 13 months and he had some fine motor difficulties. Hadi is toilet trained. Hadi had received psychomotor and speech therapy since the age of 3.

Hussein: Hussein was a 5-year-old boy (at intake) diagnosed with autism with a moderate level of disability, Hussein has three brothers, and they are typically developing children. Hussein's parents are both educated with Baccalaureate. There is a history of mental retardation and speech delay in Hussein's family. As for his behavior, Hussein engaged in self-stimulatory behaviors such smelling food and objects, flapping hands, gazing, and flickering fingers. As for his medical history, Hussein did not suffer any of the childhood illnesses. He was not breastfed. As for his diet, he has an excess of sugar, artificial sweeteners, dairy and wheat products. As for his language, Hussein is a verbal child (uses one single word); however, he requests his needs by crying or sometimes by pulling hands and leading adults to the desired items. His language skills were characterized as being moderately to severely delayed. As for his development history, Hussein walked at the age of 14 months and he had some fine and gross motor difficulties. Hussein is toilet trained. Hussein had received psychomotor and speech therapy since the age of 2.

Mahdi: Mahdi was a 5-year-old boy (at intake) diagnosed with autism with a moderate level of disability, He has a twin brother who also has autism, Mahdi's parents are both educated with Baccalaureate. There is a history of mental retardation and speech delay in Mahdi's family. As for his behavior, he engages in self-stimulatory behaviors such as flapping hands, and gazing. As for his medical history, he did not suffer any of the childhood illnesses. He was breastfed for few months. As for his diet, he has an excess of sugar, artificial sweeteners, dairy and wheat products. As for his language, Mahdi is a verbal child (uses two-word sentences). His language skills were characterized as being moderately delayed. As for his development history, Mahdi walked at the age of 13 months and he had some fine motor difficulties. Mahdi is toilet trained. He had received psychomotor and speech therapy since the age of 3.

Mariam: Mariam was a 4-year-old girl at intake, diagnosed with autism and mild learning difficulties, she has one sibling her twin sister who also is diagnosed with autism. There is no history of autism or any mental disabilities in the family. Both parents are educated with Baccalaureate. Mariam uses two-word sentences and she had acquired some spontaneous requests (mands), some labels (Tacts), and some limited conversational skills (Intraverbals). Her language skills were characterized as being moderately delayed. She had met all her milestones at the appropriate age of 18 months. She was not toilet trained.

Sami: Sami was a 5-year-old boy (at intake) diagnosed with autism with a moderate to severe level of disability, Sami has two siblings, and they are typically developing children. Sami's parents are both educated with Baccalaureate. There is a history of mental retardation and speech delays in Sami's family. As for his behavior, he is aggressive towards himself and others, he engages in self-stimulatory behaviors such as mouthing objects, flapping hands, and flickering fingers. As for his medical history, Sami did not suffer any of the childhood illnesses. He was not breastfed. As for his diet, he has an excess of sugar, artificial sweeteners, dairy, crisps, chocolate, and wheat products. As for his language, he is a nonverbal child (uses some sounds and few meaningful words), he requests his needs by crying or sometimes by pulling hands and leading adults to the desired items. His language skills were characterized as being severely delayed. As for his development history, he walked at the age of 16 months. Sami is not toilet trained. Sami had received psychomotor and speech therapy since the age of 3.

Sarah: Sarah was a 4-year-old girl at intake, diagnosed with autism and moderate learning difficulties, she has one sibling her twin sister who also is diagnosed with autism. There is no history of autism or any mental disabilities in the family. Both parents are educated with Baccalaureate. Sarah uses single words to communicate for very few things, she uses crying and screaming for communication, and her language skills were characterized as being severely delayed. As for her behavior, Sarah engaged in self-stimulatory behaviors such as hand mannerism, vocal stim, rocking, and mouthing objects. As for her medical history, Sarah had some frequent ear infections. She had met all her milestones at the appropriate age of 18 months. She was not toilet trained.

Youssef: Youssef was a 7-year-old boy (at intake) diagnosed with autism with a moderate to severe level of disability, Youssef has two siblings, and they are typically developing children. Youssef's parents are both educated with secondary degrees. There is a history of mental retardation and speech delays in Youssef's family. As for his behavior, he is aggressive towards himself and others, he engages in self-stimulatory behaviors such as flapping hands, and flickering fingers. As for his medical history Youssef did not suffer any of the childhood illnesses. He was breastfed for eight months. As for his diet, he has an excess of sugar, artificial sweeteners, dairy, crisps, chocolate, soda, and wheat products. As for his language, he is verbal child (two-word sentences). His language skills were characterized as being moderately delayed. As for his development history, he walked at the age of 14 months. Youssef is toilet trained. he had received psychomotor and speech therapy since the age of 3.

Procedures

Ten children, ranging in age from 4 to 7 years, participated in this study. Each child was diagnosed with autism by a child psychiatrist according to DSM 5 and was referred to ALI for ABA Center, in Ain Anoub Lebanon, for intervention. In addition, the researcher screened each child symptoms of ASD prior to the start of the study. As well, each child was screened by their teachers.

The students spent 5 hours per day, 5 days per week for a total of 25 hours per week in school, over 2 years.

ABA/VB intervention

- This research was conducted at the Autism Learning Institute for Applied Behavior Analysis (ALI for ABA) to study the effects of Applied Behavior Analysis/Verbal Behavior in teaching children with autism and associated learning difficulties.
- ABA/VB is the main teaching method at the center. It is a structured teaching program built on a discipline devoted to the understanding and improvement of human behaviors. ALI for ABA uses ABA/VB program to deliver a broad comprehensive curriculum in line with each child's IEP.
- Applied Behavior Analysis (ABA) is the science of applying experimentally derived principles of behavior to improve socially significant behavior. It takes what we know about behavior and uses it to bring about positive changes (Applied). Behaviors are defined in observable and measurable terms in order to assess change over time (Behavior). The behavior is analyzed within the environment to determine what factors are influencing the behavior (Analysis) (Cooper, Heron, & Heward, 2007; Lovaas, 1987).

Aims and objectives

The aims of this study were threefold: (1) to evaluate the use of the ABA/VB approach as a comprehensive means of managing core and associated ASD features; (2) to assess the long-term efficacy of such an approach; and (3) to evaluate levels of parental stress throughout the intervention.

ABA/VB is the main teaching method at the center. It is a structured teaching program built on a discipline devoted to the understanding and improvement of human behaviors. ALI for ABA Center uses ABA/VB to deliver a broad curriculum in line with each child's IEP.

Each element of the teaching process is continuously charted and assessed. This enables staff to identify strengths and weaknesses and to help the child progress in a positive and targeted direction.

The Center's curriculum also includes art, music, and dance and there are regular activities for indoor and outdoor play.

Staff and parents at ALI for ABA received intensive training using the ABA/VB manual:

Teaching Language to Children with Autism or Other Developmental Disabilities by Sundberg and Partington (1998a, 1998b). The staff's skills are assessed on an ongoing basis to ensure that the standards are maintained.

This study tracks these children over a period of 2 years, monitors their performances at fixed intervals, and provides a summative overview of the progress made by each individual child in response to the program.

This research was the author's attempt to study the effects and the impacts of implementing an ABA/VB program on children with autism. Children's performance on specific skills were assessed, evaluated, and reported by four parties:

- the researcher;
- the independent psychologists;
- the teachers; and
- the parents.

This study was set out with two aims:

- The first aim is to study the effects of implementing an Applied Verbal Behaviors (AVB) approach on children with autism regarding the children's academic functioning, language functioning and adaptive functioning.
- The second aim is to study the effects of implementing the AVB program on the children's parents by measuring their stress level before and after the AVB intervention.

Outcome measures and assessment tools

The purpose of the research is to study the effects of implementing an ABA/VB program on children with autism regarding their academic, language and communication, behaviors, and adaptive functioning in addition to the teachers' and parent's evaluation. It is important to define "the unit of analysis" as (Yin, 1994) suggests. The intervention study is therefore children with autism who are attending classes at ALI for ABA center. The participants of this study are 10 children. The study was done over 2 years. All the children are diagnosed with autism by an outside agencies and the researcher had the chance to confirm the diagnosis using the Diagnostic and Statistical Manual of Mental Disorders, Fifth Edition (DSM 5) (American Psychiatric Association, 2013).

Multiple baseline design

- The research used a combination of quantitative and some qualitative methods. The ABA/VB intervention used for this study was based on multiple baseline design across behavior, participants, and settings. The different use of methods for this research has contributed to the methodology, by using different methods to collect data and involving many parties who can evaluate the children's performance and report their progress from their own perspectives.

Triangulation

Triangulation may be defined as the use of two or more methods of data collections in the study of some aspect of human behavior (Cohen, Manion, & Morrison, 2000). This is also called "cross examination" (Cheng, 2005, p. 72.). Children's performance on specific skills were assessed, evaluated, and reported by four parties:

- the researcher;
- the independent psychologists;
- the teachers; and
- the parents.

For this research, the following assessments were used:

- Childhood Autism Rating Scales (CARS) (Schopler, Reichle, & Rochen Renner, 1988). CARS was conducted separately by an independent psychologist and the researcher twice pre and post ABA/VB intervention.

- The Behavioral Language Assessment (BLAF) (designed by Sundberg & Partington, 1998a, 1998b). The BLAF was conducted by the researcher twice, pre and post ABA/VB intervention.
- The Assessment of Basic Language and Learning Skills (ABLLS) (Sundberg & Partington, 1998a, 1998b). The ABLLS was conducted by the researcher twice, pre and post ABA/VB intervention.
- Evaluation Form by teachers and parents. The evaluation forms by teachers and parents were conducted twice, pre and post ABA/VB intervention.
- Parenting Stress Index (PSI) Short Form ("Parenting Stress Index (PSI) Short Form", 1995). This was filled by the child's mother twice, pre and post ABA/VB intervention.

The data were collected by direct observations on a daily, weekly, and periodical basis by the teachers, and the researcher had access to the children's records, such as daily, weekly: written notes on the communication book (between parents and teachers), periodically and annually. The researcher was present at the center on a daily basis.

Results: ALI for ABA research

The results of this study showed that ABA/VB intervention was effective at improving social communication skills for children with autism. The children participating in this study demonstrated greater gains in their communication and social skills, academic, play, self-help skills, and fine and gross motor skills.

The present study did incorporate the parents, where it was helpful to assess the effect of the intervention from their perspective alongside the teachers.

The outcomes of this present study yielded better results than the previous study (Gharbieh, 2009) as 8 out of 10 children were placed in regular schools after ABA/VB intervention, whereas in the previous study only 4 out of 10 children were placed in regular schools after the ABA/VB intervention.

The present study demonstrated the efficiency of the AVB program with 10 children with autism. Its effects have been clear on the emergence of speech, collateral gains in social communicative behaviors, and decrease of problems behaviors, as well as the decrease of parental level stress. Eight children out of ten were placed in a regular school following the national curriculum.

Discussion

Summary of results

Parenting stress index

PSI Short Form is a questionnaire which contains 36 statements (a standardized test by "Parenting Stress Index (PSI) Short Form", 1995), where parents are instructed to read each statement carefully. For each statement, the parent is instructed to focus on the child who they are most concerned about (the child participating in the study), and the parents were requested to circle the response that best represented their opinion. The reader is advised that only the mothers agreed to participate in this study.

It can be seen from analyzing the PSI Short Form (Fig. 12.1), that the parental stress level was decreased significantly. The results of the PSI indicate that the improvement and progress of the children using the ABA/VB program have influenced and decreased their mothers' stress levels which allowed a better parent to child relationship.

Childhood autism rating scales by Schopler et al. (1988)

The CARS was designed by Schopler et al. (1988). It was developed to identify children with autism and to distinguish them from developmentally handicapped children without the autism syndrome (Schopler et al., 1988). CARS distinguishes children with autism in the mild to moderate range from children with autism in the moderate to severe range.

As for the CARS assessment which was conducted by an independent psychologist, in addition to the researcher analyzing CARS pre and post AVB intervention, all the children had made noticeable progress and they showed a decrease in the degree of autism. Four children had made significant improvement: Ali A, Hadi, Hussein, Mahdi, and Mariam, whose scores were in the nonautistic category (Figs. 12.2 and 12.3).

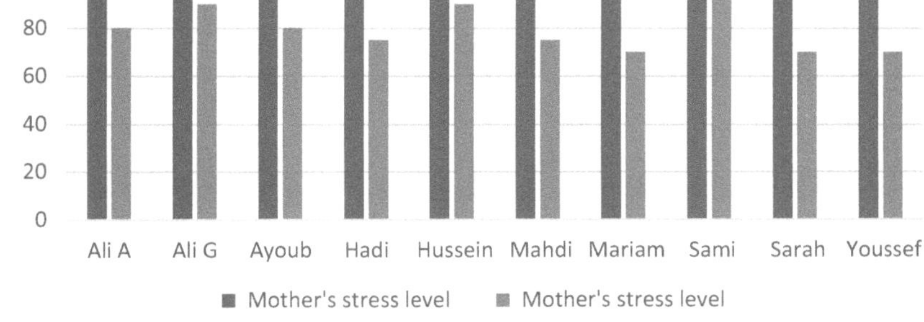

Figure 12.1 Mother PSI percentage of improvement, out of maximum score. High percentage indicates high stress level.

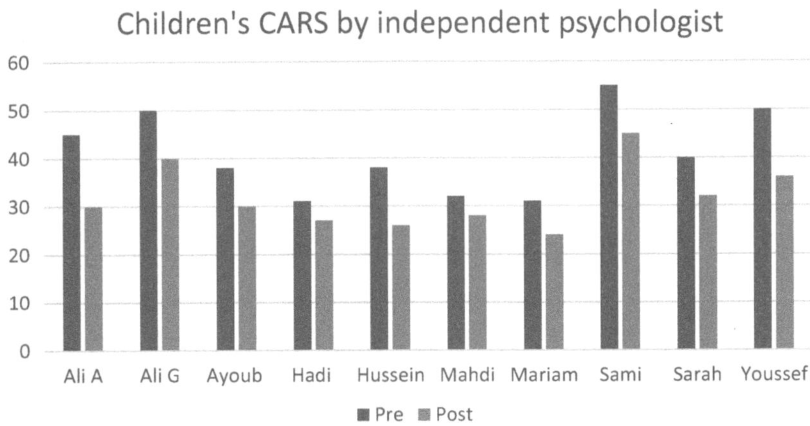

Figure 12.2 CARS by an independent psychologist, out of maximum score. High scores indicate severity of symptoms.

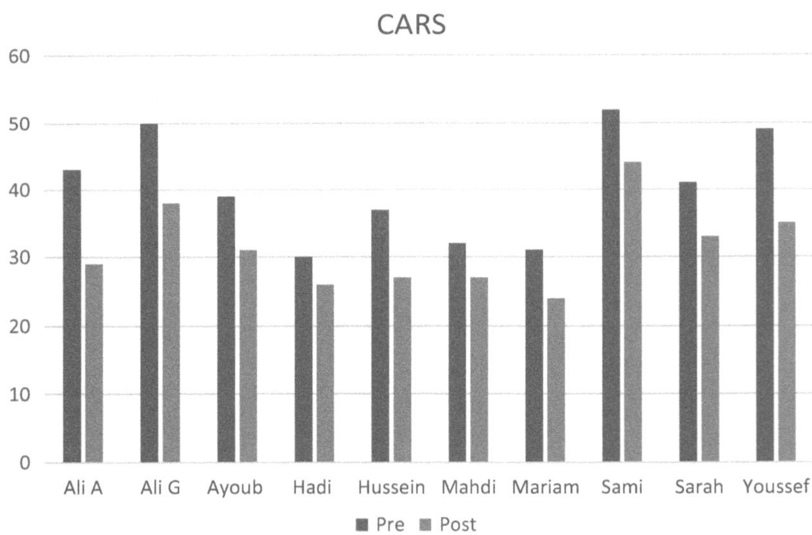

Figure 12.3 CARS by researcher, out of maximum score. High scores indicate severity of symptoms.

The behavioral language assessment form by Sundberg and Partington (1998a, 1998b)

The BLAF is an introductory assessment. Initial data were taken on children to measure their performance using the BLAF. The assessment is designed to reflect the average performance of typical 2- to 3-year-old children. Most of these typically developed children would have received a score of five on each of the areas in the assessment (with the exception of the numbers and letters sections). This level of linguistic performance allows typical children to learn from their everyday experiences, while children with autism might have some difficulties to acquire the simplest levels of communication and to learn without an intervention program. The BLAF is a simple scale which is used in an initial meeting with each child, in order to assess their current functioning level.

The BLAF is used to examine the children in different areas. It contains 12 different sections which cover a variety of early language skills and related areas. Each section is broken down into five levels. For this test, high scores indicate better outcomes.

In the BLAF, which is used to examine the children's skills in different areas such as cooperation, requesting, imitation, matching, labeling, receptive language, conversation, academic and social skills, the children showed noticeable improvement in all areas. Examining the pre and post scores of the BLAF, it is clearly indicated that all the children (10 out 10 children) had improved significantly. In addition, three children were able to score the maximum scores on the BLAF: Ali A, Hussein, and Mariam (Fig. 12.4).

The assessment of basic language and learning skills

The ABLLS is an assessment, curriculum guide, and skills tracking system for children with language delays. The ABLLS contains a task analysis of the many skills necessary to communicate successfully and to learn from everyday experiences.

The use of the ABLLS will enable teachers and professionals to conduct an assessment of a learner's current skills levels across all main areas of functioning social language, communications, academic, behavioral, and functional living skills.

The implementation of an ABA/VB program is comprehensive and covers many areas that the children need in order to function in the real world. The ABLLS (Sundberg & Partington, 1998a, 1998b) is an assessment used by the ABA/VB program; it is a criterion reference test which has been used to determine the children's

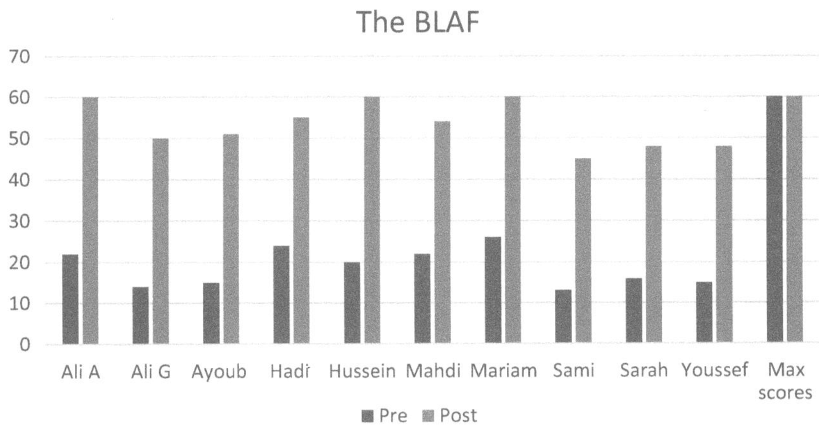

Figure 12.4 The BLAF by researcher, out of maximum score. High scores indicate improvement.

skills in each of the 25 areas of the assessment. The ABLLS has four sections, basic learner skills section, academic skills section, self-help section, and motor skills section.

The ABLLS assesses the strengths and weaknesses of an individual in each of the 25 skill sets. Each skill set is broken down into multiple skills, ordered by typical development or complexity. So, a skill of F1 (requests by indicating) is a simpler skill than F12 (requesting help). Usually, lower level skills are needed before proceeding to teach higher skills. However, many individuals display splinter skills that are above their practical level.

Examining the ABLLS results (Figs. 12.5 and 12.6), it can be seen that all the children (10 out 10 children) have made significant progress in the cooperation program, play and leisure, social interactions, group instructions, class-room routines, and generalized responding, dressing, eating, and grooming programs. As for the toileting program 9 out of 10 children had shown significant progress while Sami is the only child who still needs assistance to be consistently toilet trained as he still has a couple of minor accidents during the day.

All the children have made significant progress in the visual performance program except for three children who had made moderate progress. As for the receptive language program, imitation program, and spontaneous vocalization program, 8 out of 10 children had made significant improvements while the remaining two have made moderate progress. As for the vocal imitation, request program, 8 out 10 children have made significant improvement while the remaining two had made moderate progress. As for the labeling program and the intraverbals program, which is a very advanced program for verbal children, only six children had made noticeable progress while the rest had shown minor to moderate progress.

Names of the children	Pre ABA/VB	% Pre	Post ABA/VB	% Post	% Rate of improvement
Ali A	150	11.73	935	73.16	61.43
Ali G	140	10.90	830	64.94	54.04
Ayoub	80	6.25	900	70.42	64.17
Hadi	148	11.58	929	72.69	61.11
Hussein	145	11.34	1000	78.24	66.90
Mahdi	150	11.73	899	70.34	58.61
Mariam	200	15.64	1009	78.95	63.31
Sami	60	4.69	400	31.29	26.60
Sarah	75	5.86	450	35.21	29.35
Youssef	111	8.68	460	35.99	27.31
Max scores	**1278**	**100**	**1278**	**100**	**100**

Figure 12.5 Pre and post ABLLS rate of improvement of the children.

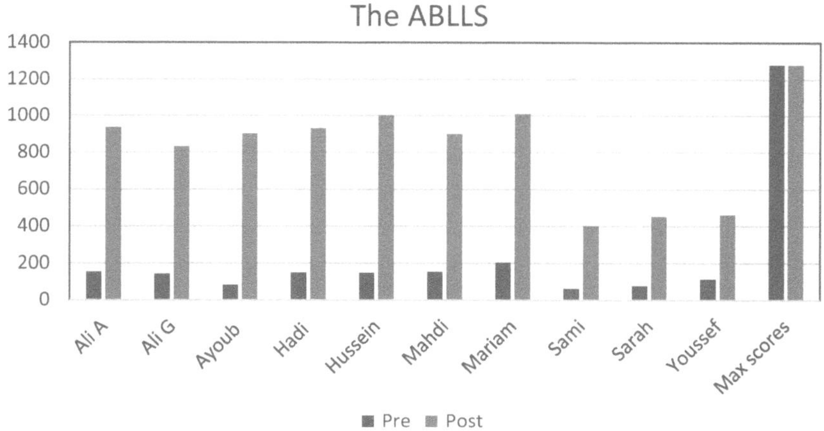

Figure 12.6 The ABLLS by researcher, out of maximum score. High scores indicates improvement.

Evaluation forms by teachers and parents

The evaluation form is a semistructured questionnaire which was designed by the researcher for both parents and teachers in order to investigate the effects of implementing an ABA/VB program on children with autism.

There are four sections in the questionnaires where children were evaluated by their teachers and parents. The reader is reminded that the evaluations by the teachers and the parents are quantitative (performing skills, tests) and qualitative judgments which are based on overall knowledge of each child:

- Section 1 looks at the child's personal details such as age and the degree of the child's disability from the teachers' or parents' perspectives.
- Section 2 looks at behavior such as self-injurious or aggressive behaviors and self-stimulatory activity.
- Section 3 looks at the progress and development of the children which might be attributed to the ABA/VB program. It covers the areas of: behavior; compliance; waiting; performing skills in different situations; receptive language; receptive and expressive behavior; social intraverbals; nonverbal imitation; matching and sorting; plays skills; objects labeling; verbal imitation; abstract concept; sentence structure; academic works; social repertoire; and self-help skills.
- Section 4 is related to the teachers or parents' personal view (Figs. 12.7 and 12.8).

On a scale from 1 to 8, the teachers and the parents are judging the degree to which each child is affected by his/her disability. The reader is advised that "1" means the child is mildly affected by disability and "8" means the child is severely affected by disability.

The children have made significant improvement from pre-ABA/VB intervention scores as shown in Fig. 12.9 by teachers, and Fig. 12.10 by parents in exception to Sami, who made a mild to moderate improvement.

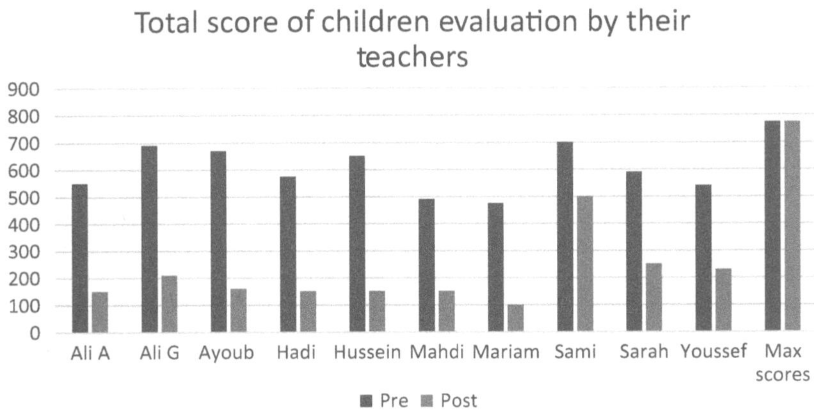

Figure 12.7 Teachers' evaluation, out of maximum score. High scores indicate severity of symptoms, low scores indicate improvement.

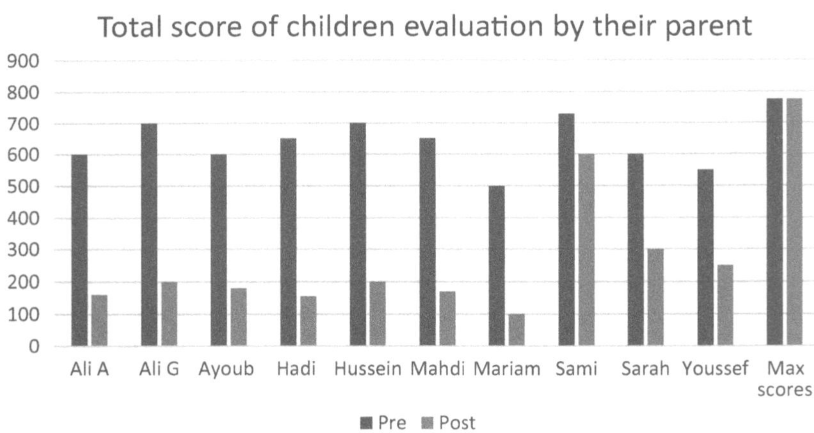

Figure 12.8 Parents' evaluation, out of maximum score. High scores indicate severity of symptoms, low scores indicate improvement.

In the aggressive and self-injurious behaviors, only three children did exhibit these types of behaviors. The children have made significant improvement from pre-ABA/VB intervention scores, as shown in Figs. 12.11 and 12.12.

Regarding the self-stim behaviors of the children participating in this study,

It can be seen from Figs. 12.13 and 12.14 that the children have made significant improvement in this field. Both teachers and parents have noticed the great improvement with the exception of Sami's parent where they reported a moderate improvement in this area.

In summary, all the children participating in this study have shown significant improvement by their teachers' and parent's evaluation, from comparing the

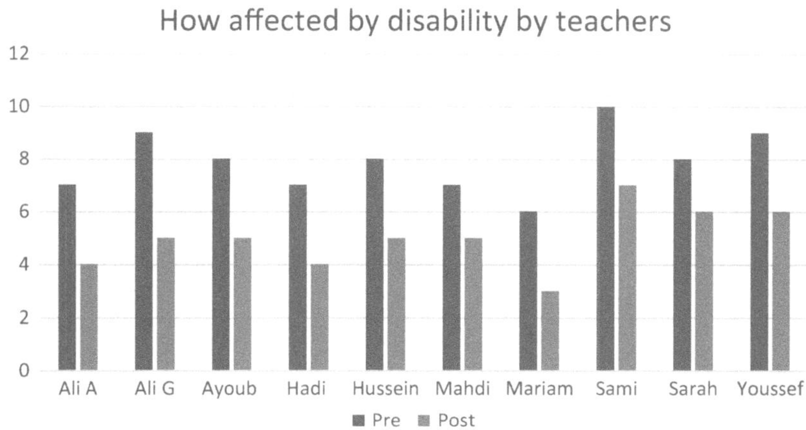

Figure 12.9 Children affected by their disabilities—teachers' evaluation out of maximum score. High scores indicate severity of symptoms, low scores indicate improvement.

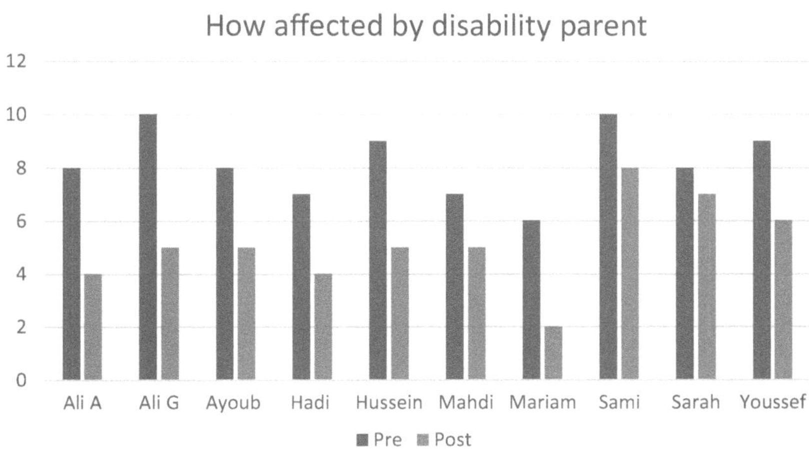

Figure 12.10 Children affected by their disabilities—parents' evaluation out of maximum score. High scores indicate severity of symptoms, low scores indicate improvement.

children's performance of specific skills pre and post ABA/VB intervention, which is indicated in Figs. 12.7 and 12.8.

The result of the comparison was very interesting, where most of the findings were almost identical. Hence, the measurements of the children's progress by their teachers and their parents were justified.

Analyzing all the above tests, it clearly indicates that the improvement the children had shown can be attributed to the implementation of the ABA/VB program. Some children have made noticeable and significant improvements, while others

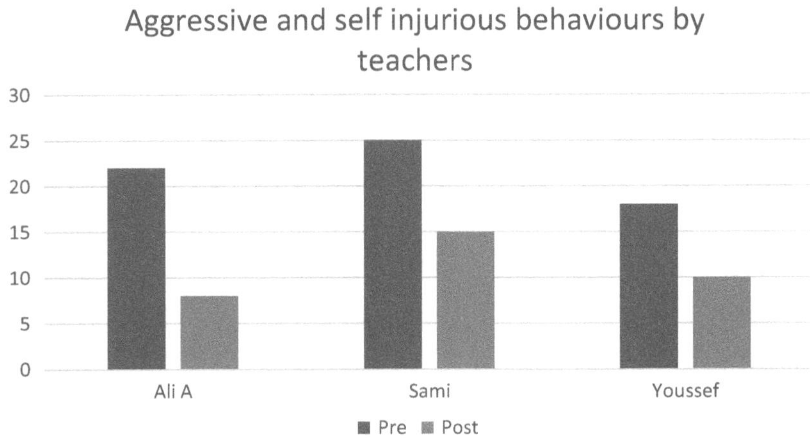

Figure 12.11 Aggressive and self-injurious behaviors—teachers' evaluation out of maximum score. High scores indicate severity of symptoms, low scores indicate improvement.

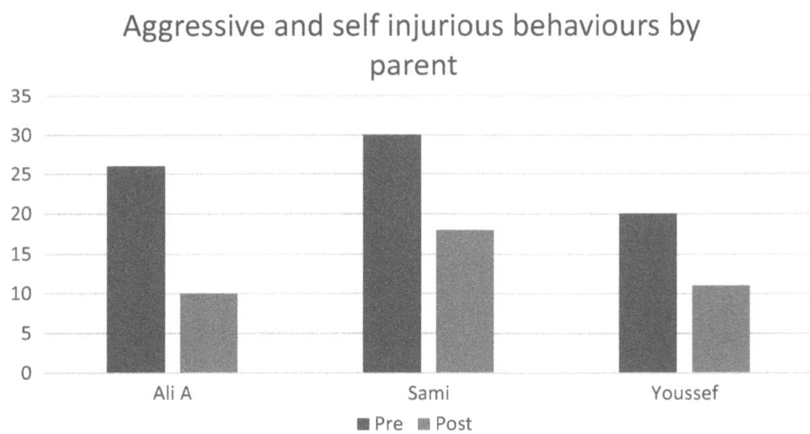

Figure 12.12 Aggressive and self-injurious behaviors—parents' evaluation out of maximum score. High scores indicate severity of symptoms, low scores indicate improvement.

had shown moderate progress. Children with autism differ in their ability and capabilities. However, all the children have shown significant progress in their performances in the areas that concern behavior, the attending skills, social and play skills. The children have become more cooperative and the parent stress level was decreased and the independent psychologist has noticed the progress in the children's performances, which were documented to all of the children who participated in this study.

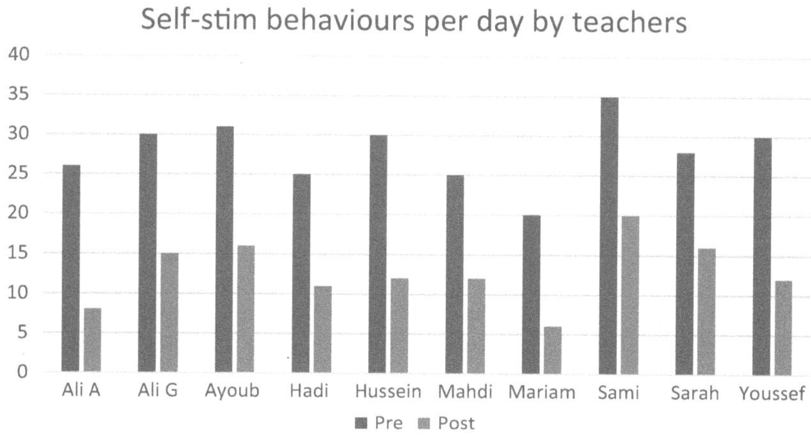

Figure 12.13 Self-stim behaviors—teachers' evaluation out of maximum score. High scores indicate severity of symptoms low scores indicate improvement.

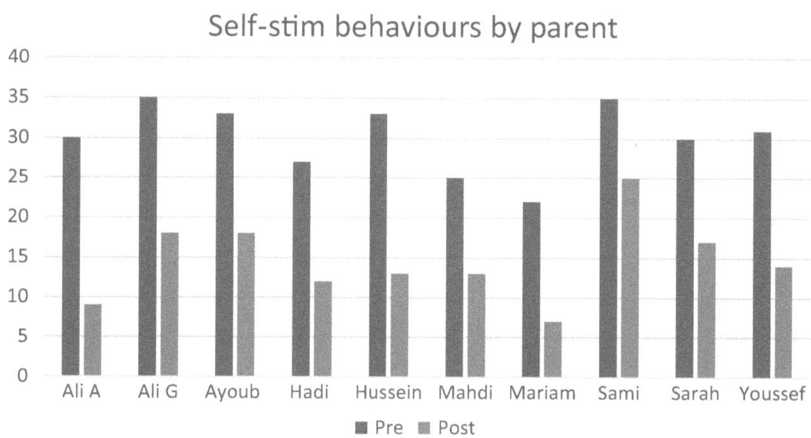

Figure 12.14 Self-stim behaviors—parents' evaluation out of maximum score. High scores indicate severity of symptoms, low scores indicate improvement.

It seems that implementing the ABA/VB program influenced all parties involved in this study, parents and children alike.

The research demonstrated clear collateral gains in speech and social communicative behaviors, as well as significant reductions in problem behaviors associated with decreased parental stress levels. The research has developed successful tools to allow children with autism to learn new concepts and ideologies, helping them to lead a happier and more independent lifestyle.

Limitation of the study

This study was limited by several factors:

- ABA/VB intervention requires a large number of well-trained individuals to administer the intervention with a high degree of coordination and supervision of the individuals administering the interventions.
- ABA/VB can be expensive for poorly financed families, thus all the participated children come from middle to upper class families.
- A specific technique should be used to train for generalization skills.
- Absence of randomized group to demonstrate that superiority of one program over another. This study has not used randomized group comparison designs because of the practical and ethical difficulties in randomly assigning children and families to treatment groups.
- Small sample of children, at young age, thus this research cannot comment on the efficacy of intervention in older persons with autism.
- ABA/VB requires treatment fidelity for successful implementation, thus parents and educators should be adequately trained prior to treatment intervention.
- Data collected by the staff may introduce a potential confounding effect. This confounding effect may be countered by having daily performance data for this study.

Implications

- The efficacy of interventions such as ABA/VB implies that this strategy should form the basis and foundation of special education for ASD.
- Many children with ASD will attend a school/center.
- Regular parent/carer awareness or teaching sessions would be valuable for generalizing these effective strategies to the home setting.
- Ongoing support and education is vital for the success of such a comprehensive approach.

Suggestion for further research

This study has raised some important questions which encourages further exploration of them for future research:

- Can a regular school with an attached unit replicate similar results findings?
- Can older children with autism with no prior educational intervention benefit from the ABA/VB intervention at the same rate as younger children?
- Can ABA/VB intervention be applied by trained paraprofessionals, such as parents and others?
- Can the effects of AVB be maintained in the longer term?
- Language limitations? Does language ability have an impact on the success of the intervention.
- Treatment hours? More work is needed to identify the ideal treatment intensity which provides maximal progress whilst also avoiding child, parent, and caregiver burnout.

References

American Psychiatric Association. (2013). *Diagnostic and statistical manual of mental disorders* (5th ed.). Washington, DC.

Cheng, L. (2005). *Changing language teaching through language testing: A washback study*. Cambridge University Press.

Cohen, L., Manion, L., & Morrison, K. (2000). *Research methods in education* (5th ed.). London: Routledge Falmer.

Cooper, J., Heron, T. E., & Heward, W. (2007). *Applied Behaviour Analysis* (2nd edition). Englewood Cliffs, NJ: Prentice Hall.

Dillenburger, K., & Keenan, M. (2009). None of the As in ABA stand for autism: Dispelling the myths. *Journal of Intellectual and Developmental Disability*, *34*(2), 193–195.

Eldevik, S., Hastings, R. P., Hughes, J. C., et al. (2009). Meta-analysis of early intensive behavioral intervention for children with autism. *Journal of Clinical Child & Adolescent Psychology*, *38*(3), 439–450.

Foxx, R. M. (2008). Applied behavior analysis treatment of autism: The state of the art. *Child and Adolescent Psychiatric Clinics of North America*, *17*(4), 821–834.

Gharbieh, C. (2009). *Studying the effects of implementing an applied behaviour analysis/applied verbal behaviour "ABA/AVB" on children with autism and related disorders* (Published Ph.D. thesis). United Kingdom: Brunel University.

Hanley, G. P., Iwata, B. A., & McCord, B. E. (2003). Functional analysis of problem behavior: A review. *Journal of Applied Behavior Analysis*, *36*(2), 147–185.

Lovaas, O. I. (1987). Behavioral treatment and normal educational and intellectual functioning in young autistic children. *Journal and Consulting and Clinical Psychology*, *55*, 3–9.

Mohammad Zaheri, F., Koegel, L. K., Rezaee, M., & Rafiee, S. m. (2014). A randomized clinical trial comparison between pivotal response treatment (PRT) and structure applied behaviour analysis (ABA) intervention for children with autism. *Journal of Autism and Developmental Disorders*, *44*(11), 2769–2777.

O'Brien, G., & Pearson, J. (2004). *Autism and Learning Disability*, *8*(2), 125–140. Available from https://doi.org/10.1177/1362361304042718.

Parenting Stress Index (PSI) Short Form. (1995). Psychological Assessment Resources Inc.

Reichow, B., & Wolery, M. (2009). Comprehensive synthesis of early intensive behavioral interventions for young children with autism based on the UCLA young autism project model. *Journal of Autism Developmental Disorders*, *39*, 23–41.

Schopler, E., Reichle, R. J., & Rochen Renner, B. (1988). *Childhood* autism rating scales C.A.R.S. CA: Western Psychological Services WPS.

Sundberg, M. L., & Partington, J. W. (1998a). *Teaching language to children with autism or other developmental disabilities*. Pleasant Hill, CA: Behavior Analysts Inc, version 7.1.

Sundberg, M. L., & Partington, J. W. (1998b). *The assessment of basic language and learning skills*. Danville, CA: Behavior Analysts Inc.

Tassé, M. J., Havercamp, S. M., & Lecavalier. (2002). Differential reinforcement of other behavior. *Editors-in-Chief*, 633–639.

Yin, R. (1994). *Case study research* (2nd edition). London: Sage.

Further reading

Sigmund, E., Richard, P. H., Carl, J. H., Erik, J., Svein, E., & Scott, C. (2010). Using participant data to extend the evidence base for intensive behavioral intervention for children with autism. *American Journal on Intellectual Developmental Disabilities*, *115*(5), 381–405. Available from https://doi.org/10.1352/1944-7558-115.5.381.

Center for Disease Control and Prevention *CDC Data and Statistics on Autism Spectrum Disorder | CDC*. (2019). <https://www.cdc.gov/ncbddd/autism/data.html>.

National Institute for Health and Clinical Excellence. (2016). *Autism: Recognition, referral, diagnosis and management of adults on the autism spectrum*. Available from: <http://www.nice.org.uk/guidance/cg142/chapter/guidance> Accessed November 2, 2017.

Persicke, A., Bishop, M. R., Coffman, C. M., Najdowski, A. C., Tarbox, J., Chi, K., et al. (2014). *Evaluation of the concurrent validity of a skills assessment for autism treatment* (8, pp. 281–285). Research in Autism Spectrum Disorders, Elsevier.

Wittke, K., Mastergeorge, A. M., Ozonoff, S., et al. (2017). Grammatical language impairment in autism spectrum disorder: Exploring language phenotypes beyond standardized testing. *Frontiers in Psychology*, *8*, 532.

13 Reconceptualizing training as professional formation in the fields of autism and infant mental health

Gerard Costa
Center for Autism and Early Childhood Mental Health, College of Education and Human Services, Montclair State University, Montclair, NJ, United States

What matters is not methods or techniques but a sensitivity to problems, and a consuming passion for them; or as the Greeks said, the gift of wonder.
Karl Popper (1963/1989)

Use of language and pronouns in this chapter. The author alternately uses male and female pronouns (he/she, him/her) as a convenience. In discourse about autism, the author employs person-first language ("PWD"—person with disability), "individual with autism." The author also honors the language of many self-advocates in which "autistic individual" is preferred, reflecting autism as a unique expression of neurodiversity.

The teaching and helping professions must continually evolve in their discernment of effective models of pedagogy and epistemology, by attempting to answer two principal questions: "How do we best teach our multidisciplinary workforce about our discipline?" and "How do learners come to know what they know?"

In this chapter, common methods of professional development are challenged as being inadequate at best, and ineffective at worst. These approaches to professional development frequently rely on "trainings" that focus on the transmission of knowledge which is viewed as fundamental to the discipline. Such trainings also seek to develop skills that are viewed as derivatives of that core knowledge.

Delineating the scope of this chapter on formation

Before we begin, it is important to acknowledge some limitations in this chapter. We will address, in a limited way, the distinctions among the different scientific perspectives or "world views" in our fields (e.g., DeWitt, 2010; Overton, 1984, 2013; Pepper, 1942/1970; Popper, 1959). Such a deep discussion about the many

Emerging Programs for Autism Spectrum Disorder. DOI: https://doi.org/10.1016/B978-0-323-85031-5.00008-6

perspectives that spawn different ideas, research, methods, and interventions (which constitute the field of "philosophy of science") demand a much fuller exploration than we can cover in this chapter. These different "world views" generate different metatheoretical beliefs and suppositions about human development, and in the fields of infant mental health and autism, generate different theories, methods, and ideas about research, education, remediation, and intervention. Costa and Witten (2009) examined the different underlying beliefs, concepts, methods, theories, and practices in the field of autism. These differences are noted and they must be addressed in any comprehensive discourse about professional development, because knowledge and skills, as well as the ways in which research and therapeutics are conceptualized, are significantly different depending on one's underlying metatheoretical views. Nonetheless, core philosophy of science will be presented as constituting the larger context of discourse in professional development in infant mental health and autism.

This is clearly evident, for example, by contrasting how the nature of autism is understood and how individuals with autism are supported and treated in Applied Behavioral Analysis (ABA) approaches (e.g., Cooper, Heron, & Heward, 2019; Lovaas, 1981), and the Developmental, Individual-difference, Relationship-based framework (e.g., Greenspan & Wieder, 1998, 2006). For professional development, these implications are profound because the differences in what is viewed as core knowledge, skills, and process of change, lead to vastly different professional development goals, content of educational curricula, related "trainings," and required experiences. Scientific inquiry is quite different depending on one's "world view." With regard to education research, Thomas (2012) argued for a new "science of education" and lamented that educational research, and education about the field, have taken a turn toward a "narrow view" and, as he quotes Lagemann (2000), "excessive quantification" (Thomas, 2012, p. 26).

While the field of infant health encompasses significant differences in how infancy and socioemotional development are examined (e.g., think about the different literature addressing "socioemotional development" versus "social-emotional learning"), most would agree that there is a high degree of agreement on what constitutes the major concepts and practices in the field. For example, the author is currently working with a team of editors on a book of multidisciplinary contributions about the ways in which "Infant Mental Health" (clinical origins) and the "Pyramid Model of Early Care and Education" (educational origins) can be seen through a common lens (e.g. Nenide, Wasserman, Costa, Corso, & Horen, In preparation). With more than 35 years in the fields of infant and early childhood mental health and autism, the author asserts that the level of unity and agreement in infant mental health is significantly greater, than is the case in the field of autism.

Accordingly, there is no "one way" to teach about autism, and this simple truth has resulted in decades of contentious debate and confusion among the multidisciplinary sciences, advocates, legislators, funders, and mostly families (e.g., Broderick, 2009; Claypool & McLaughlin, 2017). There is no question that any examination of professional development, and on how we best prepare a multidisciplinary workforce, must address the underlying philosophical, metatheoretical, theoretical, and applied differences that exist in the field. This has been addressed in other works (e.g., Overton & Reese, 1973; Overton, 1998) and continues to be needed as we apply these insights in the fields of infant mental health and autism.

There are a number of challenging questions to pose amidst the contention in the field of autism: Does the education of multidisciplinary professionals in one way of "knowing" and "doing" to the exclusion and denigration of others, constitute education? Propaganda? Indoctrination? Can we understand how the uses, and perhaps misuses, of the terms "science" and "evidence" further complicate the discourse? Is there a way to discern common ground so that each professional development provider can convey the same knowledge, skills and, as we will ask, result in the same "formation"? Can we understand the ways in which different "world views" and approaches have created economic and political differences that have both interfered with and formed scientific process? (e.g., see Kuhn, 1962/1970 for a broader examination of the shifts in scientific "paradigms" in history).

These questions are raised as necessary topics in the larger context of *what* we teach and *how* we teach. Here, we will discuss current practices that have, unfortunately, in Thomas' (2012) words, "narrowed" the process and goal of professional development. Reconceptualizing professional development as "formation" is one way to widen the discourse about how we prepare professionals.

In this chapter we will critically examine the adequacy and effectiveness of training approaches that primarily focus on "knowledge" and "skills." An argument will be made and justification offered, that such approaches fail to adequately recognize and apply the science of interpersonal processes and the relational context of education in professional development. In so doing, the development of the "full person" is thwarted. Professional development that focuses on knowledge and skills will alone never be sufficient.

Introduction to formation

The concept of "Formation" is proposed and explained as a model that expands and extends the importance of "knowledge" and "skills" in professional development, to include the critical importance of relationships and "being-with" as essential to the professional development process, and as a necessary component of multidisciplinary work in infant mental health and autism.

Costa (2016) and Costa and Mulcahy (2015, 2018) discussed this notion of "formation" as intrinsic to professional development. Use of this term "formation" originates from fields outside of the usual social sciences. A Google search of the term "formation" is revealing. A search conducted on August 22, 2020 yielded nearly 1.5 billion hits, with the song of that name ("Formation") by the American artist Beyonce (2016), and references to geological formations as the top "hits." When the search is expanded to "Professional Formation," the most common sites refer to "knowledge" and "skills" (e.g., Society for Education and Training: https://set.et-foundation.co.uk/professionalism/qtls/professional-formation/). While "personal development" and occasionally "reflection" were sometimes mentioned, the most notable "hits" were seen in two areas: (1) "Faith and Clergy Formation," and a (2) series of studies conducted by the Carnegie Foundation that will be reviewed below. These come closest to the meaning of "formation" proposed in this narrative. Both areas reflect the need for development beyond "knowing" and "doing"—and in fact address the critical importance of personal "unfolding" and relationships!

As formation will be described here, professional development and the goal of professional "training" will be understood as involving a full integration of what is known by the professional, what "doing" by professionals entails, and "who and how" they are—their ways of "being-with" and relating. (The significance of "how you are" in infant mental health work was the title and topic of a seminal monograph by Pawl and Saint-John (1998).)

In this regard, professional development is inseparable from personal development. "Formation" requires that professional growth involve the development of the whole person such that education integrates their intellectual prowess, life experiences, and the many layers of "self" that humans are. Self-reflection is part of the process which brings the professional to an understanding of how his *whole self intersects with the learned materials and her work with infants, children, and families.*

Ultimately, an education focused on formation encourages students and professionals to discover who they are called to be, and to have the foundational capacities necessary to live out that vision. Kohut and Seitz (1963/1978) said this eloquently "In actual (clinical) practice (however), the theoretical knowledge of the experienced psychoanalyst has become so fully integrated into his total observational attitude that he is usually no longer aware of a dichotomy between theory and observation..." (p. 341). Kohut might have stated this as a principle: *If you are thinking about your theory and knowledge when you are with your patient, you are not thinking about your patient!*

In a series of studies sponsored by the Carnegie Foundation and published beginning in 2007, the concept of "professional formation" was examined within certain professions, including "lawyers, engineers, clergy, nurses and physicians" (Cooke, Irby, & O'Brien, 2010; Sullivan, 2015). In the foreword to the Cooke et al. (2010), Schulman (2010) wrote, "The most overlooked aspect of professional preparation was the *formation* of a professional *identity* with a moral core of service and responsibility" (italics added, p. v). The connection among the listed helping professions and "clergy" formation is not accidental. The notion of "formation" therefore presupposes that our work in the fields of infant mental health and autism need to be guided by a deep sense of mission, integrity, and service, and relies on the development of personal well-being and a clear sense of identity in the provider—articulated above as the "...formation of a professional identity with a moral core of service and responsibility."

Within the field of Infant Mental Health, a long-standing requirement of providing support, education, and intervention to families with infants, children, and families is the requirement of "reflective practices"—a specialized kind of self-awareness, reflection, introspection, and discourse that necessitates the practitioner to examine their own subjective responses to the work and the relationships they form with infants, children, and families—and themselves (e.g., Costa & Sullivan,

2009; Fenichel, 1992; Shahmoon-Shanok, 2009). This necessity emerged from the strongly supported assertion that affect (feelings) and ideas (intellect) and actions (behavior) are inextricably linked, and cannot be separated, but can be understood (e.g., Siegel, 2010a, 2010b; Greenspan & Shanker, 2004).

Costa (2006) quoted a frequent admonition by a valued supervisor, Dr. Davis Peters, "We need supervision to save our patients from ourselves" (p. 127). Thea Bry, another supervisor's reminder was more colloquial: "Get in Cahoots with yourself." Michael Trout (1988), reflecting on the field of infant mental health, moving into the 21st century, proposed that infant mental health specialists must consider a personal psychotherapy to ensure that their personal material not intrude on the efforts to help their clients. Trout wrote, "(I)t is critical that we offer assessments, engage in treatment, conduct our research, and do our teaching free of uncontrolled contamination by our own unresolved childhood experiences, our idealizations, our needs for control: in short, that we be truly open to the data and truly available to the families. …(A) call is made for careful transdisciplinary training, supervision, individual psychotherapy, and collegial monitoring for infant mental health clinicians, researchers, and educators, alike "(p. 191). Adding gravitas to this conviction, he observed that Donald Winnicott, pediatrician, turned psychoanalyst and author, proposed that all pediatricians be psychoanalyzed; an idea likely met with resistance. So here we see the connections among what we know, who we are, and how we act—all necessary domains for examination in formation.

For this reason, the field of infant mental health has emphasized the importance of "reflective practice," the integration of affect and intellect and the requirement to ensure that services to families are not weakened by the failure to pay attention to these practices. This creates an obligation that the field must focus on professional "formation," not just "training" (knowledge and facts) or "skills" (what to "do" with an infant, child, or family).

In this chapter, a proposal is offered that professional education and "training" are better conceptualized by the concept of "FORMATION." As part of the Carnegie Foundation initiative, Hamilton (2011) wrote about professional formation in the legal profession with a similar focus on one's internal landscape and personhood: "Professional formation refers to the fostering of students' formation of an ethical professional identity. *This change from a focus on educational inputs* like a course on professional responsibility to a focus on clearly-articulated learning outcomes relating to each student's ethical development that are assessable is a major paradigm shift in legal education" (p. 765, italics added)

From this perspective, "formation" conveys the notion of a personal unfolding, reflects a way of becoming, of being, and of "being with," and implies that knowledge and affect are intertwined. It emphasizes the transactional and experiential nature of development—not only training as transmission of knowledge or teaching skills, but an expectation that the learner be actively engaged, and that authentic growth of "self"—personal development and awareness—are fundamental to creating an intuitive sense of service to others.

This notion of formation, therefore addresses three interrelated "ways" of developing: *Knowing, Doing, and Being With.*

Ways of knowing

This represents the traditional focus of training programs. Knowledge from theory, research, and practice MUST occur. BUT, in and of itself, such knowledge is insufficient, and is tantamount to the practitioner becoming a "technician"—a skill builder, not necessarily a promoter of human development, as human engagement, particularly with infants and young children is fundamentally affective and relational. Equally important as the accumulation of knowledge, is the adoption of a "*posture of wondering*" in the infant, child, and family worker. This suggests that the process of coming to know and understand a child must involve an awareness that many forces influence what we observe and encounter. These forces are within the child and his/her life AND within the worker. If we fail to "wonder" and search for possible factors involved (hypothesis-generation), we run the risk of "prematurely closing" on answers, "confirming" that we are correct, applying what we "know," and indeed we may miss the mark. Authentic knowledge from science and practice is essential in all practitioners, but alone it is inadequate.

Ways of doing

When professionals, at all levels and across disciplines, attend trainings and workshops, the goal expressed by many participants is often some variation of, "Just tell me what to do!" or "I have a child who hits and bites. How should I handle that?" or "I have a child with autism in my class who runs and screams. I have tried everything. I think she does not belong in my class. I need to find a way to convince our program director." In these cases, staff are looking for the "magic" technique that applies to any child with apparently similar behavior. In fact, many training programs are wonderful at teaching "techniques" and "skills" to manage behavior, but since similar behaviors originate for varying reasons, these strategies often fail to help children, and staff often complain that the technique "didn't work."

Here is where professional formation must engage not in the endless search for tactics of techniques (as the opening quote by Karl Popper states), but to develop the suspension of judgement and impart the gift of "wonder." It is certainly important to support the development of a range of observational, assessment, and education/interventions skills, but if these skills are viewed as the agents of therapeutic or change (e.g., the method is the effective agent) then whomever and however the method, or tactic, or technique is delivered should not matter! But consider "how" a technique is delivered and imagine it was implemented in a way that is insensitive to the individualized needs of a particular child, or in a way that is without regard to the child's availability or readiness for growth, learning or change. To press this issue *reductio ad absurdum*, imagine it were delivered with a harsh, emotionless, and frightening way, we might predict that it is likely to fail. In fact, the argument being made here is that the "doing" of an intervention by a provider is *never void of human delivery*, certainly in the psychological and developmental sciences.

Further, and this is an assertion we will revisit later, "how" the intervention is delivered can be conceptualized as a variable worth study—and if a researcher chooses only to research a "technique" (e.g., as in a reinforcement paradigm–ABA) and does not look at the "how" it is delivered (the interpersonal space), the possibility of discerning the value of the technique is obscured by the failure to unconfound the other potential agents of effectiveness outside of the 'technique." To state the logical conclusion: if a practitioner or researcher fails to examine the host of variables, the actual outcome may be due to reasons *other than* what is postulated. The "technique" in question is, in fact, rendered unexamined. The point here is to recognize that the intrinsic interrelatedness among the ways of development that are being examined, require that both our professional development programs, as well as our research and intervention protocols recognize the context within which research and intervention occurs.

So, if the "right" words and techniques are used, but are delivered with a harsh and angry affect, "mean" voice, impatiently delivered and in a rushed, punitive and demanding way, the negative response to the nonverbal context will far outweigh the intent and possible success of the words and technique employed. More on this later.

This means that emphasis on "solution-focused" therapy and the preoccupation with educational testing and measurement, are iterations of the larger emphasis in the field on "doing" and the emphasis on "products" and "justification," rather than the context and process of "discovery." The associated focus on intervening and developing strategies, tactics and programs to address problems in development, learning and behavior, are only part of the context.

This preoccupation with methods and technique has been accompanied by a failure to wonder about the nature of the problem, and instead places emphasis on "fixing" it. This has generated a volume of "empirical" research that iteratively demonstrates that certain procedures (e.g., ABA in autism) leads to behavioral change. In fact, an assertion like, "consequences change behaviors" can be regarded as an indisputable statement and a tautology. The assertion has nothing to do with the nature of the behavior being modified—that is, the underlying causes and functions of the behavior.

The focus on "doing," then conducting "research" that examines the effects of such "doing," has led the field to regard a "method" (e.g., ABA) as a "discipline," and in fact, universities now offer doctoral degrees in ABA (e.g., Caldwell College in New Jersey, USA). These patterns have violated critical tenets in "philosophy of science," by emphasizing the "context of justification" (Pepper, 1942/1970), where researchers brand their data collection as "empirical," or as the only empirical approach. However, the critical nature of scientific inquiry, deeply held guiding principles in philosophy of science, the sense of wonder, and the "context of discovery" (Popper, 1959; Reichenbach, 1951) have been abandoned. There is little authentic inquiry into the wide multidisciplinary literature that should inform "discovery" and dialectically transform "justification." When we focus on "doing," in line with the wish that many practitioners voice about wanting to "know what to "do," the process of discovery and wonder are inhibited.

Ways of being-with: the orphan of professional development

Consider this oversimplified, and admittedly artificial illustration: imagine that I (the "teacher") wanted to instruct you (the "learner") on how to "act," not a role in a play or a movie, but as a human being. Imagine that I were to insist that you emulate what I do and say, and that when you were behaving in a way that I considered right or "normal," I would encourage you—give you a tangible reward, a smile and praise, or an embrace. Now suppose the plot thickens, and I try to teach you how to show "care"—the desire to help someone. Maybe I would direct you to give food to a child who is hungry, give a hug to someone who is upset, and teach you about "good actions" that have effects on others who are in need. Soon, you begin to behave in ways that I planned for, and you show care when someone is in need, and do so even when I was not present to prompt you.

A fair question is, "What were the mechanisms that resulted in this change?" The argument could be made that you began to "know" what behaviors were acceptable, and how to "do" those things considered "caring" by others. So, were the mechanisms of change, the *knowing* of what is expected and learning the *doing* of actions that reflect that knowledge? In the case of "care," were the mechanisms, seeing someone in distress, knowing this as a trigger for caring and then doing the actions that were learned? There are, in fact epistemological formulations that, in the interest of parsimony would suggest these are sufficient explanations (e.g., "mechanistic" models, Overton & Reese, 1973). Nothing is inferred about "internal" processes, such as a cognitive state like "intentionality" (e.g., "I showed care because I intended to"), or emotional states like "empathy" (e.g., "When I saw that child crying, I felt distressed as if I could feel what the child was feeling"). If there is more going on as discovered in the sciences, isn't there an obligation to address more than what is observed?

This analysis is artificial because thinkers of all epistemological approaches acknowledge there are "feelings" that humans have, in addition to what they know and do. But does that acknowledgment actually show up, and are internal states considered in their theory and epistemology? So, this simplified analysis illustrates an important inquiry central to this discussion on "formation": can we promote development of multidisciplinary professionals in the fields of infant mental health and autism, primarily through imparting knowledge about the field and promoting the development of "skills" that involve learning and practicing strategies, techniques, tactics, and prescribed, even protocolized interventions? Are these ways of developing (Knowing and Doing) sufficient? Can professional development authentically happen when the internal experiences of the teacher and learner are not attended to?

Now, let's expand the meaning of "internal states" to include knowledge from the multidisciplinary sciences about cognitive, emotional, biological (neurosensory, neurodevelopmental, stress systems), and social/interpersonal studies. Exclusion of the growth and findings in these multidisciplinary sciences over the last quarter century could now be seen as significant omissions from the science of inquiry.

Surprisingly, an argument can be made that this is often what happened, especially in the field of autism—where the internal features (cognitive, emotional, biological, stress, and individual differences) of the teacher and learner are not a focus of inquiry and education, particularly in the dominant paradigm of ABA.

Continuing the analysis of the above illustration, the omission of any consideration of internal states and interpersonal processes (examined later) renders the analysis inadequate at best, and in the worst, obscures the identification of actual change agents. Drawing conclusions about change when significant domains of the multidisciplinary sciences are excluded, ensures the inadequacy of scientific inquiry. Furthermore, without exploring other domains, the findings are confounded by unexamined variables. So, in the example above, instructions in knowledge and doing are offered as the agents of change, but it is quite possible that change occurred due to reasons *other than* those articulated in the illustration. *In therapeutics, the intervention may work and help due to variables other than those proposed in the theory and therapeutic protocol.* The variables that were left unexamined may be the actual potent mechanisms.

Forgive this limited analysis of a complex process in logic and science, but let's consider another example: suppose you go to your car one morning and it fails to start. You call your local mechanic and she arrives, raises the hood of your car, looks around, and declares the problem is a dead battery. She recommends a new battery and you pay US$ 130. She installs the new battery—and your car starts up! All is fine with the world and the process of diagnosis and treatment (of your car) were flawless! Ah! Not so fast to that conclusion. Why? Suppose the "real" problem was the acid corrosion that developed on the wires that attached your car battery to the starter of your car. In the process of changing your battery, your mechanic cleaned the terminals on the battery and the wires to the car. Your car may have restarted with your old battery if the terminals and wires were cleaned! What happened? A diagnosis was made without examining all of the relevant variables, and an intervention was mounted which accomplished the desired effect. But NOT for the reason the mechanic identified! *The intervention was effective for a reason other than the one described!* This is an example of a common error in all areas of life: the "confirmation error" (e.g., O'Brien, Costa, & Overton, 1986; Wason 1960). If an outcome is consistent with what was predicted, individuals erroneously conclude that this is "proof" that the method or intervention worked! It may be so, but it may not be as well! This "confirmation bias" occurs in science, education, therapeutics, in parenting, and very obviously in politics—we tend to interpret as "evidence" a finding that is consistent with one's theory or belief. Costa (1988) found that when domains were more familiar and the content better known, confirmation bias is significantly reduced.

When the author was growing up in a small city in New Jersey (USA), he learned a wise lesson via a local political saying: "*If you drop a coin in the middle of the block, you don't look for it on the corner where the light is better.*" This can be adapted as a truism in science: you tend to look where you shine your light. If your inquiry (light) does not look at certain domains of human development, those will never be available as agents of interest and change. The mechanistic (ABA) paradigm, has been looking on the "corner" based on a long-standing paradigm in philosophy and in theories and frameworks in psychology and the behavioral sciences that originated at least in the late 19th and mid-20th centuries (e.g., Thorndike, 1898, 1901; Skinner, 1953; Lovaas, 1981).

Ideas and instruments—opening the multidisciplinary inner domains

Since that time, new conceptual frameworks and the findings from the multidisciplinary sciences, have made the primary focus on knowledge and doing, and the omission of internal (unobservable) processes, functionally inadequate. In the last three decades, two important forces long critical to the unfolding progress in the sciences, have continued to challenge the dominant ways of understanding the nature of autism. These forces are the two critical "I"s: *Ideas* and *Instrumentation.* Similar to the revolution in science that followed Galileo's use of the telescope to explore space, our understanding of autism has grown through the development of new ideas and new instruments.

Two ideas that support interest in "ways of being with" as essential to formation are illustrated by the field of interpersonal neurobiology (Siegel, 2010a, 2010b; Schore, 2019) and Polyvagal Theory (Porges, 2011). These "ideas" have been supported, even made possible, by the development of new *instrumentation*, notably in the brain sciences (CAT scans, MRIs, PET scans, and others) that have lifted the artificial veil of preoccupation only on what can be seen and observed with the eye. The artificiality of attending to only what can be seen and observable has long been abandoned in medicine where temperature and blood pressure measurement, and X-rays have been available for decades. Lister (1867) identified the need to protect patients from unseen bacteria and "germs" over 150 years ago. We cannot rely only on what can be seen with the eye, so instrumentation in the "hard" sciences (e.g., medicine, astronomy, and physics) has contributed to the revolution of thought for centuries.

Consider how we "see" light: A simple glass instrument (a prism) permits us to see the spectrum of light, including ultraviolet and infrared at the ends of the spectrum. We would not deny the existence of ultraviolet light simply because we cannot see it with the naked eye, in the same way we know there are frequencies of sound that humans cannot hear. Reliance only on what can be observed limits the science by the limitations of the human senses. That is the proverbial "tail wagging the dog." We need other ways to observe, and this has not occurred in the field of autism as organized by the dominant paradigm.

We will examine two ideas that make the "Ways of Being With" an essential ingredient of formation.

Interpersonal neurobiology

The field of interpersonal neurobiology examines, and documents the anatomical, physical, chemical, and functional changes that occur in the brain when two living beings interact with each other (e.g., Cozolino, 2014). Nearly two decades ago, Schore (2001) examined the empirical connection between attachment style and the development of the infant's orbitofrontal cortex, finding that the organization of the cortex was enhanced through a secure relationship with the parent. In a much earlier series of studies and publications, Giacomo Rizzolatti and his colleagues (Rizzolatti, 2005; Rizzolatti & Craighero, 2004; Rizzolatti, Fadiga, Fogassi, & Gallese, 1996; Rizzolatti, Fogassi, & Gallese, 2001) described the functioning of a certain set of brain cells they first discovered in the motor cortex of monkeys nearly 25 years ago, which they named "mirror neurons." Rizzolatti (2005) wrote, "Mirror neurons are a particular type of neurons that discharge when an individual performs an action, as well as when he/she observes a similar action done by another individual" (p. 419). (This was first discovered when one of their monkey subjects underwent parallel brain changes when the animal observed a lab assistant eating a peanut), so it seems to occur cross-species at least in mammals. Siegel (2010a) refers to "mirror neurons," as "sponge neurons," and he describes "resonance" or "we" circuits (p. 60), which are activated when two individuals are in proximity, and where the observer actually infers intentionality in the actor. While unable to explore here the deeper implications of these phenomena, it is sufficient to note that we are changed by mere observation and more so by interactions with others—and these occur at the neurological level and are largely below our level of awareness, on "autopilot" (Eagleman, 2011, p. 5), meaning that the neurological and unconscious processes actually lead to behaviors of which we are not fully aware.

In the field of infant mental health, Schore (2001) described the mother's limbic system as communicating directly to the infant's limbic system (subcortical system associated with emotionality and responding to danger)—akin to Rizzolatti's mirror neuron system and Siegel's (2010a) "resonance circuits." Trevarthen, Aitken, Nage, Delafield-Butt, and Vandekerckhove (2006) described a "Protoconversation" between the mother and preverbal infant as "Synrhythmic regulation...(a) mutual psychological engagement by exchange of expressions of interest and emotional feelings," and the "synrhythmic frontier" between them as the "living 'socioemotional space' between the expressive actions of the two human beings and their minds" (p. 49–50). The multimodal expressions in voice, facial expressions, movement, and pacing, are seen as a kind of "musicality" (Trevarthen, 2009) that changes both—in brain, mind, and emotion. Similarly, Tronick's (2007) "Mutual Regulation Model" describes the reciprocal, interactive process between parent and infant that serves to connect and modulate the connection to its optimal level.

So why is this important to our discussion of "being-with" in formation? Because the consensus in the developmental brain sciences is that we need to pay attention to what the "autopilot" is leading us to think and do, and *feel*! In my earlier illustration, there was no room in the analysis for this inquiry—neither in the "teacher" nor the "learner." Now anyone with a rudimentary understanding of psychoanalysis and general psychodynamic theory will infer from what I have said, that these processes were part of psychological theories for most of the 20th century—known as unconscious process, and in clinical work as the operation of "transference," "countertransference," and of "projection." But these are now understood as also having a neurobiological component in the "hard" science or neurology, and cannot be ignored as unworthy of study or as an inconvenient notion that does not fit into more positivist views. These findings can be regarded as the kind of evidence in the history of science that Kuhn (1962/1970) would suggest will eventually result in a "paradigm shift."

It is sufficient here to argue that the history and philosophy of science, the influence of underlying paradigms and world views, and the *existence* of differing models of thought, aside from the dominant paradigm which determine the nature of research questions, the nature of what are regarded as "data" and "evidence," and the frameworks of intervention, *must* be part of the ways of knowing and wondering in professional development. With regard to our discussion of "Ways of Being-With," we have argued that in professional formation, we must explore the workings of what happens within us and between us, both teacher and learner, similar to the need for supervision that is reflective for the practitioner and his mentor.

Polyvagal theory

We will examine one further theory about interpersonal processes: *Polyvagal Theory* (Porges, 2011, 2015). Polyvagal Theory was developed by the neuroscientist, Stephen Porges. The theory assigns new interpersonal functions to the 10th cranial nerves—the Vagus nerves. Porges states that "coregulation" (the capacity for an individual to help calm activation and stress in another) begins with the mother–infant relationship and extends throughout the life span with other significant partners. In mammals, the vagal pathways originate from a part of the brainstem that regulates the heart but also regulates the striated muscles of the face and head—a face to heart connection, that "...forms an integrated *social engagement system* that provides and senses signals of safety" (Porges, 2015, p. 4). This allows mammals (humans) to convey physiological state *via facial expression and prosody (intonation of voice), enabling facial expression and voice to calm physiological state*. Physiological state is signaled by changes in the face and voice, and this happens often below our level of awareness (neuroception vs perception). Think "autopilot." Furthermore, Porges (2015) theorizes that in the evolutionary transition from reptiles to mammals, *social behavior* emerged as the "prepotent regulator of physiology" (p. 3, italics added).

Stated plainly, mothers can calm fussy babies with a smile, soft voice, and touch —and these are psychological and physiological changes. We have known this from eons of being human. We know that our affect, voice, movement, pacing—and of course words—can coregulate or coescalate another's demeanor. Surprisingly though, in interactions conveying the social and emotional meaning of an exchange, and safety, *words* are the least important! In an oft reported analysis of the relative importance of verbal and nonverbal factors when individuals communicate feelings and attitudes, Mehrabian (1972, 1981) reported that 55% of the communicative intent is conveyed by facial expressions, 38% by vocal tone, and only 7% by the words themselves. So, when a message is "inconsistent," the nonverbal cues win out. This is particularly the case for infants (especially preverbally), but in fact Porges proposes that the functions of the many ("poly") nerves of the Vagus system convey safety and coregulation, throughout life. Shanker (2016) refers to the regulatory capacity of the relationship as the "interbrain," similar to Trevarthen's notion of the living 'socioemotional space' between the expressive actions of the two human beings, cited earlier.

Porges goes further in Polyvagal Theory by proposing that the most primitive need humans has from birth is to feel safe, and that with the emergence in evolution of social behavior as the primary regulator of stress, that humans have a "biological imperative" of "connectedness." He wrote, "...(H)umans are on a quest to calm neural defense systems by detecting features of safety. This quest is initiated at birth when an infant's need to be soothed is dependent on the caregiver" (Porges, 2015, p. 2). Porges asserts that our nervous system needs to feel safe, and that from birth we seek and expect features of safety to be present, such as caring face-to-face interactions with warmly modulated voices. If these are not detected, our "safety" brain (the fight, flight, or freeze response) becomes activated, and this deactivates our "thinking" brain; we become "defensive" and this limits learning, growth, and restoration. He notes that in all cultures, "... prosodic acoustic stimulation, whether vocal or instrumental, is an effective strategy for signaling safety and calming infants" (p. 6). Building on the foundational importance of is an effective strategy for signaling safety and calming, and cognitive development (e.g., Greenspan & Wieder, 1998, 2006; Shanker, 2016), Porges add the critical need for *safety*, and in the formulation proposed here, Porges argues that the first task of social interactions is to feel safe. The "he inerues tha that the first task of social interactions is to feel safe.task of social i safe. This is the first and foremost responsibility of the teacher and practitioner. However, the important take-away from our discussion about influential ideas is that *safety and regulation are conveyed interpersonally*, pre- and nonverbally, and are driven both by the mind (intention and purpose) and the at itioner." f the brain.

Shanker (2016) builds on MacLean's model of the "triune" brain (MacLean & Kral, 1973), segmenting the brain into three hierarchically organized "brains: the 'reptilian' ('brown') brain, the 'paleomammalian' or 'limbic' brain ('red') and the 'neocortex' ('blue') brain" (p. 14–17). Shanker proposes that we do our best when the "red" brain is relatively calm (meaning the "red" brain is needed for excitement and passion, but it must not lead to chronic activation of the stress systems) and the "blue" brain is fully available and engaged. What helps the "red" brain stay calm, is the "interbrain"—the connected, coregulating other. This, of course, adds to the premise of why we must attend to "ways of being-with."

In the ending summary of this chapter, the author will present a framework called "AGILE" to remind the practitioner of the affective and interpersonal forces, the pre- and nonverbal forces at play, that are frequently ignored in science, theory, and practice.

Before ending this section, Stern's (1995) notion of "a schema of being with" as the experience of an infant in relationship to his mother, was a clear influence in the selection of the language and concepts underlying the "Ways of Being-With" described in this chapter on "Formation."

Putting the "Ways" together as formation

Five conclusions emerge from this discussion:

1. This chapter proposes that we need to replace the term, Professional Development" and similar terminology, with the concept of "Formation" in the multidisciplinary helping sciences and practices.
2. Arguments have been offered that, especially in the field of autism, there is no one way to "teach" and intervene. The current dominant "mechanistic" paradigm has for some time ignored the multidisciplinary and neurodevelopmental sciences which have challenged as untenable, key features of the ABA expression of that paradigm, notably the failure to attend to the interpersonal processes between practitioner and client, and the reliance on observable phenomena when new ideas and instruments offer ways of thinking, observing, and measuring. The implication for growth is that these must also be considered in the formation of the professional.
3. Three "ways" of promoting professional growth under the umbrella of "formation" are offered: knowing, doing, and being-with. Efforts to cultivate "ways of knowing" must include educating the multidisciplinary workforce in infant mental health and autism, in the multiple ways of understanding, researching, and intervening, that are represented by different "world views" and paradigms. Such an education in the "Ways of Knowing" must include an examination of "Philosophy of Science" (e.g., DeWitt, 2010; Kuhn, 1962/1970; Pepper, 1942/1970; Popper, 1959; Reichenbach, 1951).
4. Professional "Development" is often conflated with terms like training, skill-building, education, problem-solving, etc., and these are often seen as focusing on knowledge and skills that derive from that knowledge. The interpersonal process is omitted. The development of intervention "skills," strategies, techniques, and tactics is insufficient in the preparation of the multidisciplinary workforce, because interventions are delivered by humans, whose inner lives and neurology must be the subject of understanding and development, as these are significant influences to the development of attitudes, beliefs, and ideas that are formed "below the radar"—our "autopilot." Skills, even those which are standardized and protocolized, will necessarily be delivered in differing ways reflecting the inner life and individual histories of the practitioner.
5. We must identify the necessary experiences in professional growth and the three interrelated ways of development can serve as a model for the development of curricula and "formative" offerings and programs.

The developmental/relational paradigms (e.g., Overton, 2013) offer alternate perspectives, and the multidisciplinary sciences have been shining the light in a growing number of areas that matter in human development including:

- developmental/relational interventions that address the missing areas in the above discussion (e.g., Greenspan & Wieder, 1998, 2006; Solomon, Van Egeren, Mahoney, Quon Huber, & Zimmerman, 2014; Solomon, 2016);
- neurosensory systems and sensory processing (e.g., Miller, 2014);
- stress systems in autism (e.g., Whitman, Shanker, 2016); and
- the motor sciences (e.g., Torres, 2018; Trevarthen & Delafield-Butt, 2013). Torres (2018), for example, developed a range of biometric sensors that detect subtle movements indicating intentionality in individuals with autism who do not demonstrate responses in any observable way (new "instruments").

For years in the field of autism, the dominant paradigm promoted a discourse which diminished interest and value in nondominant frameworks (e.g., Broderick, 2009; Claypool & McLaughlin, 2017) and in the multidisciplinary sciences. We have examined this before but the omissions include the advances in developmental neurobiology of autism (e.g., Courchesne, Campbell, & Solso, 2011; Khan et al., 2015), and frameworks that examine the comprehensive ecological and environmental forces that form the larger context and discourse of autism (e.g., Herbert & Weintraub, 2012). These perspectives have broadened the relevant content and discourse on which to shine the light of inquiry. These are absent in most autism curricula. The "light" simply does not shine in these areas, so what is unexamined is then omitted from thought and ideas, and what is taught is based on an implicit demarcation of limited concepts.

"Ways of being-with" address the capacity to form attuned, empathic, contingent, coregulating, caring relationships with the infants, children, and families to whom professionals provide service. This is the "how you are" with families in addition to the "what you know and do." A repeated theme in this chapter has been that services are provided within the context of relationships. The author argues that this is now indisputable—even if many approaches ignore relationships! But we cannot ignore relationships in the development of our multidisciplinary workforce!

The necessity to support awareness of, and growth in "ways of being-with" are essential to the development of professionals in infant mental health and autism. This means that the nature of the teacher–learner relationship must also be a primary focus of professional growth.

Formation

The concept of "formation" embodies a perspective that requires that the practitioner be fully integrated, as Kohut (1984) suggested, and in so doing, provide a "corrective emotional experience" (p. 153) through the nature of "being with" (author's interpretation) the client, integrating what the practitioner knows and does. Of course, it comes as no surprise that the "self-psychological" perspective of Kohut with his psychoanalytic roots (a world view quite different from the dominant paradigm) would lead him to focus on the inner life of the practitioner and client, but it appears that this is exactly the message coming from the interpersonal neurosciences as well. The language and interpretations that Kohut would employ are, of course, quite different, but in this attempt to articulate the essential elements of "formation," we are "landing" in a similar place.

"Formation" here is being used as a term encompassing the development of the fully human practitioner! This means that the "ways" of knowing, doing, and being-with are actually experienced and expressed as inseparable. The practitioner, *in the moment of interaction* with her client is NOT thinking about what she knows and does, and even may be unaware of what is "going on inside." These of course are "grist for the mill" of reflection and supervision. True formation is about being *fully present in the moment*, and this includes "presence" and "attunement," carefully articulated and illustrated by Dan Siegel (2010b). This is not at all to suggest that the process of intervening is mindless. It is just the opposite: what the practitioner knows and does, and their awareness of "being-with" has been cultivated through education, reflection, and supervision, so that what occurs in the practitioner's relationship flows together. This is of course an idealized vision of the therapeutic relationship, but it is what we strive for, in *formation.*

So "formation" implies that our goals are to support professional and personal growth, and the later includes growth of our awareness of, and care for, our "inner life," our "well-being," and our neurobiological "autopilot"—a practice Siegel (2010a) calls "mindsight." Formation calls us as practitioners to promote personal "unfolding" meaning that as we developmentally and professionally become who we are, our knowledge, actions, and experiences "unfold" and become integrated.

The journey of formation entails at the least four components of preparation in the "teaching" and "learning" about the fields of infant mental health and autism. These are:

1. The development and delivery of a curriculum of "knowing" as described earlier that covers not only the dominant paradigms and approaches in the fields, but a deep education about the philosophy of science and its implications. Such a curriculum should promote knowledge and understanding about the historically different metatheoretical ideas and theories, the definition of data, the varying models of change, the articulation of research methods, the identification of what "data" are and "evidence" is, and the varying explanation on human development and interventions. Maddi (1968/1980/1995) offers an extraordinary framework for comparative analyses of approaches, and Overton and Reese (1973) and Reese and Overton (1970) present a comparison of the philosophical traditions that undergird present developmental theories. Costa and Witten (2009) applied these frameworks to the field of autism.
2. The identification and implementation of *critical experiences* that create an interest in new ways of thinking about development and autism. In an initial formulation of these experiences that grew out of a *Post Baccalaureate Certificate in Developmental Models of Autism Intervention*, rooted in this formation framework at the Center for Autism and Early Childhood Mental Health (Montclair State University, New Jersey/USA) (https://www.montclair.edu/center-for-autism-and-early-childhood-mental-health/), developed by them, Costa and Catalano (2014) presented a representative list of five such critical experiences. These included: (1) An exploration of the learner's "sensory" systems through an experiential survey. This served as a portal to explore the "hidden" autopilot of what happens "inside;" (2) Reading of "first person" literature: autobiographical account of individuals with autism. *Carly's Voice* (Fleischmann & Fleischmann, 2012) was particularly vision-changing for the learners. *Look Me in the Eye* (Robison, 2007) was equally effective in challenging notions about autism only being seen as a disability, and the need for education by individuals with autism. For example, John Robison (2007) wrote, "All those child psychologists who said John prefers to play by himself were dead wrong. I played by myself because I was a failure at playing with others" (p. 211). These efforts to create "disequilibrium" in the learner by challenging what they "knew" about autism, also broadened the discourse to include an understanding of an emerging perspective in disabilities in general and specifically in autism, about "neurodiversity" (e.g., Silberman, 2016); (3) View Ed Tronick's "still face" experiment video and discuss. This now famous experiment (see Tronick, 2007 for a review of the history and research program that emerged from this research that began in the 1970s) serves as a model of what occurs when a relationship is changed by the

unavailability of one partner. In the "still face," a parent of a young infant (usually between 3–8 months) interacts playfully with the child, and is then asked to become silent and to create a "still-face" with no gestures and movement. This results in almost immediate distress in the infant. The learner is asked to reflect on, "*What if the baby is the still face?*" opening the discourse into the interactive and interpersonal processes that occur in all human relationships. The "still face" offers a view on the parent's perspective and encourages an understanding of the interpersonal process that is changed in a child with autism; (4) Examine Stern's (1984) notion "Affect Attunement." This critical experience reveals the deep connectedness between the field of infant mental health and autism, rooted in the awareness of the importance of reciprocal processes. In examining the "feeling states" of a child with autism, who might have limited or no language, what might occur when the child's "feeling" cannot be attuned to or "felt with" by the parent? Students are asked to explore the "meanings" of certain behaviors often seen in individuals with autism, especially those without language (e.g., gaze aversion, and-flapping, screaming, or running). This critical experience offers the learner to wonder about the inner life of the child with autism, not just the observables. Often such behaviors are viewed in the dominant paradigm as noncompliant and unacceptable behaviors, and this exercise offers the learner the opportunity to reflect on what might happen if she had a feeling or idea that could not be expressed and could not be shared and "attuned to" another. In Shanker's (2016) formulation, the "misbehavior" might better be understood as "stress" behavior (p. 2); and (5) Explore science as a field of inquiry, guided by different "paradigms." This has been addressed in earlier sections. Catalano, Fives, McKeating, & Barnes, 2020, using these critical experiences developed in the *Developmental Models of Autism Intervention* (DMAI) graduate program at Montclair State University (see earlier section) examined self-efficacy and views on autism among preservice teachers. They reported higher levels of self-efficacy for teaching in general and more specifically, for teaching children with ASD in inclusive settings. They also reported a significant reduction in regarding children with autism as different from how children in general should be regarded.

3. A rigorous commitment to exploring interpersonal/relational processes that are involved in all therapeutic relationship. This includes the necessity of reflective supervision and consultation for all multidisciplinary professionals during formation, and therapeutic experiences as part of clinical training.

Fig. 13.1 offers a framework of conceptualizing the many aspects of human experience building on the idea that we can consider each individual as having three levels of "self": The "Public Self," which is the "you" that you live out in public as you meet others in casual, everyday settings. The "Private Self" is the "you" that those closest to you (e.g., your family and close friends), come to know. Then there is the "Secret Self," the inner self that others, and even "you" do not always have access to.

In Fig. 13.1 these "Three Selves" are seen as emerging from the "self" that you and others "know" and the "self" you and others, don't know. This 2×2 grid produces a unique area for exploration and reflective process, consistent with the critical importance of understanding "ways of being-with."

a. The "self" you know and that others know, constitutes the "Public Self" we described above. In a real sense this is our "lived life" moment-to-moment, often on "autopilot" and with a minimal of reflection and introspection. Ways to cultivate formation here, can occur by openly discussing yourself with others and acknowledging your style, appearance, habits, and behaviors

b. The self you know that others don't know. We have referred to this as the "private life." The formative tools we have are: cultivating introspection and self-awareness,

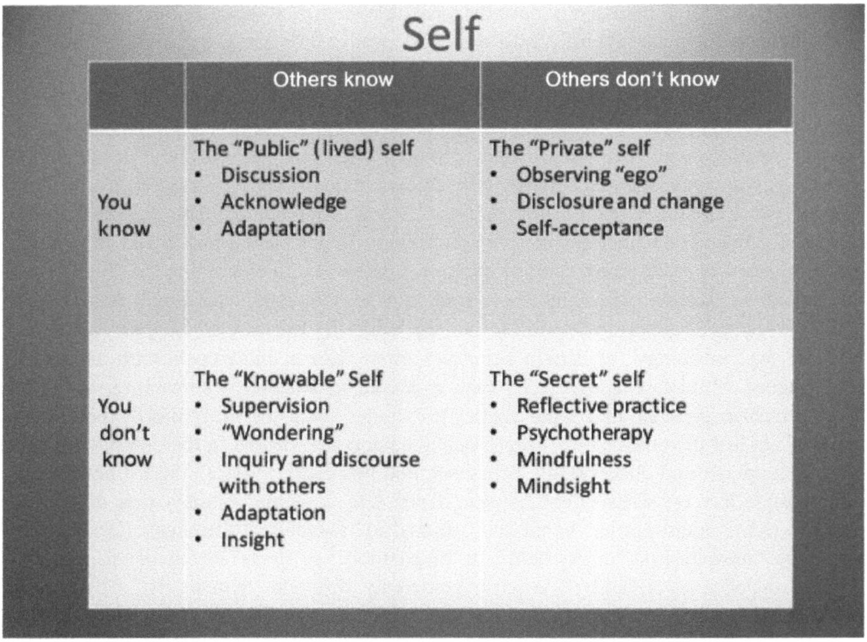

Figure 13.1 Aspects of the "three selves" and strategies for formation.

working on seeing yourself as others might ("observing ego"), disclosing with candor and comfort, things about yourself that you either try to change or accept.

c. The self that you and others don't know. We have labeled this the "secret life." (Note that in cases of early childhood experience and trauma, an individual might not recall events that happened while others might. This is considered in the final fourth cell of the grid.) This is an area of great opportunity in Formation, because through an examination of the secret life, individuals, explore, contain and alter, those unconscious and "autopilot" forces that can lead them to feel and act in ways that might not be helpful. Activities including "Reflective Practices," cultivating mindfulness, practicing "mindsight" (Siegel, 2010a), and engaging in psychotherapy. These are all paths to examining our secret lives, and address a set of influences that are often ignored and disregarded. Yet they constitute an essential component of promoting "ways of being-with."

d. Finally, the fourth cell refers to the self that you don't know about yourself, but others might know. We have labeled this the "Knowable" self. Ways to develop in this domain can be cultivated by supervision, reflection and self-wondering, safe conversations, and developing insight.

The cultivation of an informed, educated, sensitive, and responsive multidisciplinary workforce is the goal of Formation. All of us choose our work, professions, and careers do so on the basis of *all three* selves! Formation must engage all three!

4. The opportunity to engage in supervision, within and cross-disciplinary experiences guided by mentors who themselves are in a reflective supervision. This requirement emerges from our discussion above. This is a variant of the admonition: "Physician, heal thyself" (New Testament, Luke 4:23), and was echoed in Winnicott's recommendation mentioned earlier that pediatricians should consider psychoanalysis. It is important to note that psychoanalysis was not only viewed as a treatment for mental illness, but also as a recommended method of self-exploration and self-understanding. So, while Winnicott undoubtedly did not regard pediatricians as a class of physicians as pathological, his insistence that the helping professional must be committed to rigorous self-examination and self-awareness was evident. This view is consistent with the formation framework discussed throughout this chapter. In his chapter on "Training for Child Psychiatry," Winnicott (1965) wrote, "It is generally accepted that the case conference is of no value unless afterwards someone carries over into a *personal relationship* the new understanding that that discussion has brought. *New understanding does nothing by itself*" (p. 194, italics added). In other words, knowledge (i.e., understanding) in and of itself is meaningless until it is reflected in a change in the "personal relationship" between the clinician and the client—in the "doing" and "being-with" the client. So, *formation, must engage all three selves*, as stated earlier, and psychoanalysis/psychotherapy is a journey worth taking for those of us in the helping professions.

Closing

Our premise throughout this chapter has been to consider the best ways to prepare the multidisciplinary workforce to understand and work in the fields of infant

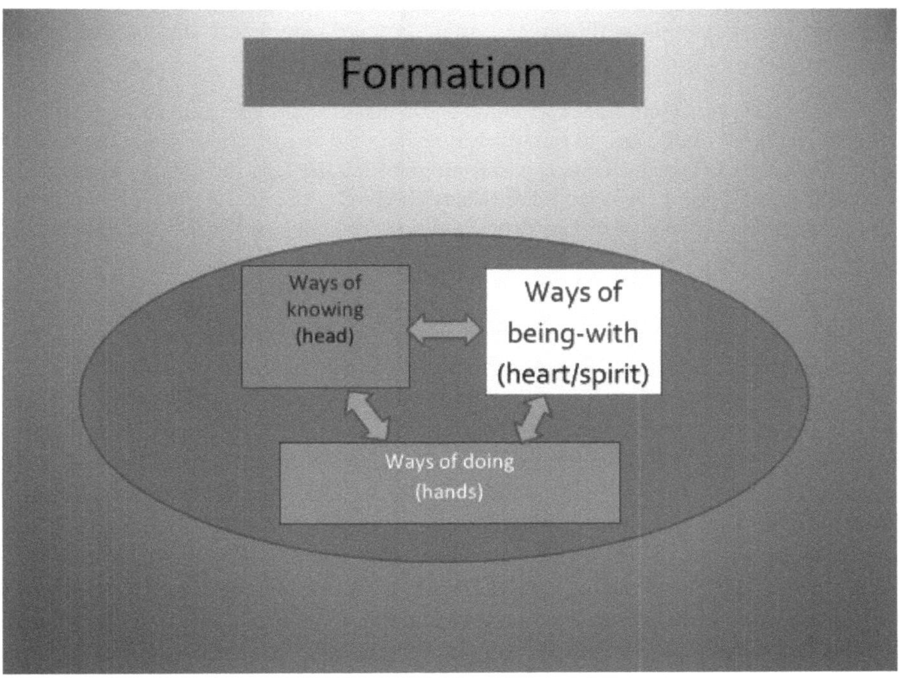

Figure 13.2 An integrated framework for formation.

mental health and autism, and to honor the ways that learners best grow as a result of professional development efforts. Understanding and responding to infants, children, families, and individuals with autism, must be rooted in its relationship to "ways of knowing" (what does the broad, multidisciplinary field and sciences lead me to know and how can I cultivate a sense of "wonder" so as not to see my "theory" when I am with my client?), "ways of doing" (what can I do to be of most help?) and "ways of being-with" (how can I understand the nature of my relationship with the client?), including what I am feeling and how can I best use my "self."

Fig. 13.2 presents these three "ways" of development that must be attended to in formation. The domains mutually influence each other as we develop through our continuous encounters and growth. This figure employs a colloquial way of considering professional growth and helping by the integrated employment of our "Head" (knowing), or "Hands" (doing), and our "Heart" (being-with).

Summary

In this chapter, a framework for professional development has been described that cultivates growth in the multidisciplinary workforce in three interrelated ways: knowing, doing and being-with, together conceptualized as *Formation*. Those who are responsible for the professional development of the multidisciplinary helping workforce, must grapple with two essential "knotty"—complex, intertwined, cross-disciplinary—questions about our educational endeavors:

1. What are the educational and experiential encounters that are foundational for staff at all levels and in all disciplines, to form their capacities for empathy and care in the fields of infant mental health and autism; how can we best form the capacities for professionals for educating and *forming*, their multidisciplinary charges?
2. Is emphasizing acquisition of knowledge and skill, enough, and if not, what else must be attended to in *formation*?

This chapter offered answers to these questions, and challenges those charged with the responsibility to grow and educate our multidisciplinary workforce, to create transformative educational experiences.

In the end, most professionals who have been engaged in professional development know of the importance of "knowing" and "doing," although the discussion about these "ways" of development here considerably broadened, we hope, the meaning and scope of what they entail. However, while the field of infant mental health is rooted in "relationship-based" approaches, it is largely absent in the discourse about autism in the dominant mechanistic paradigm. Developmental/relational approaches are growing, and the science in interpersonal neurobiology and interpersonal processes clearly demand attention to the nature of the helping relationship and what happens "inside" the practitioner and the client.

As a tool to support the sensitivity to the nonverbal dimension of relationships in multidisciplinary work, Costa (2020) developed an "AGILE" framework to help

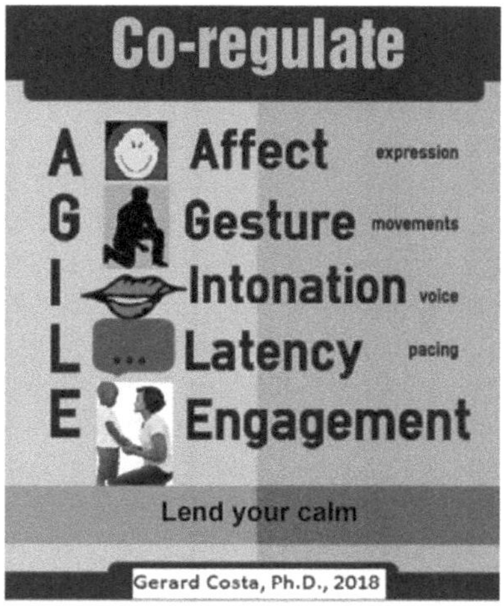

Figure 13.3 The AGILE framework for interpersonal process. *AGILE*, Affect, Gesture, Intonation, Latency (Wait), Engagement.

practitioners "in the moment" as they are working with children and families. This is not meant in any way to circumvent the required experiences that constitute formation, but merely as a memorial aid to support reflection about the operation of the practitioner's "inner life" and autopilot.

The AGILE framework is presented in Fig. 13.3, which was developed as a laminated "pocket card."

The AGILE acronym stands for:

- Affect—this is what a child experiences first and most!
- Gesture—modulate and be attuned in face, hands, movement, and pacing
- Intonation—modulate the tone of your voice as this conveys affect
- Latency (Wait)—wait and allow the child time to "take you in"
- Engagement—before you continue, be sure you have engaged the child

Collectively

Sullivan, Colby, Wegner, Bond, and Shulman (2007), writing about lawyers in the Carnegie Foundation reports on professional formation, stated clearly what is regarded as the key conclusion of this chapter on Formation. They wrote, "Identity formation trumps information transmission" (p. 6).

We cannot be satisfied with transmission of knowledge and skill alone. We must consider who the individuals are that we are being called upon to FORM! Professional development must engage what is often regarded as personal and private domains—not requiring disclosure of personal narratives, but recognizing that they exist—because they INFLUENCE how we are and what we do.

Formation requires that those who "form" others must do so through a relationship that is felt as safe. We need to cultivate a shared sense of wonderment, self-awareness, and the capacity for reflectivity.

There are also aspects of our multidisciplinary work that involve authentic human engagement and care. This is expressed when the practitioner holds a deep sense of modesty and connectedness to human frailty, the capacity to suspend judgment, and a deep sense of caring.

As we have described "formation" as an integrated expression of the three interrelated ways of knowing, doing, and being-with, it emerges as a unified expression of the unfolding personhood of the practitioner. It becomes both a mind and a brain process. Knowledge is integrated and expressed in "ways of doing" with others, and "ways of being-with." It integrates affect and intellect, and as Mary Gordon (Gordon, 2009) said about "empathy," it is not "taught" as much as it is "caught" in the formation process.

References

Beyonce (2016). *Formation* (Song/lyrics). <https://genius.com/Beyonce-formation-lyrics>

Broderick, A. A. (2009). Autism, "recovery (to normalcy)," and the politics of hope. *Intellectual and Developmental Disabilities*, *47*(4), 263–281.

Catalano, C. G., Fives, H., McKeating, E., & Barnes, N. (2020). Preservice early childhood teachers' sense of efficacy for teaching children with autism spectrum disorder. *Journal of Early Childhood Teacher Education*. Available from http://doi.org/10.1080/10901027.2020.1806152.

Claypool, M. K., & McLaughlin, J. M. (2017). *How autism is reshaping special education: The unbundling of IDEA*. Lanham, MD: Rowman and Littlefield.

Cooke, M., Irby, D. M., & O'Brien, B. C. (2010). *Educating physicians: A call for reform of medical school and residency* (1st ed.). San Francisco, CA: Jossey-Bass, The Carnegie Foundation for the Advancement of teaching.

Cooper, J. O., Heron, T. E., & Heward, W. L. (2019). *Applied behavior analysis-3rd edition*. London: Pearson.

Costa, G. (1988). *A confirmation-disconfirmation synthesis in the development of deductive reasoning*. (Unpublished dissertation). Philadelphia, PA: Temple University.

Costa, G. (2006). Mental health principles, practices, strategies and dynamics pertinent to early intervention practitioners. In G. M. Foley, & J. D. Hochman (Eds.), *Mental health in early intervention: Achieving unity in principles and practice*. Baltimore: Paul T. Brookes Publishers.

Costa, G. (2016). Reconceptualizing training as "professional formation" in the field of autism. In *Invited plenary presentation at the first annual Cyprus international conference on autism treatment and research: Actions not words. . .love autism*. Paphos, Cyprus.

Costa, G. (2020). Expert voice: On autism. In S. Shanker, & S. Hopkins (Eds.), *Self-reg for schools: A handbook for educators* (pp. 58–61). North York, Ontario: Pearson Canada.

Costa, G. & Catalano, C. (2014). Formative and transformative processes in professional development: What are the critical experiences that engender new ways of thinking about development and autism. In *Oral presentation at annual conference of the interdisciplinary council on developmental and learning disorders*. Boston, MA.

Costa, G. & Mulcahy, K. (2015). *Framework for the formation of the transdisciplinary infant-family workforce*. Zero to Three National Training Institute. Seattle, WA.
Costa, G. & Mulcahy, K. (2018). Ways of knowing, doing and being in professional formation. In *Oral presentation at the 16th annual world association for infant mental health world congress*. Rome, Italy.
Costa, G., & Sullivan, L. (2009). What staff development activities can be used to build reflective capacity? In S. S. Heller, & L. Gilkerson (Eds.), *A practical guide to reflective supervision*. Washington, DC: ZERO TO THREE Press.
Costa, G., & Witten, M. R. (2009). Pervasive developmental disorders (Chapter 4). In B. Mowder, F. Robinson, & A. Yasik (Eds.), *Evidence based practice in infant and early childhood psychology* (pp. 467–499). Hoboken, NJ: John Wiley & Son, Publishers.
Courchesne, E., Campbell, K., & Solso, S. (2011). Brain growth across the life span in autism: Age-specific changes in anatomical pathology. *Brain Research*, *1380*(138-45), 2011.
Cozolino, L. (2014). *The neuroscience of human relationships: attachment and the developing social brain (2nd ed.)*. New York: W.W. Norton and Company, Norton series on interpersonal neurobiology.
DeWitt, R. (2010). *Worldviews: An introduction to the history and philosophy of science 2nd Edition*. Hoboken, NJ: Wiley-Blackwell.
Eagleman, D. (2011). Incognito: The secret lives of the brain-*illustrated edition*. New York: Pantheon Books.
Fenichel, E. (1992). *Learning through supervision and mentorship to support the development of infants, toddlers and their families: A source book*. Washington, DC: ZERO TO THREE Press.
Fleischmann, A., & Fleischmann, C. (2012). *Carly's voice: Breaking through autism*. New York: Touchstone, Simon and Schuster.
Gordon, M. (2009). *Roots of empathy: Changing the world child by child*. Toronto, Canada: Thomas Allen Publishers.
Greenspan, S. I., & Shanker, S. G. (2004). *The first idea: How symbols, language, and intelligence evolved from our primate ancestors to modern humans*. New York, NY: Da Capo Press.
Greenspan, S. I., & Wieder, S. (1998). *The child with special needs: Encouraging Intellectual and Emotional Growth*. Cambridge, MA: A Merloyd Lawrence Book.
Greenspan, S. I., & Wieder, S. (2006). *Engaging autism: Using the floortime approach to help children relate, communicate, and think*. Cambridge, MA: A Merloyd Lawrence Book.
Hamilton, N. (2011). Fostering professional formation (professionalism): Lessons from the Carnegie foundation's five studies on educating professionals. *Creighton Law Review*, *45*, 764–798.
Herbert, M. R., & Weintraub, K. (2012). *The autism revolution: Whole body strategies for making life all it can be*. MA: Ballantine/Harvard Health Publications.
Khan, A. J., Nair, A., Keown, C. L., Datko, M. C., Lincoln, A. J., & Müller, R.-A. (2015). Cerebro-cerebellar resting-state functional connectivity in children and adolescents with autism spectrum disorder. *Biological Psychiatry*, *78*(9), 625–634.
Kohut, H. (1984). *How does analysis cure?* Chicago: The University of Chicago Press.
Kohut, H., & Seitz, P. F. D. (1963/1978). Concepts and theories of psychoanalysis. In P. H. Orstein (Ed.), *The search for the self: selected writings of Heinz Kohut: 1950-1978* (Vol. 1), pp. 337–374). Madison, CN: International Universities Press, Inc.
Kuhn, T. (1962/1970). *The structure of scientific revolutions—2nd ed. Enlarged*. Chicago: University of Chicago Press.

Lagemann, E. C. (2000). *An elusive science: The troubling history of education research.* Chicago: University of Chicago Press.

Lister, J. (1867). On the antiseptic principle in the practice of surgery. *British Medical Journal*, *2*(351), 246–248.

Lovaas, O. I. (1981). *Teaching developmentally disabled children: The me book.* Australia: Pro-Ed.

MacLean, P. D., & Kral, V. A. (1973). *A triune concept of the brain and behavior.* Toronto: University of Toronto Press.

Maddi, S. (1968/1980). *Personality theories: A comparative analysis.* Homewood, IL: The Dorsey Press.

Mehrabian, A. (1972). *Nonverbal communication.* Chicago: Aldine-Atherton.

Mehrabian, A. (1981). *Silent messages: Implicit communication of emotions and attitudes.* Belmont, CA: Wadsworth currently distributed by Albert Mehrabian. Available from am@kaaj.com.

Miller, L. J. (2014). *Sensational kids: Hope and help for children with sensory processing disorder (SPD).* New York: Penguin Books.

Nenide, L., Wasserman, K., Costa, G., Corso, R., & Horen, N. (In preparation). *Provisional title: Two perspectives, one child: Unifying the pyramid model and infant mental health.* In discussions with. Baltimore: Paul T. Brookes Publishers.

O'Brien, D. P., Costa, G., & Overton, W. F. (1986). Evaluations of causal and conditional hypotheses. *The Quarterly Journal of Experimental Psychology*, *38A*, 493–512.

Overton, W. F. (1984). World views and their influence on psychological theory and research: Kuhn–Lakatos–Laudan. In H. W. Reese (Ed.), *Advances in child development and behavior* (Vol. 18, pp. 191–226). New York: Academic Press.

Overton, W. F. (1998). Developmental psychology: Philosophy, concepts, and methodology. In R. M. Lerner (Ed.), *Theoretical models of human development: (Vol. 1). Handbook of child psychology 5th ed* (pp. 107–188). New York: Wiley.

Overton, W. F. (2013). Relational developmental systems and developmental science: A focus on methodology. In P. C. M. Molenar, R. M. Lerner, & K. Newell (Eds.), *Handbook of developmental systems: Theory and methodology* (pp. 19–64). New York: Guilford.

Overton, W. F., & Reese, H. W. (1973). Models of development: Methodological implications. In J. R. Nesselroade, & H. W. Reese (Eds.), *Life-span developmental psychology: Methodological issues* (pp. 65–86). New York: Academic Press.

Pawl, J., & Saint-John, M. (1998). *How you are is as important as what you do in making a positive difference for infants, toddlers and their families.* Washington, DC: ZERO TO THREE.

Pepper, S. C. (1942/1970). *World hypotheses.* Los Angeles: University of California Press.

Popper, K. (1959). *The logic of scientific discovery.* Basic Books.

Popper, K. (1963/1989). *Conjectures and refutations: The growth of scientific knowledge -2nd edition.* London: Routledge.

Porges, S. (2011). *The Polyvagal theory: neurophysiological foundations of emotions, attachment, communication, and self-regulation.* New York: W. W. Norton & Company, Norton series on interpersonal neurobiology.

Porges, S. (2015). Making the world safe for our children: Down-regulating defence and up-regulating social engagement to "optimise" the human experience. *Children Australia*, 1–9.

Reese, H. W., & Overton, W. F. (1970). Models of development and theories of development,". In L. R. Goulet, & P. B. Baltes (Eds.), *Life-span developmental psychology.* New York: Academic Press.

Reichenbach, H. (1951). *The rise of scientific philosophy*. California: University of California Press.

Rizzolatti, G. (2005). The mirror neuron system and its function in humans. *Advances in Anatomy, Embryology, and Cell Biology, 210*, 419–421.

Rizzolatti, G., & Craighero, L. (2004). The mirror neuron system. *Annual Review of Neuroscience, 27*, 169–192.

Rizzolatti, G., Fadiga, L., Fogassi, L., & Gallese, V. (1996). Premotor cortex and the recognition of motor actions. *Cognitive Brain Research, 3*, 131–141.

Rizzolatti, G., Fogassi, L., & Gallese, V. (2001). Neurophysiological mechanisms underlying the understanding and imitation of action. *Nature Reviews. Neuroscience, 2*, 661–670.

Robison, J. E. (2007). *Look me in the eye: My life with Asperger's*. New York: Crown Publishers.

Schore, A. N. (2001). Effects of a secure attachment relationship on right brain development, affect regulation, and infant mental health. *Infant Mental Health Journal, 2001*(22), 7–66.

Schore, A. N. (2019). *Right brain psychotherapy*. New York: W.W. Norton and Company, Norton series on interpersonal neurobiology.

Schulman, L. S. (2010). Forward: On the shoulders of Flexner. In M. Cooke, D. M. Irby, & B. C. O'Brien (Eds.), *Educating physicians: A call for reform of medical school and residency* (1st ed.). San Francisco, CA: Jossey -Bass. v-xii., The Carnegie Foundation for the Advancement of teaching.

Shahmoon-Shanok, R. (2009). What is reflective supervision? In S. S. Heller, & L. Gilkerson (Eds.), *A practical guide to reflective supervision*. Washington, DC: ZERO TO THREE Press.

Shanker, S. (2016). *Self-reg: How to help your child (and you) break the stress cycle and successfully engage with life*. New York: Penguin Press.

Siegel, D. J. (2010a). *Mindsight: The new science of personal transformation*. New York, NY: Bantam.

Siegel, D. J. (2010b). *The mindful therapist*. New York: W.W. Norton.

Silberman, S. (2016). *Neurotribes:* The legacy of autism and the future of neurodiversity. New York: Penguin Random House.

Skinner, B. F. (1953). *Science and human behavior*. New York: MacMillan.

Solomon, R. (2016). *Autism: The potential within: The PLAY Project approach to helping young children with autism*. Morrisville, NC: Lulu Publishing.

Solomon, R., Van Egeren, L. A., Mahoney, G., Quon Huber, M. S., & Zimmerman, P. (2014). PLAY Project home consultation intervention program for young children with autism spectrum disorders: A randomized controlled trial. *Journal of Developmental & Behavioral Pediatrics, 35*(8), 475–485.

Stern, D. (1984). Affect attunement. In J. Call, E. Galenson, & R. Tyson (Eds.), *Frontiers of infant psychiatry*. New York, NY: Basic Books.

Stern, D. N. (1995). *The motherhood constellation: A unified view of parent-infant psychotherapy* (1st Edition). New York: Basic Books.

Sullivan, W. M., Colby, A., Wegner, J. W., Bond, L., & Shulman, L. (2007). *Educating lawyers: Preparation for the practice of law*. California: The Carnegie Foundation for the Advancement of Teaching-Jossey-Bass/Wiley.

Sullivan, W. (2015). Professional formation as a social movement. The professional lawyer. *American Bar Association, 23*(1), 1–8.

Thomas, G. (2012). Changing our landscape of inquiry for a new science of education. *Harvard Educational Review, 82*(1), 26–50.

Thorndike, E. L. (1898). Some experiments on animal intelligence. *Science (New York, N.Y.), VII*, 818–823.

Thorndike, E. L. (1901). Animal intelligence: An experimental study of the associative processes in animals. *Psychological Review Monograph Supplement*, *2*, 1–109.

Torres, E. B. (2018). *Objective biometric methods for the diagnosis and treatment of nervous system disorders 1st edition*. Amsterdam, The Netherlands: Elsevier.

Trevarthen, C. (2009). The functions of emotion in infancy: The regulation and communication of rhythm, sympathy, and meaning in human development. In D. Fosha, D. Siegel, & M. F. Solomon (Eds.), *The healing power of emotion: Affective neuroscience, development & clinical practice* (pp. 35–85). New York: W.W. Norton & Company.

Trevarthen, C., Aitken, K., Nage, E., Delafield-Butt, J., & Vandekerckhove, M. (2006). Collaborative regulations of vitality in early childhood: Stress in intimate relationships and postnatal psychopathology. In D. Cicchetti, & D. J. Cohen (Eds.), *Developmental psychopathology, Second Edition* (pp. 2–78). Hoboken, NJ: John Wiley & Sons.

Trevarthen, C., & Delafield-Butt, J. T. (2013). Autism as a developmental disorder in intentional movement and affective engagement. *Frontiers in Integrative Neuroscience*, *7* (49), 1–16.

Tronick, E. (2007). *The neurobehavioral and social-emotional development of infants and children*. New York: W.W. Norton & Company, Norton series on interpersonal neurobiology.

Trout, M. (1988). Infant mental health: Monitoring our movement into the twenty-first century. *Infant Mental Health Journal*, *9*, 191–200.

Wason, P. (1960). On the failure to eliminate hypotheses in a conceptual task.". *Quarterly Journal of Experimental Psychology*, *12*(3), 129–140.

Winnicott, D. W. (1965). *The maturational processes and the facilitating environment*. CN: International Universities Press, Inc.

Parenting and autistic child

14

Alexandra Harrison[1,2,3,4] *and Ed Tronick*[5]
[1]Boston Psychoanalytic Society and Institute, Boston, MA, United States, [2]Psychiatry, HMS, Boston, MA, United States, [3]UMB IPMHPGCC, Boston, MA, United States, [4]SCC Cambridge, United States, [5]Psychology CDU UMB, Boston, MA, United States

Overview of parental reactions to their autistic child

Let's begin with parents' first suspicion that there might be something wrong with their child. Parents' perception occurs in the context of parents' typical concerns and anxiety for their child, which are now exacerbated by the current heightened general awareness of autism, particularly in pediatrics and the media. It is not uncommon these days for parents to consult pediatricians or child psychiatrists with the worry that their child is autistic as their primary concern, a very unlikely concern just 15 or 20 years ago (Lord & Cook, 2000). Sometimes parents will not acknowledge this fear initially, as if the clinician coming to this conclusion without the parents suggesting it would make it more legitimate, or as if not speaking the word "autistic" would make it not so.

The fear is magnified, of course, when the parents have an older child on the autistic spectrum, or if they have a relative such as the child of a sibling with autism (Ozonoff, Young, & Carter, 2013). One parent of a child who was on the autistic spectrum, told the psychiatrist that she worried about autism when her newborn daughter did not meet her gaze. Another parent who had an older child with severe autism defended against her terrified suspicion by forcefully denying that her younger son, who had clear signs of autism, was autistic.

The behavior of a child with autism spectrum disorder (ASD) can be puzzling for the parent. Some parents who have spectrum-like behavior of their own see the signs of autism in their child as temperamental characteristics—nothing to be concerned about—and resist professional consultation. In one instance, when concern was expressed to a mother about her 18-month-old's ASD-like behavior—flapping, lack of language, repetitive play—said not to worry because he was just like his father, an engineer who could work on his computer literally for days on end without a break and without engaging with anyone in the family. Further confounding the situation is the wide range of symptomatology in autistic spectrum children that often confuses the parents; children who are severely affected seem very different from those who have milder symptoms, but are still compromised. Finally, there is the complex situation of children on the autistic spectrum who have extraordinary intellectual gifts—in mathematics, music, drawing or painting, or language. Parents

Emerging Programs for Autism Spectrum Disorder. DOI: https://doi.org/10.1016/B978-0-323-85031-5.00030-X

of one gifted child were shocked by the consultant's identification of a language disorder. The child taught himself to read at 3 years old but had characteristic problems with the prosody of his speech and with auditory processing.

Generally, concern about their child's behavior is what leads parents to consult a child therapist. Parents of children with autism are no exception. It is common for children on the autistic spectrum to exhibit noncompliant and aggressive outbursts, typically related to problems with regulation—for example, inattentiveness and impulsivity (Mazefsky, Pelphrey, & Dahl, 2012). This problematic behavior, stressful enough at home or in the car, can be even more challenging when it occurs in public—where it is often misinterpreted by others as simple noncompliance or poor parenting—or at school, when it may provoke numerous "bad news" phone calls from the school to the parent. Other times it is embarrassing to parents and siblings, such as taking a bite out of a stranger's hamburger at a restaurant. Since these problems are public, the stress parent's experience from them is exacerbated by the shame they experience.

Other behaviors provoke fear for the future of their child in the parents. The child may lack the "skills of daily living." Some behaviors are self-destructive to a greater or lesser degree—such as an ASD child who wanders away from home, or is hurtful to others—such as biting a child at a birthday party. Parents—even quite young parents—ask, "Who will get him dressed in the morning when I am gone?" (Velikonja, Fett, & Velthorst, 2019).

These behavioral issues are often compounded by the difficulty parents have communicating with their child and making realistic expectations for their ASD child's behavior. These difficulties often arise from the atypical developmental capacities of ASD children. ASD children may have widely varying areas of competence—for example, precocious verbal ability but poor apprehension of social cues, or exceptional mathematical intelligence but poor language production. They also may have associated developmental problems—for example, auditory processing problems, sensory hypersensitivities, or chronic gastrointestinal distress. Unrealistic expectations of the ASD child lead—as they do with any child—to disappointment and frustration on both the part of the parent and the child. These emotions can also diminish motivation, which can interfere with learning. Difficulties communicating with the child and making realistic expectations derive from parents' difficulty understanding the child's emotions and intentions and the child's difficulty communicating them.

This disruption in the parent–child connection can lead to a subjective sense of disconnection (Singletary, 2015). From time to time and at some level of awareness, parents feel something missing in their relationship with their child and may fear that they are unable to attune to the child's feelings, unable to coordinate intentions with him, and that the child is, in effect, lost to them. It recalls the still-face paradigm, in which the infant is faced with contradictory behavior and violated expectations when interacting with the still-faced noninteractive parent (Tronick, 2007). In this case, however, it may it is the parent who is confronted with the child's "still face," and it is the parent rather than the infant who is stressed by the contradictory behavior and violated expectations in interactions with their child.

Parents describe the loneliness, or even grief, they feel when the child looks beyond them, or the lack of response when they greet him or call his name. Parents who have had to place their child in a residential school talk about their emotional pain when their child does not greet them when they come to visit. This sense of lost connection—whether it is severe or relatively small—may be the greatest pain parents of ASD children feel. We think of this experience of pain as difficulty of the parent and child being able to cocreate meaning.

Co-creating meaning with an autistic child

While many hold to the view that the interactions of parents and children should be smooth and attuned most of the time, this view is misguided (Tronick & Gold, 2020; Winnicott, 1965). The normal interaction of a parent and a child is typically messy, in the sense that there are periods of their matching intentions and emotions along with periods of mismatching. On average, mismatching periods make up as much as 70% of the interaction. However, these mismatches are quickly repaired to matching states. (Tronick & Gianino, 1986). Repairs not only resolve the stress of the mismatch. Perhaps even more important, they generate positive emotions, feelings of connection and agency in the child, as well as in the parent. The experience of repairs helps develop coping skills and a core implicit knowing that negative affect can be transformed into positive affect. Successful repairs lead to moments of meeting or to a dyadic state of consciousness in which child and parent make new meanings about their relationship to each other and their own sense of self in the world (Tronick, 2008).

For the parent and child with autism the meaning-making process of match–mismatch–repair is disrupted and derailed to various degrees. The child's communicative and regulatory disturbances disrupt the communicative process (Slade, 2006). Mismatches are more frequent, they last longer, and repairing them becomes increasingly difficult (Baron-Cohen, 1995; Tronick & Beeghly, 2011). Paradoxically, interactions become increasingly and highly contingent. They lack messiness, but the contingency is made up of the repetitive mismatch of intentions and negative behaviors. Negative emotions come to predominate in both the child and the parent. The meanings made are ones of mutual failure and disconnection. Over time these meanings self-amplify and interactive distortions become more rigid.

An obvious experiential consequence for parents is physical and psychological exhaustion (Greenspan & Wieder, 2006). A case in point is offered by a child on the spectrum seen in psychotherapy by one of the authors. Although very fond of the child, the therapist found herself feeling exhausted after the sessions with her. Searching for a means of understanding her subjective sense of exhaustion, she decided to videotape a session and use an adaptation of Beebe's technique of analyzing vocal rhythm coordination, to explore the microprocess (Beebe & Lachmann, 2002; Harrison & Beebe, 2018). When she first viewed the videotape, she noticed confusion in two domains of their interaction. In the domain of spoken language, the clinician confirmed that she struggled to make sense of the narrative the child was trying to tell her. Then, when she analyzed the microprocess—a domain in which the increments of time are too small to form language or to be aware of—a more striking finding emerged.

The second-by-second analysis first revealed that the therapist was attempting—again out of her awareness—to coordinate her vocal turns with those of the child. For example, when the child spoke, the therapist waited a second or two and then followed with a vocalization of the more or less the same duration of the child's. Then, the therapist identified a pattern in which the child interrupted her just before she completed her vocalization. This was particularly disruptive. Had the child interrupted her at the beginning of her communication, she could have stopped and not continued. Had the child interrupted her in the middle of her communication, she could have paused and perhaps continued later. However, when the child interrupted her just before the end of her communication, she had the subjective sense of the meaning being cut off, almost lost. The effect this pattern of communication had on the therapist was one of lack of coordination, a disturbance in their connection, and a disruption of making any kind of shared meaning. This detailed analysis by the therapist revealed patterns she was not aware of and point to the enormous difficulty parents face in trying to gain traction on understanding their reaction to their child.

The therapist brought this this discovery to the child's mother, who responded with a strong expression of surprise and relief. She said that she had a similar subjective experience of disruption, and that she had wondered what it was that was so exhausting and stressful about her efforts to communicate with her daughter. In the therapy, once the therapist recognized the pattern, she could allow it to exist, releasing herself somewhat from the expectation of "matching" her young patient and tolerating the disruptions. It was not, however, as easy for the child's mother, for whom the disruption of connection was a constant strain.

These experiential effects also have developmental consequences. In a typical situation, parents utilize their resources to scaffold the child's engagement and regulation of themselves and others and their engagement with others and the inanimate world of things. This parental investment leads to growth and development of the complexity and coherence of the child's sense of self in the world. Many factors function to enhance or deplete this input or resources. High levels of parental work stress, poverty, or mental illness deplete parental resources. On the other hand, social support, high social status, and well-being enhance parental resources. Most often, parent–child interactions "give back" to parents, in other words, are more enhancing of parental resources than depleting. Moreover, parents buffer the child from stressors that would otherwise deplete the resources the child needs for growth and development (Tronick, 2017).

For the parent and child with autism the balance is shifted. Other factors aside, their engagement with each other can be intensely demanding of resources. The parent–child interaction is more likely to be disturbed and stressful. Parents' must deploy more physical and psychological resources to engage and regulate their child. They are less able to buffer the child from both internal and external disruptions. The child, in turn, is also stressed. The child's resources, resources that should be used for growth and development, are redirected to self-regulation, and coping with stress. The derailment of resources is self-amplifying in the context of the child's already limited capacities and progressively increasing interactive distortion. Thus not only is development sacrificed, but the child's problems are exacerbated—especially the meaning the child with autism makes of himself in the world.

Conclusion

What are the consequences of the parents' reactions to their autistic child? The parents' stress will necessarily influence their mental and physical health and may contribute to high blood pressure or other medical conditions, or to mental health problems such as anxiety disorder or depression. It is not unusual for the stress of parenting an ASD child to result in marital strain or even divorce, and for the family situation to promote mental health problems in siblings. And though a different issue than presented here, keep in mind the siblings face many of the problems parents face in interacting with their sibling on the spectrum. In response to this stress, parents may tend to withdraw or to become more intrusive and controlling in the context of their child's vulnerability and impairment.

Yet, not everything about parenting an autistic child is traumatic. Each ASD child is an individual, and the challenge of joining the child, of meeting the child where he is, can generate otherwise unreachable creative responses in the parents and can result in an enhanced perspective that can open up and grow parents' personal values and beliefs. Consider the child described in the above case example. The recognition of a pattern of disruption in the communication with the therapist led to a new awareness in the mother that the fragmentation of her child's communication required a different kind of listening. Over time, as she lowered her expectations both of herself and of her child, she—as had the therapist—found a different way of communicating. This way of communicating involved greater tolerance of "not knowing" and more patience with repetition. The mother realized a new creativity in her child that matched her own creative personality. This example illustrates how the challenges involved in parenting an autistic child can result not only in greater acceptance and appreciation of the child but also in enhanced satisfaction in the parents' personal lives.

References

Baron-Cohen, S. (1995). *Mindblindedness: An essay on autism and theory of mind.* Cambridge, MA: MIT Press.

Beebe, B., & Lachmann, F. (2002). *Infant research and adult treatment: Co-constructing interactions.* Hillsdale, NJ: The Analytic Press.

Greenspan, S., & Wieder, S. (2006). *Engaging autism: Using the floortime approach to help children relate, communicate, and think.* Cambrdige, MA: Da Capo Press.
Harrison, A., & Beebe, B. (2018). Rhythms of dialogue in infant research and child analysis: Implicit/explicit therapeutic action. *Psychoanalytic Psychology, 35*(4), 367–381.
Lord, C., & Cook, E. (2000). Autism spectrum disorders: Review. *Neuron, 28*, 355–363.
Mazefsky, C., Pelphrey, K., & Dahl, R. (2012). The need for a broader approach to emotion regulation. *Child Development Perspectives, 6*(1), 92–97.
Ozonoff, S., Young, G., Carter, A., et al. (2013). Recurrence risk for autism spectrum disorders: A baby siblings research consortium study. *Pediatrics.* Available from https://doi.org/10.1542/peds.2010-2825.
Singletary, W. (2015). An integrative model of autism spectrum disorder of experienced environmental deprivation, early life stress and allostatic overload. *Neuropsychoanalysis, 17*(2), 81–119.
Slade, A. (2006). Reflective parenting programs: Theory and development. *Psychoanalytic Inquiry, 26*, 640–657.
Tronick, E. (2007). *Neurobehavioral and social emotional development of the infant and young child.* Norton Press.
Tronick, E. (2008). Multilevel meaning making and dyadic expansion of consciousness theory: The emotional and the polymorphic polysemic flow of meaning. In D. Fosha, M. Solomon, & D. Siegel (Eds.), *The healing power of emotion: Affective neuroscience, development, clinical practice.* New York: Norton.
Tronick, E. (2017). The caregiver–Infant dyad as a buffer or transducer of resource enhancing or depleting factors that shape psychobiological development. *Australian and New Zealand Journal of Family Therapy, 38*(4), 561–572.
Tronick, E., & Beeghly, M. (2011). Meaning making and infant mental health. *American Psychologist*, 107–119.
Tronick, E., & Gianino, A. (1986). Interactive mismatch and repair: Challenges to the coping infant. *Zero to Three, 3*, 1–6.
Tronick, E., & Gold, C. (2020). *The power of discord.* Sparks, NY: Little Brown.
Velikonja, T., Fett, A.-K., & Velthorst, E. (2019). Patterns of nonsocial and social cognitive functioning in adults with autism spectrum disorders: A systematic review and meta-analysis. *JAMA Psychiatry.* Available from https://doi.org/10.1001/jamapsychiatry.2018.3645.
Winnicott, D. W. (1965). *Maturational processes and the facilitating environment.* New York: International Universities Press.

Further reading

Hastings, R. (2008). Stress in parents of children with autism. In E. McGregor, M. Nunez, K. Cebule, & J. Gomez (Eds.), *Autism: An integrated view from neurocognitive, clinical, and intervention research* (pp. 303–324). Oxford, UK: Blackwell Publishing.
Slade, A. (2009). Mentalizing the unmentalizable: Parenting children on the spectrum. *Journal of Infant, Child, and Adolescent Psychotherapy, 8*, 7–21.

Movements and development. Art-therapy approach in the complex rehabilitation of children with intellectual disorders, including autism spectrum disorder

15

Olga G. Safonicheva and Marina A. Ovchinnikova
Department of Sports Medicine and Medical Rehabilitation, Institute of Clinical Medicine, I.M. Sechenov First Moscow State Medical University (Sechenov University), Moscow, Russia

> *The challenge of our society, if it is interested in its future existence, is to find new forms of introducing a healthy lifestyle and health culture into everyday practice in the shortest possible time, to develop a new system of values in which health will be one of the main personal priorities.*
>
> *Leo Bokeria*

The most important tasks of modern schools, in line with sustaining a high level of education, the disclosure of creative abilities, and familiarization with the cultural heritage of children and adolescents, are to improve their physical and mental health, as well as the formation of their active life position. Almost all forums devoted to education talk about the priority of health in the system of social and spiritual values, the need to introduce health-saving and health-forming technologies and innovative interdisciplinary models of education for the younger generation in children's institutions.

Health, educational, developmental, and further social adaptation issues are particularly relevant for special correctional schools of the VIII type, where children with intelligence disorders, including autism spectrum disorder (ASD), are trained. At present, the social structure of society is becoming more complex, the flow of information is increasing, and requirements for a child entering school and for a graduate choosing his life trajectory are increasing. The pedagogical situation is complicated by the fact that the number of children with disabilities is growing and all children without exception are included in the learning process, even those who were previously considered "untrained," but only "tutored." According to the data of Russian scientists and observations of experienced speech pathologists, children

Emerging Programs for Autism Spectrum Disorder. DOI: https://doi.org/10.1016/B978-0-323-85031-5.00019-0

with multiple sensory, intellectual, emotional, and volitional disorders with combined coordination and motor disorders make up on average up to 40%–50% of the contingent of special educational institutions. Deviations in the development of the motor sphere among children with a delay in mental and intellectual development create certain difficulties in educational activities: the underdevelopment of voluntary movements can be realized in violation of purposeful types of actions—when drawing, writing, and manual labor. Experts claim that the generally accepted psychological and pedagogical methods that were supposed to effectively correct a particular child's deficit using a "symptom-target" method in many cases failed to bring results both in the learning process and in the process of directed correction (Belov, Pitchers, & Brain, 2006; The draft law, 1995). In this situation, a systematic approach to correction and habilitation of the child's psychophysical development is optimal; cognitive and motor methods should be applied in a certain hierarchical complex, taking into account their complementary influence. In the last decade special correctional schools focused more on children's education through the integration of cognitive and motor centers of the brain to purposefully overcome motor deficiencies, improve movement, and promote overall health. Thus the modern school increases the requirements for the development of new curricula, as well as for changing the content of education with the introduction of developing classes and technologies, and for interdepartmental cooperation. In addition to physical education, educational programs also include music and rhythmic classes that allow children to develop in a new sociocultural environment.

Music for health

There is a long history of the use of music and music therapy services to help individuals with ASD achieve nonmusical goals, including social skills (Reschke-Hernandez, 2011). Music therapy currently is taking a more important place among various alternative therapies around the world. The American Music Therapy Association defines this area as "the clinical and scientific use of musical interventions to achieve individualized therapeutic outcome goals by a certified professional who has completed an approved music training program." Music therapists develop music programs that help people with ASD develop social, communication, motor/sensory, emotional, cognitive, and musical skills. Music therapy technologies can be used to treat people of different socioeconomic status, culture, and age (American Music Therapy Association, 2005, 2015, 2017). Such technologies are widely used in schools, at home, in music therapy clinics, or in hospitals. Scientific research on the influence of music on health is represented by the works of G.-G. Decker-Voigt, J. Campbell, A. Tomatis, and K. Schwabe. The works of R.O. Benenzon describe the positive effect of using music for therapeutic purposes for children suffering from neurosis. Musical stimuli are used for the development of the "emotional brain" and social adaptation of children suffering from early childhood autism and other intellectual disabilities (A Blythe LaGasse, 2017). Therefore there are many different approaches and interventions that can be used to target social skills in music therapy. One commonality between these approaches is the use of musical stimuli and musical engagement to provide a foundation for enhanced socialization in children with ASD, leading to improved nonmusic social skills.

Music therapy is a unique treatment approach that uses music experiences that can engage children in meaningful interactions with others. Many children with ASD respond positively to music experiences, making music a safe and structured stimulus for social engagement and the practice of social skills. There are several reasons that musical stimuli may help with developing social skills. Music has been demonstrated to activate neural networks involved in similar musical and nonmusical tasks (e.g., speech and singing both activate the left inferior frontal gyrus) (Özdemir, Norton, & Schlaug, 2006; Peretz & Zatorre, 2005) and further has the ability to optimize target behaviors through synchronized neural firings (Thaut & McIntosh, 2010).

Music therapy is performed using classical and folk compositions in the form of improvisations, for the development of cognitive, communicative abilities, and social interaction. Music therapy was officially included in the register of technologies and tools for healthcare in the Russian Federation in 2003 (Shushardjan). Currently, therapeutic music pedagogy is gradually taking its place in the system of measures to optimize development and training (Petrushin, 2019).

The development of innovative research-based programs for the development, rehabilitation, and socialization of children with disabilities is attracting more and more attention from researchers around the world (Russia, United States, Germany, United Kingdom, Poland) and requires interdisciplinary approaches from neurophysiologists, psychologists, neurologists, psychiatrists, and educators.

A comprehensive program of interdepartmental cooperation aimed at improving and developing technologies in the educational process was implemented in the Urban experimental site created by the Division of Psychosocial Support for children under the Department of Education of the city of Moscow together with doctors from I.M. Sechenov First MSMU and the teaching staff of the correctional school VIII type of Moscow. The pilot project program was approved by the Interuniversity Ethics Committee of the Association of Medical and Pharmaceutical Universities. Research and innovation work was carried out in the following areas: medical rehabilitation; psychological support of children, taking into account the development of modern neuropsychology; socialization of pupils, which involves a gradual complication of measures in accordance with the age of the pupils (Safonicheva & Ovchinnikova, 2019).

The aim of this pilot clinical study was to develop scientifically based technologies of the phased rehabilitation and socialization of pupils of special correctional school VIII type, capable of self-adaptation, integration, and fulfillment in society within their psychophysical possibilities.

The research objectives included:

1. To study causes of the development of a complex structure of the intellectual disabilities in students of correctional schools.

2. To study features of psychomotor and speech disorders in children, to correlate with functional biomechanical changes in the cervical–thoracic spine and cranial vertebral zone, which can affect the state of cerebral blood flow and oxygen supply of cognitive, speech, and motor centers.
3. To develop a research protocol for evaluating the metabolic supply of the brain in children with intellectual disabilities.
4. To create a program of comprehensive rehabilitation of children with the inclusion of non-medicinal methods, physical exercises, and musical and rhythmic classes in the traditions of folk art to activate the "emotional and cognitive brain" and develop neuroplasticity.
5. To evaluate the effectiveness of nondrug treatment methods in children with disabilities.

Research materials

We examined 118 primary and secondary school students aged 8–14 years with intellectual disabilities, including ASD, hyperactivity, and attention deficit disorder (as part of the F-70, F-71 ICD-10 diagnoses) (Classification of mental and behavioral disorders, 1994; DSM-IV 35 Diagnostic and Statistical Manual of Mental Disorders Washington, 1990; International Statistical Classification of Diseases and Health Related Problems, 1992; Sartorius et al., 1988). Clinical research and rehabilitation activities were conducted in an educational institution without breaks in educational process and changing daily routines of primary school children. The purpose and objectives of the study were agreed with the psychological and pedagogical staff of the school and reported at the school parent meeting. Parents and guardians signed an "informed consent" to participate in the pilot project.

Protocol and research methods

1. Neuropsychological research was conducted by school psychologists to assess the cognitive and emotional sphere in children, as well as thought processes and psychospeech functions (Bardenshtein, Molodetsky, Kurashov, & Shcherbakov, 2009).
2. Clinical neurological and kinesthetic research was conducted to identify biomechanically significant changes in the cervical–thoracic spine, muscle spasms, as well as compression–tunnel neuropathies in the cranial vertebral zone that affect the state of cerebral blood flow (Janda, 1983, 1985; Kipervas, 1991; Safonicheva, 2007; Safonicheva & Ovchinnikova, 2019; Skoromets, 2000; Trevell and Simons, 1989; Vasilyeva, 1996).
3. The purpose of the neurophysiological examination of children by the neuro-energo-cartography (NEC) method was to assess the cerebral metabolism and adaptive capabilities of the brain, as well as interhemispheric interactions in the initial state and after the rehabilitation measures. The check was carried out on a computer software system NEC, created in the laboratory of age physiology of the brain Research Center of Neurology (under the guidance of professors V. F. Fokin and N.V. Ponomareva, patent no. 2135077 A61B5/04, 08.27.1999). It is known that one of the main links in the development of pathological processes can be a deficit in the delivery of energy substrates and violation of the oxygen supply of brain structures, as well as a change in the acid–base balance at the border of the blood–brain barrier. The NEC method registered the constant potential level (CPL)—the slow electrical activity—reflecting the integrated metabolism of various brain zones (Fokin & Ponomareva, 1999, 2002). The detector of material energy processes

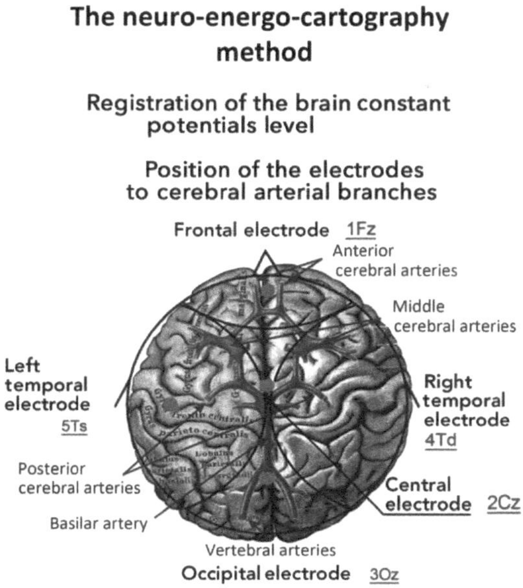

Figure 15.1 Constant potential level scheme registration.

in the brain was considered to be the CPL—the magnitude of the stable difference in the mV range, which is recorded between the brain and the referred area. According to CPL amplitude, we could measure the degree of acidosis in the brain tissues. Sources of CPL were the potentials of the blood–brain barrier and vascular potentials in the referred area. The registration was carried out at the NEC computer–software complex (Fig. 15.1).

Results of the research and further discussions

Social development of the individual occurs in three dimensions: educational, cultural, and emotional. If attention is paid to all these areas in working with a child, they have a chance to independently build an adequate adaptive emotional relationship with the environment. The formation of the child's emotional sphere is the basis of communication, emotions are enabling the child to explore the world outside. To identify the causes of intellectual disabilities, a survey and analysis of the course of pregnancy in mothers of boarding school students were conducted. Of the 48 women surveyed, 42 noted an unfavorable course of pregnancy and complicated labor (rapid labor, birth stimulation at the birth of a large fetus, cord entanglement around the neck, asphyxia of the newborn). The neuropsychological study revealed features in the emotional–volitional, cognitive sphere, and behavior of correctional school students: weak and scattered attention, motor disinhibition, and impulsive behavior were noted; it was difficult for children to concentrate, understand and remember the new material. There was also a decrease in memory, the level of voluntary memorization of words and movements and poor vocabulary. Cognitive disorders in younger students were expressed in slowness, inertia, and difficult adaptation to new conditions. According to the results of modern research, there is a direct correlation between speech and behavioral disorders. Disorders during intrauterine development, birth pathology, and slowness in the development of the nervous system in the first months of a child's life can lead to emotional and behavioral problems at an early age, which in middle childhood will manifest in communication disorders and, as a result, disorders of school skills: counting, writing, reading (Ratner, 1990, 1995).

When assessing the neurological status of children, the following symptoms were registered: headache, muscle tension in the cervical spine, meteosensivity, distracted attention, increased exhaustion, sleep disorders.

The clinical study revealed multilevel biomechanical changes in the musculoskeletal system of different degrees of severity in all children. The musculoskeletal changes were manifested by violations of posture (including kyphotic and scoliotic settings). There was hypertonicity of the shoulder girdle muscles, postural muscle imbalance with involvement of muscle groups—synergy—in the pathological process, with a violation of coordination, sequence of movements, and spatial representations. The main biomechanical changes in the examined children were sympathetic "muscle" stress: myofascial and muscle-tonic syndromes of the cervical–thoracic spine and shoulder girdle, elevation of the structures of the upper aperture of the chest, shortening of the large pectoral muscles, spasm of the respiratory diaphragm. Multilevel "tunnel" disorders supporting compression of the main vessels of the neck were also identified, which had an impact on hemaliquorodynamics and led to brain hypoxia. Some children also had disorders of chest movement, respiratory frequency, depth, and rhythm disorders (Safonicheva, 2001, 2002, 2006; Safonicheva & Ovchinnikova, 2019).

Results of neurophysiological research on NEC showed the presence of individual signs of deviations both from the age norm and stable pathological manifestations. According to the results of NEC in 43 children (aged 8 to 11 years), changes in cerebral metabolism were detected with manifestations of brain hypoxia on the background of varying degrees of acidosis or alkalosis.

The digital indicators of the acid–base balance in the NEC method were translated into color. The acid–base balance shift in the direction of acidosis (lowering the pH and increasing the CPL) was painted in a yellow–red–brown range of colors. When the brain used more of the reserve mechanism of energy exchange, the more red was painted on the picture, and the higher the CPL registered (Fig. 15.2).

The acid–base balance shift in the direction of alkalosis (raising the pH, lowering the CPL) was painted in the NEC picture in blue tones (Fig. 15.3). The normal level and type of neurometabolism was colored green with yellow on NEC. Normal indicators were calculated by the device, based on age, gender, and the dominant hemisphere in the studied child (Safonicheva & Ovchinnikova, 2019).

There was a connection of disorders of cerebral metabolism with the state of tone of the shoulder girdle muscles and the shift of the center of gravity from the vertical axis. It was suggested that the cause of the development of such pathological processes in the brain could be "tunnel" muscle-tonic syndromes of natal or postnatal origin, leading to compression of the main vessels of the neck. In 50% of

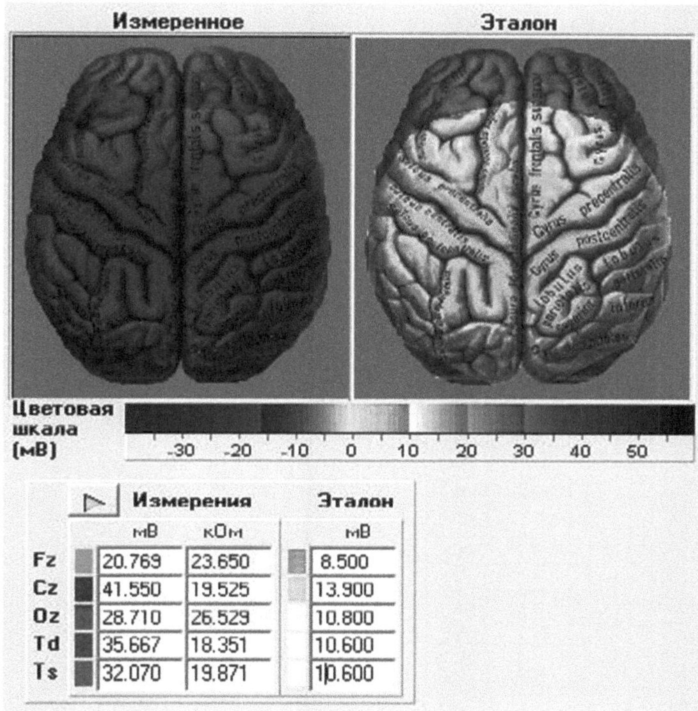

Figure 15.2 Boy D.; age: 11 years; diagnosis—autism spectrum disorder.

cases, there were signs of weakening of interhemispheric relationships (Safonicheva, 2001, 2002, 2006; Safonicheva & Ovchinnikova, 2019). The analysis of indicators of functional disorders of the balance function, neurological syndromes, vegetative dysregulation, perinatal risk factors, and natal damage to the craniovertebral region indicated the common mechanisms of their formation and the neurogenic nature of the delay in psychomotor development of the child.

Balance of the body in space, mechanisms of movement organization, role of the nervous system in providing motor acts as well as impact of movements on health and quality of life have been studied by scientists of various specialties for a long time. But only in the first half of the 19th century, the English scientist Charles Bell found that muscles are suitable for both motor and "feeling" nerves (History of Psychology in Persons: Personalities). The scientist showed the value of afferent innervation of muscles as a "feedback" that carries information from the periphery to the center and creates the basis for making corrections in the execution of movement as the basis for human interaction with the environment. I.M. Sechenov at the end of 19th century in his fundamental work "Brain Reflexes" clearly pointed to the influence of thought and motive on the formation of voluntary movements. He

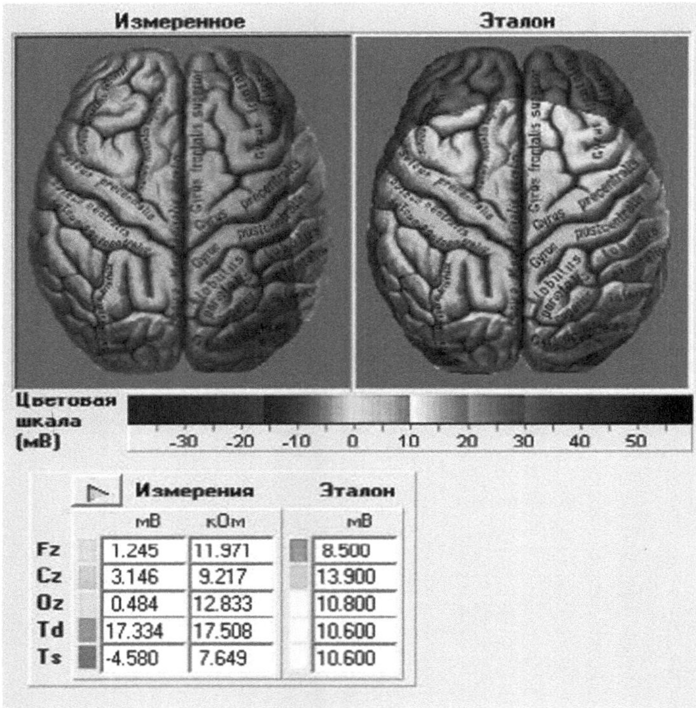

Figure 15.3 Girl A.; age: 9 years; diagnosis—autism spectrum disorder.

wrote: "All the infinite variety of external manifestations of brain activity is finally reduced to a single phenomenon—muscle movement" (Sechenov, 1863).

Several areas in the human sciences—biomechanics, physiology, psychology, and cybernetics—were represented by the outstanding Russian scientist N.A. Bernstein. By studying the special aspects of each of the directions, he was able to combine these directions under a common interdisciplinary, integral beginning of a unified psychophysiological theory of movement construction; a complete analysis of which has yet to be carried out by neurologists, psychiatrists, psychologists, and artists. Thanks to a comprehensive study of movements, biomechanics—the science of the laws of body positions and movements in three-dimensional space—developed into biodynamics, and the latter was synthesized by N.A. Bernstein with the neurophysiology and psychology of movements. The apogee of this period was the monograph "On the construction of movements," published in 1947, in which movement was first presented as a mental action (Fig. 15.4).

As noted by contemporaries, N.A. Bernstein was connected with psychology through its "higher floors," which do not affect highly specialized interests. In his works, there were only extremely psychological concepts: image, semantic structure, action, meaning, skill, activity. Research by Bernstein (1947) showed that human interaction with the environment is determined by a motor task that is

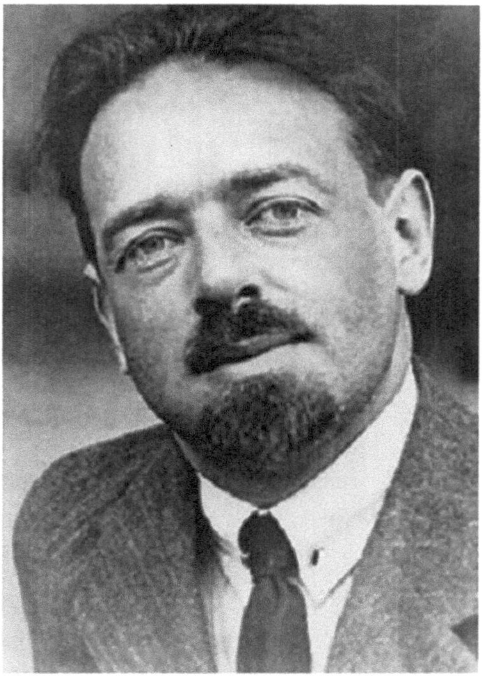

Figure 15.4 N.A. Bernstein (1896–1966).

formed at different levels of motor regulation. The degree of movement control depending on the tasks (walking, writing, speech) will be different. Bernstein developed the concept of level organization of movements, which allows one to decompose a complex motor act, as well as to identify the state and role of cortical levels of central nervous system in the regulation of positions, movements, and actions (Bernstein, 1947, 2001, 2004).

N.A. Bernstein identified the following levels of movement construction:

A—The level of paleokinetic regulation, also known as the rubrospinal level of the central nervous system (CNS).

B—The level of synergies, it is also known as the thalamopallidary level.

C—The level of the spatial field, also known as the pyramidal–strial level, which is divided into two sublevels (C1, strial, belonging to the extrapyramidal system; C2, pyramidal, belonging to the group of cortical levels).

D—The level of actions (subject actions, semantic chains, etc.), also known as the parietal-premotor level.

E—Group of higher cortical levels of symbolic coordination (associated with the II signal system—writing, speech).

Thus the cortical levels of movement organization D and E provide an optimal motor stereotype, which is built on the basis of an optimal metabolic stereotype and represents a set of sequential, smooth, economically feasible, coordinated, conscious, completed movements (Bernstein, 1947, 2001, 2004). After the completed movement associated with contraction (concentric, eccentric, isometric), muscles should return to a neutral normotonic state, and balanced multidirectional muscle pulls ensure the preservation and maintenance of the vertical axis of the body (Safonicheva, 2007). Such movements performed with a high degree of harmony, leading to the realization of the goal in any direction of activity, are perceived as art, and the result of such activities are works of art.

The relationship of cognitive and motor centers was studied by A.R. Luria. Neuropsychological studies conducted by him showed that the frontal lobes of the brain are part of the cortical departments of the motor analyzer. The motor cortex is responsible for the organization, "programming," and implementation of arbitrary motor activity of the body—a complex process that relies on the areas that are part of the cortical departments of the motor analyzer. According to Luria (2009), the whole brain takes part in the development of any mental function, but the role of different brain structures and hemispheres is ambiguous. The role and functions of brain structures can change and be supplemented depending on the task that mental activity is aimed at and the structure of its organization (Luria, 2009).

Academician P.K. Anokhin, the founder of the "Theory of functional systems," pointed out that the "intellectual" frontal cortex is not related to individual brain functions—memory, perception, motivation, emotions—but it integrates them into purposeful, plastic behavioral responses (Anokhin, 1973).

According to the teachings of Vygotsky (1999), behavioral regulation depends on the learned speech, which later becomes a thought. Speech is an important component in the ordering of acts of behavior and cognition. Motor and speech centers are located in adjacent parts of the major hemispheres of the cerebral cortex, which can cause a potential connection between speech and motor function. Therefore speech disorders significantly reduce the level of socialization, which makes a significant contribution to the formation of "vicious circles" of the pathogenesis of the "complex structure of the defect" in students of special correctional schools (Vygotsky, 1999).

The human brain consists of many neurons that differ from each other in their genetic development program: speech, thinking, goal setting, and their implementation are all neuropsychological functions. It is known that out of 15 billion nerve cells available in the cerebral cortex, humans use no more than 15% (Wayne, 2001). This leads to the presence of large reserve capabilities of the nervous system, which must be taken into account when developing programs for the development and rehabilitation of children with congenital and acquired disorders of the neuropsychological sphere and disabilities.

In a state of pathology, nondifferenciation of brain cells is the basis for compensation for impaired functions. Developing with the help of new recovery technologies the preserved links of cortical structures and adapting them to perform qualitatively new tasks (Astapov & Mikadze, 2008) it is possible to achieve sustainable success in the formation of weakened or lost health and mental capabilities (Astapov & Mikadze, 2008).

A major breakthrough in the history of neuroscience in the 21st century is associated with the theory of neuroplasticity, which changed the perception of the brain. According to the author of the theory, Professor Norman Jones, the brain is not a set of specialized parts, each of which has a specific place and function, but is a dynamic organ that can reprogram and rebuild itself if necessary. The recognition that the brain is plastic and can change itself through training and cognition is the foundation of modern neurorehabilitation: the ability to reorganize themselves by forming new neural connections, both in childhood and throughout life, can help children overcome learning difficulties, and improve concentration and memory (Doidge, 2007).

The program of the pilot project

Based on the theory of neuroplasticity and the results of the study, a program for comprehensive rehabilitation of children of a special correctional school was developed. It was attended by specialists of the Department of Integrative Medicine of the First Sechenov Moscow State Medical University and the school's psychological and pedagogical staff.

The program included medical rehabilitation, which was implemented on the basis of the school (the status of the pilot site allowed to conduct medical procedures without disrupting the educational process), and developmental activities in the form of physical culture and music–rhythmic classes. Those activities were later integrated into the mandatory school program. Federal Law of the Russian Federation No. 329–FL of December 4, 2007 *On physical culture and sport in the Russian Federation* states, "Physical culture is a part of culture that is a set of values, norms and knowledge created and used by society for the purpose of physical and intellectual development of human abilities, improving their motor activity and forming a healthy lifestyle, social adaptation through physical education, physical training and physical development" (Federal Law of the Russian Federation No. 329–FL of December 4, 2007; Khadartsev, Fudin, Zilov, Safonicheva, & Smolensky, 2015).

Health, culture, education, and social adaptation are the most important tasks of any teaching staff.

The medical unit included finger and postural gymnastics ("lateral-cross" therapy with the intersection of the midline: a set of exercises for integrating the hemispheres and "passing" the child successive age levels of building movements), which were not formed in early childhood. Special developmental exercises were aimed at correcting the sensorimotor development of children with psychophysical development problems. Methods of teaching motor skills included showing, describing, performing, repeating, and fixing. We found out the sequence of muscle activation and smoothness when performing flexor, extensor, and rotational movements (fingers–hands–elbow–shoulder joints; ankle–knee–hip joints) on the homolateral side and taking into account cross-patterns for the development of hemispheric laterality and interhemispheric connections. It took 3–4 weeks to work out the exercises.

Fixing of sensorimotor coordination is the most important step in the development of the "emotional–cognitive brain" and intellectual abilities, and the friendly activity of the visual, auditory, and kinesthetic analyzers when performing exercises ensures an adequate perception of the surrounding world (space, time, your social role).

We also applied soft-tissue manual therapy aimed at relaxing spasmodic and shortened muscle-fascial structures of the shoulder girdle, cervical spine, and cervical–cranial junction. The main techniques of soft-tissue connective-tissue therapy were: skin-fascial, muscle-fascial, and postisometric muscle relaxation (Janda, 1983, 1985; Kipervas, 1991; Safonicheva, 2007; Safonicheva & Ovchinnikova, 2019; Skoromets, 2000; Trevell and Simons, 1989; Vasilyeva, 1996).

When the restriction of fascia kinetics, trigger points in shortened muscles, and multilevel tunnel syndromes supporting brachiocephalic vascular compression were detected, tissue relaxation was performed in the craniovertebral region, the cervical spine, and the shoulder girdle. These measures were aimed at eliminating the "vicious circles" of the pathogenesis of the "complex structure" of the defect in children and multiple deficits—cognitive, speech, and motor. We used nondrug treatments with the aim of creating optimal conditions for realization of the processes of plasticity and brain development in children. The treatment methods were used for normalization of blood circulation, oxygen supply of stem and cortical structures of the brain, normalization of cerebrospinal fluid dynamics, improvement of cerebral metabolism in general, and also the integration of intra- and interhemispheric connections.

The course of treatment consisted of six to eight procedures, each child was given two to three courses of general health and rehabilitation measures. The duration of the procedure was 15–20 minutes.

All the methods used—soft muscle techniques of manual therapy, special massage, physical and respiratory exercises—have been widely used in the rehabilitation of muscle and tonic syndromes with impaired posture and diseases of the musculoskeletal system. The developed program took into account various mechanisms of development of pathology of the spine, muscles, and brain structures, and had a more pronounced and stable effect than each of the listed methods applied separately. Correction schemes were selected individually, taking into account the psychophysical status of the child. Parents should be involved in the correction process to repeat the exercises at home and consolidate the results (Safonicheva & Ovchinnikova, 2019).

Musical and rhythmic classes in the traditions of folk art were included in the correctional unit of the pilot project and were an important part of the educational program of the correctional school of the VIII type. The general developmental disorder in children enrolled in such schools is a complex process involving all aspects of speech. Delayed speech development is characterized by persistent phonetic underdevelopment, poor vocabulary, as well as a marked decrease in speech activity and interest in speech communication. Another important feature of children with intellectual disabilities, in comparison with their normally developing peers, is that the period of walking and babbling begins later, and sometimes does not exist at all; the process of pronouncing the first words is difficult or slowed down. Therefore children are deprived of the infant link of "nursery rhymes," which affects their emotional and social and personal development.

The formation of skills of voluntary self-regulation is one of the main tasks of correctional work with primary school students, who were distinguished not only by the delay in speech development, but also by the underdevelopment of rhythmic hearing. They almost did not feel a strong beat, did not feel the metrorhythm, so they could not organize their own movements to the music. Children with intellectual disabilities, with poorly developed motor skills, were characterized by insufficient coordination of movements; especially noticeable were the difficulties in quickly switching from one type of movement to another. The series of movements necessary for learning dances were formed for a longer time. The abovementioned violations affecting the intellectual and emotional spheres, as well as the sociocultural development of the student, could be corrected in the musical and rhythmic classes in the traditions of the folk art.

In these classes, students learned to correctly pronounce lines of poetry, achieving a clear reproduction of rhythmic structures (texts of jokes, counting, which were distinguished by the brevity of the syllable and a simple clear rhythm). Listening to music of different genres (lullaby, joke, dance, game) helped to develop coordination of movements and plasticity. Music classes also had a corrective effect in terms of speech disorders, since rhyming riddles, stanzas, couplets, etc. required more precise articulation, and also assumed repetitions, which eventually fixed the accuracy of pronunciation (Vlasenko, 2007; Yevtushenko, 2003).

Movements with musical accompaniment (games, choreography elements, exercises with noise instruments) had a positive effect on the development of hearing, attention, and memory. The interaction of words, music, and rhythmic movements caused a coordinated response and integration of the entire body (respiratory and cardiac systems, muscle activity), including the emotional response of the psyche, which contributed to the overall health of children with intellectual disabilities.

The main task of a teacher who conducted music and rhythmic classes with children was to comprehensively solve the problems of psychophysical and emotional gaps in the development of the student and their socialization. Socialization of the younger generation is one of the core challenges of any society and is a two-sided process. On the one hand, the individual learns social experience by entering the social environment, the system of social connections; on the other hand, social connections are changed due to the activity of entering the environment. Thus the child is not only enriched by experience, but also realizes himself as a person, influencing life circumstances and the world around him. Socialization factors are an environment that is not something spontaneous. It should be designed, well organized, and further created. The main requirement for a developing environment is to create an atmosphere in which humane relationships, trust, security, the possibility of personal growth, and the emotional harmony of children and teachers will prevail.

Work on the organization of musical and rhythmic classes with students of the correctional school was carried out in stages, with the complication of semantic tasks.

In the first quarter the theme was worked out: "Children's musical folklore" (Fig. 15.5).

The purpose of the lessons was to include in the passive vocabulary of children samples of rhythmic intonation on the example of proverbs and sayings, and to teach children to perform elementary movements consistent with the rhythm of short poems (Fig. 15.6).

The task of this block of classes was to develop the ability to think of imaginary objects and images (in nursery rhymes and short poems "Shadow-shadow," etc.).

During the lesson children learned to listen to and reproduce the sounds of their native language, to understand its expressiveness and beauty. Nursery rhymes are a form of speech communication that is present in infancy and is necessary for development. The teacher taught the child to catch the rhythm of speech, characteristic sound combinations, rhymes. The development of phonetic hearing, the formation of the ability to detect subtle sound differences prepared students to master the correct sound pronunciation.

The theme of classes in the second quarter: "Folk children's songs."

Purpose: To form students' ideas about the content and sphere of existence of folk songs, to teach children to recognize the folk songs of a certain holiday by their characteristic features.

The objectives of the classes were to introduce to students the content of folk songs, their symbolic images in order to develop imagination, as well as to teach them to express emotional experiences and images through facial expressions, intonation, gestures, and plastic movements.

During the lessons, students were introduced to the poetry of folk holidays: the Intercession of the Holy Mother of God, the Nativity of Christ, Maslenitsa, Easter,

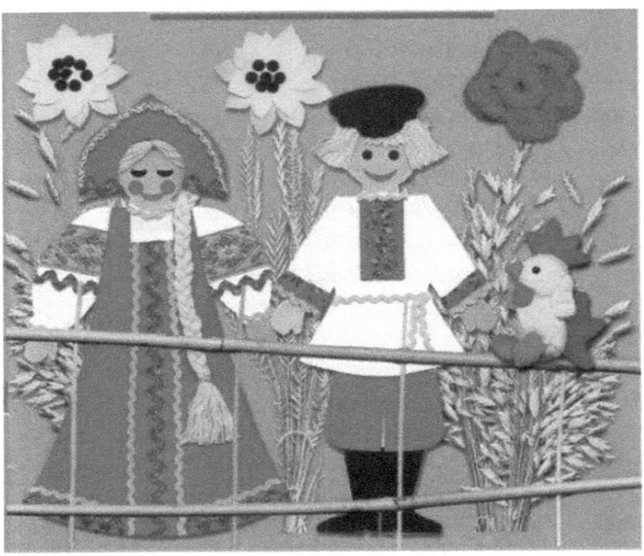

Figure 15.5 Children's musical folklore. Introduction.

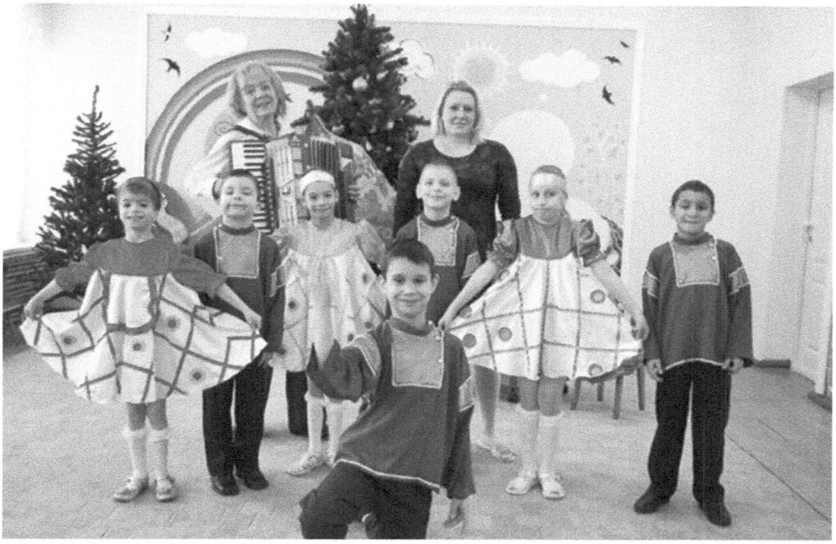

Figure 15.6 Movements with the rhythm of short poems.

and Trinity. The teacher teaches children to transform into specific characters of the festive folk action in the process of working on the text—its intonation, rhythm, image. Folk rites served as the material here: "Goat," "Holy night," "The burning of the carnival," etc. (Figs. 15.7 and 15.8).

Folk rites assumed a close relationship of figurative, poetic words and various choreographic movements—special actions and plastic in-round dances, dances, and gatherings. This helped to form the students' skills of speech support of their actions.

By mastering this material, students learned to perform a certain sequence of movements in the rhythm of the verse and in time with the music, to see their peers as partners, to develop independence, and to enter into a system of interpersonal communications.

The third quarter was devoted to the theme: "Children's play folklore."

Goal: To form students' positive motivation to play together, role-playing skills related to emotional and volitional development.

The objectives of this quarter were to teach children to express a variety of feelings and emotions in the game; to foster interest in the game "by the rules," in which each participant respects the partners and acts in accordance with a sense of justice; to form students' speech communication skills in the game; and to teach them to improvise within the game scenario.

For example, in the game "the kite and the hen" we can see the connection between words and music:

Burn, burn clearly, so that it does not go out! Look at the sky-the birds are flying!

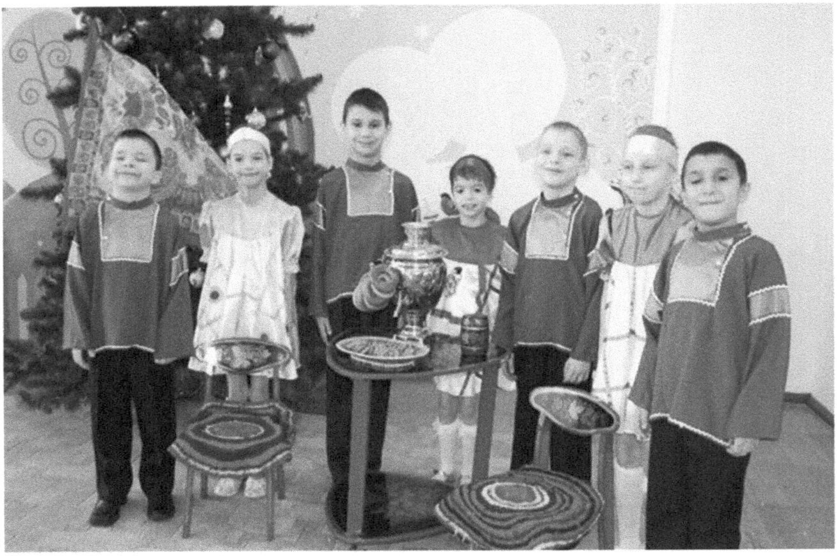

Figure 15.7 Holy night.

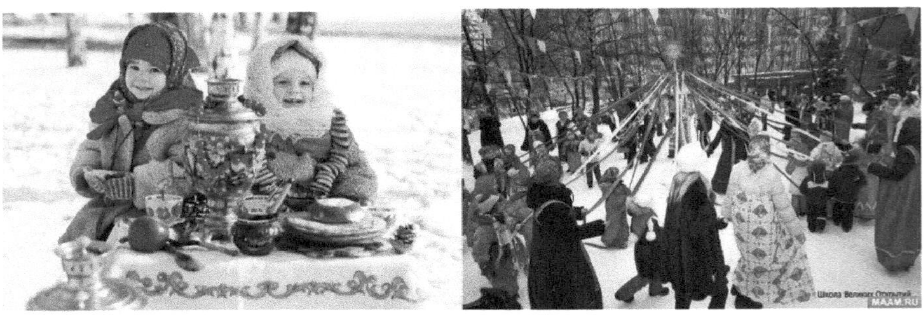

Figure 15.8 The holiday "Maslenitsa."

The bells are ringing!

Participation in the game involved performing certain rhythmic movements to the music and playing various characters (a kite, a hen, chickens). Such games evoked an emotional response of children, promoted development of creative imagination and developed drama skills.

In the fourth quarter the theme was revealed: "The children's ritual folklore."

An example of a lesson in this topic is the holiday "Maslenitsa," which presents the entire complex of elements of folklore ritual action.

The purpose of the lesson was to introduce students to the poetic and symbolic content of Maslenitsa—a traditional Russian folk holiday—festivities.

Tasks: Create a festive atmosphere for students, and teach them to consistently perform actions of the holiday scenario based on traditional folk actions; introduce students rules of behavior at the festival and etiquette; and help children to see the poetic and artistic beauty of folk traditions and Maslenitsa events.

The beauty of Russian Maslenitsa is in fun games, fun, and witty proverbs. In the course of classes, the teacher alternately draws students' attention to the words (lyrics, nursery rhymes, riddles), movement (musical and choral games), and the story that connects them (festive action).

The purpose of this lesson is to achieve greater emotional openness of children, their readiness to communicate, to play together, to show everyone their irreplaceable role in the whole action, the significance of each participant.

Technical support of the lessons at the beginning included baby books, audio recordings, reproductions of paintings, drawings. Then there were added folklore costumes, decorations, stuffed Shrovetide, and attributes of the holiday fair (Fig. 15.9).

Music and rhythmic classes in many ways echoed lessons of physical culture and singing. The difference between rhythmics and physical culture was that classes in rhythmics were held with music, and allowed to think in symbols and images; so rhythmics complemented physical education and did not replace it. Singing formed proper breathing, developed speech, diction, and improved quality of sound reproduction. Rhythmic classes contributed to better coordination of movements,

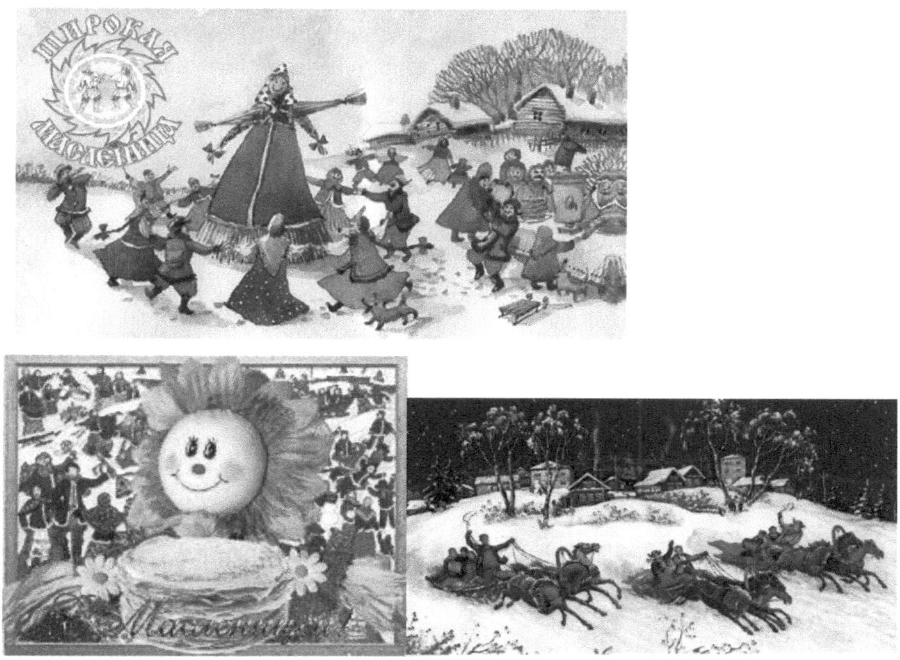

Figure 15.9 Baby books, reproductions of paintings.

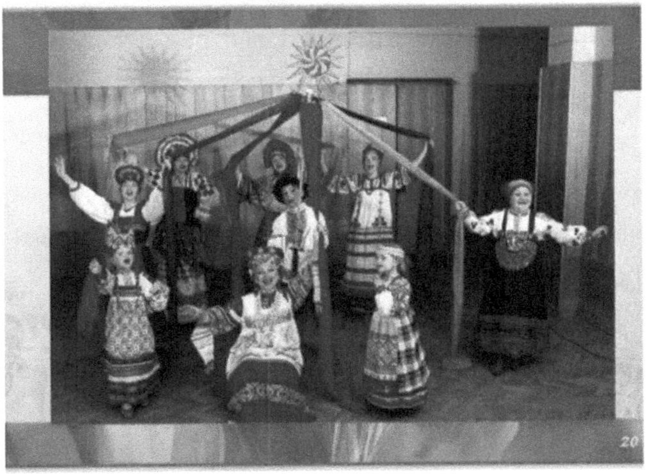

Figure 15.10 Musical and rhythmic classes.

development of correct posture, learning of a sense of aesthetic beauty (plasticity) of movements. In addition, they reduced psychoemotional stress and smoothed affective states (Fig. 15.10).

Music and rhythm taught the child to understand and express emotions. Feelings caused by music colored movements emotionally, and influenced plasticity and expressiveness of gestures. Musical and rhythmic classes contributed to intonation and auditory development; trained the rhythmic sense and corresponding motor skills that ensure consistency of movements. Such studies formed the speech and music attention; they taught joint actions, promoted the establishment of interpersonal contacts in the children's team, and gradually instilled aesthetic taste. In general, classes were aimed at consistently restoring motor abilities—coordination (tone, muscle strength, flexibility), conditioning (accuracy, dexterity), constructive (household, sports skills), and creativity.

The curriculum of musical and rhythmic classes in the traditions of folk art was based on the principle of interconnected concentric circles: the chosen topic gradually acquired new subjects, semantic and value connections for the necessary repetition of the material passed, which contributed to the strengthening of knowledge, skills, and involvement of all levels of movement organization.

Conclusion

Research has shown the need for scientific justification of a comprehensive systematic approach of doctors, psychologists, and teachers to the development of interdisciplinary programs that will allow children with disabilities to improve their physical and mental health and improve the quality of education (Momot, 2007; Mozgovoy, 2008). Pilot studies conducted in correctional schools have shown the ambiguity of the problem of poor academic performance of children and the inability to solve it solely by psychological and pedagogical forces. The medical aspect of the issue showed all the possible depth of the problem, reaching periods of prenatal, natal, and postnatal management of motherhood and childbirth. Early detection of hypoxic–traumatic injuries in childbirth and the postnatal period remains relevant. Therefore, for maximum effectiveness of rehabilitation measures (therapeutic, psychological, pedagogical and social), timely personalized diagnostics and the earliest possible start of these measures are necessary—at the stage of forming a motor stereotype and sequential construction of movements, starting from spinal reflexes and ending with coordinated, smooth, consistent, conscious movements "with meaning," in the organization of which cortical structures participate.

Despite the rather "late" start of rehabilitation activities in the pilot project (children of primary and secondary classes of correctional schools aged 8–14 years), the results showed a significant improvement in the clinical picture and psychoemotional status. Teachers noted improvements in concentration, perseverance, memory, and cognitive functions. Muscle "tunnels" in the cervical spine were eliminated, coordination improved, and there was a tendency to normalize the center of gravity.

According to the NEC data, there was an improvement in cerebral metabolism: the number of children with normal indicators of cerebral metabolism increased, which proved the positive impact of the treatment on the oxygen supply and adaptive capabilities of the brain (Safonicheva & Ovchinnikova, 2019) (Fig. 15.11).

There was an equalization of interhemispheric asymmetry and a uniform distribution of rhythms in power between the hemispheres. Changes occurred mainly in the parietal–central and occipital regions and could be associated with improved blood circulation in the vertebrobasilar pool and posterior brain parts.

The pilot project allowed integrating into the school curriculum musical and rhythmic classes in the traditions of folk art, which include several important components: sociocultural, communication, wellness, and neuroplastic elements. Medical professionals evaluated the effectiveness of such classes and noted the

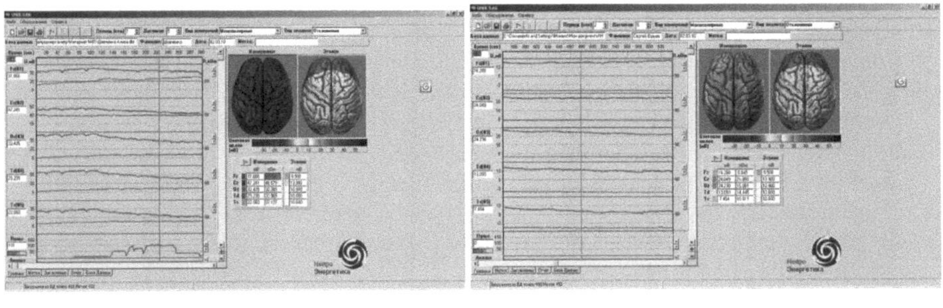

Figure 15.11 Dynamics of cerebral metabolism parameters: significantly increased acidosis (before), tendency to middle level of acidosis (after treatment) in boy N., aged 10 years.

important role in the development of children's "emotional and social" intelligence, and familiarization with cultural values. Adaptive physical exercise, music and rhythmic lessons in the traditions of folk art—not just contributed to better coordination, but also helped to develop proper posture, nurtured a sense of aesthetic beauty of the movements, music, and rhythm; taught the child to understand and express emotions and to balance the functions of the higher nervous activity; and integrated locomotor, cardiovascular, respiratory, and cognitive centers to reorganize the brain and improve its plasticity (Safonicheva & Ovchinnikova, 2019).

The regularities, described by Bernstein (1947, 2001, 2004), have to be taken into account when organizing the rehabilitation and recovery process: when a person learns something new, he uses the highest levels of movement organization, creating new neural connections both intra- and interhemispheric. Therefore for optimal development of the child, for example, after a birth trauma, hypoxic–traumatic process, it is necessary to set the highest goals that he can realize, but it is necessary to start restoring damaged functions from the very initial levels of A and B (with finger exercises, cross movements). Next, it is important to connect movements with movement in the "spatial field" of level C. And at the next stage of rehabilitation, the most effective may be musical and rhythmic dance movements, for the development and coordination of which the cortical levels D and E are responsible.

Music and rhythm give movements an emotional color and affect the expressiveness of gestures. This approach will combine art and creativity with the art of healing to restore health.

These studies have just begun recently, but we are full of confidence that a systematic approach, scientific justification of best practices, and their early implementation in children's institutions will improve the physical and mental health of children with disabilities, unlock their creative potential, and improve the quality of education and socialization in society.

References

A Blythe LaGasse. (2017). Social outcomes in children with autism spectrum disorder: a review of music therapy outcomes. *Patient Relat Outcome Meas*, *8*, 23–32. Available from https://doi.org/10.2147/PROM.S106267, Published online Feb 20, 2017.

American Music Therapy Association, (2005). [webpage on the Internet] *What is music therapy?* [Accessed 11.12.2016]. Available from <http://www.musictherapy.org/about/quotes/>.

American Music Therapy Association. (2015). *Fact sheet: Music therapy and autism spectrum disorder*. Silver Spring, MD: American Music Therapy Association, [Google Scholar].

American Music Therapy Association [webpage on the Internet] Professional requirements for music therapists. [Accessed 16.01.2017]. Available from <http://www.musictherapy.org/about/requirements/>.

Anokhin, P. K. (1973). *Essays on the physiology of functional systems*.

Astapov, V. M., Mikadze, Y. V. *Psychology of children with disorders and deviations of mental development: an anthology*, 2nd ed. (384 p). St. Petersburg, 2008.

Bardenshtein, L. M., Molodetsky, V. A., Kurashov, A. S., Shcherbakov, I. V. (2009). *Psychopathology of cognitive activity (violation of sensations, perception, memory, thinking, attention)* (p. 64). M.: GEOTAR-Media.

Bernstein, N.A. (1947). *On the construction of the movement: Scientific publication*. M.: Medgiz. 255 p.

Bernstein, N. A. (2001). *Selected works on biomechanics and cybernetics*. M.: Sport-academpress, (p. 296).

Bernstein, N. A. (2004). Biomechanics and physiology of movements. In V. P. Zinchenko (Ed.), *Selected psychological works* (2nd ed.)-M.: MODEK, 668 s.

Classification of mental and behavioral disorders (1994). *Clinical descriptions and guidelines for diagnosis*, L. Nuller Yu, Tsirkina S.Yu (Ed.), (p. 304), WHO/Translated from English, St. Petersburg, Russia: ADIS.

Doidge, N. (2007). *The brain that changes itself: stories of personal triumph from the frontiers of brain science*. ISBN 9781101147115/.

DSM-IV (1990). Diagnostic and Statistical Manual od Mental Disorders. Washington.

Federal Law of the Russian Federation No. 329–FL of December 4, (2007). *On physical culture and sport in the Russian Federation*." Available from <www.consultant.ru/document/cons_doc_>.

Fokin, V. F. & Ponomareva, N. V. (1999). *A method for assessing the energy state of the brain*. The patent of the Russian Federation No. 2135077 A61B5/04.

Fokin, V. V. & Ponomareva, N. V. (2002). *Energetic physiology of the brain*. Moscow.

History of Psychology in Persons: Personalities. (2005). *Psychological vocabulary. Encyclopedic dictionary in six volumes/edition*, L. A. Karpenko (Ed.).

ICD -10 International Classification of Diseases (10 revision). (1988). Psychiatric classification in an international perspective. With special reference to Choper V (F) of the recision of the international classification of diseases—mental, behavioral and developmental disorders/, Sartorius, N., Jablensky, A., et al. *British Journal of Psychiatry* (Suppl. I), 152.

International Statistical Classification of Diseases and Health Related Problems. (1992). *In three volumes, 10th revision*. Geneva: WHO.

Janda, V. (1983). On the concept of postural muscles and posture in men. *Australian Journal of Physiotherapy*, *29*, 83–84.

Janda, V. (1985). Muskelfunktions diagnostik (2 Aufl, p. 160 s). Berlin: Volk U. Ges.

Khadartsev, A. A., Fudin, N. A., Zilov, V. G., Safonicheva, O. G., & Smolensky, A. V. (2015). Psychology of movements and perception in sport. *Physiotherapy exercises and sports medicine*, *4*(130), 47–56, S.

Kipervas, I. P. (1991). *Peripheral tunnel syndromes*. MMA them. THEM. Sechenov, 32s.

Luria, A.R. (2009). *Fundamentals of neuropsychology: A textbook for students of higher. Studies. Institutions* (7th ed., p. 384 c). Moscow: Publishing Center Academy.

Momot, V. A. (2007). *Medical, psychological and pedagogical rehabilitation of children and adolescents with disabilities in a specialized institution*. In Bulletin of restorative medicine No. 4 (pp. 11-13). Moscow.

Mozgovoy, V. M. (2008). *Creating a health-saving educational space in the system of physical education of students with intellectual disabilities. international scientific and practical conference "Correctional development work with children in a multifunctional interactive environment"*. Book of articles (Vol. 2, pp. 81–85). M.: MSPU.

Özdemir, E., Norton, A., & Schlaug, G. (2006). Shared and distinct neural correlates of singing and speaking. *Neuroimage.*, *33*(2), 628–635, [PubMed] [Google Scholar].

Peretz, I., & Zatorre, R. J. (2005). Brain organization for music processing. *Annual Review of Psychology*, *56*, 89–114.

Petrushin, V. I. (2019). *Music therapy. New frontiers: From therapy to coaching. The integrated approach* (p. 512). M.: Gorodets: Publishing House.

Ratner, A. Y. (1990). *Late complications of birth damage to the nervous system* (p. 310) Kazan: Kazan University.

Ratner A.Y. (1995). *Neurology of newborns*. Kazan, 367 p.

Reschke-Hernandez, A. E. (2011). History of music therapy treatment unterventions for children with autism. *J Music Ther, 48*(2), 169–207, [PubMed] [Google Scholar].

Safonicheva, O. (2006). The syndrome of upper aperture of the chest (A new view of pathogenesis and treatment). *Doctor, No. 13*, 68–70.

Safonicheva, O. G. (2001). *The method of correction of functional state of the human body*. Patent 2163795 C1. 61 No. 39/04, published March 10, 2001 in Bl.7.

Safonicheva O.G. 2002. *Rehabilitation method of patients with diseases of the musculoskeletal system*. Patent 2187293 C1. 61 No. 9/04, published 20.08.2002 in Bl.23.

Safonicheva, O. G. (2007). *Rehabilitation and treatment of structural-functional disorders of the musculoskeletal system (pre-nosological diagnostics and complex treatment for emotional and affective disorders)*. Thesis for the degree of Doctor of Medical Sciences/ Tula State University. Tula.

Safonicheva, O. G., & Ovchinnikova, M. A. (2019). New approaches to the development of personalized rehabilitation programs for the children with disabilities, including autism spectrum disorders. In U. Das, N. Papaneophytou, & T. El-Kour (Eds.), *Autism 360* (pp. 427–475). Elsevier Academic Press. Available from <https://www.elsevier.com/books/autism-360/das/978-0-12-818466-0>.

Sechenov, I. M. (1863). *Reflexes of the brain*. Available from <www.litres.ru>.

Shushardjan, S. V. Doctor Art. Available from <http://www.doctor-art.ru/shushardjan-sergei>.

Skoromets, A. A. (2000). *Topical diagnosis of diseases of the nervous system. L.: Medicine.*, 320.

Thaut, M. H., McIntosh, G. C. (2010). *How music helps to heal the injured brain: therapeutic use crescendos thanks to advances in brain science. Cerebrum*. [Accessed 31.01.2017]. Available from <https://www.dana.org/article/how-music-helps-to-heal-the-injured-brain/>.

The draft law (1995). *On special education*. Defectology. No. 1 (pp. 3-16).

The program of special (correctional) educational institutions of type VIII. Preparatory, grades 1-4/V. M. Belov, V. S. Pitchers (2006). Brain (pp. 136-148). V. V. Voronkova (Ed.). M.: Education.

Trevell, D. G., Simons, D. G. (1989). *Myofascial pain. Translated from from English* (Vol. 1). *M.: Medicine*, 256s.

Vasilyeva, L. F. (1996). *Visual diagnosis of violations of statics and dynamics of the musculoskeletal system of a person* (p. 112). Ivanovo: MIK.

Vlasenko, O. P. (2007). *Musically-aesthetic education in correctional classes* (p. 9) Publisher "Teacher,", 10,15,19.

Vygotsky, L. S. (1999). *Questions of child psychology*. SPb.

Wayne, A. M. (2001). *Lectures on the neurology of non-specific brain systems* (3rd ed., p. 112)M: MEDPress-Inform.

Yevtushenko, I. V. (2003). *Musical education of mentally retarded children* (78, p. 26). Publishing Center Academy.

Robotics and autism: a review of current applications of robotics for autism spectrum disorder

16

Pericles Cheng
Department of Computer Science and Engineering, School of Sciences, European University Cyprus, Nicosia, Cyprus

Introduction

Robotics has been used in many areas other than manufacturing for many years now, ranging from educational areas, smart home applications, to medical implementations such as rehabilitation. Using robotics in education provides a wide range of skills for young students from elementary school all the way to university students and even further than that (Johnson, 2003). Robotics in education allows children to gain problem-solving skills, enhances their creativity, and promotes social communication and teamwork (Eguchi, 2015; Johnson, 2003). The Diagnostic and Statistical Manual of Mental Disorders (American Psychiatric Association, 2013) highlights the symptoms that may indicate a child is in the Autism Spectrum but the National Autism Society indicates three areas related to autism: social communication, social integration, and imagination (Dautenhahn & Werry, 2020). It is these social communication and integration skills that make robotics a powerful tool in autism treatment.

Using robotics in the diagnosis and treatment of autism spectrum disorder (ASD) has several benefits. Since the robots are programmed to perform specific tasks and record the responses of the person interacting with them there is no need for a healthcare expert to always be present, thus making them ideal for use in a home setting (Jain, Thiagarajan, Shi, Clabaugh, & Matarić, 2020; Matarić & Scassellati, 2016). Socially assistive robots (SAR) also allow the healthcare expert to define social interactions that are not frequent in real life and also be able to adjust them accordingly while at the same time keeping the child engaged and motivated (Boucenna et al., 2014; Dickstein-Fischer, Crone-Todd, Chapman, Fathima, & Fischer, 2018; Scassellati, 2005).

Recently, a number of survey studies were done on the effectiveness of robotics in autism treatment (Boucenna et al., 2014; DI Nuovo et al., 2020; Ntaountaki et al., 2019; Valentine et al., 2020). This chapter is not an exhaustive review of all the research done on robotics and autism but focuses more on presenting current research trends and providing a guide for people interested in the subject. The following section presents the use of robotics in helping healthcare providers in the

Emerging Programs for Autism Spectrum Disorder. DOI: https://doi.org/10.1016/B978-0-323-85031-5.00012-8

diagnosis of ASD. The next section introduces the use of robotics in autism treatment and the following section presents some of the robots used in the studies. Finally, the chapter concludes with a discussion on the current state of robotics for ASD and what are possible trends and opportunities for research in the area.

Robotics and autism spectrum disorder diagnosis

Early diagnosis of ASD can increase the chances of helping children with early intervention treatment (Bradshaw, Steiner, Gengoux, & Koegel, 2015; Zwaigenbaum et al., 2015). One of the areas where robotics can be used for ASD is in helping with the early screening of the condition. Social robotics technology is considered one of the most promising areas in ASD diagnosis since ASD is considered a behavioral condition and there are no blood, genetic, or imaging tests for the diagnosis (Matarić & Scassellati, 2016). ASD is usually diagnosed during the second year of life, although sometimes it can be diagnosed earlier in severe cases and later in more subtle cases (American Psychiatric Association, 2013).

The Diagnostic and Statistical Manual of Mental Disorders (American Psychiatric Association, 2013) presents four main criteria in diagnosing Autism Spectrum Disorders. The first criterion is an impairment of social communication and interaction while the second criterion is "restrictive repetitive patterns of behavior, interests or activities" (American Psychiatric Association, 2013). In a 1997 survey of more than 1200 families with children diagnosed with ASD, the authors discovered that diagnosis was too lengthy therefore placing the age of diagnosis at an average of 6 years (Howlin & Moore, 1997). In a more recent survey of more than 1000 families, there was a delay of 3.5 years from the first time a parent contacted a healthcare professional to receiving the diagnostic results (Crane, Chester, Goddard, Henry, & Hill, 2016). This was further delayed because parents took a year to observe the developmental problems of the child before reaching out to the healthcare professional making the delay in diagnosing ASD 4.5 years. The study found that the parents were the first ones to note the problems with the child's development and on average that occurred between the second and fifth year after birth. It is important to note that the results of the study in comparison to the 1997 study had very few changes in the diagnosis delay. For this end a review of diagnostic methods using robotics is being done in this chapter.

In one study at the Yale Child Study Center, the clinic was fitted with various sensors, such as cameras and microphones, in order to record and analyze subjects as they are going through a clinical evaluation (Scassellati, 2005). The sensors were able to detect changes in the subject's gaze, patterns in voice, and how they moved around the examination room. Computer vision using artificial intelligence has been shown to improve the traditional methods of ASD diagnosis (Noris, Benmachiche, Meynet, Thiran, & Billard, 2007; Piccardi et al., 2007; Ramírez-Duque, Frizera-Neto, & Bastos, 2019). Recent research on eye-contact detection using deep learning models has shown that diagnosis using a camera is on a par with diagnosis made by human experts (Chong et al., 2020). Body movement is also considered a way to help experts diagnose ASD and research has been conducted that shows almost 83% accuracy in predicting ASD in a child (Raya et al., 2020).

In addition to the passive data gathering, robots can be used for a more interactive test of ASD (Scassellati, 2005). In his study, Scassellati (2005) used a device called Playtest, which consisted of two buttons that the child could press, and one of two predefined sounds were played, and lights turned on. The device recorded the interactions of the child with the machine and these were later analyzed to identify auditory preferences in the child. Even though research exists that supports the method as a diagnostic tool (Klin, 1991; LePage & Courey, 2019), auditory preferences are more prevalent in older children and not in 2–3-year-old children (Paul, Chawarska, Fowler, Cicchetti, & Volkmar, 2007).

Autism treatment using robotics

In the past years, a number of research papers were involved in the area of robot use for treating people with ASD (Ntaountaki et al., 2019; Pennisi et al., 2016; Valentine et al., 2020). There are different ways that robots can be used in ASD treatments such as using robots to initiate social interactions with other children (Huskens, Palmen, Werff, Lourens, & Barakova, 2015) or using robots that can help children with ASD with specific tasks (David, Costescu, Matu, Szentagotai, & Dobrean, 2020). There is also a belief that people with ASD are more keen to follow a Science, Technology, Engineering, and Mathematics field of study due to the systematic nature of the field (Baron-Cohen, Wheelwright, Burtenshaw, & Hobson, 2007). To this end, the use of robots in ASD treatments has been considered beneficial.

One of the research studies had children with ASD work with typically developing siblings of around the same age to construct specific models using LEGO pieces (Huskens et al., 2015). The children would be given cards which would indicate who would build a specific part of the construction and a NAO robot was placed near them to mediate any social behavior between the children. The study did not find strong evidence of collaborative play using robot-mediated LEGO therapy, but the overall study does support the effectiveness of robotic interventions for children with ASD. In another study, two NAO robots were used in order to provoke specific social behaviors from children that a single robot would not be able to achieve (Amanatiadis, Kaburlasos, Dardani, Chatzichristofis, & Mitropoulos, 2020). The robots in the study would begin playing a game amongst themselves with the children watching and then the robots would engage the children in playing the game with them. The study found positive effects in several areas such as communication and interaction skills and cognitive flexibility.

Robotics can also assist in the treatment of autism through the involvement of children with ASD in robotics clubs. This inclusion has been shown to help children with ASD in forming closer relationships with other peers and enhancing their social communication skills (Bellini, Peters, Benner, & Hopf, 2007; Kasari, Locke,

Gulsrud, & Rotheram-Fuller, 2011). A study in two schools in Australia, placed typically developing children along with children diagnosed with ASD in two robotics clubs (Hinchliffe, Saggers, Chalmers, & Hobbs, 2016). The children learned how to program robots using the LEGO MINDSTORMS EV3 platform and after a year they were given a survey which assessed their social interactions. The results of the pre and post surveys showed that children with ASD felt isolated from other students before the intervention but after the 12-week program they felt more included. There was also an increase in social network centrality which indicates the amount of integration of a person within a social network. In another study, a group of two children with ASD and two typically developing children, the researchers noticed that even though the children with ASD were motivated to use robotics, they exhibited disruptive behaviors (Tsiomi & Nanou, 2020). Due to this reason, the researchers believed that the cooperative learning strategy was not effective.

In addition, to detecting and responding to user actions, research shows that robots should be able to detect moods and adapt to those changes accordingly in real time (Matarić & Scassellati, 2016; Dautenhahn and Werry, 2020). New machine learning algorithms are being developed so that robots will automatically analyze a child's behavior by capturing various inputs from facial expressions, body movements, and voice changes. The robots will then be able to trigger various actions and also learn when these actions are appropriate through a deep learning framework (Rudovic, Lee, Dai, Schuller, & Picard, 2018).

Robotic platforms used with autism spectrum disorder

Several robotics platforms have been used in the past years to help in diagnosing and treating ASD. In this section we will introduce some of these platforms that are widely used in research and have provided some experimental results.

One of the most commonly used humanoid robots for research in autism treatment and diagnosis is NAO. NAO was developed in 2006 from Aldebaran, later renamed to Softbank Robotics. A recent report from Softbank robotics states that their robots can "reduce shyness, reluctance, un-confidence and frustration, improving social skills and self-esteem" (Softbank Robotics, 2020). RobotLab (https://www.robotlab.com) provides a special education package which includes a NAO robot and a specialized software for autism to help in the treatment of children with ASD.

In 2013 Robokind developed a robot named Milo and a set of instructional material for people with ASD. Robots4Autism (https://robots4autism.com/) provides a curriculum designed for children 5–17 years old with an emphasis on developing social behaviors and emotional identification. Milo (Fig. 16.1) is a humanoid robot with the ability to walk, talk, and show emotions through facial expressions. In a case study in 2016 in Spartanburg, South Carolina, 8 of the 17 students taking part showed improvements in their GARS-3 scale while another 4 showed a reduction

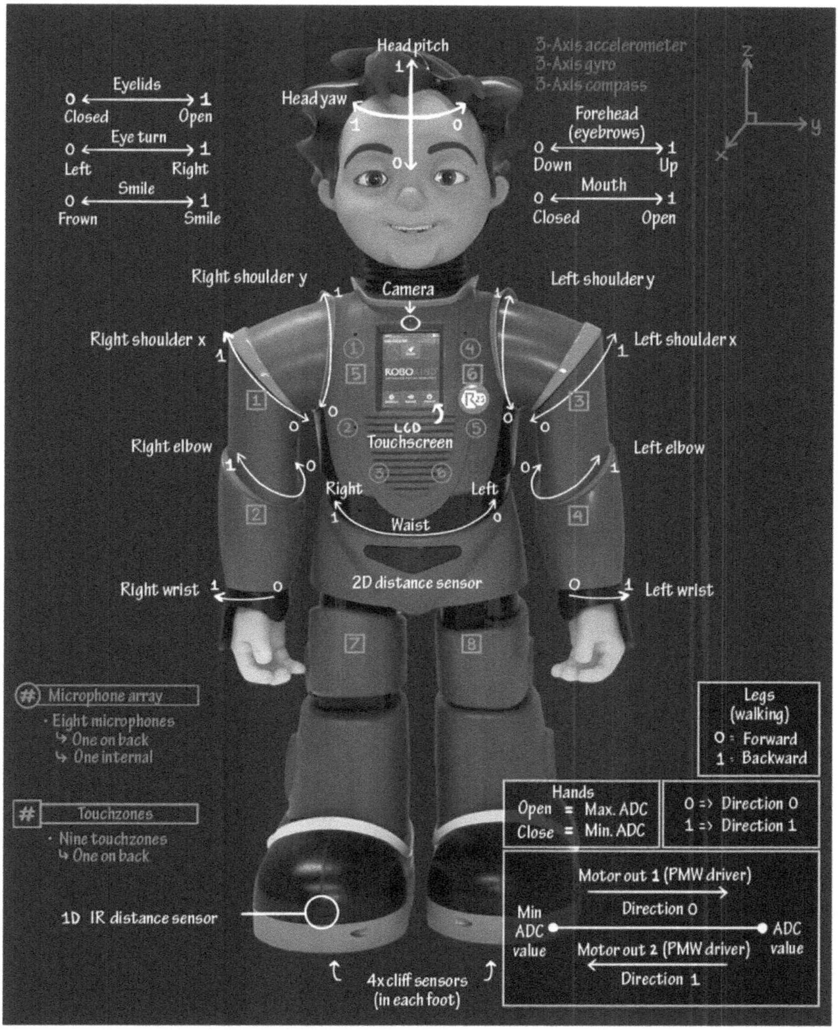

Figure 16.1 Robokind's humanoid robot Milo.

of restrictive repetition behavior and most of the students exhibited an increase in social communication after their treatments with Milo (Anon, 2016).

Another humanoid robot that is used in Autism treatment is Kaspar (https://www.herts.ac.uk/kaspar/the-social-robot). Kaspar was developed by the University of Hertfordshire's Adaptive Systems Research Group in 2005 after several years of research on how to develop robots for use in therapy of children with autism.

There are several other platforms that are currently being researched for use in ASD treatments, such as Keepon (https://beatbots.net/keepon-pro), Hanson Robotics Zeno (https://www.hansonrobotics.com/zeno/), Buddy Emotional Companion Robot (https://buddytherobot.com/en/buddy-the-emotional-robot/), and Bandit, a socially assistive Humanoid robot built by the University of Southern California Interaction Lab (http://robotics.usc.edu/interaction/domains/desc.php?name = asd).

Conclusion

Recent reviews of applications of robotics with regard to the diagnosis and treatment of people with ASD have shown a need for more diversity in research focus, and more research on the effectiveness of robotic interventions and on their contributions toward autism impairments (Dickstein-Fischer et al., 2018; Ismail, Verhoeven, Dambre, & Wyffels, 2019). Even though most of the research studies indicate substantial benefits in the use of robotics for children with ASD, there are some studies that did not observe major changes in collaborative abilities (Huskens, Palmen, Werff, Lourens, & Barakova, 2015; Tsiomi & Nanou, 2020). There is also a need for more research on what types of treatments are most effective, like free or semistructured interactions, and the type of SAR system that is most suited for the application.

One of the biggest issues with robotics for autism though, is the cost of the equipment. Currently robots are so expensive that it is hard for most healthcare providers to purchase them and maintain them let alone parents who would like to use a SAR system at home. As the cost of robotic equipment drops there is a chance to develop more affordable solutions that children can take home and use rather than relying on occasional treatments at the healthcare office. In addition, the development of more efficient and accurate artificial intelligence will allow the robots to learn and interact with children autonomously, thus reducing the need for a healthcare expert to handle the robot.

Using robotics for people with ASD is an area that has been researched but there is still a large area where researchers can pursue. It is a subject that I believe has a huge potential for research and an even greater impact on helping healthcare professionals diagnose and treat people with ASD.

References

Amanatiadis, A., Kaburlasos, V. G., Dardani, C., Chatzichristofis, S. A., & Mitropoulos, A. (2020). Social robots in special education: creating dynamic interactions for optimal experience. *IEEE Consumer Electronics Magazine*, *9*(3), 39–45.

American Psychiatric Association. (2013). *Diagnostic and statistical manual of mental disorders*.

Anon. (2016). *IESD case study: Children on the autism spectrum show improvement with Robot4autism in Spartanburg*.

Baron-Cohen, S., Wheelwright, S., Burtenshaw, A., & Hobson, E. (2007). Mathematical talent is linked to autism. *Human Nature*.

Bellini, S., Peters, J. K., Benner, L., & Hopf, A. (2007). A meta-analysis of school-based social skills interventions for children with autism spectrum disorders. *Remedial and Special Education*.

Boucenna, S., Narzisi, A., Tilmont, E., Muratori, F., Pioggia, G., Cohen, D., & Chetouani, M. (2014). Interactive technologies for autistic children: A review. *Cognitive Computation*, *6*(4), 722–740.

Bradshaw, J., Steiner, A. M., Gengoux, G., & Koegel, L. K. (2015). Feasibility and effectiveness of very early intervention for infants at-risk for autism spectrum disorder: A systematic review. *Journal of Autism and Developmental Disorders*, *45*(3), 778–794.

Chong, E., Clark-Whitney, E., Southerland, A., Stubbs, E., Miller, C., Ajodan, E. L., & Rehg, J. M. (2020). Detection of eye contact with deep neural networks is as accurate as human experts. *Nature communications*, *11*(1), 1–10.

Crane, L., Chester, J. W., Goddard, L., Henry, L. A., & Hill, E. (2016). Experiences of autism diagnosis: A survey of over 1000 parents in the United Kingdom. *Autism: the International Journal of Research and Practice*, *20*(2), 153–162.

Dautenhahn, K., & Werry, I. (2020). Issues of robot-human interaction dynamics in the rehabilitation of children with autism. *From Animals to Animats 6*.

David, D. O., Costescu, C. A., Matu, S., Szentagotai, A., & Dobrean, A. (2020). Effects of a robot-enhanced intervention for children with ASD on teaching turn-taking skills. *Journal of Educational Computing Research*, *58*(1), 29–62.

Di Nuovo, A., Bamforth, J., Conti, D., Sage, K., Ibbotson, R., Clegg, J., & Arnold, K. (2020). An explorative study on robotics for supporting children with autism spectrum disorder during clinical procedures. In *ACM/IEEE International Conference on Human-Robot Interaction*, (pp. 189–191). New York, NY: Association for Computing Machinery.

Dickstein-Fischer, L. A., Crone-Todd, D. E., Chapman, I. M., Fathima, A. T., & Fischer, G. S. (2018). *Socially assistive robots: current status and future prospects for autism interventions*, . *Innovation and Entrepreneurship in Health* (5, pp. 15–25).

Eguchi, A. (2015). Educational robotics as a learning tool for promoting rich environments for active learning (REALs). *Human-Computer Interaction*, 740–767.

Hinchliffe, K., Saggers, B., Chalmers, C., & Hobbs, J. (2016). *Utilising robotics social clubs to support the needs of students on the autism spectrum within inclusive school settings*.

Howlin, P., & Moore, A. (1997). Diagnosis in autism-a survey of over 1200 patients in the UK. *Autism: the International Journal of Research and Practice*.

Huskens, B., Palmen, A., Werff, M. Vd, Lourens, T., & Barakova, E. (2015). Improving collaborative play between children with autism spectrum disorders and their siblings: The effectiveness of a robot-mediated intervention based on Lego® therapy. *Journal of Autism and Developmental Disorders*, *45*(11), 3746–3755.

Ismail, L. I., Verhoeven, T., Dambre, J., & Wyffels, F. (2019). Leveraging robotics research for children with autism: A review. *International Journal of Social Robotics*, *11*(3), 389–410.

Jain, S., Thiagarajan, B., Shi, Z., Clabaugh, C., & Matarić, M. J. (2020). Modeling engagement in long-term, in-home socially assistive robot interventions for children with autism spectrum disorders. *Science Robotics*, *5*(39), 1–39.

Johnson, J. (2003). Children, robotics, and education. *Artificial Life and Robotics*, *7*(1–2), 16–21.

Kasari, C., Locke, J., Gulsrud, A., & Rotheram-Fuller, E. (2011). Social networks and friendships at school: Comparing children with and without ASD. *Journal of Autism and Developmental Disorders*.

Klin, A. (1991). Young autistic children's listening preferences in regard to speech: A possible characterization of the symptom of social withdrawal. *Journal of Autism and Developmental Disorders*.

LePage, P., & Courey, S. (2019). Characteristics of children with autism. *Teaching Children with High-Level Autism* (1), 19–34.

Matarić, M. J., & Scassellati, B. (2016). Socially Assistive Robotics. In B. Siciliano, & O. Khatib (Eds.), *Springer Handbook of Robotics* (pp. 1973–1994). Springer International Publishing. Available from https://doi.org/10.1007/978-3-319-32552-1_73

Noris, B., Benmachiche, K., Meynet, J., Thiran, J. P., & Billard, A. G. (2007). Analysis of head-mounted wireless camera videos for early diagnosis of autism. *Advances in Soft Computing, 45*, 663–670.

Ntaountaki, P., Lorentzou, G., Lykothanasi, A., Anagnostopoulou, P., Alexandropoulou, V., & Drigas, A. (2019). Robotics in autism intervention. *International Journal of Recent Contributions from Engineering, Science & IT (IJES), 7*(4), 4.

Paul, R., Chawarska, K., Fowler, C., Cicchetti, D., & Volkmar, F. (2007). 'Listen my children and you shall hear': Auditory preferences in toddlers with autism spectrum disorders. *Journal of Speech, Language, and Hearing Research, 50*(5), 1350–1364.

Pennisi, P., Tonacci, A., Tartarisco, G., Billeci, L., Ruta, L., Gangemi, S., & Pioggia, G. (2016). Autism and social robotics: A systematic review. *Autism Research, 9*(2), 165–183.

Piccardi, L., Noris, B., Barbey, O., Billard, A., Schiavone, G., Keller, F., & Hofsten, C. V. (2007). WearCam: A head mounted wireless camera for monitoring gaze attention and for the diagnosis of developmental disorders in young children. *In Proceedings-IEEE International Workshop on Robot and Human Interactive Communication* (pp. 594–598). IEEE.

Ramírez-Duque, A. A., Frizera-Neto, A., & Bastos, T. F. (2019). Robot-assisted autism spectrum disorder diagnostic based on artificial reasoning. *Journal of Intelligent and Robotic Systems: Theory and Applications, 96*(2), 267–281.

Raya, M. A., Marín-Morales, J., Minissi, M. E., Garcia, G. T., Abad, L., & Giglioli, I. A. C. (2020). Machine learning and virtual reality on body movements' behaviors to classify children with autism spectrum disorder. *Journal of Clinical Medicine, 9*(5), 1260.

Rudovic, O., Lee, J., Dai, M., Schuller, B., & Picard, R. W. (2018). Personalized machine learning for robot perception of affect and engagement in autism therapy. *Science Robotics, 3*(19).

Scassellati, B. (2005). Scassellati, B. (2005). Quantitative metrics of social response for autism diagnosis. *In ROMAN 2005, IEEE International Workshop on Robot and Human Interactive Communication* (pp. 585–590). IEEE.

Softbank Robotics. (2020). *World autism awareness day : Humanoid robots helping children with autism.* [Press Release]. Retrieved from: <https://www.softbankrobotics.com/emea/en/world-autism-awareness-day-nao>.

Tsiomi, E., & Nanou, A. (2020). Cooperative strategies for children with autism spectrum disorders in inclusive robotics activities. In SOCIETY. INTEGRATION. EDUCATION. *Proceedings of the International Scientific Conference, Vol. 4*, 148–156.

Valentine, A. Z., Brown, B. J., Groom, M. J., Young, E., Hollis, C., & Hall, C. L. (2020). A systematic review evaluating the implementation of technologies to assess, monitor and treat neurodevelopmental disorders: A map of the current evidence. *Clinical Psychology Review, 80*, 101870.

Zwaigenbaum, L., Bauman, M. L., Choueiri, R., Kasari, C., Carter, A., Granpeesheh, D., ... Natowicz, M. R. (2015). Early intervention for children with autism spectrum disorder under 3 years of age: Recommendations for practice and research. *Pediatrics, 136* (Supplement), S60–S81.

The importance of motor assessment, and current motor assessment tools available for individuals with autism spectrum disorder

17

Natalia Neophytou
Faculty of Health Science, Centre for Exercise Science and Sports Medicine, University of the Witwatersrand, Johannesburg, South Africa

Introduction

According to the Diagnostic and Statistical Manual of Mental Disorders (DSM-5), (Association AP, 2013) in order for an individual to be diagnosed with autism spectrum disorder (ASD), an individual must experience "persistent deficits in social communication and social interaction across multiple contexts," "have restrictive, repetitive patterns of behavior, interests, or activities," "their symptoms must be present in the early developmental period," and "should cause clinically significant impairment in social, occupational, or other important areas of functioning." The diagnostic criteria however, make no mention of motor impairments, which are commonly found in ASD.

Although the precise etiologic and pathophysiologic mechanisms of ASD have not been determined, it has been suggested that abnormal neurotransmission in the brain may result in impaired motor performance (Ming, Brimacombe, & Wagner, 2007). Unfortunately, the incidence of motor impairments is poorly documented and there are no studies to date to provide concise, multivariable, overall motor impairment incidence rates within this population. In a study by Ming et al., however, it was documented that 43% of individuals demonstrated hypotonia, 41% apraxia, and 9% gross motor delay for the age group 2–6 years (n = 154), suggesting there are likely different incidences for various motor impairments (Ming et al., 2007).

Common motor impairments, experienced by individuals with ASD include problems with fine and gross motor skill development, gait and coordination difficulties, abnormalities in posture, as well as impairments in motor control, imitation, and planning. These impairments are common and are consistent across both low- and high-functioning individuals (Ferguson, 2010).

Emerging Programs for Autism Spectrum Disorder. DOI: https://doi.org/10.1016/B978-0-323-85031-5.00006-2

Over time there has been a shift toward addressing these motor impairments through various interventions (Allenn, 1980; Bass, Duchowny, & Llabre, 2009; Casey, Quenneville-Himbeault, Normore, Davis, & Martell, 2015; Ehleringer, 2010), since it has been shown that a reduction in motor impairments has resulted in a better quality of life for these individuals (Badia et al., 2014). Nevertheless, there remains an obvious need for further research to determine the extent to which various motor variables are compromised within the population. The main hindrance for this research is the lack of appropriate motor assessment tools for this population. Furthermore, the motor deficits within this population are often disregarded or not readily tested globally, due to the motor impairments not being listed as a core deficit according to the diagnostic criteria in the population.

Current research indicates that a number of modified assessment tools are being used to determine the motor proficiency of individuals with ASD (Section on pediatrics, 2015). Although these modified tools may seem to be appropriate initially, there have been studies to comment on the inappropriateness of certain test items after a tool has been used (Neophytou, 2016; Tidy, 2016).

According to the American Physical Therapy Association, the most common tools used to assess physical activity related items in individuals with ASD (although the majority have not been specifically designed for individuals with ASD) include:

1. The Miller Function and participation scale (M-FUN) (Miller, 2006) which looks at motor skills for games and play in context. Although visual, fine motor, and gross motor skills are evaluated in this test, the test does not measure overall motor proficiency needed for everyday tasks.
2. The Test of Gross Motor Development, second edition (TGMD-2) (Ulrich, 2000), which identifies children who are significantly behind their peers in gross motor development. This test only measures gross motor skills (which may not be appropriate for individuals with ASD), therefore a holistic motor proficiency profile of participants may not be obtained using this test solely.
3. The Movement Assessment Battery for Children, second edition (MABC-2) (Henderson, Sugden, & Barnett, 2007), which measures manual dexterity, aiming and catching, and balance. This test may be a challenge for some children due to the large number of repeated trials.
4. The Bruininks–Oseresky Test of Motor Proficiency, second edition (BOT-2) test measures running speed, agility, balance, bilateral coordination, strength, upper limb coordination, response speed, visual motor control, and upper limb speed and dexterity. According to the American Physical Therapy Association the test is not recommended for children with significant motor disabilities and may have to be administered over multiple sessions due to fatigue experienced by the child.
5. The Help 3–6 (second edition), helps guide observations and review expectations for play skills expected of children at 3–6 years. This test does not physically measure motor proficiency, but rather checks whether individuals are able to perform specific tasks. The test is also not standardized.
6. The Assessment, Evaluation, and Programming System tests simple gross motor tasks expected of children up to age 6 years. Similarly to the Help 3–6 (second edition), this test does not physically measure motor proficiency. The test rates skills on a 3-point scale

were individuals are scored as doing a task as "consistently," "inconsistently," or "does not meet criterion." This test is also not standardized.

7. The Early Start Denver Model Checklist for Young Children with Autism, is used for tracking progress and goal setting with one of the domains out of eight being fine and gross motor skills. This test does not therefore provide a holistic motor proficiency assessment.

The lack of an appropriate tool for motor assessment is, however, not the only problem facing individuals with ASD. Assessments have often, in the past looked at particular motor deficits in isolation. For example, in a study by Rinehart et al. (2006), gait disturbances were assessed in newly diagnosed individuals with ASD, yet coordination necessary for optimal gait was not measured (Rinehart et al., 2006). Following this, often targeted interventions are developed to improve single motor variables. Although this may have improved the specific motor impairments at the time, other motor impairments (in equal disarray) may have been neglected. For example, in a study by Kern, Koegel, and Dunlap (1984), an alternating exercise intervention (jogging for 15 minutes and ball playing for 15 minutes) was used to determine whether stereotypic behaviors decreased in individuals following the intervention, however, no other variables were measured and documented to see if the intervention would influence them (Kern et al., 1984). A standardized tool measuring a variety of motor variables would therefore help combat this problem.

Autism diagnosis

It is imperative that a diagnosis of autism is made as early as possible. The benefit of timeous early diagnosis is twofold: (1) the sooner the individual is diagnosed the sooner appropriate intervention can ensue to improve disease specific outcomes, and more likely the less their stereotyped behaviors would be, and (2) it allows time for counseling, and help with future family planning from the parents perspective (Zwaigenbaum et al., 2007).

In 2013 the American Psychiatric Association released the fifth edition of its DSM-5 which is considered the standard reference that healthcare providers use to diagnose autism. The DSM-5 demonstrates good sensitivity and specificity for various instruments for the criteria (Frazier et al., 2012; Huerta, Bishop, Duncan, Hus, & Lord, 2012; Kent et al., 2013).

Although an autism diagnosis can be made as early as 18 months, in general a valid, reliable, and stable diagnosis of ASD can be given to an individual from 20 to 24 months, (Guthrie, Swineford, Nottke, & Wetherby, 2013). At present, however, most individuals are diagnosed with ASD after the age of 4 years (Christensen et al., 2016). This delay in diagnosis may hinder early implementation of necessary treatment/therapy interventions, thus this is a critical area for future improvement in ASD diagnosis. Furthermore it has been described by Christensen et al. (2016) that not all ASDs subtypes are diagnosed at similar rates. In fact he reports that autistic disorder is generally reported sooner at a mean age of 3 years, 10 months; while

Pervasive developmental disorder—not otherwise specified (PDD-NOS) is reported slightly later at a mean age of 4 years, 1 month; and lastly Asperger's disorder is reported far later at a mean age of 6 years, 2 months (Christensen et al., 2016). Furthermore, Christensen et al. (2016) reports that hearing and vision problems are generally some of the first problems to be reported within the first few months of an individual's life coupled, while fine motor skills, communication, and social difficulties are generally reported from 6 months of the individuals life (Christensen et al., 2016).

Since there are no discrete neuroanatomical abnormalities or definite biomechanical markers that define ASD, diagnosis is purely based on clinical and behavioral assessment (Landrigan, 2010). According to the Centers of Disease Control and Prevention (CDC) children are recommended to undergo broad developmental screenings at 9, 18, and 24 months, which assess if the individuals have any developmental delays (Centre of Disease Control, 2019). More specific ASD screenings are recommended by the CDC at 18 months should the child have a higher risk of ASD based on family history or abnormal behaviors noted from general screenings. The process should follow the pediatric developmental screening protocol recommended by the CDC. The starting point for diagnosis would be parents completing a relevant screening questionnaire for their child. Follow-up comprehensive diagnostic evaluations would be conducted if any impairments are observed in the screening observations.

Common screening tools used for general development and ASD may include the following:

1. The Ages and Stages Questionnaires (ASQ), which is a parent-completed general developmental screening questionnaire. It comprises 19 age-specific questionnaires screening personal adaptive skills, communication, gross and fine motor skills and results in a pass or fail score for domains.
2. The Parent Evaluations of Developmental Status, which is a general development parent-interview screening form. It comprises 10 items, which detect behavioral and developmental problems in children from birth to 11 months.
3. The Communication and Symbolic Behavior Scale, which is a norm-referenced, standardized, one page parent-completed checklist-screening tool. It comprises a 15 minute questionnaire and videotaped behavior sample, which measures communication and communicative behaviors in children 8–24 months (up to 72 months if developmental delays are present).

Specific ASD screening tools include:

1. The Screening tool for Autism in Toddlers and Young Children, which is an interactive screening tool designed to identify children between the ages of 24 and 36 months who may be on the autism spectrum. It comprises 12 activities assessing play, communication, and imitation skills and takes approximately 20 minutes to administer.
2. The Modified Checklist for Autism in Toddlers, which is a parent-completed screening questionnaire. It comprises 20 questions regarding a child's behavior and is intended for toddlers aged 16 to 30 months of age.
3. Gilliam Autism Rating Scale- Second Edition (GARS-2), which is a norm-referenced instrument used to assess individuals who have severe behavioral problems that may be

indicative of autism. It comprises 42 items categorized into three main areas, namely, stereotyped behaviors, communication, and social interaction, as well as containing developmental history questions (Montgomery, Newton, & Smith, 2008). It may be used by teachers, parents, and clinicians in a variety of settings including the home or school and is used to assess individuals aged 3 to 22 years (Montgomery et al., 2008). To the researchers knowledge, sensitivity and specificity data are not available for the GAR-2. However, good internal consistency reliability (0.94 total test) as well as good test–retest reliability (0.84 for Autism Index) has been reported (McClintock and Fraser, 2011; Montgomery et al., 2008). There is reportedly evidence for construct and content validity (Montgomery et al., 2008), however, it has been suggested that further research on differentiation of the subscales is needed (Montgomery et al., 2008).

4. The Childhood Autism Rating Scale (CARS); which is a brief 15 item rating scale used to identify individuals with ASD and distinguish them from those with severe cognitive deficits. CARS can also distinguish between mild-to-moderate and severe autism. CARS includes items drawn from five prominent systems for diagnosing autism, including social communication, emotional reactivity, social orientation, cognitive and behavioral consistency, and odd sensory exploration. It takes approximately 10 minutes to administer. It has been reported by Nebel-Scwalm & Matson (2008) that the CARS has good internal consistency reliability 94%, average test–retest reliability for diagnoses of 64%, and good test–retest reliability for CARS scores 81%. They also report that there was acceptable interrater reliability (0.71) (Nebel-Scwalm & Matson, 2008). One hundred percent sensitivity was reported for children with autism when CARS was compared to with DSM-IV criteria (Rellini, Tortolani, Trillo, Carbone, & Montecchi, 2004); this would need to be confirmed for the more recent DSM-5 criteria. One of the critiques for CARS is that CARS does not include "some constructs considered important to the diagnosis of autism due to the items being derived from five different theoretical perspectives of autism, including Kanner's description of the syndrome to the DSM-IIIR" (McClintock and Fraser, 2011; Ozonoff, Goodlin-Jones, & Solomon, 2005).
5. The Social Communication Questionnaire (SCQ), is based on the DSM-IV and the content of the Autism Diagnostic Interview-Revised (ADI-R) (McClintock & Fraser, 2011). It is a rating scale developed to assess symptoms associated with ASD comprises yes/no questions and involves two formats: the lifetime and current behavior formats. The lifetime form includes an account of developmental history over the individuals' lifetime, while the current behavior form includes an account of behaviors observed in the last 3 months (McClintock & Fraser, 2011). The SCQ was previously termed the ASQ and can distinguish between children with ASD and children with other disabilities. It takes approximately 10 minutes to administer. Sensitivity and specificity (differentiating ASD from other diagnoses) for a cut-off score above 15 have been reported as 85% and 75% respectively, and for a cut-off score of 22 has been reported as 75% and 60%, respectively (Berument, Rutter, Lord, Pickles, & Bailey, 1999). It has also been reported that internal consistency is good, and ranges from 81%–93% (Berument et al., 1999).
6. The Social Responsiveness Scale (SRS), which is a screening questionnaire comprising 65 items, which fall under three domains, namely, social behavior, communication, and repetitive behaviors associated with ASD. Parents and teachers are required to complete separate forms after which scores are added together to form an overall score (McClintock & Fraser, 2011). The SRS may be administered to individuals between the ages of 4 and 18 years and takes approximately 20 minutes to complete. Sensitivity and specificity (differentiating ASD from other diagnoses) are reported to be 85% and 75%, respectively. Internal consistency has been reported to range between 93% and 97%

(McClintock & Fraser, 2011). A difference however, in terms of test−retest reliability has been reported between males 85% and females 77% (Constantino, Hudziak, & Todd, 2003).

It needs to be highlighted that the ASD-specific screening tools, seem to lack fundamental motor assessment elements and thus generally would need to be coupled with general development tools such as the ASQ to acquire this information. This may not be cost- nor time-effective. From the researchers experience, in most instances, this is not usually done and further gross and fine motor skill assessment does not generally occur in this population. Thus gross and fine motor therapy interventions are generally delayed, which can impair the quality of life of the individual. Development of appropriate motor assessment/screening tools or optimal combination of screening and diagnostic tools could potentially remedy this problem.

Furthermore, it should be noted that screening tools do not provide conclusive evidence or in-depth information regarding developmental delays and thus further thorough investigations using specific diagnostic tools need to be conducted in order for a diagnosis to be made (Centre of Disease Control, 2019).

Autism diagnostic tools

Following the screening process, if ASD is suspected, an ASD-specific diagnostic tool should be used to confirm diagnosis. It has been suggested that, although there are many ASD diagnostic tools, no single tool should be used as the basis for diagnosis but rather a combination of a few to confirm the diagnosis (Centre of Disease Control, 2019). In general ASD diagnostic tools depend on two main sources of information: parents' or caregivers' reports of their child's development, as well a clinical professional's assessment of the child's behavior (Centre of Disease Control, 2019). Following diagnosis there may be referral to specialists for further investigation and management.

The DSM-5 provides the standardized criteria to help diagnose ASD and is used as a reference for all ASD-specific diagnostic tools. Current ASD-specific diagnostic tools include the following:

Gold standard

1. The Autism Diagnostic Observation Schedule-Generic (ADOS-G), which is a "semistructured, standardized assessment of social interaction, communication, play, and imaginative use of materials for individuals suspected of having ASD. The observational schedule consists of four 30-minute modules, each designed to be administered to different individuals according to their level of expressive language. The Autism Diagnostic Observation Schedule-Generic (ADOS-G) is a semistructured, standardized assessment of social interaction, communication, play, and imaginative use of materials for individuals suspected of having autism spectrum disorders" (Lord et al., 2000). The observational schedule consists of four 30-minute modules, each designed to be administered to different individuals according to their level of expressive language. The ADOS-G has been reported to have

excellent interrater and test-retest reliability for individual items, excellent interrater reliability within domains and excellent internal consistency (Lord et al., 2000). Sensitivity and specificity for the ADOS-G is reported to be greater than 90% and 80%, respectively. According to Lord et al., internal consistency for all domains and modules ranged from 47% to 94%, while interrater reliability within each module ranged from 65% to 78% and test−retest reliability ranged from 59%−82% over an average period of nine months (Lord et al., 2000).

2. The Autism Diagnostic Interview-Revised (ADI-R), which is a clinical diagnostic structured interview, whereby an experienced clinical interviewer questions a parent or caretaker regarding the developmental history and current behavior of the individual being evaluated (Lord, Rutter, & Le Couteur, 1994). The ADI-R comprises 93 items, and evaluates three functional domains including language/communication, reciprocal social interactions, and restricted, repetitive, and stereotyped behaviors and interests—as per the three core traits of ASD. The ADI-R usually takes between 60−90 minutes to administer and is appropriate for children and adults with mental ages above 18 months (Lord et al., 1994). "For each domain, a range of sensitivity (86%−100%) (Lord et al., 1994) and specificity (75%−96%) (Lord et al., 1994) values are reported for various combinations of score (either total score or cut-off score) and language ability of the individual assessed" (McClintock & Fraser, 2011). Internal consistency over the four domains ranges from 69%−95% (Lord et al., 1994).

Nongold standard

1. The Autism Behavioral Checklist (ABC) comprises a list of 57 questions regarding a child's behavior. Questions fall under five main categories, namely, sensory behaviors, relating behaviors, body and object use behaviors, and language behaviors. The ABC was designed to be answered independently by a parent, teacher, or caregiver after which a trained clinician would score and analyze the findings. The checklist takes approximately 10−20 minutes to administer and analyze and can be used in individuals aged 2−14 years of age. The checklist has been considered useful in the screening of individuals suspected of having autism, yet has been reported to have poor psychometric properties (Marteleto & Pedromônico, 2005).
2. The high-Functioning Autism Spectrum Screening Questionnaire (ASSQ) is a 27 item informant report questionnaire assesses characteristic symptoms of Asperger's and other high-functioning Autism Spectrum disorders. The ASSQ comprises of five main domains namely: social interaction, communication problems, restricted and repetitive behaviors, motor clumsiness, and associated behaviors. The ASSQ takes approximately 10 minutes to administer and score and comes in parent and teacher formats. It may be administered to individuals from birth 7−16 years of age and takes approximately 10−15 minutes to administer. The ASSQ is reported to have good specificity in correctly identifying non-Asperger's disorder (Ehlers, Gillberg, & Wing, 1999) as well as good sensitivity (91%) and specificity (86%) (Posserud, Lundervold, & Gillberg, 2009).
3. The Development And Well-Being Assessment (DAWBA) comprises a mixture of structured and open-ended questions, which was developed to assess children for psychiatric disorders (Aebi et al., 2012). It can be administered in person or via a secure internet connection. The DAWBA items refer to ICD-10 and DSM-IV diagnostic criteria and inbuilt diagnostic algorithms provide useful guides to the likelihood of different diagnoses. It takes 20 minutes to administer.

4. The Developmental, Dimensional and Diagnostic Interview (3di) is a computerized parent-interview comprising 183 items assessing overall ASD symptomology in terms of extent of impairment, which takes into account demographics, family, developmental history, and motor skills. The 3di also determines comorbidity across a full range of child psychiatric disorders. Of the 557 questions, 266 relate to disorders on the autism spectrum, while 291 questions relate to mental state relevant to other diagnoses. The interview takes 90 minutes to administer. Sensitivity and specificity (differentiating ASD from other diagnoses) are reported to be 100% and 97%, respectively (McClintock & Fraser, 2011; Skuse et al., 2004). Furthermore according to Skuse et al. (2004), test–retest and interrater reliability are reported to be excellent, for the tool with the majority of correlation coefficients being greater than 0.9 (Skuse et al., 2004).
5. The Diagnostic Interview for Social and Communicative Disorders (DISCO) is a semi-structured interview which comprises three domains, namely, social interaction, social communication and social imagination, and repetitive behaviors associated with ASD. It assesses areas of impairment in each domain to create a profile of the individual, and is one of the few tools which may be used for both children and adults on the spectrum (Wing, Leekam, Libby, Gould, & Larcombe, 2002). The interview takes 2–3 hours to complete. The questions are flexible, and may be adapted according to the individual's level of functioning, previous assessment, and cultural background. The authors of the DISCO report high interrater reliability of greater than 75% (Wing et al., 2002).

It has been suggested by McClintock and Fraser (2011) that there may be potentially preferable instrument combinations for the screening and diagnosis of autism, as illustrated in Table 17.1 (McClintock & Fraser, 2011). Again a real concern is that three of the six combinations suggested would result in motor skills not being assessed.

It should be noted that according to McClintock and Fraser (2011) option 6 is postulated to be the lowest cost option. This option also makes use of the 3di which therefore

Table 17.1 Potentially preferable instrument combinations for the screening and diagnosis of autism as per McClintock and Fraser (2011).

Combination number	Screening instrument	Diagnostic instrument		Motor assessment (Yes/no)
		Interview type	Observational type	
1	SCQ	AD1-R	ADOS	No
2	SCQ	AD1-R	CARS	No
3	SCQ	3di[a]	ADOS	Yes
4	SCQ	3di[a]	CARS	Yes
5	CARS	AD1-R	ADOS	No
6	CARS	3di[a]	ADOS	Yes

ADI-R, Autism Diagnostic Interview-Revised; *ADOS*, The Autism Diagnostic Observation Schedule; *CARS*, The Childhood Autism Rating Scale; *SCQ*, The Social Communication Questionnaire; *3di*, The Developmental, Dimensional and Diagnostic Interview.
[a]Motor skills assessed.

means motor skills would be assessed in the process, and thus this combination may be preferred in low-income settings and for those with suspected motor deficits.

Current ASD diagnosis processes are currently by no means perfect. In fact, although there has been an expansion of the current diagnostic criteria (DSM-5), some argue that some clinically important characteristics are still missing from the criteria (Murray-Slutsky & Paris, 2000). Poor postural control, general motor deficits, an inability to process sensory stimuli, impaired imitation skills, as well as low levels of attention and arousal are some of the common characteristics noted in individuals with ASD, yet have failed to be included in the criteria (Murray-Slutsky & Paris, 2000). It is thought that one of the reasons motor impairments are not included in the criteria is that in most cases the motor impairments found are not pervasive (Page & Boucher, 1998). However, recent research suggests that these impairments are much more common than previously thought.

Actually, according to Teitelbaum et al., it was found that motor impairments, for example, movement asymmetries, are present at birth, and it was suggested that they could therefore contribute to the early identification of ASD (Teitelbaum, Teitelbaum, Nye, Fryman, & Maurer, 1998). Similarly, Baraneck also reported that the assessment of motor activity may play a part in the early identification of ASD (Baranek, 1999). In addition, Pan, Tsai, and Chu (2009) found that children with ASD obtain lower scores in motor tests compared to typically developing counterparts, and suggested that impaired motor performance may be an early sign of autism, therefore being important to screen for early on in life (Pan et al., 2009).

The lack of motor skill screening and assessment is an area of great concern as individuals with ASD often display numerous motor impairments, which will be elaborated on in the next section. In most instances, these motor deficits may severely impair quality of life.

Furthermore another concern is that there is increasing evidence that current diagnostic processes may "fail to capture the female manifestation of ASD" (Ratto et al., 2018), which has been said to skew the prevalence rates seen amongst boys and girls diagnosed with ASD. Furthermore, there have been questions raised regarding the sensitivity of gold standard autism diagnostic tools for females (Ratto et al., 2018). This issue needs to be investigated, and possibly the development of more sensitive tools for the female population needs to be undertaken.

In summary

While numerous screening tools and diagnostic tools for ASD exist, there remains a concern that critical impairments are not being assessed and as a result not being effectively managed/treated. Although some combinations of screening tools and diagnostic tools are better and may catch motor deficits, overall early motor assessment in the population is lacking. Overall, the development of specific ASD motor screening tools, as well as the inclusion of motor skill proficiency tests in current ASD diagnostic tools should be pursued.

References

Aebi, M., Kuhn, C., Metzke, C. W., Stringaris, A., Goodman, R., & Steinhausen, H.-C. (2012). The use of the development and well-being assessment (DAWBA) in clinical practice: A randomized trial. *European Child & Adolescent Psychiatry*, *21*(10), 559–567.

Allenn, J. (1980). Jogging can modify disruptive behaviours. *Teaching Exceptional Children*, *12*(2), 66–70.

Association AP. (2013). *Diagnostic and statistical manual of mental disorders*. Arlington, VA: American Psychiatric Publishing.

Badia, M., Riquelme, I., Orgaz, B., Acevedo, R., Longo, E., & Montoya, P. (2014). Pain, motor function and health-related quality of life in children with cerebral palsy as reported by their physiotherapists. *BMC Pediatrics*, *14*, 192.

Baranek, G. T. (1999). Autism during infancy: A retrospective video analysis of sensory-motor and social behaviors at 9–12 months of age. *Journal of Autism and Developmental Disorders*, *29*(3), 213–224.

Bass, M., Duchowny, C., & Llabre, M. (2009). The effect of therapeutic horseback riding on social functioning in children with autism. *Journal of Autism and Developmental Disorders*, *29*, 1261–1267.

Berument, K, Rutter, M, Lord, C, Pickles, A, & Bailey, A (1999). Autism Screening Questionnaire: Diagnostic Validity. Br J Psychiatry. 1999;173:444–51. *British Journal of Psychiatry*, *175*(5), 444–451. Available from https://doi.org/10.1192/bjp.175.5.444.

Casey, A., Quenneville-Himbeault, G., Normore, A., Davis, H., & Martell, S. (2015). A therapeutic skating intervention for children with autism spectrum disorder. *Pediatric Physical Therapy*, *27*(2), 170–177.

Christensen, D., Baio, J., Braun, K., Bilder, D., Charles, J., Constantino, J. N., et al. (2016). Prevalence and characteristics of autism spectrum disorder among children aged 8 years —Autism and Developmental Disabilities Monitoring Network, 11 Sites, United States, 2012. *MMWR. Surveillance Summaries: Morbidity and Mortality Weekly Report. Surveillance Summaries/CDC*, *65*(SS-3), 1–23.

Centre of Disease Control. (2019). *Screening and diagnosis of autism spectrum disorder for healthcare providers*. United States, [cited 12.02.2019]. Available from: <https://www.cdc.gov/ncbddd/autism/hcp-screening.html>.

Constantino, J. N., Hudziak, J. J., & Todd, R. D. (2003). Deficits in reciprocal social behavior in male twins: Evidence for a genetically independent domain of psychopathology. *Journal of the American Academy of Child and Adolescent Psychiatry*, *42*, 458–467.

Ehleringer, J. (2010). Yoga therapy in practice. Yoga for children on the autism spectrum. *International Journal of Yoga Therapy*, *20*, 131–139.

Ehlers, S., Gillberg, C., & Wing, L. (1999). A screening questionnaire for Asperger syndrome and, of oh-fasdisac. *JAaDD*, 129–141.

Ferguson, L. (2010). *The effect of an adapted physical activity program on motor performance and behaviour of children with autism spectrum disorder* (Masters Disertation, Stellenbosch University). Retrieved from <https://www.semanticscholar.org/paper/THE-EFFECTS-OF-AN-ADAPTED-PHYSICAL-ACTIVITY-PROGRAM-Ferguson/cf1c356d988e2598f263707e6432bbe91b8ada3b>.

Frazier, T., Youngstrom, E., Speer, L., Embacher, R., Law, P., Constantino, J., et al. (2012). Validation of proposed DSM-5 criteria for autism spectrum disorder. *Journal of the American Academy of Child and Adolescent Psychiatry*, *51*, 28–40.

Guthrie, W., Swineford, L., Nottke, C., & Wetherby, A. (2013). Early diagnosis of autism spectrum disorder: Stability and change in clinical diagnosis and symptom presentation. *Journal of Child Psychology and Psychiatry, 54*, 582–590.

Henderson, S. E., Sugden, D. A., & Barnett, A. L. (2007). *The movement assessment battery for children* (Second edition (MABC-2). London: Pearson Education, Inc.

Huerta, M., Bishop, S., Duncan, A., Hus, V., & Lord, C. (2012). Application of DSM-5 criteria for autism spectrum disorder to three samples of children with DSM-IV diagnoses of pervasive developmental disorders. *The American Journal of Psychiatry, 169*, 1056–1064.

Kent, R., Carrington, S., Le Couteur, A., Gould, J., Wing, L., & Maljaars, J. (2013). Diagnosing autism spectrum disorder: Who will get a DSM-5 diagnosis? *Journal of Child Psychology and Psychiatry, 54*, 1242–1250.

Kern, L., Koegel, R., & Dunlap, G. (1984). The influenece of vogorous versus mild exercise on autistic stereoptyped behavious. *Journal of Autism and Developmental Disorders, 14*, 57–67.

Landrigan, P. (2010). What causes autism? Exploring the environmental contribution. *Current Opinion in Pediatrics, 22*, 219–225.

Lord, C., Risi, S., Lambrecht, L., Cook, H., Edwin, H. J., Leventhal, B., et al. (2000). The autism diagnostic observation schedule-generic: A standard measure of social and communication deficits associated with the spectrum of autism. *Journal of Autism and Developmental Disorders, 30*(3), 205–223.

Lord, C., Rutter, M., & Le Couteur, A. (1994). Autism diagnostic interview-revised: A revised version of a diagnostic interview for caregivers of individuals with possible pervasive developmental disorders. *Journal of Autism and Developmental Disorders, 24*(5), 659–685.

Marteleto, M. R. F., & Pedromônico, M. R. M. (2005). Validity of Autism Behavior Checklist (ABC): preliminary study. *Brazilian Journal of Psychiatry, 27*, 295–301.

McClintock, J. M., & Fraser, J. (2011). *Diagnostic instruments for autism spectrum disorder: A brief review New Zealand Guidelines Group.*

Miller, L. J. (2006). *Miller function and partcipation scales.* San Antonio, TX: Harcourt Assessment Inc.

Ming, X., Brimacombe, M., & Wagner, G. C. (2007). Prevalence of motor impairment in autism spectrum disorders. *Brain and Development, 29*(9), 565–570.

Montgomery, J. M., Newton, B., & Smith, C. (2008). Test review: Gilliam, J. (2006). GARS-2: Gilliam autism rating scale—second edition. Austin, TX: PRO-ED. *Journal of Psychoeducational Assessment, 26*(4), 395–401.

Murray-Slutsky, C., & Paris, B. (2000). *Exploring the spectrum of autism and pervasive developmental disorders.* TX: Therapy Skill Builders.

Nebel-Scwalm, M. S., & Matson, J. L. (2008). Differential diagnosis. In J. L. Matson (Ed.), *Clinical Assessment and Intervention for Autism Spectrum Disorder* (pp. 91–129). Burlington: Elsevier.

Neophytou, N. (2016). *The efficacy of a 12 week intervention in 11-16 year old adolescents with autism spectrum disorder* (Masters Dissertation). Retrieved from <http://wiredspace.wits.ac.za/bitstream/handle/10539/21201>.

Ozonoff, S., Goodlin-Jones, B., & Solomon, M. (2005). Evidence-based assessment of autism spectrum disorders in children and adolescents. *Journal of Clinical Child and Adolescent Psychology, 34*, 523–540.

Page, J., & Boucher, J. (1998). Motor impairments in children with autistic disorder. *Child Language Teaching and Therapy, 14*(3), 233–259.

Pan, C. Y., Tsai, C. L., & Chu, C. H. (2009). Fundamental movement skills in children diagnosed with autism spectrum disorders and attention deficit hyperactivity disorder. *Journal of Autism and Developmental Disorders*, *39*, 1694–1705.

Posserud, M. B., Lundervold, A. J., & Gillberg, C. (2009). Validation of the autism spectrum screening questionnaire in a total population sample. *Journal of Autism and Developmental Disorders*, *39*(1), 126–134.

Ratto, A. B., Kenworthy, L., Yerys, B. E., Bascom, J., Wieckowski, A. T., White, S. W., et al. (2018). What about the girls? Sex-based differences in autistic traits and adaptive skills. *Journal of Autism and Developmental Disorders*, *48*(5), 1698–1711.

Rellini, E., Tortolani, D., Trillo, S., Carbone, S., & Montecchi, F. (2004). Childhood autism rating scale (CARS) and autism behavior checklist (ABC) correspondence and conflicts with DSM-IV criteria in diagnosis of autism. *Journal of Autism and Developmental Disorders*, *34*, 703–708.

Rinehart, N., Bruce, J., Tonge, B., Iansek, R., Mc Ginley, J., Brereton, A., et al. (2006). Gait function in newly diagnosed children with autism: Cerebellar and basal ganglia related motor disorder. *Developmental Medicine and Child Neurology*, *48*(10), 819–824.

Section on Pediatrics. (2015). *Selected assesment tools for evaluation of children with autism spectrum disorder in school-based practice (fact sheet)*. American Physical Therapy Assosiation, [cited 1.11.2016]. Available from: <https://pediatricapta.org/includes/fact-sheets/pdfs/15%20Selected%20Assess%20Tools%20for%20ASD.pdf>.

Skuse, D., Warrington, R., Bishop, D., Chowdhury, U., Lau, J., Mandy, W., et al. (2004). The Developmental, Dimensional and Diagnostic Interview (3di): A Novel Computerized Assessment for Autism Spectrum Disorders. *Journal of the American Academy of Child & Adolescent Psychiatry*, *43*(5), 548–558.

Teitelbaum, P., Teitelbaum, O., Nye, J., Fryman, J., & Maurer, R. G. (1998). Movement analysis in infancy may be useful for early diagnosis of autism. *Proceedings of the National Academy of Sciences*, *95*(23), 13982–13987.

Tidy, C. (2016). *Autism spectrum disorders*, EMS Group. [cited 01.11.2016]. Available from: <http://patient.info/doctor/autistic-spectrum-disorders-pro>.

Ulrich, D. A. (2000). *Test of gross motor development. Examiners manual* (2nd ed.). Austin, TX: ProED.

Wing, L., Leekam, S. R., Libby, S. J., Gould, J., & Larcombe, M. (2002). The diagnostic interview for, social and communication disorders: Background, inter-rater reliability and clinical use. *Journal of Child Psychology and Psychiatry, and Allied Disciplines*, *43* (3), 307–325. Available from https://doi.org/10.1111/1469-7610.00023.

Zwaigenbaum, L., Thurm, A., Stone, W., Baranek, G., Bryson, S., Iverson, J., et al. (2007). Studying the emergence of autism spectrum disorders in high-risk infants: methodological and practical issues. *Journal of Autism and Developmental Disorders*, *37*, 466–480.

Autism and employment: challenges and strategies for a bright future

18

Tibor N. Farkas, Niko Kargas and John Mendy
University of Lincoln, Lincoln, United Kingdom

"Ever since Richard has left school, he has always wanted to do work and make sure his skills and talents will be recognized and valued by his future employers. First, he found it difficult to highlight his experience and aptitude when he completed job applications or when he needed to express himself well at job interviews, possibly due to some of his characteristics, associated with autism. Nonetheless, when he started volunteering at a local charity shop, he felt great pride, which only increased when he secured his first paid position as a customer assistant at a grocery store, especially since he did not access any additional support from governmental bodies or from other support services. All seemed well for a while until several complaints were made both by customers and Richard's colleagues, making remarks about his manner, communication style and behavior. Ultimately, it turned out that while Richard enjoyed the day-to-day tasks and the opportunity to better himself, in contrast with a customer-facing environment, he preferred to be outdoors in nature, where the dynamic with visitors was very different. Therefore, changing jobs had a particularly positive effect on Richard and it helped him find a more suitable career pathway".

Similar challenges, underlying or associated causes, and potential solutions, like the ones in Richard's case, can be easily and frequently found in our work with autistic young adults, preparing to enter the job market, and with jobseekers, employees, employers, and retirees with autism. Usually, these difficulties—whether they are happening during the application process or to do with the retention of a position—arise not from an extraordinary, inexplicable source but as a result of the interplay between several ordinary and typical factors. In Richard's story the work environment and the job itself limited how his skills, abilities, and personal characteristics could be demonstrated; in other words, they were unsuitable to match his strengths, interests, and needs. A report from The British Psychological Society reflects and adds to this fundamental aspect:

A successful interaction between the individual and their workplace needs to take into account needs linked to physical and social settings. (Weinberg & Doyle, 2017, p. 70)

Emerging Programs for Autism Spectrum Disorder. DOI: https://doi.org/10.1016/B978-0-323-85031-5.00015-3

> *... work is not a universally positive experience. Poorly designed jobs, work that is not organized well, difficult work environments, poorly trained managers and a lack of understanding of human behaviour in the workplace can create or exacerbate mental health conditions. For some people with physical or mental health conditions or disabilities, a lack of the right support at the right time from employers can make finding and keeping a meaningful job difficult. (Weinberg & Doyle, 2017, p. 3)*

The picture we often see in these employment narratives is that while the façade, the presentation of the difficulties might be, or might seem atypical, the root of the problem is anything but uncommon or exclusive. In fact, each story is truly unique, valuable, and greatly important not only to the person going through it, but also to their wider communities and to society as a whole as the conclusions of these lived experiences need to be integrated or even better to have a leading role in employment policy and employment service provision development.

This chapter offers a view into some of the difficulties faced by autistic people in the area of employment and aims to showcase three initiatives, which utilize a community-based participatory research (CBPR) approach to overcome these challenges and to provide a framework through these examples on how this strategy could be used to design and evaluate employment-focused interventions. In addition, the use of CBPR provides a unique and greatly valuable opportunity (1) to learn more about the everyday challenges of autistic jobseekers, employees, and employers; and (2) to actively involve them in offering effective, evidence-based advice and Human Resource Management (HRM) solutions to all stakeholders.

Autism and employment: where are we now?

Work has a central role in most people's lives, offering rewards beyond that of income. Employment provides not only a monetary recompense but also "latent" benefits—nonfinancial gains to the worker which include social identity and status; social contacts and support; a means of structuring and occupying time; activity and involvement; and a sense of personal achievement (Shepherd, 1989). The benefits of employment and/or regular work on people with autism spectrum conditions (ASC) can be immense, improving independence, well-being, reducing isolation promoting better mental health, as well as providing many employers with a loyal and productive employee.

While finding employment conveys a number of confirmed cognitive benefits and remunerative packages, lack of employment is associated with declining mental health, increased social exclusion, and poor quality of life in autistic people (e.g., Billstedt, Gillberg, & Gillberg, 2011). In fact, in the United States and the United Kingdom, only 10%–20% of adults with ASC are employed compared to 80%–95% of nondisabled people, and most often they only work part-time, despite established figures that approximately 50% of people with ASC have an IQ in the average to high range and do not have any additional physical needs (Griffiths, Giannantonio,

Hurley-Hanson, & Cardinal, 2016). Furthermore, studies conducted in the United Kingdom, United States, Canada, and Australia showed that the unemployment rates in ASC are considerably higher than those observed in other disability groups (Hedley et al., 2017).

Studies have also revealed it is more difficult for people with ASC than for non-autistic individuals to secure employment, whereas those who do enter the work-force find it hard to retain their positions, switch work often, have difficulties adjusting to work environments, and find it challenging to fit within traditional job descriptions and person specifications (e.g., Baldwin, Costley, & Warren, 2014; Hurlbutt & Chalmers, 2004). The unfolding autism prevalence in the UK and other developed countries has led to an increase in demand for employment support mechanisms (Hedley et al., 2018; Hendricks, 2010). Although both US and UK government legislation recommends the development of evidence-based needs-led services for people with ASC, there is limited research to guide employment service provision (Hedley et al., 2017; Summer & Brown, 2015). It is estimated that autism costs at least £32 billion per year and $236 billion per year in treatment, lost earnings, care, and support for autistic children and adults in the United Kingdom and the United States, respectively (Buescher, Cidav, Knapp, & Mandell, 2014). In parallel, unemployment rates for people with ASC remain high, while access to employment support services are of varying quality with little coordination between some key agencies.

The transition to adult life for people with autism is complex and fraught with difficulty. Recent research suggests that young adults with autism struggle to develop significant social relationships, to live independently, and to find and retain employment, which may result in the emergence of anxiety and/or depression (Graetz, 2010; Trembath, Germano, Johanson, & Dissanayake, 2012). These findings are of particular concern as there are unprecedented numbers in this cohort, leading to a need for more adult services, such as supported tenancies, employment support, dietary support, etc.

The unemployed consult their General Practitioners more often than the general population and those who have been unemployed for more than 12 weeks show 4–10 times the prevalence of depression and anxiety (Waddell & Burton, 2006). Unemployment is also associated with increased rates of suicide. It is estimated that one to four people experience mental health problems during the course of their lives and that the prevalence rate of a diagnosable mental health disorder is approximately three times higher in people with autism and/or Learning Disabilities than that of typically developing people (Hatton, Emerson, & Glover, 2016).

Challenges and difficulties in employment

Making effective job applications and dealing successfully with the day-to-day occurrences within the work environment requires a number of flexible skills. Social difficulties associated with autism may include the avoidance of eye contact and the use of atypical communicative measures, which could make both gaining and retaining employment more difficult, for example, by creating a communication barrier at a job interview (Gal, Landes, & Katz, 2015). Autistic people may also struggle with sensory sensitivity, such as oversensitivity to sound, which may involve a difficulty to block out or filter background noise, making conversations difficult. Some of these atypicalities associated with autism can be debilitating at interviews, which rely heavily on the individual's social capabilities. While informing employers prior to the interview about possible characteristics of autism is uncommon (similarly to disclosure) and potential solutions (notional, practical, or technical) to any difficulties may also be scarce at the workplace, alternatives to the interview process, for example, work trials, where skills and personal characteristics can be tested, are available to accommodate for the needs of autistic individuals (Barnham & Martin, 2017).

Moreover, autistic people may not be matched to a job based on their skill set (Lattimore, Parsons, & Reid, 2006). High-functioning autistic people often have specific skills they are exceptionally talented at. Happé (2018) suggested that superior skills are more common in autistic people yet they still have difficulties finding employment. Emphasizing the assets of autism and showcasing individual talents could help finding the right job for the right people, using a strength-based perspective (Lorenz, Frischling, Cuadros, & Heinitz, 2016). This may also aid employers by enabling them to recruit people with specialized skills (Simone, 2010). High-functioning autistic people, for example, tend to be interested and engage in STEM subjects (Science, Technology, Engineering, and Mathematics), although their numbers in STEM-related careers still need to increase drastically (Wei, Yu, Shattuck, McCracken, & Blackorby, 2013).

Furthermore, autistic individuals can find job retention difficult and leave jobs frequently (Hurlbutt & Chalmers, 2004). These observations may be explained by ineffective adjustments to work environments, which may also lack adequate support and extensive understanding (Baldwin et al., 2014; Milton, 2017). Ultimately, in order to ensure true, complete, and comprehensive societal inclusivity, both physical and conceptual environments will need to incorporate principles of universal design (Milton, Martin, & Melham, 2016). However, currently many employers do not understand the varied symptomatology of autism, leading to a further barrier to employment: the failure of employers to make reasonable adjustments in the workplace (López & Keenan, 2014).

To implement accommodations effectively, employers need to have a good understanding of both autism and of the autistic individual, who should benefit from these adaptations, therefore asking the autistic person about potential ways to help them work to the best of their ability can be the first and most important strategy to implement. Reasonable adjustments are a requirement following the Equality Act 2010 in the United Kingdom, yet workplaces often find it difficult to create appropriate, creative, and beneficial accommodations for autistic people. Thus efficient means to inform and implement reasonable adjustments and accommodations (if they are needed or if they may be beneficial) must be person-centered because every autistic individual is unique with different strengths, preferences, and difficulties

(Griffith, Totsika, Nash, & Hastings, 2012). This approach incorporates and promotes the general principles of the UK Government's Autism Act, and the Fulfilling and Rewarding Lives and the Think Autism strategies; however, more precise, detailed guidance within particular employment contexts could be useful both for the autistic community and for those supporting them.

For instance, little is known about how to support autistic individuals to gain and retain employment, even though the unemployment rate of autistic adults consistently demonstrates the need for increased support and awareness. Focusing attention on long-term assistance and informing organizations on helping autistic people in the workplace could contribute to improving job success (including both securing and retaining jobs) and enable continuous professional development and career formation (Harmuth et al., 2018).

CBPR: a way to connect autism and effective policy development?

It is argued that employment policies, practices, and interventions, which aim to support people with ASC, should take account of the many affected parties and actively involve them in the full process of design and development (e.g., Hedley et al., 2017). Reviewing the literature shows that at present, to a great extent this population does not have a meaningful active role in the process of conceptualization, design development, or implementation of policy interventions. To put it simply, they are left out of key research process stages as they are perceived to be a passive group, whose interests are best represented by nonautistic others.

> *Fortunately, there has been increasing recognition internationally that this situation needs to change, with autistic advocates, academics and activists being some of the strongest voices to speak to these issues. (Fletcher-Watson et al., 2019, p. 944)*

Therefore engaging the autistic community in the research processes to develop needs-led services and practices in a manner that is mutually beneficial and meaningful is of great importance (see also Jivraj, Sacrey, Newton, Nicholas, & Zwaigenbaum, 2014).

CBPR and its foundation, participatory design (PD) are inspired by phenomenological approaches, which acknowledge the importance of bottom-up decision-making, for example, to improve work conditions and adhere to the principles of emancipatory practices (Nicolaidis & Raymaker, 2015). It has been suggested that these methods can be promising in engaging autistic communities in the research process such as in the identification of barriers to access health services (Raymaker et al., 2017) and the associated mental and economic difficulties (Neri & Kroll, 2003), in the development of innovative technologies and in investigating the shortened life expectancy of people with ASC (Hirvikoski et al., 2016).

Previous research indicates CBPR can inform PD to help understand the views of marginalized stakeholders and low-resource communities, for example, about their experiences as they transition into work (Racadio, Rose, & Kolko, 2014). In fact, CBPR appears to be a useful strategy to engage autistic communities in a meaningful way as it requires the involvement of stakeholders in all aspects of the research process, from the exploratory stage to dissemination (Hedley et al., 2018). For instance, CBPR has already been used to investigate the healthcare experiences of autistic adults (e.g., Nicolaidis et al., 2015).

On the other hand, additional considerations should be made to benefit the development of CBPR and the ASC communities it serves. These include defining what/who constitutes to be the autistic community, where it is located (i.e., virtually or in situ) and how CBPR is actually implemented and communicated to autistic people, whose atypicalities often make it difficult to convey their position and opinions via culturally accepted (neurotypical) interpersonal means (e.g., Jivraj et al., 2014). Furthermore, there is limited guidance on how the implementation of CBPR research can be translated from healthcare settings into the context of employment and autism (Jivraj et al., 2014; Nicolaidis et al., 2015). To be specific, further insight must be gained about how autistic jobseekers' perspectives can be gathered; and in what way they can influence research design.

In the following sections we are describing three projects as individual but interconnected initiatives to actively involve the autistic community using a CBPR approach within the context of employment. These projects are already supporting people with ASC in their journeys to find, retain, or change employment, to continue their personal development and to advance in their careers.

Video-curriculum vitaes

Project background and design

It has already been shown that there may be better alternatives to the traditional textual curriculum vitae (CV), which may present individuals' skills, experience, and personability more effectively (Lee & Cavanaugh, 2016). Moreover, written CVs may not be appropriate or effective measures of employability for autistic people, for example, because they heavily rely on education and employment history. Some autistic individuals prefer to showcase their strengths and skills, instead of highlighting their qualifications or experience, which often means their job applications get rejected. In fact, most credible, professional sources, for example, National Institute for Health and Care Excellence (NICE) guidelines for people with ASC (2012), various policy documents and reports (e.g., "*The disability and health employment strategy: the discussion so far*"; "*Improving Lives—The Work, Health and Disability Green Paper*"; "*Psychology at work: Improving wellbeing and productivity in the workplace*"), and the Supported Employment Model—to only name a few—highlighted that employment-related initiatives and instruments aiming to support autistic people need to focus and be based on individual strengths. Without any alternatives being actively used, the written CV may be contributing to the autism employment gap.

An alternative to the written CV is the video-based CV (video-CV), which is a new assessment tool that could improve HRM policies that are currently being used in the framework of autism. Video-CVs contain a prerecorded message allowing applicants' personality and communication skills to be shown (Nguyen & Gatica-Perez, 2016). This aims to improve autistic people's employment success by providing information in an accessible way both for employers and for employees (Galdino & Gotway, 2005). Autistic individuals can speak about and demonstrate their strongest skills and interests; this is something that is difficult to communicate in a written CV compellingly because the skills are often not reinforced with evidence from prior work experience.

Our project evaluated a video-CV on its ability to provide information about employability skills, including potentially beneficial reasonable workplace adjustments, as well. The sample video-CV was provided by Generating Opportunity, a community interest company that specializes in producing video-CVs and developing creative solutions to find employment for people with additional support needs that matches their strengths, interests, and needs. Video-CVs were created in collaboration with autistic jobseekers with and without learning difficulties, the Autism Research Innovation Centre (ARIC) of the University of Lincoln, and funded by the National Lottery Community Fund and the European Regional Development Fund. The video-CV showed an autistic individual talking about and demonstrating his interests and skills, as well as jobs that he would enjoy doing. It covered sections such as employment, education, and topics which relate to the employability skills discussed earlier.

The video-CV's informativeness was evaluated using questions about how well the video-CV provided information about employability skills. These questions were chosen because of their connection to autism and they were based on some of the skills outlined in the Employability Skills Framework (Curtin, 2004), including teamwork, communication, self-management, enthusiasm and willingness to learn, and job-specific skills. Participants were also asked about potentially beneficial reasonable adjustments in the workplace.

Both teamwork and communication relate to the social difficulties associated with autism. Additionally, while oral comprehension and expression were ranked as particularly important in Deloitte's report (2017) demonstrating their dominance in employability, autistic people may communicate in unique ways or utilize atypical communication styles (American Psychiatric Association, 2013).

With regards to enthusiasm, Baldwin et al. (2014) suggested that many autistic people want to learn at and contribute to their workplace. However, Schriber, Robins, and Solomon (2014) found they tended to be less open to new experiences than control participants, suggesting that their enthusiasm may be reduced in novel environments such as the workplace.

Self-management skills were outlined in the United Kingdom Commission for Employment and Skills (2009) report, emphasizing the importance of these competences. Often autistic individuals are reliant on routine, but sometimes find planning and organization difficult (Gaus, 2011). However, autistic individuals are often more focused and display enhanced local processing performance, which may give productivity advantages in some workplaces, for example, in coding and computer programming (Grandin & Duffy, 2008; Happé & Frith, 2006).

Finally, job-specific skills may relate to the exceptional skills that some individuals with high-functioning autism exhibit. For example, some individuals show savant skills, for example, exceptional memory for small details, which could be greatly beneficial in relevant workplaces. In addition, the hypersensitivity frequently associated with ASC often results in superior attention to detail (Baron-Cohen, Ashwin, Ashwin, Tavassoli, & Chakrabarti, 2009) which is desirable in a number of job sectors, for example, design, finance, and retail.

Furthermore, learning job-specific skills whilst at work is important; various theories implicate experience in learning. Kolb's (2014) experiential learning theory explains why those with more experience are usually more advanced—every experience allows for improvement. For example, studies show that experienced entrepreneurs are more likely to be successful with their businesses than inexperienced entrepreneurs (e.g., Delmar & Shane, 2006). This may be the result of learning valuable lessons over time; they understand what works and what does not.

Findings and implications

Results and feedback from our participants (autistic and nonautistic, employers and university students) suggested that the video-CV was seen as accessible and effective in conveying key personality traits and employability skills. In other words, the video-CV enabled the portrayed person to speak about their interests and demonstrate their strengths and best qualities. Furthermore, the video-CV's overall ability to provide information on employability skills was positively connected to the observer's autism knowledge. More specifically, increased autism knowledge was linked to greater informativeness about enthusiasm and willingness to learn, job-specific skills, and reasonable adjustments, while employers' understanding of autism was also linked to greater information gain about self-management.

These results regarding knowledge can be explained by the notion of transfer of learning (Perkins & Salomon, 1992). Information learned can be applied to different contexts, suggesting why those with more knowledge of autism gained more information from the video-CV. Improving knowledge of autism could enable individuals to utilize their knowledge in various contexts, such as different workplaces and cultures (Leberman, McDonald, & Doyle, 2016). In addition, participants with more knowledge of autism are likely to have had more experience surrounding it, which may explain why they gained more information from the video-CV than participants who understood less about autism (Kolb, 2014).

In terms of applying the findings of this study, the video-CV was found to be accessible for employers and employees, both autistic and neurotypical. This was shown as employers gained considerable information about employability skills. For employers, understanding ways to progress and improve on employing autistic individuals could be an advancement in disability awareness with potential widespread benefits. For example, securing a job, which is meaningful to an autistic individual could increase their independence, as well as reduce the risk of mental health problems (Burke, Andersen, Bowen, Howard, & Allen, 2010). Using video-CVs as a new recruitment strategy could provide autistic people with more opportunities to apply for work and gain employment, which contributes to better quality of life. In addition, the use of video-CVs could facilitate efficient job matching within the context of supported employment.

Alongside direct benefits to autistic individuals, there are considerable benefits to employers when hiring autistics. For example, some autistic people have particular strengths and skillsets (Happé, 2018), meaning that if they are placed into the correct position, their work could be exceptional. Also, some autistic people may particularly enjoy the completion of unique or repetitive tasks due to their work and social preferences.

With reference to future employment strategies, these results have shown that knowledge of autism was a key factor in terms of retrieving information from the video-CV. This suggests that in order to successfully employ autistic people increased knowledge about the condition could be beneficial and may be necessary, highlighting the importance of relevant autism training programs and peer-support mechanisms (e.g., Farkas, Mendy, & Kargas, 2020). These programs may enable employers (and colleagues) to correctly assess an autistic individual's employability skills, to appreciate the value and importance of having autistic employees, to use a truly objective and fair recruitment framework to employ autistic people, and to provide effective and beneficial reasonable workplace adjustments, if they are needed. Furthermore, greater knowledge about autism could reduce stigma alongside increasing opportunities available to the autistic community.

The Autism Work Peer Support Group

Project background and design

Understanding that autistic jobseekers, employees, and employers may experience a number of employment-related difficulties and barriers, it is also clear that they need considerable inner strength and efficient adaptations (resilience) to develop positive strategies and attitudes to deal with- and overcome adversities. On the other hand, HRM policies and procedures rarely consider the concepts of resilience and resilience-building, especially within the context of autism. Thankfully, we also know that having a sense of belonging—for example, to family, communities, peer groups—plays a particularly significant role in promoting resilience amongst autistic adults (Lai & Szatmari, 2019).

Building on these findings, we codeveloped and established the Autism Work Peer Support Group (AWPSG) with the UK Department for Work and Pensions' Jobcenter Plus in Lincoln and in Grantham with the aim to "assist jobseekers in generating and sharing thoughts, opinions, and concerns, and making comments on intervention measures in a relaxed, comfortable setting, where the engagement of discussion partners (other autistic jobseekers and employees) could motivate others and help in expressing their views" (Farkas et al., 2020, p. 11).

In our initial meeting with the peer support group members (24 autistic jobseekers with various employment histories within diverse job sectors, 90% with secondary education up to A-levels and 10% with Higher National Diploma or above, and two disability employment advisors, familiar to the group members' employment and health related issues, who acted as the AWPSG facilitators) we agreed on the "peer support sessions' structure and format (e.g., accessible location, convenient times and frequency of meetings, group size, choice of facilitators, range of topics and activities, alternative format to participate in discussions) in order to ensure that these will be accessible and fit for purpose" (Farkas et al., 2020, p. 11). For some key agreements and accommodations we made with AWPSG members please see Table 18.1 (Farkas et al., 2020, p. 11).

The potential benefits of AWPSG as an intervention was evaluated 1 year after its conception by asking members to reflect on (1) measures introduced at the peer support sessions to "accommodate the needs of autistic jobseekers and to facilitate active participation" and on (2) any changes in members' "perspectives on employment, employability skills, self-esteem and social network, to reflect on overall quality of CBPR implementation and on the potential increase in member's resilience, respectively" (Farkas et al., 2020, p. 12).

Findings and implications

One of the key findings indicated that the implemented considerations regarding the AWPSG sessions' structure and format was successful at accommodating the members' needs and requirements, and members' active participation increased their self-esteem, social connections, employability skills, and conviction in securing and

Table 18.1 Examples of key decisions and joint solutions to showcase the creation of accessible Autism Work Peer Support Group sessions.

Key decisions	Joint solutions
Main type of peer support	In person group support
Additional, complementary peer support	Online peer support group (e.g., Digital Forum)
Location	Familiar environment (e.g., local Jobcenter Plus)
Frequency	Twice per month
Duration	90 minutes
Membership type	Closed membership (e.g., restricted to specific autistic jobseekers)
Facilitation and coordination	Organizational support (e.g., selected facilitators were knowledgeable about autism and familiar with the members' individual circumstances)
Focus of peer support	Employment-related issues and experiences

Note. Key agreements and accommodations. Adapted from Farkas et al., 2020.

retaining paid employment. "These findings combine to support the efficacy of the AWPSG program and provide a successful framework for delivering employment-focused peer support interventions to this population" (Farkas et al., 2020, p. 13). This indicates that interventions and support programs aiming to develop autistic people's educational (Hillier, Fish, Cloppert, & Beversdorf, 2007; McCurdy & Cole, 2014) and vocational characteristics should be complemented with social- and/or community-focused initiatives (Lai & Szatmari, 2019). For more information about members' views on the intervention measures implemented in the AWPSG sessions please see Table 18.2 (Farkas et al., 2020, p. 12)

> *"With regards to designing accessible AWPSG sessions, involving autistic members in its development was crucial in creating a relaxed and safe environment to foster the emergence of a subjectively meaningful community group. There, through a sense of connectedness, members could openly share experiences and learn from*

Table 18.2 Agreement of Autism Work Peer Support Group (AWPSG) members with the community-based participatory research (CBPR) implementation-quality items.

CBPR implementation-quality items	Agreement of AWPSG members			
	Strongly agree	Agree	Disagree	Strongly disagree
By taking part I was able to express my views and opinions.	70%	30%	0%	0%
Having regular meetings helped me feel comfortable and relaxed during discussions with the other members.	45%	50%	5%	0%
Having regular meetings helped me discuss difficult topics with the other members.	35%	65%	0%	0%
Having a facilitator from the Department for Work and Pensions at the meetings helped me discuss difficult topics with the other members.	50%	50%	0%	0%
I feel my opinions and views changed how other members thought about the discussed topics.	30%	60%	10%	0%
I feel other members' opinions and views changed how I think about the discussed topics.	30%	60%	10%	0%
It is good to have the option to express my opinions and views online through the Digital Forums instead of sharing them in person.	35%	50%	15%	0%

Note. Views on implemented accommodations. Adapted from Farkas et al., 2020.

one another about potential ways to overcome challenges, which they may encounter during the process of finding and keeping employment and which may be magnified by their autism profile (e.g., managing unpredictable changes in the work environment, forming effective work-relationships)." (Farkas et al., 2020, p. 14)

It was also of great importance that group members developed new social connections with each other, which continued outside the AWPSG, in some cases enabling the pursuit of entirely new employment opportunities. This also supports the suggestion that sense of belonging greatly and positively influences resilience-building capacities, for example, within inclusive educational settings, personalized environmental accommodation, and supported employment (Lai & Szatmari, 2019; Szatmari, 2018). For more information about members' views on their social network, self-esteem, employability skills, and employment please see Table 18.3 (Farkas et al., 2020, p. 13).

The Individualized Career Development Action Plan

Project background and design

Interventions such as Individual Placement and Support (IPS), which is a vocational rehabilitation programme designed in the USA to improve employment outcomes for people with severe mental health problems, have been shown to double the chances of individuals gaining competitive employment compared to traditional vocational rehabilitation. These interventions have been used in the UK, although such an approach requires more intensive support. The Improving Lives

Table 18.3 Agreement of Autism Work Peer Support Group (AWPSG) members with the resilience items.

Resilience items	Agreement of AWPSG Members			
	Strongly agree	**Agree**	**Disagree**	**Strongly disagree**
I have made friends with members.	10%	70%	20%	0%
Participation has increased my confidence in my skills.	35%	65%	0%	0%
Participation has made me feel better about myself.	45%	55%	0%	0%
Participation has made me feel more positive about employment.	45%	55%	0%	0%
Participation has made me more confident in finding employment.	25%	75%	0%	0%
Participation has made me more confident in retaining employment.	25%	60%	15%	0%

Note. Views on self. Adapted from Farkas et al., 2020.

> *Green Paper suggests extra provision, but concerns have been expressed about the adequacy of support available to claimants, including overload on Disability Employment Advisors and the limits on training of work coaches, as well as the toll of work pressures on the mental health of psychological support staff. (Weinberg & Doyle, 2017, p. 70)*

In addition, the British Psychological Society promotes the use of holistic, individualized, biopsychosocial approaches, for example, when assessing an individual's eligibility for benefits, such as for Employment and Support Allowance, however, these person-centered tools and strategies should also be implemented in employment support service provision and supported employment initiatives. On the other hand, as noted above, Individual Placement and Support (IPS) requires both extensive and intensive support from work coaches, disability employment advisors, support workers, and other support staff, who also require specialized and continuous training to be able to provide autistic people insightful, well-informed advice and help, and perform signposting to other available services effectively. Alternatively, professionals, supporting people with ASC in employment-related matters, need to have access to a centralized, automated system, which could help them make informed decisions more efficiently.

The aim of the Individualized Career Development Action Plan (ICDAP) project is to create an effective, easy-to-use, time- and cost-efficient supported employment tool that incorporates and builds on relevant guidelines and strategies. In order to develop such an instrument, which can serve as a framework for offering and coordinating supported employment services, it is indicated and emphasized by various professional bodies, policy documents, and academic research findings (e.g., Chen, Leader, Sung, & Leahy, 2014; Hedley et al., 2017, 2018) that supported employment services, programs and tools need to incorporate a focus on individual strengths, vital training in employability skills, efficient procedures and models to perform job matching to establish high-quality job opportunities, bespoke, person-centered support for current and potential future employees with ASC and their employers, clear guidance on creating effective reasonable adjustments, and multidisciplinary and multiagent collaboration.

The vision behind the ICDAP project embodies is to ensure everyone can realize their full potential in the world of employment and to increase well-being and quality of life, reduce social isolation, promote better mental health, and improve independence. Getting people with ASC with or without learning difficulties into employment can be complex and challenging. To do it successfully requires a holistic, person-centered approach, with key specialized employment services, employers, supporting organizations, and service provision agencies working together to provide a 360° supported employment strategy. In order to achieve this, through the close collaboration between Linkage Community Trust (LCT) and the University of Lincoln's ARIC, ICDAP, an online employment support tool was developed.

Embracing the ethos above and building on existing empirical research findings, ICDAP aims to achieve social and economic impact by guiding people with ASC in their journey to paid employment and beyond, providing the support they need to achieve higher levels of job security, highlighting their potential for career progress, and overall helping them live meaningful lives and reducing unemployment rates. Through involving and reflecting on the perspectives of all stakeholders in the design and evaluation process, ICDAP focuses on the three interconnected layers of supported employment. It recognizes and underlines clients' strengths, skills, and job preferences; it assists support services, work coaches, and disability advisors in matching the right jobs for the right people; and it helps employers make effective reasonable workplace adjustments.

Specifically, ICDAP is a job matching and career development tool that assesses and reflects the strengths, aspirations, interests, preferences, skills, needs, and difficulties (individual characteristics) of people with ASC; it enables those supporting people with ASC to match clients' individual characteristics, educational background, work history, and experience (employment profile) to particular employment opportunities more effectively; it identifies opportunities for person-centered training and for skill and experience building to bridge potential gaps in employment profiles; it provides informed recommendations to employers, thereby enabling them to create reasonable adjustments, optimal conditions, and work environments for clients' with ASC/LD; and it establishes potential career pathway(s) for clients, based on their employment profiles.

> *Ultimately, ICDAP guides clients to achieve greater independence and enables the fade-out of direct support systematically and strategically, when it is no longer needed*

Findings and implications

The ICDAP system and its elements were introduced to autistic people, to LCT staff members, and to key partners—private, public, and third sector organizations, and local community groups. Feedback collected from the stakeholders showed they all praised ICDAP for its accessibility, usability, efficiency, and flexibility. They found the design, content, and structure of this online tool valuable and effective, while establishing individual career pathways with ICDAP was found to be both enjoyable for our clients and time-efficient for the work coaches. More specifically, a focus group was established, consisting of people with ASC and their support staff, who actively participated in piloting the ICDAP system and in informing the tool's development by making significant contributions to ensure the system is valid, user-friendly, and thorough.

> *All feedback received from stakeholders were overwhelmingly positive about the format and contents of the ICDAP system's elements.*

Three strands, one common goal: bringing it all together

While each of these initiatives convey their individual conclusions on the different ways they aimed to support autistic people within the context of employment, by showcasing these projects our ambition was to demonstrate particular means to implement CBPR to promote the employability of people with ASC and to develop effective HRM procedures and policies together, with the inclusion of all stakeholders.

We would also like to highlight the importance of understanding autism, and what the condition entails, to be able to fairly and successfully recruit autistic individuals. There are government policies that are aiming to broaden the nonautistic population's knowledge of the condition, but these need to be expanded on to support autistic people in finding and securing the jobs they are interested in and developing their careers.

With more research, empirical evidence, and allocated resources, alternative strategies such as the use of video-CVs, the creation of work-focused peer support groups and networks, and the application of online systems, such as ICDAP, could become more prevalent and work toward offering truly equal employment opportunities for autistic individuals.

References

American Psychiatric Association. (2013). Diagnostic and statistical manual of mental disorders (5th ed.). American Psychiatric Association.

Baldwin, S., Costley, D., & Warren, A. (2014). Employment activities and experiences of adults with high-functioning autism and Asperger's disorder. *Journal of Autism and Developmental Disorders*, *44*, 2440–2449.

Barnham, C., & Martin, N. (2017). Considering employment of young people with intellectual impairments and autism leaving school and college. *Autism and Intellectual Disability*, *2*, 51–53.

Baron-Cohen, S., Ashwin, E., Ashwin, C., Tavassoli, T., & Chakrabarti, B. (2009). Talent in autism: Hyper-systemizing, hyper-attention to detail and sensory hypersensitivity. *Philosophical Transactions of the Royal Society B: Biological Sciences*, *364*, 1377–1383.

Billstedt, E., Gillberg, I. C., & Gillberg, C. (2011). Aspects of quality of life in adults diagnosed with autism in childhood: A population-based study. *Autism: the International Journal of Research and Practice*, *15*, 7–20.

Buescher, A. V., Cidav, Z., Knapp, M., & Mandell, D. S. (2014). The cost of autism spectrum disorders in the United Kingdom and the United States of America. *Journal of the American Medical Association of Pediatrics*, *168*, 721–728.

Burke, R. V., Andersen, M. N., Bowen, S. L., Howard, M. R., & Allen, K. D. (2010). Evaluation of two instruction methods to increase employment options for young adults with autism spectrum disorders. *Research in Developmental Disabilities*, *31*, 1223–1233.

Chen, J. L., Leader, G., Sung, C., & Leahy, M. (2014). Trends in employment for individuals with autism spectrum disorder: A review of the research literature. *Review Journal of Autism and Developmental Disorders*, *2*, 115–127.

Curtin, P. (2004). Employability skills for the future. In J. Gibb (Ed.), *Generic Skills in Vocational Education and Training: Research readings* (pp. 38–52). National Centre for Vocational Education Research.

Delmar, F., & Shane, S. (2006). Does experience matter? The effect of founding team experience on the survival and sales of newly founded ventures. *Strategic Organization*, *4*, 215–247.

Deloitte. (2017). Power Up, The UK Workplace. <https://www2.deloitte.com/content/dam/Deloitte/uk/Documents/international-markets/deloitte-uk-power-up.pdf>.

Farkas, T. N., Mendy, J., & Kargas, N. (2020). Enhancing resilience in autistic adults using community-based participatory research: A novel HRD-intervention in employment service provision. *Advances in Developing Human Resources*, *22*(4), 370–386.

Fletcher-Watson, S., Adams, J., Brook, K., Charman, T., Crane, L., Cusack, J., ... Pellicano, E. (2019). Making the future together: Shaping autism research through meaningful participation. *Autism: the International Journal of Research and Practice*, *23*, 943–953.

Gal, E., Landes, E., & Katz, N. (2015). Work performance skills in adults with and without high functioning autism spectrum disorders (HFASD). *Research in Autism Spectrum Disorders*, *10*, 71–77.

Galdino, G. M., & Gotway, M. (2005). The digital curriculum vitae. *Journal of the American College of Radiology*, *2*, 183–188.

Gaus, V. L. (2011). Cognitive behavioural therapy for adults with autism spectrum disorder. *Advances in Mental Health and Intellectual Disabilities*, *5*, 15–25.

Graetz, J. E. (2010). Autism grows up: Opportunities for adults with autism. *Disability & Society*, *25*, 33–47.

Grandin, T., & Duffy, K. (2008). *Developing talents: Careers for individuals with Asperger syndrome and high-functioning autism*. Autism Asperger Publishing Co.

Griffith, G. M., Totsika, V., Nash, S., & Hastings, R. P. (2012). 'I just don't fit anywhere': Support experiences and future support needs of individuals with Asperger syndrome in middle adulthood. *Autism: the International Journal of Research and Practice*, *16*, 532–546.

Griffiths, A., Giannantonio, C., Hurley-Hanson, A., & Cardinal, D. N. (2016). Autism in the workplace: Assessing the transition needs of young adults with autism spectrum disorder. *Journal of Business and Management*, *22*, 5–22.

Happé, F. (2018). Why are savant skills and special talents associated with autism? *World Psychiatry: Official Journal of the World Psychiatric Association (WPA)*, *17*, 280–281.

Happé, F., & Frith, U. (2006). The weak coherence account: Detail-focused cognitive style in autism spectrum disorders. *Journal of Autism and Developmental Disorders*, *36*, 5–25.

Harmuth, E., Silletta, E., Bailey, A., Adams, T., Beck, C., & Barbic, S. P. (2018). Barriers and facilitators to employment for adults with autism: A scoping review. *Annals of International Occupational Therapy*, *1*, 31–40.

Hatton, C., Emerson, E., & Glover, G. (2016). *People with learning disabilities in England 2015*. Public Health England. Available from https://www.gov.uk/government/uploads/system/uploads/attachment_data/file/613182/PWLDIE_2015_main_report_NB090517.pdf.

Hedley, D., Cai, R., Uljarević, M., Wilmot, M., Spoor, J. R., Richdale, A., & Dissanayake, C. (2018). Transition to work: Perspectives from the autism spectrum. *Autism: The International Journal of Research and Practice*, *22*, 528541.

Hedley, D., Uljarević, M., Cameron, L., Halder, S., Richdale, A., & Dissanayake, C. (2017). Employment programmes and interventions targeting adults with autism spectrum disorder: A systematic review of the literature. *Autism: The International Journal of Research and Practice*, *21*, 929–941.

Hendricks, D. (2010). Employment and adults with autism spectrum disorders: Challenges and strategies for success. *Journal of Vocational Rehabilitation*, *32*, 125–134.

Hillier, A., Fish, T., Cloppert, P., & Beversdorf, Q. D. (2007). Outcomes of a social and vocational skills support group for adolescents and young adults on the autism spectrum. Focus on Autism and Other Developmental. *Disabilities*, *22*(2), 107–115.

Hirvikoski, T., Mittendorfer-Rutz, E., Boman, M., Larsson, H., Lichtenstein, P., & Bölte, S. (2016). Premature mortality in autism spectrum disorder. *The British Journal of Psychiatry, 208*, 232–238.

Hurlbutt, K., & Chalmers, L. (2004). Employment in adults with Asperger syndrome. *Focus on Autism and Other Developmental Disabilities, 19*, 215–222.

Jivraj, J., Sacrey, L. A., Newton, A., Nicholas, D., & Zwaigenbaum, L. (2014). Assessing the influence of researcher-partner involvement on the process and outcomes of participatory research in autism spectrum disorder and neurodevelopmental disorders: A scoping review. *Autism: The International Journal of Research and Practice, 18*, 782–793.

Kolb, D. (2014). *Experiential learning: Experience as the source of learning and development*. Pearson Education.

Lai, M.-C., & Szatmari, P. (2019). Resilience in autism: Research and practice prospects. *Autism: The International Journal of Research and Practice, 23*, 539–541.

Lattimore, L. P., Parsons, M. B., & Reid, D. H. (2006). Enhancing job-site training of supported workers with autism: A reemphasis on simulation. *Journal of Applied Behavior Analysis, 39*, 91–102.

Leberman, S., McDonald, L., & Doyle, S. (2016). *The transfer of learning: Participants' perspectives of adult education and training*. Routledge.

Lee, J. W., & Cavanaugh, T. (2016). Self-branding reflection through the use of infographic résumés. *Sport Management Education Journal, 10*, 78–85.

López, B., & Keenan, L. (2014). *Barriers to employment in autism: Future challenges to implementing the adult autism strategy*. Autism Research Network. Available from http://www.autismrpphub.org/sites/default/files/articles/employment_report.pdf>.

Lorenz, T., Frischling, C., Cuadros, R., & Heinitz, K. (2016). Autism and overcoming job barriers: Comparing job-related barriers and possible solutions in and outside of autism-specific employment. *PLoS One, 11*, e0147040.

McCurdy, E. E., & Cole, C. L. (2014). Use of a peer support intervention for promoting academic engagement of students with autism in general education settings. *Journal of Autism and Developmental Disorders, 44*, 883–893.

Milton, D. (2017). Employment: A reflective review. In D. Milton, & N. Martin (Eds.), *Autism and intellectual disabilities in adults* (Vol. 2). Pavilion Press.

Milton, D., Martin, N., & Melham, P. (2016). Beyond reasonable adjustment: Autistic-friendly spaces and universal design. In D. Milton, & N. Martin (Eds.), *Autism and intellectual disabilities in adults* (Vol. 1, pp. 81–86). Pavilion Press.

National Institute for Health and Care Excellence (NICE). (2012). *Autism spectrum disorder in adults: Diagnosis and management (Clinical guideline [CG142])*. Retrieved from <https://www.nice.org.uk/guidance/cg142>.

Neri, M. T., & Kroll, T. (2003). Understanding the consequences of access barriers to health care: experiences of adults with disabilities. *Disability and Rehabilitation, 25*, 85–96.

Nguyen, L. S., & Gatica-Perez, D. (2016). Hirability in the wild: Analysis of online conversational video resumes. *IEEE Transactions on Multimedia, 18*, 1422–1437.

Nicolaidis, C., & Raymaker, D. M. (2015). Community based participatory research with communities defined by race, ethnicity, and disability: Translating theory to practice. In H. Bradbury (Ed.), *The SAGE handbook of action research* (pp. 167–179). SAGE.

Nicolaidis, C., Raymaker, D. M., Ashkenazy, E., McDonald, K. E., Dern, S., Baggs, A. E. V., & Boisclair, W. C. (2015). "Respect the way I need to communicate with you": Healthcare experiences of adults on the autism spectrum. *Autism: The International Journal of Research and Practice, 19*, 824–831.

Perkins, D. N., & Salomon, G. (1992). *Transfer of learning*. Pergamon Press.

Racadio, R., Rose, E. J., & Kolko, B. E. (2014). Research at the margin: Participatory design and community based participatory research. In *ACM International Conference Proceeding Series*, 2, (pp. 49–52).

Raymaker, D. M., McDonald, K. E., Ashkenazy, E., Gerrity, M., Baggs, A. M., Kripke, C., & Nicolaidis, C. (2017). Barriers to healthcare: Instrument development and comparison between autistic adults and adults with and without other disabilities. *Autism: The International Journal of Research and Practice*, *21*, 972–984.

Schriber, R. A., Robins, R. W., & Solomon, M. (2014). Personality and self-insight in individuals with autism spectrum disorder. *Journal of Personality and Social Psychology*, *106*, 112–130.

Shepherd, G. (1989). The value of work in the 1980s. *Psychiatric Bulletin*, *13*, 231–233.

Simone, R. (2010). *Asperger's on the job: Must-have advice for people with Asperger's or high functioning autism, and their employers, educators, and advocates*. Future Horizons.

Summer, K. E., & Brown, T. J. (2015). Neurodiversity and human resource management: Employer challenges for applicants and employees with learning disabilities. *The Psychologist-Manager Journal*, *18*, 77–85.

Szatmari, P. (2018). Risk and resilience in autism spectrum disorder: A missed translational opportunity? *Developmental Medicine & Child Neurology*, *60*, 225–229.

Trembath, D., Germano, C., Johanson, G., & Dissanayake, C. (2012). The experience of anxiety in young adults with autism spectrum disorders. *Focus on Autism and Other Developmental Disabilities*, *27*, 213–224.

United Kingdom Commission for Employment and Skills. (2009). *The employability challenge*. <http://www.ukces.org.uk/tags/employability-challenge-full-report>.

Waddell, G., & Burton, A. K. (2006). *Is work good for your health and well-being?* The Stationery Office.

Wei, X., Yu, J. W., Shattuck, P., McCracken, M., & Blackorby, J. (2013). Science, technology, engineering, and mathematics (STEM) participation among college students with an autism spectrum disorder. *Journal of Autism and Developmental Disorders*, *43*, 1539–1546.

Weinberg, A., & Doyle, N. (2017). *Psychology at work: Improving wellbeing and productivity in the workplace*. The British Psychological Society. <https://www.bps.org.uk/sites/www.bps.org.uk/files/Policy/Policy%20-%20Files/Psychology%20at%20work%20-%20improving%20wellbeing%20and%20productivity%20in%20the%20workplace.pdf>.

Psychopharmacology of autism spectrum disorders and other related comorbidities

19

Eric C. Alcera[1,2], *Michelle Jaehning*[3] *and Ramon Solhkhah*[1,4]
[1]Department of Psychiatry and Behavioral Health, Hackensack Meridian School of Medicine, Nutley, NJ, United States, [2]Department of Psychiatry, Riverview Medical Center, Red Bank, NJ, United States, [3]Department of Psychiatry, Jersey Shore University Medical Center (affiliated with Hackensack Meridian School of Medicine), Neptune, NJ, United States, [4]Department of Psychiatry, Jersey Shore University Medical Center, Neptune, NJ, United States

Introduction

General overview

Autism spectrum disorder (ASD) is a neurodevelopmental disorder characterized by three core groups of symptoms: deficits in social interaction; impairments in communication; and repetitive and stereotyped patterns of behavior, interests, or activities ASHA (2020). People diagnosed with autism often have difficulties with social interactions, which can include an inability to maintain eye contact, not responding to their name when called upon or spoken to, difficulty dealing with complex or challenging social situations, an inability to share objects, the expression of inappropriate emotions at the wrong time and place, and a preference for solitary activities (Research Autism, 2020). Impaired communication in people with ASD can include delayed development of spoken language, a failure to initiate and/or sustain conversations, and abnormalities in the pitch, stress, rate, and tone of speech (Bonneh, Levanon, Dean-Pardo, Lossos, & Adini, 2010). Restricted and repetitive behaviors and interests can manifest as repetitive movement with objects, repeated body movements such as rocking and hand-flapping, and ritualistic behaviors (Sarker et al., 2018).

Various treatments are available to address these symptoms and associated comorbidities. They can be categorized as either nonmedication treatment strategies or medication treatments (Siegel and Erickson, 2016a).

Primary nonmedication treatment includes Applied Behavioral Analysis (ABA), Communication Supports, Cognitive Behavioral Therapy (CBT), Social Skills/ Social Cognitive Training, Life Skills, and Sensory Interventions (Siegel and Erickson, 2016a). This chapter will focus primarily on medication as a treatment.

Emerging Programs for Autism Spectrum Disorder. DOI: https://doi.org/10.1016/B978-0-323-85031-5.00021-9

Epidemiology/incidence/prevalence

Until 2013 Pervasive Developmental Disorders (PDDs) were split into subcategories of autistic disorder, Asperger's syndrome, childhood disintegrative disorder (CDD), and pervasive developmental disorder not otherwise specified (PDD-NOS) (King, Navot, Bernier, & Webb, 2014). In 2013 the American Psychiatric Association (APA) reclassified these disorders under a single umbrella as ASD. ASD is considered a "spectrum" disorder since there is a wide variety of symptoms and symptom severity that people may experience (NIMH, 2020).

The prevalence of ASD has been examined carefully over time, even as its categories and definitions have changed. By most reports, the prevalence in the United States has been rising. According to Baio et al. (2018), about 1 in 59 children in the United States have been identified with ASD by age 8 and this diagnosis has been reported in all racial, ethnic, and socioeconomic groups (Baio et al., 2018). The Centers for Disease Control and Prevention (CDC) released a biennial update of the estimated prevalence of ASD amongst the nation's children (Autism Speak, 2020). This new estimate had reported a 15% increase in prevalence nationally, from 1 in 68 by age 8 in 2012 to 1 in 59 children by age 8 in 2014 (Autism Speak, 2020). Two independent studies published in *Pediatrics* and *JAMA Pediatrics* estimate that 1 in 40 children between the ages of 3 and 17 has ASD, which is higher than the rate reported by the CDC in 2014 (OAR, 2019).

Thomas Frazier, chief science officer for *Autism Speaks*, suggested that the difference in estimates may be due to how the studies have been performed and notes that the "one in 40 is closer to what we see with direct prevalence studies where researchers go into a community to directly screen for autism" (OAR, 2019).

While ASD has been reported across all populations in the United States, there are demographic differences observed. ASD is three to four times more prevalent in boys than girls in the United States, according to a systematic review of 54 studies including >13,700,000 patients, with the overall male-to-female ratio of 4.2 (Essa, 2020). Severity of autism is higher in females than males, however, the prevalence of autism in boys is 3–4-fold greater than girls (Karimi, Kamali, Mousavi, & Karahmadi, 2017; Kinney, Munir, Crowley, & Miller, 2008; Werling and Geschwind, 2013). Palmer et al. (2017) found that, in the United States, younger male siblings of a child diagnosed with ADS are more often affected than younger female siblings: younger brothers of girls with ASD—17%; younger brothers of boys with ASD—13%; younger sisters of girls with ASD—8%; younger sisters of boys with ASD—4% (Palmer et al., 2017).

Global estimates of ASD prevalence tend to show a lower prevalence. In a systematic review of epidemiologic studies in 2010, the estimated global prevalence of ASD was 1 in 132 children, however, the prevalence of ASD in developing countries is less well described (Brasic and Morgan, 2019).

Overall, based on epidemiological studies conducted over the past 50 years, the prevalence of ASD appears to be steadily increasing on a global scale (Brasic and Morgan, 2019). There have been many explanations for this, including improved awareness of the disorder, better diagnostic tools, changes in diagnostic criteria that make the diagnosis easier, and improved reporting (Rice et al., 2015).

Genetic and environmental factors

Genetics plays a major role in the risk of developing autism spectrum disorder. The first autism twin study in 1977 reported that autism is highly heritable, stating that when one identical twin has autism, there is about an 80% chance that the other twin will develop the disorder as well (Folstein and Rutter, 1977). The corresponding rate for fraternal twins is around 40% (Folstein and Rutter, 1977). Researchers have found about 65 genes that they considered strongly linked to autism and more than 200 others that have weaker ties to autism (Zeliadt, 2017). Interestingly, there are several conditions associated with autism stemming from mutations in a single gene, including Fragile X and Rett syndromes (Avdjieva-Tzavella et al., 2012).

While there is a strong genetic component to a predisposition of autism, numerous studies have sought to determine the potential involvement of toxins in our environment that could play a role in the risk for developing ASD.

According to Karimi et al. (2017), both genetic and environmental factors have been involved in the pathogenesis of autism. Although no single environmental factor has been found that can individually cause autism, a collection of environmental factors may contribute together to increase the incidence of autism. These environmental risk factors have been divided into prenatal (Table 19.1), natal (Table 19.2), and postnatal risk factors (Table 19.3) (Karimi et al., 2017).

Based on genetic and environmental factors investigated by Karimi et al. (2017), a large number of risk factors have been identified that suggest both environmental and genetic contributions to the development of ASD and neurodevelopmental disorders:

- Advanced paternal age has a significant role in the occurrence of autism in the neonate and it is thus suggested that the best time to have a child (especially for the father) is under the age of 35 (Durkin et al., 2008; Karimi et al., 2017; Lee and McGrath, 2015).
- Families with more than one autistic child have an increased risk of having an affected infant, with a twofold increase in risk when there is more than one older affected sibling (Constantino, Zhang, Frazier, Abbacchi, & Law, 2010; Karimi et al., 2017; Ozonoff et al., 2011).
- Familial psychiatric history is much more common among families with autistic children (Bölte, Knecht, & Poustka, 2007; Karimi et al., 2017; Larsson et al., 2005).
- Occupational and mental stresses during pregnancy have been linked to the development of autism (Gudsnuk and Champagne, 2012; Karimi et al., 2017; Perera and Herbstman, 2011).
- Exposure during pregnancy to chemicals such as pesticides, air and water pollutants, and heavy metals can negatively affect fetal health through epigenetic alterations of gene expression and alter the neurodevelopmental process, which may increase the risk of ASD (Karimi et al., 2017; Pavanello et al., 2009; Shelton et al., 2014).
- Absence of mother–baby bonding during the postnatal period can have a negative impact on the postnatal development of neural and signaling pathways along with affecting hormone secretion such as dopamine, oxytocin, and serotonin, which may pose a risk for exacerbation of neurodevelopmental disorders (Curley, Jensen, Mashoodh, & Champagne, 2011; Gudsnuk and Champagne, 2012; Karimi et al., 2017).

Table 19.1 Prenatal risk factors (Karimi et al., 2017).

Risk factors	**Positive and negative association with autism**
Parental age	Positive
	Negative
Parental age	Positive
	Negative
Maternal age	Positive
	Negative
Birth order	Positive
	Negative
Maternal physical diseases	
Preeclampsia	Positive
	Negative
Maternal gestational diabetes	Positive
	Negative
Hypertension/edema	Positive
	Negative
Nausea/vomiting	Positive
Other maternal diseases including psoriasis, asthma, hay fever, atopic dermatitis, rheumatoid arthritis, celiac disease, and mastocytosis	Positive
Maternal bleeding during pregnancy	Positive
Infections during pregnancy	Positive
Bacterial infection	Positive
Viral infection	Positive
Influenza	
Rubella	
Cytomegalovirus	
Measles	
Mumps	
Chicken pox	
Herpes virus	
Pneumonia	
Syphilis	
Varicella zoster	
Maternal mental diseases	
Schizophrenia	Positive
Depression	Positive
Anxiety and stress	Positive
	Negative
Personality disorders	Positive
Infant gender	Positive
Existence of >1 affected sibling	Positive
Maternal prenatal medication use	Positive
	Negative
Psychotropic drugs	Positive
Antidepressant drugs	Positive

(Continued)

Table 19.1 (Continued)

Risk factors	Positive and negative association with autism
Beta 2 adrenergic agonist drugs	Positive
Paracetamol (acetaminophen)	Positive
Antipyretics	Positive
Thalidomide	Positive
Misoprostol	Positive
Exposure to certain chemicals heavy metals	Positive
Pesticides	Positive
Air pollutants	Positive
P-CB[a]	Positive
PBDE[b]	Positive
PAH[c]	Positive
Familial socioeconomic status	
Economic situation	Positive Negative
Social status	Positive
Educational level	Positive
Mother born abroad	Positive Negative
Cigarettes or alcohol addiction of one parent	Positive Negative
Maternal iron, folate, and methionine deficiency	Positive
Maternal vitamin deficiency	Positive
Weight gain during pregnancy	Positive
Threatened abortion	Positive

[a]Polychlorinated biphenyls.
[b]Polybrominated diphenyl ether.
[c]Polycyclic aromatic hydrocarbons.

- Maternal smoking and alcohol consumption can have adverse health effects that may cause fetal hypoxia and fetal brain development leading to increased susceptibility to ASD (Karimi et al., 2017; Wright, 2009; Xiao, Sorensen, Williams, & Luthy, 2003).
- An appropriate diet during pregnancy is important with regards to receiving appropriate amounts of unsaturated fatty acids, folic acid, iron, methionine, and vitamins. A deficiency or improper balance can lead to abnormal development of the embryo (Fernell et al., 2010; Haggarty, 2004; Roza et al., 2010).
- Obesity during pregnancy (>90 kg) and excessive weight gain during pregnancy have been linked to the incidence of autism (Karimi et al., 2017; Krakowiak et al., 2012; Xiao et al., 2003).
- Prolonged exposure to elevated temperature during pregnancy increases susceptibility to child autism (Gardener, Spiegelman, & Buka, 2011).

All of these, however, require further investigation, as many of them may be associated with other, unknown factors, or effects may be cumulative.

Table 19.2 Natal risk factors (Karimi et al., 2017).

Risk factors	Positive and negative association with autism
Abnormal presentation	
Preterm birth	Positive
Postterm birth	Positive
	Negative
Cesarean delivery	Positive
Fetal complications	Positive
Hypoxia (lack of oxygen)	Negative
	Positive
	Negative
Congenital anomalies	Positive
Fetal respiratory distress	Positive
Natal ulcers and bleeding	Positive
Umbilical cord complication	Positive
Maternal complications	
Maternal bleeding after childbirth	Positive
Venous thrombosis	Positive
Assisted conception (IVF)	Positive
Season of birth	
Winter	Positive
Summer	Positive

IVF, In vitro fertilization.

The study of epigenetics has helped us understand interactions between genetics and the environment in the predisposition to autism. Epigenetic alterations via methylation of genes such as MECP2 and EGR2 have been shown to play a role in the development of autism (LaSalle and Yasui, 2009; Swanberg, Nagarajan, Peddada, Yasui, & LaSalle, 2009). Especially during pregnancy, the fetus is undergoing vast neurocognitive development and exposure to harmful environmental contaminants, pesticides, or air pollution may trigger a genetic mutation or epigenetic alteration that could increase susceptibility to autism (Levy, 2015).

The question is whether these factors increase the risk overall or increase the risk for those who are genetically predisposed to this disorder (Chaste and Leboyer, 2012). The National Institute of Environmental Health Sciences (NIEHS) are funding researchers to investigate the epigenetics behind the development of autism (NIEHS, 2020). Researchers are looking into early-life exposure to air pollution, prenatal conditions, maternal factors such as problems with the mother's immune system or certain metabolic conditions or inflammation during pregnancy, prenatal exposure to contaminants (such as metals and pesticides), and perinatal nutrition (taking vitamins and supplements that may provide protective effects for fetuses that may be exposed to certain environmental contaminants during pregnancy) (NIEHS, 2020).

Table 19.3 Postnatal risk factors (Karimi et al., 2017).

Risk factors	**Positive and negative association with autism**
Postnatal complications	
Low birth weight and size	Positive
	Negative
Jaundice and hyperbilirubinemia	Positive
	Negative
Encephalopathy	Positive
Birth defects	Positive
	Negative
Early infant infections	Positive
	Negative
Meningitis	Positive
Lack of breathing and infant resuscitation	Positive
	Negative
Postnatal anemia	Positive
	Negative
Weak or no crying after birth	Positive
	Negative
Postnatal vitamin D deficiency	Positive
Feeding difficulties	Positive
Medication intervention	Positive
Low levels of primary maternal care	Positive
Postnatal chemical exposure to trihalomethanes, tetrachloroethylene, and trichloroethylene	Positive

History

The word "autism" was coined by Eugen Bleuler, a Swiss psychiatrist, in 1911, to describe a group of symptoms related to schizophrenia (Evans, 2013). Derived from the Greek word *autos*, meaning "self," it was used to describe extreme social withdrawal common with psychiatric disorders that presented with psychosis (MSEPG, 2020). During this period, ASDs were not distinguished from psychotic disorders. In the 1920s, electroconvulsive therapy (ECT) was first used to treat the symptoms of "autism" and dietary restrictions were implemented to treat the disorder. ECT had been used to treat psychiatric illnesses such as schizophrenia and bipolar disorder, and was thus thought to be of benefit to patients with autism (Applied Behavioral Analysisi Program Guide ABAPG, 2020). During this time, another school of thought was that autism may be caused by toxic dietary factors and thus this disorder could be treated through dietary changes such as through a gluten-free and casein-free diet (Applied Behavioral Analysisi Program Guide ABAPG, 2020). In 1943 Dr. Leo Kanner, an Austrian-American child psychiatrist working in the United States, was the first to characterize autism as a social and emotional disorder in children, in a published paper in the journal *Nervous Child* titled "Autistic Disturbances of Affective Contact" (Applied Behavioral Analysisi Program Guide ABAPG, 2020).

At the time, there was debate about the etiology of the disorder, and some thought that parents were the root cause of the disease. Bruno Bettelheim popularized the term Refrigerator Mother, arguing that children got autism from mothers who were especially cold toward them (Cohmer, 2014). The treatment at that time was to forcibly remove the child from their parents for long periods of time, known as parentectomy. The "refrigerator mother" concept was hotly debated at the time and subsequently overthrown with research that showed the neurodevelopmental basis for ASD and no evidence of a direct contribution from maternal or paternal affection (Cohmer, 2014).

In 1980 the American Psychiatric Association published DSM-III and established autism as its own separate diagnosis, describing it as a pervasive developmental disorder distinct from schizophrenia, with three essential features: "a lack of interest in people, severe impairments in communication, and bizarre responses to the environment, all developing in the first 30 months of life" (Volkmar and Reichow, 2013). DSM-III was revised in 1987 and broadened the concept of autism by adding diagnoses at the more mild end of the spectrum, pervasive developmental disorder—not otherwise specified (PDD-NOS), and no longer requiring the onset of symptoms before 30 months (Volkmar and Reichow, 2013). DSM-IV was released in 1994 and revised in 2000 and was the first edition to categorize autism as a spectrum disorder to include not only autism and PDD-NOS, but also Asperger's disorder (also at the mild end of the spectrum), CDD, and Rett syndrome Volkmar and Reichow (2013).

Throughout the years, it became clear that it would be impossible to find the genetic underpinnings and treatments for each of the five conditions specified in DSM-IV and little reliability and validity in these distinctions, so the DSM committees decided to group these conditions as ASDs, in a spectrum ranging from mild to severe in DSM-V, published in 2013 (Zeldovich, 2018).

Diagnostic criteria

The DSM-V criteria for Autism Spectrum Disorder (ASD) are listed below (American Psychiatric Association, 2013):

"The American Psychiatric Association's Diagnostic and Statistical Manual of Mental Disorders is the main diagnostic reference used by mental health professionals and insurance providers in the United States. The current (fifth) edition, which was published in 2013, is commonly referred to as the "DSM-V."
The Medical/Psychiatric Diagnosis of Autism: The DSM-V Criteria
A. Persistent deficits in social communication and social interaction across multiple contexts, as manifested by the following, currently or by history (examples are illustrative, not exhaustive, see text):
1. Deficits in social-emotional reciprocity, ranging, for example, from abnormal social approach and failure of normal back-and-forth conversation; to reduced sharing of interests, emotions, or affect; to failure to initiate or respond to social interactions.
2. Deficits in nonverbal communicative behaviors used for social interaction, ranging, for example, from poorly integrated verbal and nonverbal communication; to abnormalities in eye contact and body language or deficits in understanding and use of gestures; to a total lack of facial expressions and nonverbal communication.
3. Deficits in developing, maintaining, and understanding relationships, ranging, for example, from difficulties adjusting behavior to suit various social contexts; to difficulties in sharing imaginative play or in making friends; to absence of interest in peers.
Specify current severity: Severity is based on social communication impairments and restricted repetitive patterns of behavior. (See table below.)
B. Restricted, repetitive patterns of behavior, interests, or activities, as manifested by at least two of the following, currently or by history (examples are illustrative, not exhaustive; see text):
1. Stereotyped or repetitive motor movements, use of objects, or speech (e.g., simple motor stereotypies, lining up toys or flipping objects, echolalia, idiosyncratic phrases).
2. Insistence on sameness, inflexible adherence to routines, or ritualized patterns or verbal nonverbal behavior (e.g., extreme distress at small changes, difficulties with transitions, rigid thinking patterns, greeting rituals, need to take same route or eat food every day).
3. Highly restricted, fixated interests that are abnormal in intensity or focus (e.g, strong attachment to or preoccupation with unusual objects, excessively circumscribed or perseverative interest).
4. Hyper- or hyporeactivity to sensory input or unusual interests in sensory aspects of the environment (e.g., apparent indifference to pain/temperature, adverse response to specific sounds or textures, excessive smelling or touching of objects, visual fascination with lights or movement).

Specify current severity: Severity is based on social communication impairments and restricted, repetitive patterns of behavior. (See table below.)
C. Symptoms must be present in the early developmental period (but may not become fully manifest until social demands exceed limited capacities or may be masked by learned strategies in later life).
D. Symptoms cause clinically significant impairment in social, occupational, or other important areas of current functioning.
E. These disturbances are not better explained by intellectual disability (intellectual developmental disorder) or global developmental delay. Intellectual disability and autism spectrum disorder frequently co-occur; to make comorbid diagnoses of autism spectrum disorder and intellectual disability, social communication should be below that expected for general developmental level.
Note: Individuals with a well-established DSM-IV diagnosis of autistic disorder, Asperger's disorder, or pervasive developmental disorder not otherwise specified should be given the diagnosis of autism spectrum disorder. Individuals who have marked deficits in social communication, but whose symptoms do not otherwise meet criteria for autism spectrum disorder, should be evaluated for social (pragmatic) communication disorder.
Specify if:
• **With or without accompanying intellectual impairment**
• **With or without accompanying language impairment**
o (Coding note: Use additional code to identify the associated medical or genetic condition.)
• **Associated with another neurodevelopmental, mental, or behavioral disorder**
o (Coding note: Use additional code[s] to identify the associated neurodevelopmental, mental, or behavioral disorder[s].)
• **With catatonia**
• **Associated with a known medical or genetic condition or environmental factor**

In the table above for each of the two categories (A and B), the provider must specify current severity: "Severity is based on social communication impairments and restricted, repetitive patterns of behavior." See the table below for severity levels for autism spectrum disorder (ASD) (American Psychiatric Association, 2013).

Severity level	Social communication	Restricted, repetitive behaviors
Level 3 "Requiring very substantial support"	Severe deficits in verbal and nonverbal social communication skills cause severe impairments in functioning, very limited initiation of social interactions, and minimal response to social overtures from others. For example, a person with few words of intelligible speech who rarely initiates interaction and, when he or she does, makes unusual approaches to meet needs only and responds to only very direct social approaches	Inflexibility of behavior, extreme difficulty coping with change, or other restricted/repetitive behaviors markedly interfere with functioning in all spheres. Great distress/difficulty changing focus or action.
Level 2 "Requiring substantial support"	Marked deficits in verbal and nonverbal social communication skills; social impairments apparent even with supports in place; limited initiation of social interactions; and reduced or abnormal responses to social overtures from others. For example, a person who speaks simple sentences, whose interaction is limited to narrow special interests, and how has markedly odd nonverbal communication.	Inflexibility of behavior, difficulty coping with change, or other restricted/repetitive behaviors appear frequently enough to be obvious to the casual observer and interfere with functioning in a variety of contexts. Distress and/or difficulty changing focus or action.
Level 1 "Requiring support"	Without supports in place, deficits in social communication cause noticeable impairments. Difficulty initiating social interactions, and clear examples of atypical or unsuccessful response to social overtures of others. May appear to have decreased interest in social interactions. For example, a person who is able to speak in full sentences and engages in communication but whose to- and-fro conversation with others fails, and whose attempts to make friends are odd and typically unsuccessful.	Inflexibility of behavior causes significant interference with functioning in one or more contexts. Difficulty switching between activities. Problems of organization and planning hamper independence.

Table: Severity levels for autism spectrum disorder[53]

FDA approved treatment of autism

There remains a relatively small evidence base for the pharmacological treatment of ASD and its associated behaviors.

Only two medications have been approved by the Food and Drug Administration (FDA) for treating irritability associated with ASD: risperidone and aripiprazole. These antipsychotics have been shown in replicated studies to reduce irritability in youth with ASD, and can thus indirectly ease the core symptoms, including improved sociability, reducing tantrums, aggressive outbursts, and self-injurious behaviors, which are some of the most dangerous behaviors associated with ASD. Irritability and aggression, especially as children with ASD get older and stronger, can result in substantial danger for themselves and others, especially their caregivers, and can also lead to hospitalization and out-of-home placement.

According to McCracken et al. (2002), risperidone was effective and well tolerated for the treatment of tantrums, aggression, or self-injurious behavior in children with autistic disorder. A total of 101 children were randomly assigned to receive risperidone versus placebo. Treatment with risperidone for 8 weeks (dose range 0.5–3.5 mg/d) resulted in 56.9% reduction in irritability score as compared with 14.1% reduction in placebo group. Risperidone therapy as associated with an average weight gain of 2.7 ± 2.9 kg as compared with 0.8 ± 2.2 kg with placebo. Increased appetite, fatigue, drowsiness, dizziness, and drooling were more common in the risperidone group than in the placebo group ($P < .05$ for each comparison).

In Shea et al. (2004), risperidone was also seen to be well tolerated and efficacious in treating behavioral symptoms associated with Pervasive Developmental Disorder (according to DSM-IV at the time). Seventy-nine children aged 5–12 years old diagnosed with PDD were randomized to risperidone versus placebo solution over an 8-week period. Subjects taking risperidone experienced a significantly greater mean decrease on the irritability subscale of the ABC (primary endpoint) compared with those taking placebo. By the study endpoint, risperidone-treated subjects exhibited 64% improvement over baseline in irritability score, almost double that of placebo-treated subjects. Somnolence was the most frequently reported adverse event (72.5% of those taking risperidone) versus 7.7% of subjects taking placebo. Risperidone-treated subjects experienced statistically significantly greater increases in weight (2.7 kg vs 1.0 kg), pulse rate, and systolic blood pressure.

According to Marcus et al. (2009), aripiprazole was efficacious and generally safe and well tolerated in children and adolescents with irritability associated with autistic disorder. Two hundred and eighteen children and adolescents aged 6–17 years old with a diagnosis of autistic disorder were randomized to aripiprazole medication versus placebo. At all aripiprazole doses, the study showed significantly greater improvement than placebo in mean Aberrant Behavior Checklist (ABC) irritability subscale scores (5 mg/d, −12.4; 10 mg/d, −13.2; 15 mg/d, −14.4; vs placebo, −8.4).

The three most common adverse events leading to discontinuation were sedation, drooling, and tremor.

Similarly, Marcus et al., (2009), aripiprazole was also found to be efficacious in children and adolescents with irritability associated with autistic disorder and was generally safe and well tolerated (Owen et al., 2009). Ninety-eight children (aged 6-17 years old) who were diagnosed with autistic disorder were randomized to flexibly dosed aripiprazole versus placebo. Mean improvement in ABC-I subscale score was significantly greater with aripiprazole than with placebo from week 1 through week 8. Aripiprazole also demonstrated significantly greater global improvements than placebo, as assessed by the mean CGI-I score from week 1 through week 8. Clinically significant residual effects may persist for some patients and discontinuation rates as a result of adverse events (AEs) were 10.6% for aripiprazole and 5.9% for placebo. Mean weight gain was 2.0 kg on aripiprazole and 0.8 kg on placebo at week 8.

A comparison of the two FDA approved medications, risperidone and aripiprazole, was performed by Ghanizadeh, Sahraeizadeh, and Beck (2014). In this head-to-head comparison, it was concluded that these two medications should be chosen based on clinical equipoise considering the patient's preference and clinical profile. Risperidone and aripiprazole both lowered ABC-I scores during the 2 months of the study. Rates of adverse effects were not significantly different between the 2 groups. Safety and efficacy of risperidone (mean dose of 1.12 mg/d) and aripiprazole (mean dose of 5.5 mg/d) were comparable.

Related comorbidities

Mood and anxiety disorders

Anxiety and depression can occur in children diagnosed with ASD, though it may be underrecognized and undertreated. Psychotherapeutic interventions must always be a consideration, and Cognitive Behavioral Therapy (CBT) has been shown to be helpful for patients with ASD and anxiety.

Although no medication has been specifically studied for anxiety or depression in ASD, practitioners may consider the use of SSRI such as fluoxetine or sertraline (Nadeau et al., 2011). Oswald and Sonenklar (2007) states that SSRIs have continuously been used in the treatment of comorbid anxiety symptoms in patients with ASD, even though research on the effectiveness of these medications in this situation is limited. Possible adverse side effects from SSRIs for anxiety and depression could include behavioral activation (e.g., agitation, irritability, aggression, and disinhibition) according to Nadeau et al. (2011).

Anxiety is common in youth with ASD. Up to 80% of children with ASDs experience a clinically significant anxiety disorder (Leyfer et al., 2006; Muris, Steerneman, Merckelbach, Holdrinet, & Meesters, 1998; Nadeau et al., 2011; Simonoff et al., 2008). The presence of anxiety in people with ASD is a key factor linked to increased impairment beyond the core ASD symptoms, which makes it important to address, as undetected anxiety can be highly impairing and adversely affect psychosocial functioning (Nadeau et al., 2011).

Besides Cognitive Behavioral Therapy (CBT), which remains a primary therapeutic intervention for youth with ASD and comorbid anxiety, a few studies have shown that children with ASD taking the antidepressant citalopram or the antianxiety drug buspirone showed some improvement in their anxiety symptoms (Nadeau et al., 2011). A retrospective study of citalopram in 17 children and adolescents ranging from 4 to 15 years old with ASD found that 59% of participants taking citalopram daily displayed a positive treatment response, with the greatest reductions noted in anxiety and aggression (Couturier and Nicholson, 2002). Participants were treated with an initial low dose of 5 mg citalopram daily, titrated up by 5 mg weekly as tolerated and as necessary, and treated with a mean final dose of 19.7 mg citalopram daily. Citalopram was well tolerated, though four of the patients developed mild adverse effects including increased agitation, insomnia, and possible tics.

A second retrospective study of citalopram in 15 children and adolescents ranging from 6 to 16 years old with ASD found that 73% of the participants displayed a positive treatment response after taking a mean final dose of 16.9 mg citalopram daily, with the greatest reductions in anxiety, repetitive behaviors, and irritability. Side effects relating to citalopram included headaches and sedation (Namerow, Thomas, Bostic, Prince, & Monuteaux, 2003). Children with ASDs may be at higher risk for adverse side effects associated with medications that target anxiety symptoms and it is thus recommended that the use of slow-titration dosing schedules be implemented in order to safely administer pharmacotherapy (Nadeau et al., 2011).

Depression appears to occur with much greater frequency among people with ASD than in the general population and the risk for comorbid depression increases with age. Currently CBT and selective serotonin reuptake inhibitors (SSRIs) are the treatment of choice for patients with ASD and comorbid depression (Namerow et al., 2003). There is limited research that examines the efficacy of various treatments for depression in individuals with ASD, especially children and adolescents and no randomized controlled trials have been conducted to examine the safety and efficacy of treatments for depression in this population (DeFillippis, 2018).

Disruptive behavioral disorders (aggression, self-injurious behavior, inappropriate sexualized behavior)

Aggression

Aggressive behavior in patients diagnosed with ASD is of significant concern and has negative impact on the quality of life for individuals with ASD and their caregivers. Pharmacologic treatments, specifically the use of second-generation antipsychotics (SGAs), may effectively reduce aggressive behaviors in some individuals with ASD. Beyond medication treatment, therapeutic behavioral strategies and psychosocial interventions need to be implemented to help treat these patients.

A proportion of children and adults with ASD present with aggression, self-injurious behavior, and/or inappropriate sexualized behaviors. Aggression is characterized as behavior that is threatening or likely to cause harm and it may be verbal or physical. This behavior is strongly associated with negative outcomes for children with ASD including decreased quality of life, increased stress levels, and reduced availability of educational and social support (Fitzpatrick, Srivorakiat, Wink, Pedapati, & Erickson, 2016). Research has indicated that aggressive behavior may be more prevalent in individuals diagnosed with ASD than in the general population. Studies have shown that those with intellectual disability (ID) and comorbid ASD are reported to demonstrate aggression more so than individuals with ID alone. Therapeutic management of aggression includes functional behavioral assessment, reinforcement strategies, and functional communication treatment in order to reduce the frequency and severity of aggressive behaviors.

Pharmacologic treatment for aggression includes second-generation antipsychotics. Risperidone is a second-generation antipsychotic that works as a D2 receptor antagonist that was originally developed as a treatment for schizophrenia. There have been numerous research studies that have demonstrated this medication's efficacy as treatment for ASD-related aggression, self-injury, and severe tantrums.

McDougle et al. in 1998 were the first to conduct a double-blind, randomized, placebo-controlled trial of risperidone in patients with ASD (McDougle et al., 1998). Thirty-one adults aged 18–43 years old were enrolled in the study, with 24 individuals that completed the 12 weeks of treatment. The subjects in the risperidone group showed a significant global improvement measured by the Clinical Global Impression-Improvement scale (CGI-I) and a decrease in physical aggression, self-injury, and property destruction.

Serious self-injury is a debilitating behavior occurring in some children and adults with ASD. In 2002, the Research Units on Pediatric Psychopharmacology (RUPP) Autism Network published their results of an 8-week, randomized, double-blind, placebo-controlled trial of risperidone in 101 youth ages 5–17 years old with ASD and comorbid aggression (McCracken et al., 2002). These patients were treated with risperidone and had a significant decrease in the ABC-I score ($P < .001$). Sixty-nine percent of the participants treated with risperidone were treatment responders (defined as 25% improvement on the ABC-I and a rating of "much improved" or "very much improved" on the CGI-I) compared to 12% of the subjects on placebo ($P < .001$) (McCracken et al., 2002).

In 2004 Shea et al. (2004) study conducted an 8-week, randomized double-blind, placebo-controlled trial in 79 children ages 5–12 years old with ASD and replicated the finding of the efficacy of risperidone in treating irritability and aggression. Then, in 2005 as a follow-up to their 2002 study, RUPP group examined the longer-term benefits of risperidone (Research Units on Pediatric Psychopharmacology Autism Network, 2005a). Those patients from the 2002 study who had showed a positive response to risperidone and those who were placebo nonresponders were enrolled in an additional 4 months of open-label treatment to determine whether the short-term efficacy and safety of risperidone were maintained. In the 51 subjects completing the extended trial, the mean ABC-Irritability score showed a 59% reduction from mean baseline rating, consistent with the results from 2002 of the initial short-term RUPP study. Although risperidone was shown to be effective in treating aggression in patients with diagnosed ASD, adverse effects are common and include weight gain and somnolence/sedation.

However, risperidone is generally very well tolerated, and side effects may be managed by proper dosing and appropriate dosing schedule modifications as well as psychosocial and supportive interventions including dietary recommendations.

Aripiprazole is another second-generation antipsychotic, acting as a partial D2 receptor and 5-HT1A receptor agonist, and a 5-HT2A receptor antagonist. This medication has been studied extensively in patients with ASD and comorbid irritability as previously noted and may be used to mitigate symptoms of aggression.

Clozapine was the first approved second-generation antipsychotic in the United States and is currently approved for treatment-resistant bipolar disorder and schizophrenia (Lally and MacCabe, 2015; Li, Tang, Wang, & de Leon, 2015). This medication acts as a mild antagonist at D2 receptors, with additional actions at serotonin, histamine, and noradrenergic receptors. There have been several case reports demonstrating this medication's safety and efficacy in reducing aggression in ASD. Gobbi and Pulvirenti (2001) presented a case study to describe the positive effects of clozapine in a 32-year old man with autistic disorder accompanied by disruptive behavior (Gobbi and Pulvirenti, 2001). Beherec et al. (2011) reviewed the charts of six individuals with ASD (whose mean age was 23.2 ± 6.9 years who were treated with clozapine for aggressive behavior (Beherec et al., 2011). The study found that clozapine treatment was associated with a twofold reduction in aggressive behaviors. Adverse side effects did include constipation, significant weight gain, and tachycardia. Clozapine requires regular, frequent blood draws to monitor the white blood cell counts due to the potential for agranulocytosis. As blood draws are hard to obtain in highly irritable and aggressive patients, this medication is rarely used in this population.

Olanzapine works at both the D2 and 5-HT2A receptors and is a first-line FDA approved treatment for schizophrenia (CenterWatch, 2009). Hollander et al. (2006) authored a case report suggesting that olanzapine is effective treatment for aggression, along with hyperactivity, in patients with ASD. One double-blind, placebo-controlled trial studied olanzapine in patients with ASD. Eleven subjects were enrolled, and eight completed the 8 weeks of treatment with the medication. The dose of olanzapine ranged from 7.5 to 12.5 mg/d and did not reduce symptoms measured by the Overt Aggression Scale Modified irritability measure or the OAS-M aggression measure. However, the CGI-I rating scale showed significant improvement in global functioning as compared to placebo (Hollander et al., 2006). Weight gain and sedation were the most common side effects reported in this study. A 12-week open-label trial of four adolescents and four adults with ASD showed significant improvement on the CGI-I as well as reduction of aggressive symptoms on the SIB-Q after these subjects were treated with an average olanzapine dose of 7.8 ± 4.7 mg/d. Again, adverse effects included significant weight gain and sedation (Potenza, Holmes, Kanes, & McDougle, 1999). A more recent 13-week open-label study of olanzapine studied 40 adolescents diagnosed with ASD and compared to baseline scores, 13-week scores showed significant improvement on all subscales of the ABC (Fido and Al-Saad, 2008). Although studies show mixed results in patients with ASD and aggression treated with olanzapine, it is suggested that this medication is somewhat effective and is relatively safe and well tolerated.

Quetiapine is a second-generation antipsychotic that functions as a dopamine, serotonin, and adrenergic antagonist. Although double-blind, placebo-controlled trials of quetiapine in patients with ASD are limited, there are several open-label studies and case series showing efficacy of this medication to reduce aggression. One open-label study looked at nine adolescents aged 12–17 years old diagnosed with ASD and treated with quetiapine for 12 weeks with a mean dose of 292 mg/d (Findling et al., 2004). Six subjects completed the trial and two were considered responders based on the CGI-I with weight gain as the most significant reported side effect (Findling et al., 2004). Many of these open-label studies demonstrated global improvement of symptoms rather than reduction of aggression, however, quetiapine is still a medication that may still be of some benefit to patients with ASD and concomitant aggression. There is a paucity of double-blind, placebo-controlled studies of quetiapine in this population.

Paliperidone is a major active metabolite of risperidone and unlike other antipsychotics, delivery of the drug can be controlled for up to 24 hours using osmotic controlled release system technology, and thus requires only once-daily dosing (Karlsson, Dencker, & Nyberg, 2005). Although there have been no randomized, placebo-controlled studies of paliperidone in individuals diagnosed with ASD, there have been two case reports and an open-label study suggesting that paliperidone may be effective in treating aggression and that it is generally well-tolerated. The first case report was described in a 20-year-old male with ASD and severe aggression and self-injurious behavior. 8 mg/d of risperidone was changed to 12 mg/d of paliperidone while his other medications were maintained. The subject subsequently had a significant decrease in aggression, SIB, and tantrums, and a "much improved" rating on the CGI-I with no reported adverse side effects (Stigler, Erickson, Mullett, Posey, & McDougle, 2010). The limited evidence suggests that paliperidone may be effective and well-tolerated for treating aggression in ASD and could provide an alternative treatment for patients who do not respond to risperidone.

Antiepileptic medication is frequently prescribed off-label in youth with ASD to target symptoms of irritability. Valproate (VPA) has been of particular interest in ASD (Huband, Ferriter, Nathan, & Jones, 2010). Hellings et al. (2005) performed a double-blind, placebo-controlled trial of VPA to target aggressive behavior in youth with ASD. Thirty individuals with ASD aged 6–20 years old received treatment with VPA or placebo for 8 weeks (Hellings et al., 2005). There was no significant improvement reported with VPA treatment on the ABC-I primary outcome measure and it was concluded that this medication is not a viable treatment option for the youth with ASD and irritability (Hellings et al., 2005). Larger controlled trials may be indicated to fully establish any efficacy in the ASD population.

Lithium is indicated for treatment of bipolar disorder, although despite its extensive psychiatric history, it has been studied only peripherally in ASD. In 2014 Sigel et al. performed a retrospective review of lithium treatment in 30 children diagnosed with ASD. Forty-three percent of included participants had scores of "very much improved" or "much improved" on the CGI-I primary outcome measure (Siegel et al., 2014). However, its side effect profile, including vomiting, tremor, fatigue, irritability, and enuresis, the need for blood draws to ensure a therapeutic dose, and its potential for toxicity, limit its use in targeting ASD-associated aggression (Fitzpatrick et al., 2016; Siegel et al., 2014).

There is research performed on pharmacologic management of refractory aggression, aggressive behavior that does not respond to first-line psychopharmacologic treatments in patients with ASD. A recent study performed by Wink, Pedapati, Horn, McDougle, and Erickson (2015) identified combination antipsychotic treatment as a potential treatment option for patients with ASD and severe behavioral problems. Unfortunately, the psychiatric literature has consistently demonstrated increased rates of adverse effects with combination antipsychotic therapy (Gallego, Nielsen, De Hert, Kane, & Correll, 2012).

Due to the challenge of treating refractory aggression in patients with ASD, investigators are turning to novel mechanisms for treating ASD-associated aggression with glutamatergic agents and gamma-aminobutyric acid modulators. For example, amantadine, memantine, riluzole, and arbaclofen have shown promise in preliminary studies of disruptive behaviors in ASD (Erickson and Chambers, 2006; Erickson et al., 2014; Ghaleiha, Asadabadi, et al., 2013; Ghaleiha, Mohammadi, et al., 2013; Mohammadi et al., 2013; Wink, Erickson, Stigler, & McDougle, 2011).

Self-injurious behavior

Behavioral and pharmacological treatments are the two treatment options available for individuals with autism and SIB. The first step to determine which treatment approach will be most effective, a functional assessment should be conducted (Mahatmya, Zobel, & Valdovinos, 2008). If SIB has a solely social function, then drug treatment may not be appropriate, however, if SIB is determined to have a nonsocial function, then medication management may be the best option. Self-injurious behavior can occur in children and adults diagnosed with ASD and can have a devastating impact on their overall physical health, developmental outcomes, and quality of life (Summers et al., 2017). This behavior refers to actions directed toward one's self and can lead to physical harm. If this behavior continues and is pervasive, long-standing, or very severe, then medications may need to be utilized. Specific types of medications used include antidepressants such as citalopram and sertraline, antipsychotics such as clozapine and risperidone, and opioid antagonists such as naltrexone and naloxone.

A study by Carminati, Deriaz, and Bertschy (2006) proposed that SIB may be from a dysregulation of the serotonin reuptake process (Luiselli, Blew, & Thibadeau, 2001). In their study, two antidepressant medications were evaluated for efficacy: sertraline and clomipramine (Luiselli et al., 2001). These studies showed that sertraline reduced SIB in a 20-year-old male with severe mental retardation and that clomipramine (a tricyclic antidepressant) was effective in eliminating aggressive behavior in an autistic 14-year old male (Luiselli et al., 2001). SSRIs, such as fluoxetine and fluvoxamine, have been shown to decrease aggression in people with autism in a dose-dependent manner. Higher doses of SSRIs have shown to be more effective in reducing aggressive behavior according to Carminati et al. (2006). On the other hand, clomipramine (a tricyclic antidepressant) was found to decrease SIB in individuals with autism based on the exact dose used. Luiselli et al. (2001) found that clomipramine decreased SIB when dosed under 125 mg, however, at higher doses, this medication increased SIB symptoms.

Animal research has shown that dopamine receptors have been overstimulated and are supersensitive in animals displaying SIB (Canitano, 2006; Hammock, Schroeder, & Levine, 1995). Due to the adverse side effects, atypical antipsychotics are preferred in the treatment of patients with autism and SIB. Clozapine is effective in treating schizophrenia and has been found to have a dose-dependent decrease in SIB symptoms in patients with autism according to Hammock et al. (1995). Risperidone, although FDA approved for the treatment of individuals with autism and irritability, has been shown to improve SIB, often showing improvements by the second week of treatment (Barrera, Violo, & Graver, 2007). Like other antipsychotics, risperidone has shown to be dose-dependent with low to intermediate doses more effective in targeting SIB.

Studies have suggested that opioid antagonists may be an effective treatment for SIB (Mahatmya et al., 2008). Opioid antagonists can restore pain thresholds through sedation or by making SIB more aversive. Naltrexone is the most widely used opioid antagonist and may be more beneficial for certain individuals with both autism and SIB (Mahatmya et al., 2008). Those with severe SIB and those with lower B-endorphin levels are better responders to the medication (Elchaar, Maisch, Augusto, & Wehring, 2006; Taylor et al., 1991). Male patients respond better to naltrexone than their female counterparts who often require much higher doses of medication (Symons, Hoch, Dahl, & McComas, 2003). However, if used long-term, naltrexone may have negative effects leading to increased relapse rates if this medication is discontinued (Benjamin, Seek, Tresise, Price, & Gagnon, 1995; Campbell et al., 1993). Thus naltrexone has been found to be effective for autistic patients with severe SIB in the short term with very wide individual variation in response to this medication (Benjamin et al., 1995; Campbell et al., 1993).

Inappropriate sexualized behavior

Individuals with ASD typically struggle with deficits in social competence and poor communication skills and may be more vulnerable to missing social cues around sexualized behaviors in interactions and personal behaviors (e.g., not comprehending that masturbation in public is taboo). Young adults transitioning into adolescence may exhibit inappropriate sexual behaviors in tandem with hormonal surges and these behaviors can include masturbating in public, disrobing, inappropriate touching, copropraxia (obscene gestures), and pornographomania (Coskun, Karakoc, Kircelli, & Mukaddes, 2009). Many adolescents with ASD are deprived of adequate sexual education and are discouraged by their parents and society from expressing their sexuality. For inappropriate sexualized behavior (ISB), most clinicians highly suggest starting with educational and behavioral approaches before starting medications (Coskun et al., 2009).

Mirtazapine, an antidepressant, has been shown to be efficacious for ISBs as found in a case series of nine subjects with ASD conducted by Coskun et al.

(2009). Other studies have attested to the efficacy of mirtazapine for ISBs in ASD due to their antilibidinal properties (Nguyen and Murphy, 2001). A case study reported by Deepmala and Agrawal has shown that the B-blocker, propranolol, when given at a low dose (10 mg BID) has helped an adolescent patient with ASD and comorbid ISB, suggesting this is through reduction in the central sympathetic nervous system stimulation and impaired vasodilation of the corpora cavernosa (Deepmala and Agrawal, 2014; Naguy, Alrashidi, & AlShalabi, 2019). SSRIs or antipsychotics may also be helpful through reducing libido, though this has theory has remained untested. Leuprolide was described in one case report as effectively reducing ISB in a young adult male with ASD, however it had severe adverse effects of depression, seizures, and anaphylaxis (Realmuto and Ruble, 1999; Siegel and Erickson, 2016b).

ADHD

There has been growing interest in the cooccurrence of attention deficit/hyperactivity disorder (ADHD) and ASD, though relatively little research has been devoted to treatment in this area. Most of the intervention research has examined pharmacological treatment using well-established ADHD medications available to the general population, including both psychostimulants, such as methylphenidate and long-acting dextroamphetamine/amphetamine, and nonstimulant medications, such as atomoxetine or guanfacine (Davis and Kollins, 2012).

In studies, children with comorbid ASD and ADHD taking methylphenidate have experienced adverse effects such as irritability, self-injury, and stereotypy (Scahill and Pachler, 2007). The Research Units on Pediatric Psychopharmacology Autism Network conducted a randomized, placebo-controlled trial of methylphenidate with 72 children ranging from ages 5–14 years old and diagnosed with both autism and moderate-to-severe hyperactivity. Results indicated that the stimulant medication was effective at reducing hyperactivity and impulsivity in only about half of the participants, which is considerably lower than the response rates of 70%–80% found in studies of methylphenidate in children with ADHD only (Davis and Kollins, 2012; Greenhill et al., 2006; Research Units on Pediatric Psychopharmacology RUPP Autism Network, 2005b). There is only one study that directly compares methylphenidate treatment response between children and ADHD and children with ASD plus ADHD (Santosh, Baird, Pityaratstian, Tavare, & Gringras, 2006). In Santosh et al. (2006), a retrospective analysis of clinical cases and a small prospective clinical trial were performed. This study reported overall improvement in ADHD symptoms, with few differences in treatment response between children with ADHD versus children with ASD and ADHD. However, the administration of stimulant treatment of patients with ASD and ADHD need to be monitored heavily for side effects.

Nonstimulant medications have also been investigated for cooccurring ADHD and ASD symptoms, particularly atomoxetine. Atomoxetine likely functions via the norepinephrine transporters and has demonstrated better tolerability than stimulant medications in this population (Davis and Kollins, 2012; Murray, 2010). Additional research using parents and teachers as informants have also shown that there have been significant reductions in ADHD symptoms among children diagnosed with both ASD and ADHD. However, just like most of the medications for ADHD, atomoxetine is not as effective and is less well-tolerated in the ASD population than the general population.

Another nonstimulant, guanfacine, is an alpha-2 adrenergic agonist that has historically been used for hypertension and now more recently approved for use in patients with ADHD in an extended release formulation. This medication can be used alone or in combination with stimulants to treat children with ADHD. However, positive effects have been found in studies using guanfacine for treatment of children with both ASD and ADHD symptoms. In 2004 Posey et al. performed a retrospective analysis of 80 patients aged 3–18 years old treated with guanfacine within an academic specialty clinic. Charts were reviewed to determine the response of specific target symptoms such as hyperactivity, inattention, and impulsivity. It was found that guanfacine at a mean daily dose of 2.6 ± 1.7 mg over the course of 334 ± 374 days, was effective in 19 of 80 patients (23.8%). Guanfacine was well tolerated and found to have a role in the treatment of hyperactivity and inattention that cooccurs in patients diagnosed with ASD (Posey, Puntney, Sasher, Kem, & McDougle, 2004). In a prospective open trial of guanfacine in children with ASD performed by Scahill et al. (2006), the study found that children with a mean age of 9.03 ± 3.14 years after 8 weeks of treatment with guanfacine, had a parent-rated hyperactivity subscale of the Aberrant Behavior Checklist (ABC) mean of 31.3 ± 8.89 at baseline to 18.9 ± 10.37. Twelve of the children (48%) were rated as much improved or very much improved on the Clinical Global Impressions (CGI)–Improvement. Adverse effects included irritability, sedation, sleep disturbance, and constipation, however, no significant changes in pulse, blood pressure, or electrocardiogram (Scahill et al., 2006).

While these preliminary studies support the use of psychopharmacological treatments for reducing ADHD symptoms in individuals with comorbid ASD and ADHD, there need to be further studies to increase the understanding of these medications' effectiveness and adverse effect profiles in order to fully inform clinical practice.

Sleep disturbance

Individuals with ASD, especially children, tend to have sleep problems such as insomnia Siegel and Erickson, 2016b). Sleep problems can exacerbate the core and related symptoms of ASD. The reported prevalence by parents of sleep problems in children with ASD range from 44% to 83% (Krakowiak, Goodlin-Jones, Hertz-Picciotto, Croen, & Hansen, 2008). Clinicians suggest that establishing good sleep hygiene is the primary intervention, such as removing electronics and other stimulating devices and activities from the bedtime, and creating a consistent bedtime routine (Siegel and Erickson, 2016b). Good sleep hygiene includes ensuring that the child's bedroom is dark and quiet at a comfortable temperature, creating a consistent bedtime routine that should last between 20 and 30 minutes, and including relaxing activities such as reading books or listening to music, avoiding caffeine before bedtime, and ensuring that naps do not fall too late into the afternoon close to bedtime. For children who have consistent trouble falling asleep or staying asleep, melatonin may be a safe and effective option to improve sleep in children with ASD (Siegel and Erickson, 2016b).

Stereotypy/repetitive behavior

Autistic individuals may display repetitive behaviors and insist on sameness (Siegel and Erickson, 2016b). These behaviors can include repeated motor mannerisms such as hand flapping, atypical sensory interests, complex body movements, and repeating a sound, word, or phrase multiple times (Siegel and Erickson, 2016b). Interruption of these repetitive behavioral patterns may cause anxiety and aggression. Some of these persistent behavioral patterns may not cause problems or may even be helpful in the learning process, while at other times they can be interruptive and cause difficulties in academic and social settings. Since SSRIs have been known to be efficacious in patients showing repetitive symptoms of OCD, clinicians have attempted to treat autistic repetitive behaviors with SSRIs (Siegel and Erickson, 2016b). Specifically, the SSRI fluvoxamine and the SNRI clomipramine have been shown to improve repetitive behaviors in patients with autism (Ghanizadeh, 2010; McDougle et al., 1995). Antipsychotics, such as risperidone, have demonstrated efficacy in reducing stereotypies and improving the restricted, repetitive, and stereotypic behavior of children with ASD (McDougle et al., 1998, 2005). The effect of pharmacotherapy on stereotypic behaviors is not well studied unfortunately, however, SSRIs and certain antipsychotics, such as risperidone, have been shown to improve stereotypy in individuals with ASD (McDougle et al., 1998, 2005).

Psychosis

ASD and many psychotic disorders, such as schizophrenia, are neurodevelopmental disorders (Siegel and Erickson, 2016b). Psychosis is defined as abnormal perceptions (hallucinations) and distortions of reality (delusions) and are found more often in people with ASD than in the general population (Foss-Feig and Velthorst, 2019). The first pharmacological line of treating psychotic symptoms in people with ASD is antipsychotic medication, usually a second-generation antipsychotic.

Neurological disorders

ASDs are frequently comorbid with other neurological disorders, including intellectual disability (ID), global developmental delay (GDD), and epilepsy (Amiet et al., 2008). Studies have identified more than 1000 ASD risk genes and most of these have reported relationships with other neurological diseases (Xiong et al., 2019). Two clear risk factors for epilepsy in autism are the presence of intellectual disability and female gender. About one third of the population of people with autism have developed seizures in early adult life and unfortunately little is known about the treatment of epilepsy in autism (Besag, 2018).

Future direction ECT/VNS/TMS

Currently the main treatments for ASD include behavioral interventions, psychotherapies, psychosocial and educational interventions, and pharmacologic treatment targeting specific symptom clusters, comorbid psychiatric disorders, or dangerous behaviors.

Other neuropsychiatric interventions that have demonstrated some efficacy in non-ASD populations are being considered for people with ASD (Kim, Ryu, & Bahn, 2016).

Electroconvulsive therapy (ECT) is used in individuals with both ASD and catatonia; vagal nerve stimulation (VNS) is used for ASD and comorbid epilepsy; and deep brain stimulation (DBS) is used for serious self-injurious behaviors (Kim et al., 2016). There can be an excitation/inhibition imbalance that alters the brain mechanism of information processing and behavioral regulation that may be stabilized with repetitive transcranial magnetic stimulation (RTMS) (Kim et al., 2016).

Applications of neurostimulation or neuromodulation by either new or old techniques have been regarded as highly invasive treatment options restricted for use with patients with treatment-resistant disorders. ECT applies an electric stimulus to the surface of the head and induces a seizure (Kim et al., 2016). Its use has generally been limited to treating catatonia, which may occur in as many as 12%–18% of young people with ASD (Kim et al., 2016). ECT is an effective treatment option for comorbid catatonia in patients with ASD when benzodiazepine treatment is insufficient (Kim et al., 2016). It has been hypothesized that abnormalities in the gamma aminobutyric acid (GABA) system plays a role in the pathophysiology of ASD and catatonia and that ECT may enhance GABA functioning (Kim et al., 2016).

RTMS is an increasingly used treatment modality. RTMS involves safe and non-invasive neurostimulation and modulation through a series of pulsed magnetic stimuli to the brain (Kim et al., 2016). The therapeutic application of TMS in ASD is emerging and research has suggested that RTMS improves executive functioning and clinical symptoms including irritability, hyperactivity, and stereotypic behaviors in individuals with ASD (Kim et al., 2016). Extended dosing (6000 pulses) of high-frequency (such as 20 Hz) RTMS in ASD may work by stabilizing aberrant neuroplasticity and improving social and cognitive performance (Kim et al., 2016).

Vagal nerve stimulation is the intermittent repeated stimulation of the left vagus nerve with a small electrical pulse originating from an implanted neurostimulator (Kim et al., 2016). The left vagus nerve is stimulated rather than the right vagus nerve since the right nerve plays a major role in cardiac function and alteration of its function may be fatal (Kim et al., 2016). VNS was initially approved for treatment-resistant epilepsy (Kim et al., 2016). Research has shown that VNS in ASD is associated with modest behavioral improvement and seizure control in both children and adults (Kim et al., 2016).

Deep brain stimulation is a surgical procedure under stereotactic technique to implant electrodes at target regions in the brain (Kim et al., 2016). It was initially used to treat movement disorders and has therapeutic indications for depression and

OCD (Kim et al., 2016). Various case reports have shown that DBS for severe ASD can show remarkable improvement in motor stereotypies (Kim et al., 2016). Interestingly, DBS of the basolateral nucleus of the amygdala (BLA) has been shown to be a potential therapeutic intervention for refractory ASD with life-threatening SIB, since the amygdala has a central role in social cognition and its abnormality is closely linked to SIB in ASD (Kim et al., 2016).

Brain stimulation and neuromodulation are getting increased attention as new therapeutic tools for treating ASD and its comorbid symptoms (Kim et al., 2016). This treatment route is potentially effective and is a viable treatment option for patients with ASD (Kim et al., 2016).

Optogenetics is a new area of science that studies the role of specific subcortical circuits in aggression and anxiety and allows scientists to explore the prefrontal cortex in social dysfunction (Kim et al., 2016). Optogenetics uses different wavelengths of light, delivered via fiber optic cable, to control the activity of cells that send and receive information in the brain, for example, blue light activates targeted neurons and yellow light quiets them (Kim et al., 2016). This optogenetic toolbox may shed light on research and treatment of ASD and its comorbidities (Kim et al., 2016).

Currently, vasopressin is emerging as a hormone of interest in ASD research as it appears that this chemical is associated with social bonding, similar to the hormone oxytocin, and it is involved with several social and sensory processes (Carson et al., 2015).

Two chemicals, intranasal vasopressin and balovaptan, an antagonist of the vasopressin receptor, are being studied, and, although they appear to function in opposite ways, they have shown early positive results in improving social communication in patients with autism (Zeliadt, 2019).

Carson et al. demonstrated the relationship between arginine vasopressin (AVP) and social functioning in children diagnosed with autism (Carson et al., 2015). A study performed by Parker et al. in 2019 was the first clinical trial to show that intranasal vasopressin improves social deficits in children with autism (Parker et al., 2019). This was a clinical study that administered vasopressin intranasally to children diagnosed with ASD for 4 weeks and the results showed that the drug was well tolerated and that AVP treatment has the potential to treat social impairments in autistic children (Parker et al., 2019).

Balovaptan blocks the vasopressin receptor in the brain and dampens the hormone's activity (Zeliadt, 2019). There is a current clinical trial testing this substance and its efficacy in enhancing social communication in patients diagnosed with autism (Zeliadt, 2019).

Conclusion

Autism Spectrum Disorder has evolved over the years and is now recognized as a neurodevelopmental based disorder. ASD core symptoms present with medical and public health complexities which warrant more clinical trials and research. Current best practice treatment approaches utilize multimodal interventions such as applied behavioral analysis (ABA) and social skills training focusing on communicative and adaptive skills. Although pharmacologic agents do not specifically address the three core symptoms of ASD, their utility is in addressing the disruptive behavior, mood, anxiety, and other related comorbid psychopathologies associated with the disorder. Pharmacologic agents are essential in treating ASD-related comorbidities, and when used in conjunction with nonpharmacologic interventions, are the best current practice approach. Finding the correct medication combination to maximize efficacy and minimize side effects is the goal for treatment when developing an individualized treatment plan for people with autism.

References

Applied Behavioral Analysis Program Guide (ABAPG). (2020). <https://www.appliedbehavioranalysisprograms.com/history-autism-treatment/>.

American Psychiatric Association. (2013). *Diagnostic and statistical manual of mental disorders* (5th ed.). https://doi.org/10.1176/appi.books.9780890425596.

Amiet, C., Gourfinkel-An, I., Bouzamondo, A., Tordjman, S., Baulac, M., Lechat, P., ... Cohen, D. (2008). *Society of Biological Psychiatry, 64*, 577–582.

ASHA. (2020). Autism. *ASHA American Speech-Language-Hearing Association.* <https://www.asha.org/Practice-Portal/Clinical-Topics/Autism/>.

Autism Speak. (2020). CDC increases estimate of Autism's prevalence by 15 percent, to 1 in 59 children: Autism speaks calls on Nation's leaders to adequately fund critically needed research and support services. *Autism Speaks.* <https://www.autismspeaks.org/science-news/cdc-increases-estimate-autisms-prevalence-15-percent-1-59-children>.

Avdjieva-Tzavella, D., Todorov, T., Todorova, A., Kirov, A., Litvinenko, I., Hristova, D., ... Toncheva, D. (2012). The relationship between fragile X syndrome, rett syndrome, and autism spectrum disorders. *Pediatriya, 51*(1), 35–37. Available from https://www.researchgate.net/publication/286471429_The_relationship_between_fragile_X_syndrome_rett_syndrome_and_autism_spectrum_disorders.

Baio, J., Wiggins, L., Christensen, D. L., et al. (2018). Prevalence of autism spectrum disorder among children aged 8 years—autism and developmental disabilities monitoring network, 11 sites, United States, 2014. *MMWR Surveillance Summaries: Morbidity and Mortality Weekly Report Surveillance Summaries/CDC, 67*(SS-6), 1–23. Available from http://doi.org/10.15585/mmwr.ss6706a1externalicon.

Barrera, F. J., Violo, R. A., & Graver, E. E. (2007). On the form and function of severe self-injurious behavior. *Behavioral Interventions, 22*, 5–33.

Beherec, L., Lambrey, S., Quilici, G., Rosier, A., Falissard, B., & Guillin, O. (2011). Retrospective review of clozapine in the treatment of patients with autism spectrum disorder and severe disruptive behaviors. *Journal of Clinical Psychopharmacology, 31*(3), 341–344.

Benjamin, S., Seek, A., Tresise, L., Price, E., & Gagnon, M. (1995). Case study: Paradoxical response to naltrexone treatment of self-injurious behavior. *Journal of the American Academy of Child and Adolescent Psychiatry, 34*(2), 238–242.

Besag, F. (2018). Epilepsy in patients with autism: Links, risks and treatment challenges. *Neuropsychiatric Disease and Treatment*, *14*, 1–10. Available from https://doi.org/10.2147/NDT.S120509.

Bölte, S., Knecht, S., & Poustka, F. (2007). A case-control study of personality style and psychopathology in parents of subjects with autism. *Journal of Autism and Developmental Disorders*, *37*, 243–250.

Bonneh, Y. S., Levanon, Y., Dean-Pardo, O., Lossos, L., & Adini, Y. (2010). Abnormal speech spectrum and increased pitch variability in young autistic children. *Frontiers in Human Neuroscience*, *4*, 237. Available from https://doi.org/10.3389/fnhum.2010.00237.

Brasic, J. R., & Morgan, R. H. (2019). What is the global prevalence of autism spectrum disorder (ASD)? *Medscape*. <https://www.medscape.com/answers/912781-193662/what-is-the-global-prevalence-of-autism-spectrum-disorder-asd>.

Campbell, M., Anderson, L. T., Small, A. M., Adams, P., Gonzalez, N. M., & Ernst, M. (1993). Naltrexone in autistic children: Behavioral symptoms and attentional learning. *Journal of the American Academy of Child and Adolescent Psychiatry*, *32*(6), 1283–1291.

Canitano, R. (2006). Self injurious behavior in autism: Clinical aspects and treatment with risperidone. *Journal of Neural Transmission*, *113*(3), 425–431.

Carminati, G. G., Deriaz, N., & Bertschy, G. (2006). Low-dose venlafaxine in three adolescents and young adults with autistic disorder improves self-injurious behavior and attention deficit/hyperactivity disorders (ADHD)-like symptoms. *Progress in Neuro-Psychopharmacology and Biological Psychiatry*, *30*(2), 312–315. Available from https://doi.org/10.1016/j.pnpbp.2005.10.002.

Carson, D. S., Garner, J. P., Hyde, S. A., Libove, R. A., Berquist, S. W., Hornbeak, K. B., ... Parker, K. J. (2015). Argining vasopressin is a blood-based biomarker for social functioning in children with autism. *PLoS One*. Available from https://doi.org/10.1371/journal.pone.0132224.

CenterWatch. (2009). *Drug information: FDA-approved drugs*. Silver Spring, MD: US Food and Drug Administration. Available from: <http://www.centerwatch.com/drug-information/fda-approved-drugs/year/2009> Accessed April 26, 2016.

Chaste, P., & Leboyer, M. (2012). Autism risk factors: Genes, environment, and gene-environment interactions. *Dialogues in Clinical Neuroscience*, *14*(3), 281–292.

Cohmer, S. (2014). Early infantile autism and the refrigerator mother theory (1943–1970). *The Embryo Project Encyclopedia*. <https://embryo.asu.edu/pages/early-infantile-autism-and-refrigerator-mother-theory-1943-1970>.

Constantino, J. N., Zhang, Y., Frazier, T., Abbacchi, A. M., & Law, P. (2010). Sibling recurrence and the genetic epidemiology of autism. *The American Journal of Psychiatry*, *167*, 1349–1356.

Coskun, M., Karakoc, S., Kircelli, F., & Mukaddes, N. M. (2009). Effectiveness of mirtazapine in the treatment of inappropriate sexual behaviors in individuals with autistic disorder. *Journal of Child and Adolescent Psychopharmacology*, *19*(2). Available from https://doi.org/10.1089/cap.2008.020.

Couturier, J. L., & Nicholson, R. (2002). A retrospective assessment of citalopram in children and adolescents with pervasive developmental disorders. *Journal of Child and Adolescent Psychopharmacology*, *12*, 243–248.

Curley, J. P., Jensen, C. L., Mashoodh, R., & Champagne, F. A. (2011). Social influences on neurobiology and behavior: Epigenetic effects during development. *Psychoneuroendocrinology*, *36*, 352–371.

Davis, N. O., & Kollins, S. H. (2012). Treatment for co-occurring attention deficit/hyperactivity disorder and autism spectrum disorder. *Neurotherapeutics: The Journal of the American Society for Experimental NeuroTherapeutics*, *9*(3), 518–530. Available from https://doi.org/10.1007/s13311-012-0126-9.

Deepmala., & Agrawal, M. (2014). Use of propranolol for hypersexual behavior in an adolescent with autism. *Annals of Pharmacotherapy*. Available from https://doi.org/10.1177/1060028014541630.

DeFillippis, M. (2018). Depression in children and adolescents with autism spectrum disorder. *Children (Basel)*, *5*(9), 112. Available from https://doi.org/10.3390/children5090112.

Durkin, M. S., Maenner, M. J., Newschaffer, C. J., Lee, L. C., Cunniff, C. M., Daniels, J. L., et al. (2008). Advanced parental age and the risk of autism spectrum disorder. *American Journal of Epidemiology*, *168*, 1268–1276.

Elchaar, G. M., Maisch, N. M., Augusto, L. M., & Wehring, H. J. (2006). Efficacy and safety of naltrexone use in pediatric patients with autistic disorder. *The Annals of Pharmacotherapy*, *40*(6), 1086–1095.

Erickson, C. A., & Chambers, J. E. (2006). Memantine for disruptive behavior in autistic disorder. *The Journal of Clinical Psychiatry*, *67*(6), 1000.

Erickson, C. A., Veenstra-Vanderweele, J. M., Melmed, R. D., et al. (2014). STX209 (arbaclofen) for autism spectrum disorders: An 8-week open-label study. *Journal of Autism and Developmental Disorders*, *44*(4), 958–964.

Essa, M. M. (2020). *Personalized food intervention and therapy for autism spectrum disorder management. Advances in Neurology*. Switzerland AG: Springer Nature.

Evans, B. (2013). How Autism Became Autism: The radical transformation of a central concept of child development in Britain. *History of the Human Sciences*, *26*(3), 3–31. Available from https://doi.org/10.1177/0952695113484320.

Fernell, E., Barnevik-Olsson, M., Bågenholm, G., Gillberg, C., Gustafsson, S., & Sääf, M. (2010). Serum levels of 25-hydroxyvitamin D in mothers of Swedish and of Somali origin who have children with and without autism. *Acta Paediatrica*, *99*, 743–747.

Fido, A., & Al-Saad, S. (2008). Olanzapine in the treatment of behavioral problems associated with autism: An open-label trial in Kuwait. *Medical Principles and Practice: International Journal of the Kuwait University, Health Science Centre*, *17*(5), 415–418.

Findling, R. L., McNamara, N. K., Gracious, B. L., et al. (2004). Quetiapine in nine youths with autistic disorder. *Journal of Child and Adolescent Psychopharmacology*, *14*(2), 287–294.

Fitzpatrick, S. E., Srivorakiat, L., Wink, L. K., Pedapati, E. V., & Erickson, C. A. (2016). Aggression in autism spectrum disorder: Presentation and treatment options. *Neuropsychiatric Disease and Treatment*, *12*, 1525–1538.

Folstein, S., & Rutter, M. (1977). Infantile autism: A genetic study of 21 twin pairs. *Journal of Child Psychology and Psychiatry*, *18*(4). Available from https://doi.org/10.1111/j.1469-7610.1977.tb00443.x.

Foss-Feig, J., & Velthorst, E. (2019). Signs of psychosis in people with autism warrant serious concern. *Spectrum*. <https://www.spectrumnews.org/opinion/viewpoint/signs-psychosis-people-autism-warrant-serious-concern/>.

Gallego, J. A., Nielsen, J., De Hert, M., Kane, J. M., & Correll, C. U. (2012). Safety and tolerability of antipsychotic polypharmacy. *Expert Opinion on Drug Safety*, *11*(4), 527–542.

Gardener, H., Spiegelman, D., & Buka, S. L. (2011). Perinatal and neonatal risk factors for autism: A comprehensive meta-analysis. *Pediatrics*, *128*, 344–355.

Ghaleiha, A., Asadabadi, M., Mohammadi, M. R., et al. (2013). Memantine as adjunctive treatment to risperidone in children with autistic disorder: A randomized, double-blind, placebo-controlled trial. *The International Journal of Neuropsychopharmacology/Official Scientific Journal of the Collegium Internationale Neuropsychopharmacologicum (CINP)*, *16*(4), 783–789.

Ghaleiha, A., Mohammadi, E., Mohammadi, M. R., et al. (2013). Riluzole as an adjunctive therapy to risperidone for the treatment of irritability in children with autistic disorder: A double-blind, placebo-controlled, randomized trial. *Paediatric Drugs*, *15*(6), 505–514.

Ghanizadeh, A., Sahraeizadeh, A., & Beck, M. (2014). A head-to-head comparison of aripiprazole and risperidone for safety and treating autistic disorders, a randomized double blind clinical trial. *Child Psychiatry and Human Development*, *45*(2), 185–192. Available from https://doi.org/10.1007/s10578-013-0390-x.

Ghanizadeh, A. (2010). Clinical approach to motor stereotypies in autistic children. *Iranian Journal of Pediatrics*, *20*(2), 149–159.

Gobbi, G., & Pulvirenti, L. (2001). Long-term treatment with clozapine in an adult with autistic disorder accompanied by aggressive behaviour. *Journal of Psychiatry & Neuroscience: JPN*, *26*(4), 340–341.

Greenhill, L., Kollins, S., Abikoff, H., McCracken, J., Riddle, M., Swanson, J., ... Cooper, T. (2006). Efficacy and safety of immediate-release methylphenidate treatment for preschoolers with ADHD. *Journal of the American Academy of Child and Adolescent Psychiatry*, *45*(11), 1284–1293.

Gudsnuk, K., & Champagne, F. A. (2012). Epigenetic influence of stress and the social environment. *ILAR Journal/National Research Council, Institute of Laboratory Animal Resources*, *53*, 279–288. Available from https://doi.org/10.1093/ilar.53.3-4.279.

Haggarty, P. (2004). Effect of placental function on fatty acid requirements during pregnancy. *European Journal of Clinical Nutrition*, *58*, 1559–1570.

Hammock, R. G., Schroeder, S. R., & Levine, W. R. (1995). The effect of clozapine on SIB. *Journal of Autism and Developmental Disorders*, *25*(6), 611–626.

Hellings, J. A., Weckbaugh, M., Nickel, E. J., et al. (2005). A double-blind, placebo-controlled study of valproate for aggression in youth with pervasive developmental disorders. *Journal of Child and Adolescent Psychopharmacology*, *15*(4), 682–692.

Hollander, E., Wasserman, S., Swanson, E. N., et al. (2006). A double-blind placebo-controlled pilot study of olanzapine in childhood/adolescent pervasive developmental disorder. *Journal of Child and Adolescent Psychopharmacology*, *16*(5), 541–548.

Huband, N., Ferriter, M., Nathan, R., & Jones, H. (2010). Antiepileptics for aggression and associated impulsivity. *Cochrane Database of Systematic Reviews (Online)*, *2010*(2), CD003499.

Karimi, P., Kamali, E., Mousavi, S. M., & Karahmadi, M. (2017). Environmental factors influencing the risk of autism. *Journal of Research in Medical Sciences*, *22*, 27. Available from https://doi.org/10.4103/1735-1995.200272.

Karlsson, P., Dencker, E., & Nyberg, S. (2005). Pharmacokinetics, dopamine D2 and serotonin 5-HT2A receptor occupancy and safety profile of paliperidone ER, in healthy volunteers. *European Neuropsychopharmacology: The Journal of the European College of Neuropsychopharmacology*, *15*(Suppl. 3), S38.

Kim, T., Ryu, J. E., & Bahn, G. H. (2016). Brain stimulation and modulation for autism spectrum disorder. *Hanyang Medical Reviews*, *36*(1), 65–71. Available from https://doi.org/10.7599/hmr.2016.36.1.65.

King, B. H., Navot, N., Bernier, R., & Webb, S. J. (2014). Update on diagnostic classification in autism. *Current Opinion in Psychiatry*, *27*(2), 105–109. Available from https://doi.org/10.1097/YCO.0000000000000040.

Kinney, D. K., Munir, K. M., Crowley, D. J., & Miller, A. M. (2008). Prenatal stress and risk for autism. *Neuroscience and Biobehavioral Reviews*, *32*, 1519–1532.

Krakowiak, P., Goodlin-Jones, B., Hertz-Picciotto, I., Croen, L. A., & Hansen, R. L. (2008). Sleep problems in children with autism spectrum disorders, developmental delays, and typical development: A population-based study. *Journal of Sleep Research*, *17*, 197–206.

Krakowiak, P., Walker, C. K., Bremer, A. A., Baker, A. S., Ozonoff, S., Hansen, R. L., et al. (2012). Maternal metabolic conditions and risk for autism and other neurodevelopmental disorders. *Pediatrics*, *129*, e1121–e1128.

Lally, J., & MacCabe, J. H. (2015). Antipsychotic medication in schizophrenia: A review. *British Medical Bulletin*, *114*(1), 169–179.

Larsson, H. J., Eaton, W. W., Madsen, K. M., Vestergaard, M., Olesen, A. V., Agerbo, E., et al. (2005). Risk factors for autism: Perinatal factors, parental psychiatric history, and socioeconomic status. *American Journal of Epidemiology*, *161*, 916–925.

LaSalle, J. M., & Yasui, D. H. (2009). Evolving role of MeCP2 in rett syndrome and autism. *Epigenomics*, *1*(1), 119–130. Available from https://doi.org/10.2217/epi.09.13.

Lee, B. K., & McGrath, J. J. (2015). Advancing parental age and autism: Multifactorial pathways. *Trends in Molecular Medicine*, *21*, 118–125.

Levy, R. J. (2015). Carbon monoxide pollution and neurodvelopment: A public health concern. *Neurotoxicology and Teratology*, *49*, 31–40.

Leyfer, O. T., Folstein, S. E., Bacalman, S., et al. (2006). Comorbid psychiatric disorders in children with autism: Interview development and rates of disorders. *Journal of Autism and Developmental Disorders*, *36*, 849–861.

Li, X. B., Tang, Y. L., Wang, C. Y., & de Leon, J. (2015). Clozapine for treatment-resistant bipolar disorder: A systematic review. *Bipolar Disorders*, *17*(3), 235–247.

Luiselli, J., Blew, P., & Thibadeau, S. (2001). Therapeutic effects and long-term efficacy of antidepressant medication for persons with developmental disabilities: Behavioral assessment in two cases of treatment-resistant aggression and self-injury. *Behavior Modification*, *25*(1), 62–78. Available from https://doi.org/10.1177/0145445501251004.

Mahatmya, D., Zobel, A., & Valdovinos, M. G. (2008). Treatment approaches for self-injurious behavior in individuals with autism: Behavioral and pharmacological methods. *JEIBI*, *5*(1), 106–118.

Marcus, R. N., Owen, R., Kamen, L., Manos, G., McQuade, R. D., Carson, W. H., & Aman, M. G. (2009). A placebo-controlled, fixed-dose study of aripiprazole in children and adolescents with irritability associated with autistic disorder. *Journal of the American Academy of Child and Adolescent Psychiatry*, *48*(11), 1110–1119. Available from https://doi.org/10.1097/CHI.0b013e3181b76658.

McCracken, J. T., McGough, J., Shah, B., Cronin, P., Hong, D., Aman, M. G., et al. (2002). Risperidone in children with autism and serious behavior problems. *The New England Journal of Medicine*, *347*(5), 314–321.

McDougle, C. J., Holmes, J. P., Carlson, D. C., Pelton, G. H., Cohen, D. J., & Price, L. H. (1998). A double-blind, placebo-controlled study of risperidone in adults with autistic disorder and other pervasive developmental disorders. *Archives of General Psychiatry*, *55*(7), 633–641.

McDougle, C. J., Kresch, L. E., Goodman, W. K., et al. (1995). A case-controlled study of repetitive thoughts and behavior in adults with autistic disorder and obsessive-compulsive disorder. *The American Journal of Psychiatry*, *152*(5), 772–777.

McDougle, C. J., Scahill, L., Aman, M. G., et al. (2005). Risperidone for the core symptom domains of autism: Results from the study by the autism network of the research units on pediatric psychopharmacology. *The American Journal of Psychiatry, 162*(6), 1142–1148.

Mohammadi, M. R., Yadegari, N., Hassanzadeh, E., et al. (2013). Double-blind, placebo-controlled trial of risperidone plus amantadine in children with autism: A 10-week randomized study. *Clinical Neuropharmacology, 36*(6), 179–184.

MSEPG. (2020). The history of autism. *Masters in Special Education Program Guide*. <https://www.masters-in-special-education.com/history-of-autism/>.

Muris, P., Steerneman, P., Merckelbach, H., Holdrinet, I., & Meesters, C. (1998). Comorbid anxiety symptoms in children with pervasive developmental disorders. *Journal of Anxiety Disorders, 12*, 387–393.

Murray, M. J. (2010). Attention-deficit/hyperactivity disorder in the context of autism spectrum disorders. *Current Psychiatry Reports, 12*, 382–388. Available from https://doi.org/10.1007/s11920-010-0145-3.

Nadeau, J., Sulkowski, M. L., Ung, D., Wood, J. J., Lewin, A. B., Murphy, T. K., … Storch, E. A. (2011). Treatment of comorbid anxiety and autism spectrum disorders. *Neuropsychiatry (London), 1*(6), 567–578.

Naguy, A., Alrashidi, F., & AlShalabi, S. R. (2019). Mirtazapine for inappropriate sexual behaviors in autism. *American Journal of Therapeutics, 26*(6), e751–e753. Available from https://doi.org/10.1097/MJT.0000000000000908.

Namerow, L. B., Thomas, P., Bostic, J. Q., Prince, J., & Monuteaux, M. C. (2003). Use of citalopram in pervasive developmental disorders. *Journal of Developmental and Behavioral Pediatrics: JDBP, 24*, 104–108.

Nguyen, M., & Murphy, T. (2001). Mirtazapine for excessive masturbation in an adolescent with autism. *Journal of the American Academy of Child and Adolescent Psychiatry, 40*(8), 868–869. Available from https://doi.org/10.1097/00004583-200108000-00004.

NIEHS. (2020). Environmental Epigenetics. *NIH: National Institute of Environmental Health Sciences*. <https://www.niehs.nih.gov/research/supported/health/envepi/index.cfm>.

NIMH. (2020). Autism spectrum disorder. *NIH: National Institute of Mental Health*. <https://www.nimh.nih.gov/health/topics/autism-spectrum-disorders-asd/index.shtml>.

OAR. (2019). New studies estimate autism prevalence at 1 in 40. *OAR: Organization for Autism Research*. <https://researchautism.org/new-studies-estimate-autism-prevalence-at-1-in-40/>.

Oswald, D. P., & Sonenklar, N. A. (2007). Medication use among children with autism spectrum disorders. *Journal of Child and Adolescent Psychopharmacology, 17*(3), 348–355.

Owen, R., Sikich, L., Marcus, R. N., Corey-Lisle, P., Manos, G., McQuade, R. D., … Findling, R. L. (2009). Aripiprazole in the treatment of irritability in children and adolescents with autistic disorder. *Pediatrics, 124*(6), 1533–1540. Available from https://doi.org/10.1542/peds.2008-3782.

Ozonoff, S., Young, G. S., Carter, A., Messinger, D., Yirmiya, N., Zwaigenbaum, L., et al. (2011). Recurrence risk for autism spectrum disorders: A baby siblings research consortium study. *Pediatrics, 128*, e488–e495.

Palmer, N., Beam, A., Agniel, D., et al. (2017). Association of sex with recurrence of autism spectrum disorder among siblings. *JAMA Pediatrics, 171*(11), 1107–1112. Available from https://doi.org/10.1001/jamapediatrics.2017.2832.

Parker, K. J., Oztan, O., Libove, R. A., Mohsin, N., Karhson, D. S., Sumiyoshi, R. D., … Hardan, A. Y. (2019). A randomized placebo-controlled pilot trial shows that intranasal vasopressin improves social deficits in children with autism. *Science Translational Medicine, 11*(491). Available from https://doi.org/10.1126/scitransimed.aau7356, eaau7356.

Pavanello, S., Bollati, V., Pesatori, A. C., Kapka, L., Bolognesi, C., Bertazzi, P. A., et al. (2009). Global and gene-specific promoter methylation changes are related to anti-B[a] PDE-DNA adduct levels and influence micronuclei levels in polycyclic aromatic hydrocarbon-exposed individuals. *International Journal of Cancer. Journal International du Cancer*, *125*, 1692–1697.

Perera, F., & Herbstman, J. (2011). Prenatal environmental exposures, epigenetics, and disease. *Reproductive Toxicology (Elmsford, N.Y.)*, *31*, 363–373.

Posey, D. J., Puntney, J. I., Sasher, T. M., Kem, D. L., & McDougle, C. J. (2004). Guanfacine treatment of hyperactivity and inattention in pervasive developmental disorders: A retrospective analysis of 80 cases. *Journal of Child and Adolescent Psychopharmacology*, *14*, 233–241. Available from https://doi.org/10.1089/1044546041649084.

Potenza, M. N., Holmes, J. P., Kanes, S. J., & McDougle, C. J. (1999). Olanzapine treatment of children, adolescents, and adults with pervasive developmental disorders: An open-label pilot study. *Journal of Clinical Psychopharmacology*, *19*(1), 37–44.

Realmuto, G. M., & Ruble, L. A. (1999). Sexual behaviors in autism: Problems of definition and management. *Journal of Autism and Developmental Disorders*, *29*(2), 121–127.

Research Autism. (2020). Social interaction and autism. *Research Autism: Improving the Quality of Life*. <http://www.researchautism.net/issues/3/social-interaction-and-autism>.

Research Units on Pediatric Psychopharmacology Autism Network. (2005a). Risperidone treatment of autistic disorder: Longer-term benefits and blinded discontinuation after 6 months. *The American Journal of Psychiatry*, *162*(7), 1361–1369.

Research Units on Pediatric Psychopharmacology (RUPP) Autism Network. (2005b). Randomized, controlled, crossover tiral of methylphenidate in pervasive developmental disorders with hyperactivity. *Archives of General Psychiatry*, *62*(11), 1266–1274.

Rice, C. E., Rosanoff, M., Dawson, G., Durkin, M. S., Croen, L. A., Singer, A., & Yeargin-Allsopp, M. (2015). Evaluating changes in the prevalence of the autism spectrum disorders (ASDs). *Public Health Rey*, *34*(2), 1–22. Available from https://doi.org/10.1007/bf03391685.

Roza, S. J., van Batenburg-Eddes, T., Steegers, E. A., Jaddoe, V. W., Mackenbach, J. P., Hofman, A., et al. (2010). Maternal folic acid supplement use in early pregnancy and child behavioural problems: The generation R study. *The British Journal of Nutrition*, *103*, 445–452.

Santosh, P. J., Baird, G., Pityaratstian, N., Tavare, E., & Gringras, P. (2006). Impact of comorbid autism spectrum disorders on stimulant response in children with attention deficit hyperactivity disorder: A retrospective and prospective effectiveness study. *Child: Care, Health and Development*, *32*, 575–583. Available from https://doi.org/10.1111/j.1365-2214.2006.00631.

Sarker, H., Tam, A., Foreman, M., Fay, N., Dhuliawala, M., & Das, A. (2018). Detection of stereotypical motor movements in autism using a smartwatch-based system. *AMIA Annual Symposium Proceedings/AMIA Symposium*, *2018*, 952–960. Available from https://www.ncbi.nlm.nih.gov/pmc/articles/PMC6371313/.

Scahill, L., Aman, M. G., McDougle, C. J., et al. (2006). A prospective open trial of guanfacine in children with pervasive developmental disorders. *Journal of Child and Adolescent Psychopharmacology*, *16*, 589–598. Available from https://doi.org/10.1089/cap.2006.16.589.

Scahill, L., & Pachler, M. (2007). Treatment of hyperactivity in children with pervasive developmental disorders. *Journal of Child and Adolescent Psychiatric Nursing: Official*

Publication of the Association of Child and Adolescent Psychiatric Nurses, Inc, 20, 59–62. Available from https://doi.org/10.1111/j.1744-6171.2007.00080.

Shea, S., Turgay, A., Carroll, A., Schulz, M., Orlik, H., Smith, I., & Dunbar, F. (2004). Risperidone in the treatment of disruptive behavioral symptoms in children with autistic and other pervasive developmental disorders. *Pediatrics, 114*(5), e634–e641. Available from https://doi.org/10.1542/peds.2003-0264-F.

Shelton, J. F., Geraghty, E. M., Tancredi, D. J., Delwiche, L. D., Schmidt, R. J., Ritz, B., et al. (2014). Neurodevelopmental disorders and prenatal residential proximity to agricultural pesticides: The CHARGE study. *Environmental Health Perspectives, 122*, 1103–1109.

Siegel, M., Beresford, C. A., Bunker, M., et al. (2014). Preliminary investigation of lithium for mood disorder symptoms in children and adolescents with autism spectrum disorder. *Journal of Child and Adolescent Psychopharmacology, 24*(7), 399–402.

Siegel, M., & Erickson, C. (2016a). Autism spectrum disorder: Parents' medication guide. *American Academy of Child & Adolescent Psychiatry*. Available from https://medicine.tulane.edu/sites/g/files/rdw761/f/pictures/Autism_Spectrum_Disorder_Parents_Medication_Guide.pdf.

Siegel, M., & Erickson, C. (2016b). Autism spectrum disorder: Parents' medication guide. *American Academy of Child & Adolescent Psychiatry*, 1–23. Available from www.aacap.org.

Simonoff, E., Pickles, A., Charman, T., Chandler, S., Loucas, T., & Baird, G. (2008). Psychiatric disorders in children with autism spectrum disorders: Prevalence, comorbidity, and associated factors in a population-derived sample. *Journal of the American Academy of Child and Adolescent Psychiatry, 47*, 921–929.

Stigler, K. A., Erickson, C. A., Mullett, J. E., Posey, D. J., & McDougle, C. J. (2010). Paliperidone for irritability in autistic disorder. *Journal of Child and Adolescent Psychopharmacology, 20*(1), 75–78.

Summers, J., Shahrami, A., Cali, S., D'Mello, C., Kako, M., Palikucin-Reljin, A., ... Lunsky, Y. (2017). Self-injury in autism spectrum disorder and intellectual disability: Exploring the role of reactivity to pain and sensory input. *Brain Science, 7*(1), 140. Available from https://doi.org/10.3390/brainsci7110140.

Swanberg, S. E., Nagarajan, R. P., Peddada, S., Yasui, D. H., & LaSalle, J. M. (2009). Reciprocal Co-regulation of EGR2 and MECP2 is disrupted in rett syndrome and autism. *Human Molecular Genetics, 18*(3), 525–534. Available from https://doi.org/10.1093/hmg/ddn380.

Symons, F. J., Hoch, J., Dahl, N. A., & McComas, J. J. (2003). Sequential and matching analyses of selfinjurious behavior a case of overmatching in the natural environment. *Journal of Applied Behavior Analysis, 36*(2), 267–270.

Taylor, D. V., Hetrick, W. P., Neri, C. L., Touchette, P., Barron, J. L., & Sandman, C. A. (1991). Effect of Naltrexone upon self-injurious behavior, learning, and activity: A case study. *Pharmacology Biochemistry & Behavior, 40*(1), 79–82.

Volkmar, F. R., & Reichow, B. (2013). Autism in DSM-5: Progress and challenges. *Molecular Autism, 4*, 13. Available from https://doi.org/10.1186/2040-2392-4-13.

Werling, D. M., & Geschwind, D. H. (2013). Sex differences in autism spectrum disorders. *Current Opinion in Neurology, 26*, 146–153.

Wink, L. K., Erickson, C. A., Stigler, K. A., & McDougle, C. J. (2011). Riluzole in autistic disorder. *Journal of Child and Adolescent Psychopharmacology, 21*(4), 375–379.

Wink, L. K., Pedapati, E. V., Horn, P. S., McDougle, C. J., & Erickson, C. A. (2015). Multiple antipsychotic medication use in autism spectrum disorder. *Journal of Child and Adolescent Psychopharmacology*, Epub.

Wright, R. J. (2009). Moving towards making social toxins mainstream in children's environmental health. *Current Opinion in Pediatrics*, *21*, 222–229.

Xiao, R., Sorensen, T. K., Williams, M. A., & Luthy, D. A. (2003). Influence of pre-eclampsia on fetal growth. *The Journal of Maternal-Fetal & Neonatal Medicine: The Official Journal of the European Association of Perinatal Medicine, the Federation of Asia and Oceania Perinatal Societies, the International Society of Perinatal Obstetricians*, *13*, 157–162.

Xiong, J., Chen, S., Pang, N., Deng, X., Yang, L., He, F., … Peng, J. (2019). Neurological diseases with autism spectrum disorder: Role of ASD risk genes. *Frontiers in Neuroscience*, *13*, 349. Available from https://doi.org/10.3389/fnins.2019.00349, 2019 Apr 11.

Zeldovich, L. *The evolution of 'autism' as a diagnosis, explained*. 9 May 2018. <https://www.spectrumnews.org/news/evolution-autism-diagnosis-explained/>.

Zeliadt, N. Autism genetics, explained. *Spectrum*. 27 June 2017. <https://www.spectrumnews.org/news/autism-genetics-explained/>.

Zeliadt, N. Ready or not, two drugs for autism edge closer to clinic. *Spectrum*. 1 May 2019. <https://www.spectrumnews.org/news/ready-not-two-drugs-autism-edge-closer-clinic/>.

Language habilitation through typing program for nonspeaking and minimally speaking people with autism: the Phaedrus Approach

20

Daniel Orlievsky[1,2,3], *Ramiro Pérez Martín*[1,4], *Damián Borda*[1,5], *Courtney Bitting*[6,7,8] *and María Astorga*[6,9]
[1]Faculty of Psychology, Pontifical Catholic University, Buenos Aires, Argentina, [2]Andrés Bello University, Santiago de Chile, Chile, [3]Universitarie Institute of the Italian Hospital, Buenos Aires, Argentina, [4]Argentine Psychiatrists Association Board Member, Argentina, [5]Child and Adolescents Psychiatric Hospital "Dra.Carolina Tobar García", Buenos Aires, Argentina, [6]Imagine Academy for Autism, New York, NY, United States, [7]New York State Association for Behavior Analysis Membership, New York, NY, United States, [8]Association of Professional Behavior Analysts Membership, United States, [9]Profectum Foundation Professional Membership, United States

Introduction to nonspeaking and minimally speaking people with autism

It is known that difficulties in language and communication affect a significant proportion of people within the autism spectrum (AS). This problem is one of the most important disabling factors that affect their quality of life and their interactions with family, and hence has an impact on their overall prognosis.

Through the program we have developed that teaches nonspeaking or minimally speaking people on the AS to write, we have found that it is possible to enable language through typing even when oral language is not developed and that sometimes writing enables and strengthens oral language development. There are two paradigms that we challenge, the first one is that it is generally believed that children first acquire spoken language and then they learn to write. When children don't develop spoken language and seem not to understand it, nobody tries to teach them to write, but we have seen that teaching writing can be incredibly valuable and meaningful. The other paradigm is that if children don't develop spoken language by the age of 7 or 8 years old they have a bad prognosis. Through our research, we have learned that there are reasons to think that those paradigms can be wrong for many nonspeaking and minimally speaking children with autism. Before-and-after

Emerging Programs for Autism Spectrum Disorder. DOI: https://doi.org/10.1016/B978-0-323-85031-5.00003-7

brain scans of verbal students who have intensive reading intervention showed increased connectivity between areas of the brain whose coordination is important for understanding written and spoken language (Murdaugh, Deshpande, & Kana, 2016; Murdaugh, Maximo, & Kana, 2015). In addition, we have found that the bond that develops between the children and the teachers and therapists who work with them in our program is significant.

According to a review (Orlievsky & Pérez Martín, 2016a), despite being a relatively poorly studied population, the percentage of nonspeaking or minimally speaking people with AS varies between 25% and 40% of the overall number of those with autism. According to the National Autism Association, about 40% of children with autism do not speak. About 25%–30% of children with autism have some words at 12–18 months of age and then lose them. Others might speak, but not until later in childhood (National Autism Association, 2020).

Even though there is relatively little research about the nonspeaking and minimally speaking, according to Pubmed timeline results, indexed publications about the nonspeaking and minimally speaking has increased around 40%–50% in the last decade (National Library of Medicine, 2020a). That means that there is an increased interest in this large part of the spectrum. Nevertheless, there are almost no studies or articles related to writing/typing with nonspeaking or minimally speaking people on the spectrum (National Library of Medicine, 2020b). Exploring what happened over the course of the last decade with the research on nonspeaking and minimally speaking people on the spectrum, we found that there was little progress in investigating the prevalence of being nonspeaking or minimally speaking, defining exactly what it means to be nonspeaking or minimally speaking and exploring therapies for this group.

Researchers gathered by Autism Speaks in 2009 reported that very little was known about the abilities and their needs of these groups. They also concluded that one of the first challenges in studying nonspeaking autism was defining what exactly was meant by "nonspeaking" because some individuals have spoken words but do not use them functionally while others may have little spoken language but are able to use it to communicate their needs (Autism Speaks, 2009).

Four years later, AS researchers raised the issue that one of the main topics in researching the AS is what treatments or interventions are effective in improving spoken language and communication in these children and that the current state of scientific knowledge highlighted critical gaps in our knowledge, and identified research opportunities to address knowledge gaps (Kasarim, Brady, Lord, & Tager-Flusberg, 2013; Tager-Flusberg & Kasari, 2013). Although this question has been raised, it seems that it remains unanswered and that almost nothing has changed since then, so in this article we will share more than 20 years of an innovative clinic- and educational approach. Later, in the same article Kasari et al. (2013) defined the minimally speaking child as one who has a very small repertoire of spoken words or fixed phrases that are used communicatively. Speech in these children ranges from the absence of spoken words or phrases to spoken words or phrases that are often restricted by the child to limited contexts. They said:

> *Moreover, the rate of spoken language is usually very low and may include scripted phrases that have been highly trained (e.g., I want "X"). In some cases, the minimally speaking child may also use echolalic or stereotyped language that does not appear to be functionally communicative. (Kasari et al., 2013, p. 480)*

Minimally speaking children are defined as some children who understand a considerable amount of spoken language although they remain essentially nonspeaking, and both articles recognized that many minimally speaking children are able to communicate using alternative means of communication like Picture Exchange Communication System (PECS), Augmentative and Alternative Communication (AAC) devices, sign language, and written language. None of these articles responds to the problem as to why despite access to early intense interventions, they fail to acquire spoken language skills. The most important direction for future research will be to develop novel interventions that specifically target this population, but without adequate assessment tools and protocols, progress on this will remain severely limited.

Tager-Flusberg and Kasari (2013), said that "it is currently estimated that about 30% of children with autism spectrum disorder (ASD) remain minimally speaking, even after receiving years of interventions and a range of educational opportunities [...] very little is known about the individuals at this end of the autism spectrum" (p. 468). Seven years after this publication, there was no progress with the questions and the answers. Later the article said, among other conclusions:

> *It is not known how many children with ASD remain with little expressive spoken language abilities by the time they reach school age. Older statistics suggest that over half of all children with autism failed to acquire spoken language, however more recent studies suggest that this figure is now lower, at around 30%. (Tager-Flusberg & Kasari, 2013, p. 468)*

This quotation draws attention to the lack of accurate knowledge of the percentage of nonspeaking and minimally speaking people within the AS. Although the Centers for Disease Control defined the prevalence of the diagnosis of autism in the US population very precisely, at 1 in 54 in 2020 (CDC, 2020), statistics on the prevalence of nonspeaking and minimally speaking people on the AS is still imprecise. "Around" and "about" are the common words used to define the prevalence. Tager-Flusberg and Kasari (2013) said that, "we do not understand why, despite access to interventions, some children fail to make progress in acquiring language" (p. 468). They recognized that "the literature on minimally speaking children with ASD is quite sparse and there is little consistency in the definition of this group" (p. 469). According to this article, in the literature, "the benchmark of acquiring some spoken language by the age of five is considered highly significant" (pp. 469–470). They also said that, "the majority began talking between the ages 5 and 7 and some at older ages, up to age 13 [. . .] while the majority of these children increased their single word utterances, only about one-third moved into phrase speech" (p. 470). It is even suggested for this subgroup of people with AS that: "We know almost nothing about minimally speaking older children, children who despite access to these interventions fail to acquire spoken language skills" (Tager-Flusberg & Kasari, 2013, p. 476), a group of individuals who have remained at the neglected end of the autism spectrum.

A research study explored how minimally speaking children have been defined and documented the proportion of minimally speaking children in a group of 246 children with ASD receiving a community-based early-intervention program, looking at how they entered and exited this early-intervention program. The outcome is discouraging:

> *Overall, 26.3% of the children in this study exited the program using "fewer than five spontaneous and functional words" and 36.4% exited not using "two word phrases" as indicated by direct assessment. However, our findings were mixed depending on measures and definitions used, with parent reports indicating that as many as 29.4% of children were not "naming at least three objects" consistently, and 43.3% not using "phrases with a noun and verb" consistently at exit. More than half of the children who entered the program with minimal speech exited the program with a similar language profile. Despite advances in early intervention, and access to services at a younger age, around a quarter of individuals with ASD in this study exited early intervention with significant communication needs. Our findings are considered in relation to the literature and clinical implications, and future research directions are discussed. (Rose, Trembath, Keen, & Paynter, 2016, p. 464)*

As we can see in those articles, there is consensus on the lack of knowledge that exists in this area and the lack of advancement in treatments, even in early-intervention programs. Going back to one of those, Kasari et al. concluded that alternative means instead of spoken language, for example PECS, AAC devices, signed language and written language, are used with nonspeaking and minimally speaking people in the spectrum (Kasari et al., 2013). Some methods, like PECS and sign language or AAC devices are accepted, while others are controversial.

Among the controversial techniques, two are related to writing/typing, Facilitated Communication (FC) and Rapid Prompting Method (RPM). FC is a highly controversial technique because the student types with physical support given by a facilitator who holds the student's hand, wrist, arm, shoulder or back to write. The teacher in RPM does not give physical support but instead holds the letterboard in her/his hand so that the opponents claim that the teachers move it. Both techniques fail and have problems in demonstrating authorship of the messages, as well communicating unknown information to the teacher/facilitator. Trying to avoid message passing and unknown information problems are an obstacle and to demonstrate validation, two eye-tracking research studies were designed. In the most recent research published regarding RPM, the authors said:

> *Some have learned to communicate by pointing to letters of the alphabet. But this method is controversial because it requires the assistance of another person—someone who holds a letterboard in front of users and so could theoretically cue them to point to particular letters.*
>
> *[. . .] the speed, accuracy, timing, and visual fixation patterns suggest that participants pointed to letters they selected themselves, not letters they were directed to by the assistant. The blanket dismissal of assisted autistic communication is therefore unwarranted. (Jaswal, Wayne, & Golino, 2020, p. 1)*

A previous article related to FC said that:

> *A facilitated communication user with an autism spectrum disorder produced sophisticated texts by pointing, with physical support, to letters on a letterboard while their eyes were tracked and while their pointing movements were video recorded.*
>
> *The eye-tracking data present a challenge to traditional "facilitator influence" accounts of authorship, and are consistent with the proposition that this FC user does indeed author the sophisticated texts that are attributed to him; he looks for longer at to-be-typed letters before typing them, and looks ahead to subsequent letters of words before the next letter of the word is typed. (Grayson, Emerson, Howard-Jones, & O'Neil, 2012, p. 75)*

Both articles used eye-tracking analysis and despite the positive outcomes of both researches the controversy continues. As an example of the controversy, we will quote two of the most recently published ones: in Spectrum News, by Brendan Borrell (Autism Research News, 2020), parents said the so-called "rapid prompting method" unlocks hidden talents in their minimally speaking autistic children, but researchers question whether the words produced are the child's own; a similar opinion article was published in Skeptical Inquirer Magazine entitled, "Of Eye Movements And Autism: The Latest Chapter In A Continuing Controversy" (Nicaise, 2020).

It is not the interest in this chapter to polemicize about the eye-tracking researches and the articles criticizing those papers, nevertheless we find it important to update this issue because our Program is also related to writing/typing with non-speaking and minimally speaking people on the AS.

The Phaedrus Approach

The Phaedrus Approach (APh, acronym in Spanish for *Abordaje Phaedrus*), is primarily aimed at people who were diagnosed within the AS. This mental-health tool is the result of more than 20 years of uninterrupted work in public and private institutions in Argentina and abroad, presented in numerous lectures and publications. Three research projects at the School of Psychology, University of Buenos Aires, were carried out from 2002 to 2011, and received an award in 2005 (University of Buenos Aires, 2005).The APh approach is likely to impact both the prognosis and the quality of healthcare delivery through improvements in written and/or verbal communication.

The APh started at the Infantile and Adolescents Psychiatric Hospital "Dra. Carolina Tobar García" in Buenos Aires. It was 1997 and there was little information available about FC in Argentina (Google started in 1998). We heard through a patient's family about FC as an emerging therapy and we went to Syracuse University to learn it. Once there, we found out that it was highly controversial. After being trained at Syracuse University on FC we returned to Buenos Aires and we started a pilot program to study if it were possible to implement a noncontroversial literacy program in Argentina for nonspeaking and minimally speaking people with autism. We trained professionals at the hospital, combining rigorous practice with the intent of overcoming the controversy regarding FC, trying to figure out if nonspeaking and minimally speaking people with autism were capable of reliably acquiring literacy. The first title of our program was "Communicational Rehabilitation Program" because we were included in the rehabilitation unit at the Tobar García Hospital. To make a difference with FC we defined our practice as a "Critical FC Approach," focusing exclusively on independent typing. By that time we thought that FC could probably be transformed and optimized (Orlievsky & Cukier, 2013). During this process we decided to change the name of our approach due to the substantial differences with FC and we presented lectures in the United States and other countries, such as at the MIT Media Lab, Albert Einstein College of Medicine, Rutgers University, St. John 's University, Universidad Autónoma de Madrid, Universidad de Barcelona and Universitat de Girona, in addition to various conferences and clinical presentations in Argentina.

The Phaedrus Approach was introduced with this name in the First Latin American Autism Research Symposium (Orlievsky & Pérez Martín, 2016b). It comes from the Phaedrus's book of Plato's Dialogues, in which Socrates tells Phaedrus the myth of Theut, the Egyptian god of letters. Since 2013 the program has been running at the Pediatric Mental Health Unit at the Hospital Italiano, one of the most prestigious private hospitals in Argentina. The Hospital Italiano is accredited at the US Joint Commission Institution to perform complex medical care such as heart and liver transplants, robot surgery, etc., and has its own medical school and research institute. After being evaluated over many years, this Program started within Argentina and, since 2018, at Imagine Academy, School for Autism in New York City. Since it started at schools, APh is considered both a therapeutic modality and/or an educational tool aimed at working with people with AS or other neurodevelopmental disorders, particularly with nonspeaking or minimally speaking people.

This approach is taught through typing on computers or tablets that process texts, in weekly sessions managed by trained therapists or educators. In a large proportion of our patients (our practice started at hospitals), as we said already it is possible to enable language through typing even when oral language is not developed. Conversely, sometimes writing enables and strengthens oral language development. We found that even in cases where the subjects could not gain writing skills, APh enabled different types of learning. When successful, it produces behavior regulation and positive behavior modifications. Further, lately we have observed that APh produces positive behavioral changes in "verbal" adolescents and adults with autism.

Phaedrus's approach emerged from the clinical practice of trying to assist nonspeaking and minimally speaking people with autism to achieve independent writing/typing. We recognize that approaches like PECS or tablet's communicators were, are, and will be very useful to help nonspeaking and minimally speaking people to communicate. If someone arrives at our Program we never recommend abandoning these approaches, and, conversely, we use them too because they are very useful. Nevertheless, we try to encourage our patients/students to communicate through typing because if they can be literate they will be able to have richer communication.

APh is the consequence of careful search and systematization of clinical interventions. The APh network is integrated and the Program is put into practice by different professionals like psychologists, psychiatrists, speech therapists, psychoanalysts, occupational therapists, special education professionals, etc. In this chapter, we are going to share how we work with a student at a school for autism and share some of the theories that we found consistent with our findings.

Practical of Phaedrus Approach

APh is both a therapeutic and educational tool aimed at people with AS as well as other neurodevelopmental disorders, particularly with those who do not have language or when language is limited and/or not functional. APh is taught by typing using the keyboard computer, tablet, or other device that processes text in weekly sessions, ideally, but not rigidly, with two therapists/educators. These devices should be laid on a desk or table, although occasionally, in the beginning, they can be held by the therapist/teacher as part of the approach process, always focusing on arriving at independent typing. Given the impossibility of having two therapists/educators, we have worked with their caregivers as collaborators.

One of the objectives of APh, although not always fully achieved, is the emergence of subjectivity in written language serving to enhance the relationships with others (socialization). When we say written language we refer exclusively to independent typing/writing. From our experience it has become evident on the one hand that some patients are capable of independently typing phrases with high personal significance even though they cannot express them verbally. On the other hand, the contents of these typed phrases reveal their desire to share their own interests as well as to express their emotions and their close bonds, in a manner appropriate for the person and the context. In both clinical and educational situations, the therapist-educators have discovered unexpected and spontaneous abilities by not rigidly following the standard procedures. Such serendipitous deviations allowed the emergence of emotional and spontaneous communication, which implies higher quality communication, underscoring the possible therapeutic effects which are often complementary and superior to that of functional communication (e.g., physiological needs).

Our general hypothesis is the "Hypothesis of the Available and Accessible" and arises from the systematic observation and reflection of the evolution achieved by nonspeaking or minimally speaking people with autism treated with APh. This hypothesis raises the idea that there are aspects of the neurodevelopment of people with autism that exist in potential terms although it may be assumed that they are missing or are no longer recoverable. We call this "Available." When it has not yet been possible to access and optimize these aspects of neurodevelopment that are believed to be "lost," we say that these aspects are "available but not yet accessible." It is from then that a sort of virtuous circle is formed that allows the unfolding of the aspects of neurodevelopment that were there but were not accessible.

Those of us who are part of the Program's network of professionals uphold certain principles. These principles are (1) the person with autism potentially has skills not yet developed or learned (we always assume competence), among which it is possible to include fine motor skills, visuomotor coordination, language, and emotional regulation; (2) each person with autism is unique and has a rich inner world or mental life—many times richer than the one known up to that moment—and the person is connected or interacts in his own way with his relational environment (we assume mentality and relationality); and (3) we ourselves—not people with AS—take on the difficulty of enabling the "accessible" (of transforming the "available" into "accessible"). In this sense, the strategy and technique of the approaches that arise from the APh are flexible since they must be adapted to the needs and possibilities of each moment of each person and not the other way around. As part of this third principle, we consider that to achieve this qualification or transformation we need three fundamental elements: base, guide, and tool. The *base* is relational between the therapist and the person in question as well as with their family and other therapists or teachers, the *guide* is the interest of the person with AS, and the *tool* is typing (we assume our difficulty in transforming what is available into accessible, for which the base is relational, the guide is the patient/student interest and the tool is typing) (Pérez Martín, Orlievsky, & Borda, 2019). Each principle is related to the others and results in an assisted practice such as APh. The strategy and technique, as well as its adaptation to each patient/student according to their individual profile, give a concrete form to the practice and favor a highly personalized intervention, respectful of the possibilities at any given time, specifically developed for people with AS.

The ideal conditions to start working are when the patient/student is regulated, that means: calm and attentive. Many times the patient/student comes to the Program unregulated. If a patient/student is not regulated, although it is not a program specifically designed to treat or regulate behavioral disorders, we accept the challenge and try to regulate them through different means. Many people have been regulated once the process has started although that sometimes requires an interdisciplinary approach. In this case, APh has as its first objective to optimize emotional regulation in order for people on the AS to become literate and to communicate through typing.

Regarding the typing process, if necessary, according to each individual, physical support can be used as motor modeling, always orienting it to motor independence to type, which *guarantees* that the agent of the written work is the assisted person. The motor independence when typing has an emotional positive impact on the development of self-esteem and self-regulation as well as the motivation to sustain the intervention.

Phaedrus Approach at a school for autism

Imagine Academy for Autism in Brooklyn, New York, was first introduced to the Phaedrus Approach to Typing in the Fall of 2017, with full implementation of the program schoolwide in place since Fall 2018.

In order to generalize and further quantify the program, the approach was split into three main levels by one of the school's behavior analysts in collaboration with Daniel Orlievsky. First is Level 1: Applications for Regulation, where iPad and Android apps focusing on cause-and-effect, music, sound, and pointing/dragging skills are used to increase regulation and foundational scanning/attention capacities. Next is Level 2: Typing for Literacy, where students utilize spelling-based apps or copying of meaningful words in order to enhance reading skills necessary for more complex typing. Lastly, Level 3: Typing as Communication is the end objective for all individuals (Bitting & Orlievsky, 2017). This level involves typing for communication as another mode, not grammar or syntax, where students are encouraged to expand on thoughts/topics and express feelings. The main goals at this point are to increase initiations of topics, facilitate longer typed conversations through prompted extensions, and overall, connect abstract thoughts.

One student who has received support given this method since the beginning and has made great strides in regulation and functional communication will be profiled as an example of the impact that this program has had on the lives of students at the Academy:

N. is a 11 years old boy diagnosed with an ASD from the age of 2 who has attended Imagine Academy since September of 2014, where the dual methodologies of Applied Behavior Analysis (Baer, Wolf, & Risley, 1968) and DIR/Floortime (e.g., Developmental Individual Differences Relationship-based model) are implemented throughout the school day. At this transdisciplinary placement, N. receives a variety of related services including speech, occupational, physical, and creative arts therapies. Prior to this current placement, N. attended a day care center for typically developing children when he was 2 and then transitioned to an early childhood center in a self-contained classroom 5 days a week for preschool after his initial developmental diagnosis from ages 2–5. N. is supported by his mother, who is the sole provider for him, his twin brother, and twin siblings 3 years his junior. His father is deceased and so primary care of N. has been provided in the past by his maternal grandmother and now by two community habilitation aides while his mother is working.

Throughout the years, N. has built strong relationships with staff, peers, and his family. He is a very capable boy who has exceeded our expectations and achieved increasingly complex skill-building goals. N.'s individual profile is related to his sensory reactivity, regulation, visual–spatial, auditory/language processing, and communication. He often seeks quiet, predictable spaces and situations and will actively avoid or attempt to escape anything he deems anxiety producing or frustrating. Other individual differences that are addressed in N.'s typing program include motor planning to decrease distractions and circular thought patterns (e.g., repeating words said by others or that he reads, especially nouns), tapping into his visual–-spatial strengths (e.g., scanning and persistence), and increasing the complexity of his language beyond simple needs. His initial goals at Imagine involved increasing his functional communication with use of an AAC device as N. is completely non-speaking, increasing social and communicative initiations, and increasing self-regulation to decrease time spent in escape mode, which was a significant barrier to learning and growth at the time.

In 2017 when the typing program was first introduced to him, N. presented the first four Functional and Emotional Developmental Levels (FEDLs) presented by DIR (Developmental, Individual Difference, Relationship-based model) (Greenspan & Wieder, 2009). These developmental capacities correspond to his self-regulation and attention in the world, engaging and relating, purposeful emotional interaction and problem-solving in a shared way/sense of self. The goals established over the past 3 years were mainly focused in N.'s first developmental capacities since his regulation, engagement, and communication were restricted. The objective during the course of this program has been to develop a stronger, wider base of foundational support in each level more so than building upwards.

Meeting the child at his current developmental level is the primary principle of our program, which is achieved through creating significant relationships in order to promote each child's self-regulation, eye contact, and reciprocal interactions. Given this individualized work, N. started to build a greater interest in two-way relationships and shared engagement, thus opening the door to using the typing program as a mode of emotional and regulatory communication. At the outset, N. started on Level 3 at the first or highest support level at this stage involving using choices, fill-ins, and pictures about preferred activities and relevant people/events in his life as a jumping-off point for a discussion of his interests and emotions. For example, upon being given four choices of topic, N. chose blocks and staff used fill-ins to extend the conversation (e.g., "I like to build..." student responds, "block," staff adds "With blocks I make..." student responds, "tower"). We utilized N.'s device as a way to embed more typing practice, encouraging him to type words rather than using the icons. N. was able to type phrases on his own without dictation or models, but benefited from moderate to high support to expand upon topics. Sessions would last upwards of 20 minutes where only one topic would be discussed in 1–3 sentences if any topic was chosen at all as N. would change them frequently and repeat fill-in prompts from staff as we struggled to find a connection and way forward in the conversation.

Over the next year, N.'s typing goal and level remained the same as we continued to adjust our support to find a way for him to functionally express the emotions and thoughts that he was clearly experiencing. N. would frequently become stuck repeating words from staff, insisting on changing topics, or hesitating to reply as he was afraid of giving a "wrong" answer. An example of this was when N. was typing about swimming at the local pool and in an effort to move forward, said "blue" and "wet." To try to connect these nouns, staff wrote, "Something blue and wet at the pool is" to which he spent the next 5 minutes stating other bodies of water (e.g., pond, aquarium, ocean, river) rather than associating all of these with "water." He became fixated on types rather than including emotional content. A few accommodations that were provided while furthering our relationship and building problem-solving skills with N. included typing all sentence starters, topic prompts, and answer choices for him to read, process, and respond; continuing to integrate device use into the session by having him answer first on it, then transfer to typing; and furthering his reading comprehension during his reading program to then be generalized into typing sessions.

A turning point occurred toward the end of the second year when N. was becoming increasingly dysregulated by a classmate to the point of being aggressive towards her, which was never a behavior before seen by him in school. The behavior analyst and treatment team worked together to increase his regulation through use of functional communication on his device paired with proactive coping strategies. That is when the use of both his device and typing as an outlet for emotions, needs, and thoughts really became cemented for N., bringing forth increased communicative initiations involving review of his emotions, causal relationships (e.g., mad, red, trigger student's name, loud), use of vocabulary from self-management curriculums, and thoughts/concerns about the future. N.'s level of regulation increased significantly from escape-maintained behavior being exhibited throughout the day consistently if he was not in a one-to-one session, to focused and engaged instructional control being demonstrated during the majority of groups and even transitions or downtime. Periods of crying and escape occurred weekly, if at all, rather than daily as before.

At the start of the third year of N.'s inclusion in the typing program, his functional communication continued to improve and increase in complexity, while his typing goal and level remained stalled. At this point, collaboration between the behavior analyst, new classroom teacher, and DIR/Floortime coach resulted in changes to the approach to build upon the momentum from his communication progress. Word webs and "T" charts were used to help N. organize his thoughts and the focus shifted from staying on and expanding one chosen topic to allowing him to bounce around while using previously described Floortime strategies. Two months after these changes, N. had met his initial goal developed 2 years prior, began initiating topics independently, and moved on to answer WH questions surrounding his interests.

Currently, N. looks forward to typing sessions as a one-on-one social game, where he practices more independent problem-solving while engaging in wordplay with his therapists. Adult support has shifted from moderate or high in order to expand on topics to low support using the fade-in of fill-ins or choices only when N. gets stuck or becomes disengaged. A year ago, his ability to answer WH questions regarding Who or Where based questions (e.g., "Who is your teacher?" or

"Where do you cook food?") was at an average of 20% and now he has mastered and generalized the concepts of Who, Where, What, and is now working on Why (e.g., situations that trigger emotions for him) and answering comprehension-based WH questions regarding his chosen topics during typing at the average rate of 60% of the time. He is consistently including emotional content in his typed communication 90% of the time, marking a major increase from 20% at baseline and use of a variety of feeling words beyond just happy or sad. Writing examples of this type often include the following elements: N. initiating an emotion based on a topic of his choosing (e.g., stating on his device "I'm frustrated" when asked "Do you miss school?"), working to identify causes of these emotions, and then problem-solving solutions in a shared way. Future projections for N.'s growth with typing include the same trajectory of his Floortime progress involving more shared and fluent conversations with not only adults, but generalizing to his peers and siblings as well. This case is an example of how the writing process together with emotional support makes a difference with the potential that we suppose every person has.

From Phaedrus Approach to theories

Although there are different theoretical contributions that have been proposed in our team for the APh, we will review some of them below.

From language pathophysiology, we surmise that the Baillarger–Jackson phenomenon can be similar to what happens among nonspeaking and minimally speaking people with autism. This phenomenon describes the impossibility of a patient to pronounce a word at the moment when it is requested, while he can make it when he is under the effect of an emotional state (facilitation). This was conceptualized as a dissociation between the "voluntary" and the "automatic" language. For them, the importance is to enlighten them that there is a blocking for certain language functions and that some emotional states unblock (facilitate) the verbal expressions (Azcoaga, Bello, Citrinovitz, Derman, & Frutos, 1997).

From neuroscience we learned that at the brain level, the Visual Word Form Area (VWFA)—also called "letter box" of the brain in lay terms—is a cortical area located in the left lateral temporo-occipital sulcus. This area was evolutionarily adapted to visually recognize objects and faces; however, since humans invented writing relatively recently in evolution, this area has been transforming to recognize the shapes of the letters of the currently existing alphabets (not so different from other objects). That transformation or "neuronal recycling"—as the neuroscientist S. Dehaene calls it—happens every time a human being acquires writing. The brain "letter box" is activated every time we write, as when we interact with letters or written words or even imagine them (whether they are typed or handwritten, uppercase or lowercase), completely ignoring spoken words (Dehaene & Cohen, 2011). Based on our experience, we believe that this brain area, destined at birth for a different function, retains its ability to transform into the VWFA in people within the AS, emphasizing the conservation of neuroplastic capacity. "Neuroplasticity" is a term which means that the central nervous system and, specifically, neural circuits are flexible and capable of being modified by experiences (Alvano, 2016). It has been shown that the transformation of the brain "letter box" generates neuroplastic changes in key brain regions assigned to oral language (the bilateral planum temporale and the upper left temporal gyrus) (Dehaene, Cohen, Morais, & Kolinsky, 2015) This could explain the clinical evolution observed in several of our patients: first they developed the writing and then acquired a gradual but noticeable progress in speech. Thus the main difference between the spoken or auditory language and literacy or visual language would be the participation of visual brain areas in literacy, specifically the recycling of the VWFA, which also has an effect on the neurodevelopment of spoken language at the level of the temporal lobe that is typically affected in AS (Hotier et al., 2017).

From other neuroscientific research we can see and understand how some learning interventions can modify the brain connectivity. As an example, it was reported (Murdaugh et al., 2015, 2016) that 10 weeks of intensive reading intervention for ASD children strengthen the activity of loosely connected areas of their brains that work together to comprehend reading. Beyond the connectivity improvement the reading comprehension also improved. Before-and-after brain scans showed increased connectivity between areas of the brain whose coordination is important for understanding written and spoken language. The authors said that:

> *ASD children who had the most improvement in reading comprehension after intervention showed greater functional connectivity between left-hemisphere language areas, the middle temporal gyrus and inferior frontal gyrus while reading high imagery sentences. [. . .] These results suggest the potential of a strength-based reading intervention in changing brain responses and facilitating better reading comprehension in ASD children. (Murdaugh et al., 2016, p. 141)*

In another article, Murdaugh et al. also concluded:

> *Additionally, improvement in reading comprehension in the ASD experimental group was correlated with greater connectivity in both Broca's and Wernicke's area in the Group Independent Component Analysis identified reading network component. In addition, increased connectivity between the Broca's area and right postcentral and right superior temporal gyrus, and the Wernicke's area and left inferior frontal gyrus, were also correlated with greater improvement in reading comprehension. Overall, this study revealed widespread changes in functional connectivity of the brain's reading network as a result of intervention in children with ASD. These novel findings provide valuable insights into the neuroplasticity of brain areas underlying reading and the impact of intensive intervention in modifying them in children with ASD. (Murdaugh et al., 2015, p. 2965)*

From a relational perspective, we consider the establishment of a bond of trust and safety with our patients/students as the primary axis to develop our proposal. John Bowlby proposes in his attachment theory that attachment behavior is an integral part of human nature and the form it takes in us depends on our experiences (Bowlby, 1989). This behavior is characterized by being able to generate the achievement or conservation of proximity with another individual who is considered better able to face life's challenges. The biological function of attachment behaviors of the child have their correspondence with the attachment behaviors of the adult, if that relationship works well it produces joy and produces a strong feeling of security, to achieve this the caregiver will regulate their behavior to adjust to that of the child.

Human beings are not born with the ability to regulate their own emotional experience, initially emotions exceed the infant's ability to respond to them. It is there where the presence of the caregiver is necessary, who must interpret and respond appropriately to the emotional states of the baby, so that it can learn to regulate itself. He is not going to do it alone, he needs someone else to help him, at least for some time, and it will be the adult with his presence who will help the child not to get disorganized in situations where he does not have the necessary resources to be able to deal with them successfully.

Children with AS develop the full range of attachment relationships (Rozga et al., 2017; Rutgers, Bakermans-Kranenburg, van Ijzendoorn, & van Berckelaer-Onnes, 2004; Teague, Gray, Tonge, & Newman, 2017; as cited in Coughlan et al., 2019), having observed gestures, vocalizations, and preferential behaviors, including seeking proximity of caregivers in children with AS (Rogers, Ozonoff, & Maslin-Cole, 1993; Shapiro, Sherman, Calamari, & Koch, 1987; as cited in (Coughlan, Marshall-Andon, Anderson, Reijman, & Duschinsky, 2019)).

We, as part of this program, consider it essential to generate conditions to activate safe attachment behaviors which will make us trustworthy and safe for our patients/students. Sometimes we will help them regulate themselves when situations exceed them in the therapeutic process. The therapist/educator's role is very important for the success of our task, if we do not get it we will fail, but if we do it properly we will open a channel that will facilitate exploration and contribute to the development of these people with permanent feedback.

Future perspectives

Even though in the last years research in AS has increased significantly, in the field of nonspeaking and minimally speaking topics, research and advances have been very scarce. In the last decade, as we have stated, the need for more research has been recognized as well as to find new methods that allow an improvement in the communication possibilities for the "neglected end of the spectrum" (Tager-Flusberg & Kasari, 2013). Unfortunately that has not happened and the situation remains almost unchanged.

Recently, other programs have been designed to address autism through literacy (Arciuli & Bailey, 2019; Serret et al., 2017). However, while their results are interesting and the approach modalities complement ours, these programs have as their main objective to teach literacy primarily exercising reading or proposing basic exercises of literacy, always with preestablished thematic options. These programs only have few writing exercises, but they are focused only on "reproduction" and not in the patient's own original "production," promoting only the copying of preestablished words or sentences (after hearing the word or seeing it written or its image representation, depending on each program).

On the other hand, the APh is significantly different from these new approaches. APh is not only a method of teaching literacy and although literacy is essential for its implementation, special emphasis is placed on the writings of the subject's own production. Thus reproduction is considered only as a first step which progresses to later steps that focus on themes and ideas not previously established but originating from the subject's own interests. Many of our patients have proved to be capable of original and contextualized writing production (and we start from the belief that everyone with AS is). This is far from the old prejudices such as that AS patients are "disconnected," "empty," or that nothing they can or could say makes sense, and is rather very close to enabling the expression of an inner world fully existing, connected, linkable, and vital.

In recent months, there has been a research collaboration directed by Professor Elizabeth B. Torres at Rutgers University (Sensory Motor Integration Lab, http://sensorymotorintegrationlab.com). In this study, we profiled five children with a diagnosis of autism to characterize the biorhythms reflecting their heart rate variability and kinematics time series during naturalistic activities. These included pointing to communicate, typing, walking, playing (using apps), and resting, among others. We are currently planning to develop research, retrospective and prospective investigations. We hope that these investigations will lead us to find new questions in their results and that these will lead us to project new scientific investigations.

Acknowledgments

We would like to thank Serena Wieder for her support and for introducing us to Imagine Academy. Elisa Chrem for giving us the opportunity to introduce APh at the school. To Dr. Elizabeth Torres for her support and invitation to investigate at the Sensory Motor Integration Lab at Rutgers University and Manisha Lad and Akhil Autism Foundation for funding the research. To Neophytos Papaneophytou for inviting us to collaborate on this book and to Hannah Brown for reviewing and correcting our English.

References

Alvano, S. (Ed.), (2016). Trastornos del estado de ánimo y de ansiedad -aspectos neurobiológicos, clínicos y terapéuticos- *(2°)*. GS Gráfica SRL.

Arciuli, J., & Bailey, B. (2019). Efficacy of ABRACADABRA literacy instruction in a school setting for children with autism spectrum disorders. *Research in Developmental Disabilities*, *85*, 104–115. Available from https://doi.org/10.1016/j.ridd.2018.11.003.

Autism Research News. (2020). How one communication tool may fail some autistic people. Spectrum|Autism Research News. <https://www.spectrumnews.org/features/deep-dive/how-one-communication-tool-may-fail-some-autistic-people/>

Autism Speaks. (2009). Researchers focus on non-verbal autism at high risk high impact. <https://www.autismspeaks.org/.../researchers-focus-non-verbal-autism-high-risk-high>

Azcoaga, J. E., Bello, J. A., Citrinovitz, J., Derman, B., & Frutos, W. M. (1997). In Language delays in children (7th reprint, 1st edition (1981), p. 67). Paidos Editorial.

Baer, D. M., Wolf, M. M., & Risley, T. R. (1968). Some current dimensions of applied behavior analysis. *Journal of Applied Behavior Analysis*, *1*(1), 91–97.

Bitting, C., & Orlievsky, D. (2017). *Typing for regulation, typing for literacy, typing for communication*. Written Protocols.

Bowlby, J. (1989). *A secure base: Parent-child attachment and healthy human development*. Paidós.

CDC. (2020). Data and statistics on autism spectrum disorder | CDC. Centers for Disease Control and Prevention. <https://www.cdc.gov/ncbddd/autism/data.html>

Coughlan, B., Marshall-Andon, T., Anderson, J., Reijman, S., & Duschinsky, R. (2019). Attachment and autism spectrum conditions: Exploring Mary Main's coding notes. *Developmental Child Welfare*, *1*(1), 76–93. doi:10.1177/2516103218816707.

Dehaene, S., & Cohen, L. (2011). The unique role of the visual word form area in reading. *Trends in Cognitive Sciences*, *15*(6), 254–262. Available from https://doi.org/10.1016/j.tics.2011.04.003.

Dehaene, S., Cohen, L., Morais, J., & Kolinsky, R. (2015). Illiterate to literate: Behavioural and cerebral changes induced by reading acquisition. *Nature Reviews. Neuroscience*, *16*(4), 234–244. Available from https://doi.org/10.1038/nrn3924.

Grayson, A., Emerson, A., Howard-Jones, P., & O'Neil, L. (2012). Hidden communicative competence: Case study evidence using eye-tracking and video analysis. *Autism: The International Journal of Research and Practice*, *16*(1), 75–86. Available from https://doi.org/10.1177/1362361310393260.

Greenspan, S. I., & Wieder, S. (2009). *Engaging autism: Using the floortime approach to help children relate, communicate, and think* (1st Da Capo Press pbk. ed.). Da Capo Lifelong Books.

Hotier, S., Leroy, F., Boisgontier, J., Laidi, C., Mangin, J.-F., Delorme, R., ... Houenou, J. (2017). Social cognition in autism is associated with the neurodevelopment of the posterior superior temporal sulcus. *Acta Psychiatrica Scandinavica*, *136*(5), 517–525. Available from https://doi.org/10.1111/acps.12814.

Jaswal, V., Wayne, A., & Golino, H. (2020). Eye-tracking reveals agency in assisted autistic communication. *Scientific Reports*, *10*(7882). Available from https://www.nature.com/articles/s41598-020-64553-9.

Kasari, C., Brady, N., Lord, C., & Tager-Flusberg, H. (2013). Assessing the minimally verbal school-aged child with autism spectrum disorder. *Autism Research : Official Journal of the International Society for Autism Research*, *6*(6), 479–493. Available from https://doi.org/10.1002/aur.1334.

Murdaugh, D. L., Deshpande, H. D., & Kana, R. K. (2016). The impact of reading intervention on brain responses underlying language in children with autism. *Autism Research: Official Journal of the International Society for Autism Research*, *9*(1), 141–154. Available from https://doi.org/10.1002/aur.1503.

Murdaugh, D. L., Maximo, J. O., & Kana, R. K. (2015). Changes in intrinsic connectivity of the brain's reading network following intervention in children with autism. *Human Brain Mapping*, *36*(8), 2965–2979. Available from https://doi.org/10.1002/hbm.22821.

National Autism Association. (2020). About autism: Autism fact sheet [Web oficial]. <https://nationalautismassociation.org/resources/autism-fact-sheet/>

National Library of Medicine. (2020a). NLM Pubmed search: Autism AND non verbal OR minimally verbal. <https://pubmed.ncbi.nlm.nih.gov/?term = autism + AND + non + verbal + OR + minimally + verbal&sort = date>

National Library of Medicine. (2020b). NLM Pubmed search: Autism AND non verbal OR minimally verbal AND writing. <https://pubmed.ncbi.nlm.nih.gov/?term = autism + AND + non + verbal + OR + minimally + verbal + AND + writing&sort = date>

Nicaise, A. (2020). Of eye movements and autism: The latest chapter in a continuing controversy. Skeptical Inquirer. <https://skepticalinquirer.org/exclusive/of-eye-movements-and-autism-the-latest-chapter-in-a-continuing-controversy/>

Orlievsky, D., & Cukier, S. (2013). Language, writing, and activity disorder in the autistic spectrum. *Frontiers in Integrative Neuroscience*, 7. Available from https://doi.org/10.3389/fnint.2013.00042.

Orlievsky, D., & Pérez Martín, R. (2016a). Autismo, lenguaje y trastornos de la comunicación en personas no verbales y mínimamente verbales. Sistemas aumentativos y alternativos de comunicación [Conferencia]. In *Simposio Latinoamericano de Investigación en los Trastornos del Espectro Autista*. Buenos Aires.

Orlievsky, D., & Pérez Martín, R. (2016b). Phaedrus: Programa de Habilitación del Lenguaje a Través de la Escritura *[Conferencia]*. Simposio Latinoamericano de Investigación en los Trastornos del Espectro Autista, Buenos Aires.

Pérez Martín, R., Orlievsky, D., & Borda, D. (2019). Writing, subjectivity and neuroscience. *Psychological Actuality*, *44*(482), 7–11.

Rogers, S. J., Ozonoff, S., & Maslin-Cole, C. (1993). Developmental aspects of attachment behavior in young children with pervasive developmental disorders. *Journal of the American Academy of Child and Adolescent Psychiatry*, *32*, 1274–1282. Available from https://doi.org/10.1097/00004583-199311000-00023.

Rose, V., Trembath, D., Keen, D., & Paynter, J. (2016). The proportion of minimally verbal children with autism spectrum disorder in a community-based early intervention programme. *Journal of Intellectual Disability Research: JIDR*, *60*(5), 464–477. Available from https://doi.org/10.1111/jir.12284.

Rozga, A., Hesse, E., Main, M., Duschinsky, R., Beckwith, L., & Sigman, M. (2017). A short-term longitudinal study of correlates and sequelae of attachment security in autism. *Attachment & Human Development*, *20*(2), 160–180. Available from https://doi.org/10.1080/14616734.2017.1383489.

Rutgers, A. H., Bakermans-Kranenburg, M. J., van Ijzendoorn, M. H., & van Berckelaer-Onnes, I. A. (2004). Autism and attachment: A meta-analytic review. *Journal of Child Psychology and Psychiatry, and Allied Disciplines*, *45*(6), 1123–1134. Available from https://doi.org/10.1111/j.1469-7610.2004.t01-1-00305.x.

Serret, S., Hun, S., Thümmler, S., Pierron, P., Santos, A., Bourgeois, J., & Askenazy, F. (2017). Teaching literacy skills to french minimally verbal school-aged children with autism spectrum disorders with the serious game SEMA-TIC: An exploratory study. *Frontiers in Psychology*, *8*, 1523. Available from https://doi.org/10.3389/fpsyg.2017.01523.

Shapiro, T., Sherman, M., Calamari, G., & Koch, D. (1987). Attachment in autism and other developmental disorders. *Journal of the American Academy of Child and Adolescent Psychiatry*, *26*(4), 480–484. Available from https://doi.org/10.1097/00004583-198707000-00003.

Tager-Flusberg, H., & Kasari, C. (2013). Minimally verbal school-aged children with autism spectrum disorder: The neglected end of the spectrum. *Autism Research: Official Journal of the International Society for Autism Research*, *6*(6), 468–478. Available from https://doi.org/10.1002/aur.1329.

Teague, S. J., Gray, K. M., Tonge, B. J., & Newman, L. K. (2017). Attachment in children with autism spectrum disorder: A systematic review. *Research in Autism Spectrum Disorders*, *35*, 35–50. Available from https://doi.org/10.1016/j.rasd.2016.12.002.

University of Buenos Aires. (2005). Faculty of Psychology Awards—University of Buenos Aires (UBA) [Official web]. <https://www.psi.uba.ar/institucional.php?var = institucional/premio/2005/premios_otorgados/orlievsky.php>

Full circle autism care includes family relationships and dynamics: practical application

21

Ruby Moye Salazar[1,2,3,4] *and Stacy Sue Rosello*[4,5,6,7]
[1]Smith College, Northhampton, MA, United States, [2]Karen Horney Institute, New York, NY, United States, [3]Pennsylvania Lifespan Services, Dalton, PA, United States, [4]Profectum Academy, Mendham, NJ, United States, [5]Occupational Therapy, University of Pittsburgh, Pittsburgh, PA, United States, [6]Occupational Therapy, Texas Women's University, Houston, TX, United States, [7]Embrace the Child®, Ltd., Pittsburgh, PA, United States

Introduction and background

A paradigm shift is underway around the role of a family in working with an individual child. The complex interpersonal and group dynamics of a family have profound and relevant impact on the child (previously discussed in Volume 1 of this book; Salazar, 2019). Families set and change rules, and individuals within the family unit define each other. Within a family, people change, mature, and regress, so the subsystems and alliances within the family form and reorganize over one's life span. Because family forms our first group, family dynamics influence self-definition, the establishment of a sense of self, and the engagement mode we form to interact with the world. An individual simply cannot be understood without understanding the elements at play within a family.

Relationships foster healthy child development

Relationships and caregiving: attunement and attachment

For a child to develop optimally, he or she must receive sensitive, responsive caregiving, which requires that parent and child attach to each other and have quality of attunement. By learning to calibrate effectively to each other, parent and child learn to live together in life's realities. The character of a parent shapes the life of a child, yet parenthood itself is a developmental process, where the parent's support system, unconscious influences, and past relationships all impact the approach a parent will take (Provence, 1978).

Incapable of mature speech, infants primarily communicate through behavior, experience the world emotionally, and show needs though affective states. The transactional exchanges and conversations between parent and child (Tronick, 1989) rely

Emerging Programs for Autism Spectrum Disorder. DOI: https://doi.org/10.1016/B978-0-323-85031-5.00014-1

on both caregivers and baby to signal, understand, and contingently respond to one another (Bornstein et al., 2012). Over time, these repeated interactions become the organizing substrate for the developing relationship as well as the child's developmental integration and experience-dependent development of the brain and person. In their relationship, both parent and child experience reward and frustration, which helps both to be together in the imperfections of relationships and the world.

Infants and young children with autism bring strengths and appealing characteristics to the caregiving relationships. Still, they may also challenge traditional ideas of social experience with different styles of coorientation, perceiving, and processing hard-to-read or unusual behaviors, interests, or reactions. Behaviors reflect efforts at coping or adapting to underlying physiological differences particularly in moving and sensing (Torres & Whyatt, 2018).

The connections that parents nurture help his or her child develop and promote internalized feelings of trust, safety, security, independence, and empathy. Parents understand that behaviors are communicating deeper thoughts and feelings than the words their children speak. So parents who can match the emotional and pragmatic needs of their child, including difficulties, angst, limit setting, and problem solving achieve a level of attunement needed for an enduring relationship. Shaped by their own parental models, parents both acknowledge and value positive interactions and tolerate or address negative actions and feelings, and this experience orients the lives of both parent and child.

The continuous process of attunement provides the foundation for a child feeling deeply loved. Learning to be a parent is a complex demanding role which is shaped and influenced by how the parent was parented. Notions of parenting become internalized across generations as customs, practices, and culture and get handed down and experienced through trial and error. These results are not always doing everything right. By paying attention to each other's signals, both parents and child will know if they are doing well with each other. The caregiver's responses offer the child control over reactions in his or her world as maturation of the nervous and motor systems forge forward (Brazelton, 1981).

Attunement may be harder when the child has autism because the caregivers early on may experience more difficulty in being connected in ways difficult to articulate. They may sense their child needs sameness, exhibits sensitivity, or has difficulty engaging. Sensory preferences and sensitivities and motor challenges affect attunement so that misunderstandings occur which can affect the back and forth interactions, thus compromising the "we-ness" quality of their relationships. Because this behavior is typically not well-understood by the parent, they may seek support from family, friends, or independent professionals to learn how to be more attuned and present in the shared world of the family. Attuned connections support both caregivers and children to build trust and confidence, and create a foundational sense of safety and comfort.

Synchrony

Shaped by varied interpersonal experiences, children integrate themselves with the world through self-awareness, adaptation, and a sense of self (Greenspan & Wieder,

1998; Stern, 1985). Affective connectedness—knowing and being—is best practiced within our most valued relationships, thus children with autism benefit from family relationships which value and can offer synchrony.

Synchrony encompasses both the parent's and child's responsivity to each other and emotional capacity for each other. It involves a matching of behaviors, emotional states, and biological rhythms between parents and children that forms a dyad—a single relational unit. It promotes a sense of "we-ness." Other terms which have been used for synchrony include mutuality, reciprocity, rhythmicity, harmonious interactions, turn-taking, and shared affect. This dynamic and reciprocal adaptation of behaviors and affects defines the interactions between the two (Leclere et al., 2014). To understand the dimensions of synchrony, these authors conducted a longitudinal study and reviewed 63 studies on it. They concluded that child outcomes are better with caregivers-child synchrony as associated with familiarity (vs unknown partner), a healthy caregiver (vs pathological caregiver), typical development (vs psychopathological development).

Synchrony is a dynamic and reciprocal process of behaviors between caregivers and children which involves behaviors (verbal and nonverbal), emotions (gestures, postures, facial, vocalizations, gazes) with coordination between partners and intermodality. Synchrony is a "dance" that occurs day in and day out, over weeks, months, years in short intense, or playful interactions that shift and change as development requires. It builds on familiarity and depicts arousal moments of interpersonal exchange (Bebe & Lachmann, 1988).

Synchrony impacts the child's cognitive processing, school adjustment, learning of word-object relations, naming of object wholes, and IQ. It is also important in correlating better adaptation overall, capacity for empathy, symbolic play and internal state speech, relation between mind-related comments, attachment security, and mutual initiation and compliance (Leclere et al., 2014).

Synchrony requires responsivity by both child and caregivers and their emotional capacity to respond to each other. Matching behavior, emotional states, and biological rhythms is required. These experiences, over and over, build a foundation for attachment and promote developmental integration.

Synchrony and developmental integration

To promote developmental integration, child and caregivers interactions must establish, shift, and adjust for synchrony. The child must desire attunement, and caregivers must promote it through learning synchronous interactions. The developmental elements are motor, visual, cognitive, language/communication, social, emotional—and are sensorily impacted. These integrated elements become patterned and internalized—making them generalizable.

Bornstein et al. (1988) proposed classifying definitions of synchrony requiring adjustment of biological rhythms and congruence; operationalized synchrony as the quality of simultaneous behaviors; perceptual social phenomenon unificating behavioral elements into shared meaning. These definitions of synchrony and developmental integration involve body movement, gaze, smile, emotion, and how links occur (Delaherche et al., 2012).

Getting "on the same wavelength" and "feeling the connection" typically occurs in the first year of life and builds through ongoing processes over our lifetimes. This connection is not merely behavioral. Research has shown that child and adult brains "sync up" during play, showing measurable similarities in their neural activity—that is, activity rises and falls together as they play and form a feedback loop. The strongest coupling occurred in the prefrontal cortex, which is involved in learning, planning and executive functioning—even in infancy (Piazza et al., 2019). This lays an important foundation for ongoing developmental integration.

Families are essential, no matter what

Family offers positive foundations such as protection and security, development of values and morals, and a future-orientation. Family provides support and shapes the values which structure relational interactions with others, whether things are going well or not. Children depend on caregivers, siblings, and other family members to protect them, love them, teach them, and encourage them to grow up. Consequently, children internalize overarching feelings of trust and safety resulting in a deeply held view of their own capacities and individuality. The child should be able to expect of the family an environment that supports his or her development throughout the life span.

Memories are key. The experiences of creating together and family traditions form a sense of belonging. When families build together and with mutual contributions, they offer each other a chance to be important.

The family forms the foundations of crucial personality characteristics: thinking, relating, learning, succeeding, valuing joy, and navigating life's hurdles. When these essential aspects of family are compromised, lost, or absent, the child's foundation for self-awareness and capacity to navigate the world become proportionately compromised. When these foundations have cracks, the child's healthy physical and developmental growth can get diminished. Families must be helped to provide "good enough" family health. It is necessary to acknowledge that, as children become more worldly, new individuals and groups outside the family will influence them. These happenstance or selected influences can be compensatory, enhancing, and/or compromising.

Attachment, attunement, and synchrony all impact child development and the important roles caregivers have in this process. When these processes go well, the child is able to slowly separate from needing caregivers and gain a growing sense of autonomy and independence, a process which continues over the life span.

Caregiver separation and child autonomy/independence

In the process of healthy caregiving environments, children learn to act for themselves and become autonomous by building their sense of self, which is a balance of successes, organizations, and resolution of challenges which can affect organization or provoke disorganization.

Caregivers, especially parents, need to recognize the need to pull back incrementally to allow the child space to process. When caregivers pull back, they allow the child both achievements and failures in an ever evolving complexity of experiences (Brazelton, 1981). To promote behavioral competence, parents must not strip the child of choices, struggles, achievements, and failures, and must strive to create sensitivity in relations.

It is the child's inner control and sense of self that allows for the "hatching" that is important to alertness, persistence, and goal direction (Brazelton, 1981; Mahler, 2017). But, it is necessary that the parents allow the back and forth, in and out, up and down practice of letting go, coming back, and venturing out and on—over and over again. If caregivers allow and encourage separation, they are enabling movement away and individuation and individuality (Mahler, 2017). This process happens over time in the young child's development and evolves as the child internalizes the reliability of the caregiving and builds confidence in their caregiver. Families practice this construct throughout the life span, and it undergirds a happy life.

Families living with autism

Parents of children later diagnosed with Autism Spectrum Disorder (ASD) often intuitively have concerns before the child's 18 month of age. When caregivers experience a lack of interactivity and responsiveness, they may seek new ways of supplying soliciting behaviors, thus offering early help and support with attachment (Rutgers et al., 2004), attunement, and synchrony.

Maternal insightfulness with sensitivity into how the child experiences and processes—the child's particular best ways of being in the world—is essential. Mothers also need to make meaning of an ASD diagnosis for themselves and their child in the family. These two important mother–child interactional components impact for a better quality of attachment (Oppenheim, 2012).

For all children, and especially a child on the autistic spectrum, for the caregivers, it is not about always doing everything right. It is more often, the not essence of exactly what one does, but it is the exchange and feedback and its quality.

Vignette 1: Different profiles, different families, same classroom

Children and caregivers naturally seek attunement, professionals who attend to this need will be in the best position to help the child and family. The following contrasting stories of two children and their families are intended to help with practicing developmental and relational integration.

Ivan and Billy—both age 8 and diagnosed on the autistic spectrum—are in the same special needs mixed category support classroom. They spend a large part of their days in school with the same lead teacher and her assistant, and Billy has full-time aide support. Their teacher experiences them very differently: Ivan is not disruptive, is well-liked but does not interact with others much because he is quiet. Billy is a "handful" and often loud, active, and aggressive.

Ivan is an only child of parents who immigrated from Eastern Europe. Poppi is a computer analyst, and Mama was a teacher in Poland. Now, she chooses to be a full-time mom at home. Mama is sensitive and attuned to Ivan and began to be concerned about him very early: for one thing, they had difficulty with breastfeeding. Knowing her breast milk would be healthier for her baby, she was very motivated, but he had trouble latching on and maintaining strong suction. Mama sought help from her doctor's nurse, but it was her own mother who visited from home who patiently supported both mama and baby to succeed. Ivan nursed until he was two. Mama and Ivan built strong ties because of their synchrony and attunement and loving mutuality. Poppi was also able to care for Ivan, and they slowly built their own relationship with unfettered and exciting play. But, Mama recognized that Ivan was slow to initiate and late with efforts at his milestones, especially talking. In fact, friends commented on what an easy baby Ivan was because he seemed satisfied to stay in his seat or crib for long periods of time. This quiescence concerned his parents who spoke about it with their pediatrician. He suggested giving it time: "every child is different," he said. But, by 16 months, Mama, who had done her own research, would not wait any longer and insisted on a referral to early intervention. That resolve made a big difference and got the whole family on a better trajectory. They had an early childhood educator and an Occupational Therapy (OT) come to their little apartment every week who showed Mama (who then shared with Poppi) what got Ivan moving and grooving. Yes, they thought Ivan might have autism, but the ways that they shared together how to most successfully be with Ivan really encouraged his parents. Even when Mama's mother came over for a visit, she appreciated the way these practitioners helped them get the best from Ivan and understand how and why. Ivan is an underresponsive little boy who also pulls back to protect himself from sensory overload, which can easily derail him. His parents learned how to get him involved in the just right ways and he began to better initiate his ideas and interests. This quiet boy can be the leader in play when his partner knows how to match him.

Sadly, at school, his classroom has too many students and two, who are very noisy and disruptive. His teacher adores Ivan, describing him as an easy, loving little fellow. While this is nice, it worries his parents who know he needs calm and help in initiating and being involved. They are concerned he is not in the best setting for making friends and learning.

Billy lives in a single parent family with his young Mom and four siblings. They live in an unsafe high-rise project building. Mom is often overwhelmed, and the family environment can be very active and even stressful. Billy is the third child and has a brother 14 months older and a baby sister 12 months younger. Billy has adapted by acting up often and loudly because it expresses his overwhelmingness and draws in attention. This response mechanism fits with his robust, seeking, and eager demeanor.

The family has gotten early intervention services for three of the children, including Billy, but never with the same practitioners. Billy receives early intervention (EI) educational and OT services in their little apartment, but Mom rarely participates due to her household duties. She has not been supported to understand her children's behaviors and what they are communicating and how to help. She often does not understand what the therapists are telling her to do at the end when they are ready to leave. Mom often gets calls from school because Billy misbehaves and once, in *first grade*, he was *suspended* for aggression. After that, the school provided him a full-time aide, so Mom does not understand why the teacher keeps calling her. She thinks the teacher does not like Billy and maybe, sometimes, Mom does not like Billy. She does love him, but she sometimes finds him too exasperating. Mom feels he demands too much attention, so she often ignores him. He frequently escalates. She is overwhelmed and unhappy, herself feeling isolated and unsupported. Mom likes to go out at night to relax and maybe meet someone special.

Discussion: Both these boys have autism but with very different profiles. Both have families, yet Ivan's family had concerns early and recognized the need for support. This family was fortunate to receive services that practiced family-focused developmental relational principles which helped the parents grow, understand their child and how to best support him. Their challenge is now to figure out how to get the school to recognize how to best engage with Ivan and not just leave him alone because he does not demand attention.

Billy lives in a family which is overwhelmed and disorganized—everyone in this family is at risk. But, Billy has not and is not getting the healthy attachment that all children need in order to develop well. And, because of his particular neurobiopsychosocial profile, Billy is often rejected, resented, and not well-matched at home or school. This family needs so much more than just concentrating on Billy's clinical needs. Mom has little support, and she needs help to understand how to find calm within herself reflectively, to organize her home and family and meet everyone's needs.

These two stories illustrate the importance of practitioners being aware and trained to identify and make sensitive use of the following important factors:

- The parents' life experiences which may or may not prepare them for parenting.
- The caregivers' ability to make meaning of the child even when it isn't easy or clear.
- The accessibility of family supports: both pragmatic and therapeutic.
- The importance of using the parents and, especially the child's behavior, as communicative to struggles that are deeper and impacting their experience of the world as safe and reliable
- Interventions which strengthen families.
- The ability and extent of caregiver's advocacy for what their child's needs—in and out of the family environment.
- Competently trained practitioners who absorb the family context and realistically leverage useful resources.

In summary, Ivan and Billy deserve a family-focused approach to the ways in which they can strengthen themselves and their families. The impact of feeling secure with their families is far more pervasive than a top down-focused repair or fix approach.

Siblings

Siblings play a definitional role in a child's development, with several factors impacting how siblings relate to each other: age differences, gender differences, spacing, number of children in the family, income, geography, culture, education, family health, and/or stresses. Naturally, the quality of relationships is affected by the home environment and capacities for loving relationships. Addressing disharmony or hostility promotes feelings of trust, safety, loyalty, and security.

Siblings seek different roles over time. Sibling research has informed us that the first born is often more conforming and traditional, identifies with parental power and authority, and will likely defend the family culture. They are tough-minded, achievement-oriented, and organized. Subsequent siblings will seek different roles becoming agreeable/antagonistic, conscientious/careless, and eager for new experiences. Later-born siblings are more likely to question parental authority, challenge the status quo, and/or be rebellious in the family, but be perceived by outsiders as easy going, cooperative, and popular.

Differences serve a purpose. They allow for individuation, not feeling or being the same. Deep-felt love and connectedness among siblings will involve a mixture of positive and negative interactions and feelings. These relationships offer ample opportunities for practice over the life span. Parents must find ways to satisfy the needs for all children so that no child among the siblings experience being treated or feeling "second rate" (Brazelton, 1981).

Families living with autism must be aware of the tendency toward the child with autism to get too much focus. Despite the need for attention, focus, therapies in and out of the home, balance, and fairness—attention to all family member's needs is important. When too much energy is expended on one family member, the skew for the family dynamic can become problematic. Especially for the siblings, building fairness, balance in energy and activities promotes satisfaction. Children observe the joys and stresses within the family functioning (parents, siblings, and extended). Attention to creating a family environment which is able to consider everyone is essential. Sensitivity and discussion can calibrate for healthier individual and family dynamics.

Supporting families in their lives

The child's behavior is important because it communicates needs, feelings, and emotions. When parents and others look deeper than the surface behavior(s) to understand what is being communicated, sensitive, matched synchronous responses will be made. Since we understand that relationships are the means through which the child grows, then practitioners should know how to discern the individualized profile of the child, and then translate and make meaning of it to caregivers. This approach is based on ascertaining the developmental integration capacities with child strengths and challenges through observing and studying the caregivers−child interactions over time and in various environments.

The Developmental Individual-Differences, Relationship-based model (DIR) offers an easy and sensible template for doing so and will be further discussed later. (Please refer to Figs. 21.1 and 21.2.) Essential to all things healthy for the child (and caregivers) is the overarching relational approach that includes realistic

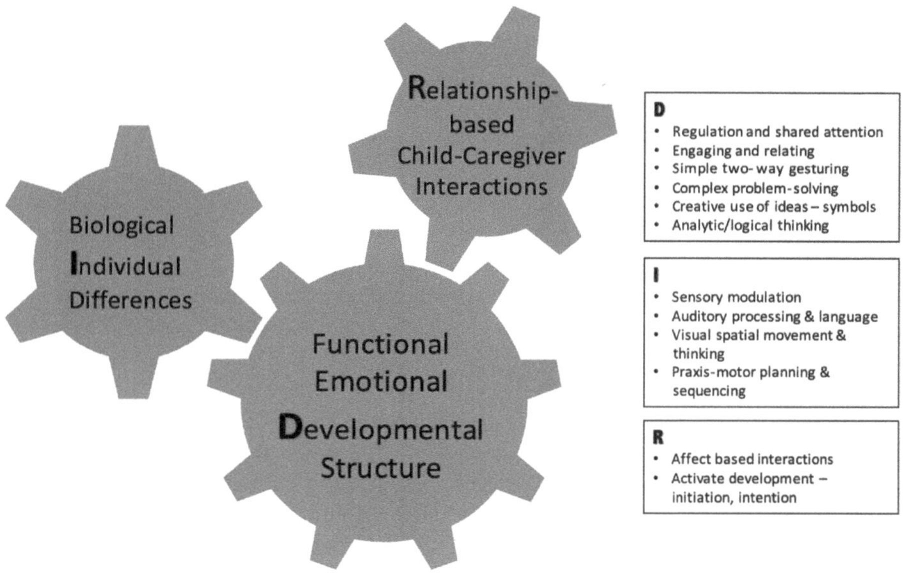

Figure 21.1 Representation of the DIR model (Developmental, Individual Difference, Relationship-based).

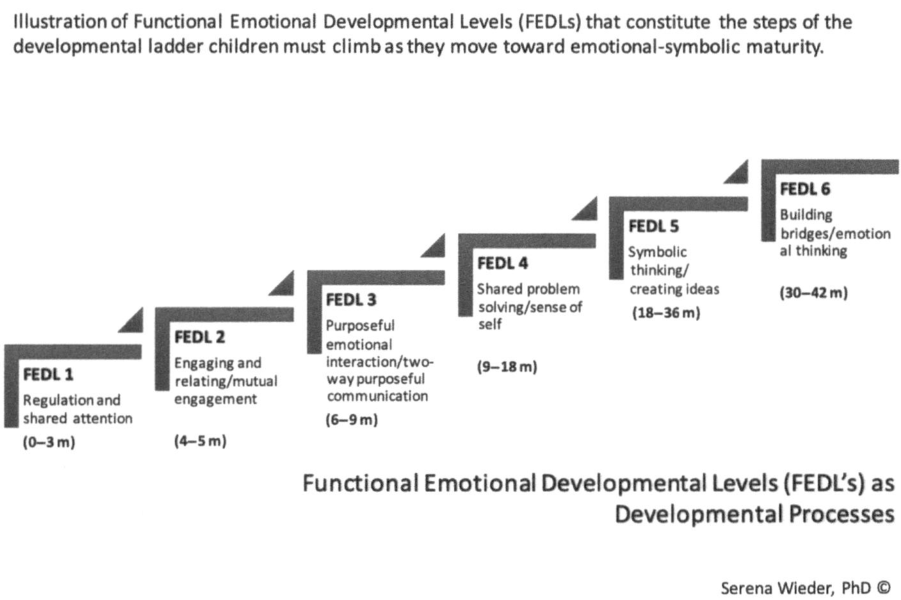

Figure 21.2 Illustration of functional emotional developmental levels (FEDLs) that constitute the steps of the developmental ladder children must climb as they move toward emotional-symbolic maturity.

support of capacity and strengths, interests, passions, and challenges. Noticing, joining, celebrating, and contributing to these engenders in the child an "I CAN" view of self as competent.

Not all families are the same, so professionals need to be ready to understand idiosyncrasies and dynamics. What is the family structure: who is in the family, where are the allegiances, how is the marriage or partnership, or how does the family function in a single parent situation, same sexed parents, or blended family? Does the family have support within the extended family, neighborhood, community, workplace? How does their economic status, educational needs, and culture impact them? What is the meaning of parental work or needs of siblings? There are more family factors that cannot all be delineated here, so it is imperative that professionals are sensitive, aware, and ready to consider and make meaning of them with and for families.

In short, practitioners need to be interested and aware of family history, how the family functions, with whom and where they live, what they hope and dream for their children and themselves. If the family is living with autism, then it becomes important to not just understand their journey, but with sensitivity support a therapeutic journey that not just considers the specific needs of the child with autism, but all individuals and family as a unit.

Impact of autism on family

The challenges and stresses of living with a child with autism in the family are still being researched. There is opportunity for the family and the individuals within the family to develop deep-felt emotional relationships and valuable life skills. There are clearly some elements to watch out for: socioeconomic disparities and stress (Delobel-Ayoub et al., 2015), getting early identification through access of services and need to clarify support/therapeutic needs, emotional, social, and financial impact on family/caregivers, especially mothers (Begum & Mamin, 2019).

Importantly, the opportunities to support families, both as a unit and the individuals within the family, are best done by use of a developmental relational paradigm further outlined below. Addressing family support, marital relationships, and participating in social activities, offering positive support and practical, well-fitted support within the family's daily life will enhance flexibility and promote individuating for family members, so that they gather increasingly positive value from each other over the life span.

Meaningful family living

Every day living and the rhythms of our days are marked by many types of activities which together define how families live. For the purposes of understanding the impact of such activities, we will carefully look at the significance of routines and rituals. Daily family life encompasses activities that are ordinary and routine, such as encouraging a child to get his shoes and put them on before going for an errand. These activities are purposeful, task-driven, and at times, mundane. Other activities have rich meaning and take the form of rituals such as snuggling for a bedtime story and a lullaby before slumber. While rituals build stronger emotional connections within relationships and deepen family bonds (DeGrace, 2003, 2004; Fiese et al., 2002; Honaker, 2007; Rosello et al., 2016; Salazar, 2012; Segal, 1999), routines can also develop and generate deeper connections (Rosello, 2020; Salazar, 2012; Segal, 1999).

The ordinary and meaningful activities

Ordinary routine activities are goal directed, predictable, and geared toward accomplishing a task. They align with neurobiopsychosocial differences for those who benefit from structure. Routines organize individual tasks and set sequences for activities within the day (American Occupational Therapy Association, 2020). They are inherently reliable and have repetition of motor sequences. For those families living with autism, routines can be very meaningful because they support individual differences. Knowing that familiarity with motor tasks elicits better motor performance (Scharoun & Bryden, 2016) and predictability of motor plans, routines provide the child and family with anchors for "doing" (DeGrace, 2003). These anchors then support a sense of safety and the potential to promote a calm and regulated state. When routines are established but also flexible to change, they can create foundations for emotional and social regulation (Chen, 2017).

While routines revolve around daily activities, rituals give rise to greater shared emotional meaning and create a sense of "being" in the family (Segal, 2004; DeGrace, 2003). The most meaningful parts of family living are the activities that foster and deepen *connectedness*. Rituals can mark meaningful daily and/or significant events. Daily or at special times, rituals are palpable emotionally experienced events. We aim for these to be positive, but sometimes they are not. When the child feels safe and connected in the ritual, the gestalt of the experience is calmer. It is in these repeated moments that relationships grow. The most important anchors within rituals are relationships.

Ordinary activities can develop into more meaningful activities (Segal, 2004). Relationships are a part of ordinary activities but are ingrained through rituals. As practitioners join in the family journey, they can slow down and identify the important factors, and use child and family's strengths to determine which spontaneous activities bring about the most emotional connection. By supporting them to recognize moments of opportunity such as a "gleam in the eye" (Greenspan, 2002), the ordinary has the potential to become valued. Slowing the pace together as the routine begins to take on characteristics of rituals, the family can find profound shared meaning. As the family evolves, additional meaningful rituals can emerge naturally and develop throughout life.

Vignette 2: Bath-Time turns into "Splash-Time" Routines turn into Rituals

The following example illustrates how, as a family discovered more about their child's uniqueness, they were better able to engage together. Their daily caregiving routine developed into a meaningful family experience.

Twenty four-month-old toddler *Roberto* is easily dysregulated and often hard to engage. He lives with his grandmother, "Abuelita" (Spanish for Grandmother), Papa, and two sisters. They put effort into teaching him how to play with his many floating toys in the tub by placing the chunky colorful people inside a boat and driving them around, shouting "WHHHHRRRRRRR." They often attempted to get his attention by calling his name loudly, but he seemed most interested only in the boat with lined red windows, sometimes splashing it in the water. Because he did not acknowledge their attempts to play, bath-time focused solely on the task of washing him. Yet, even washing him was stressful. He often cried when they quickly bathed him and wailed after bath-time; the older girls needed to be tucked into bed, and time was limited.

At 26 months, Roberto began therapy with a DIR OT clinician. With her guidance, Abuelita and Papa discovered that helping him to feel safe and secure in the world meant changing some of the ways they would interact. They began to look at him in a new way, through a *developmental lens*. They noticed that his cries and withdrawing as communicating his discomfort because he was highly sensitive to touch and recognized his disinterest was because he was feeling overwhelmed. The OT helped the family understand Roberto's interests and preferences, and the many toys were removed from the tub except for his favorite boat. Papa took more time to wash Roberto, using even and slow movements. As a result, he was more settled during the bath, and tub-time went more smoothly. After he was washed, Abuelita and Papa began to add another element, slowly singing his favorite song "Row, row, row your boat" before wrapping him tightly in a warm towel. Roberto began to show interest in not only the boat, but also Abuelita and Papa. They realized that something was changing. One day while singing they placed his favorite boat on the ledge, and he reached for it intentionally and knocked it into the water. "KERSPLASH!" He flapped his hands in excitement. His hearty belly laugh followed, and they joined in! These small bath-time moments eventually occurred more often and became fluid, filled with strong shared meaning. His sisters began to participate as well. Roberto's bath-time soon became something that the entire family looked forward to doing together: singing, joining Roberto as he knocked his boat into the water, splashing, and laughing. Knowing more about Roberto's developmental needs and how to offer support to him, the family was able to develop the ordinary into a joyful and meaningful experience. Family togetherness replaced an arduous routine of bath-time which became "SPLASH-TIME!"

Discussion: Understanding Roberto's needs and unique qualities made a powerful impact on Abuelita and Papa as they refocused their efforts to what made sense for HIM. As a result, slowly yet surely, as they changed, family life did as well. The important messages for practitioners from this vignette:

- Families can identify the moments in daily living that are either difficult or rewarding and interesting for the child with ASD.

- This information will give clues for where and how to help them begin, combining strengths, and reflecting why challenges may occur within relationships and life.
- Practitioners should help families to work through daily events of life so that they better understand their child and improve the quality of family life.

Understanding and building neurobiopsychosocial foundations in family life

Family life activities, shared in and embedded within relationships, are supported by the understanding of characteristics called "neurobiopsychosocial" profiles of the child, self, and all family members. This term encompasses the interconnectivity of the neurobiopsychosocial aspects of the mind and body which builds from Engel's (1977) biopsychosocial model. The neurobiopsychosocial nomenclature illustrates the developmental integration of all developmental elements including sensory, motor, visual-spatial, cognitive, communication/language, and social emotional and the importance of their neurological underpinnings.

Every family member's neurobiopsychosocial profile is a unique set of individual differences that intertwine and impact one another. The nervous system and sensory and motor development typically lay the foundation for these differences. However, in some cases when there are significant challenges in sensory and motor development, individuals can successfully integrate other areas of development for adequate function. Practitioners sensitively partner with caregivers to develop appreciation for the child with autism, themselves, and ALL family members and build practical ways to make sense of one another and deepen engagement.

The nervous system and relational safety in family life

Relational synchrony, attunement, and healthy attachment affect the quality of individuation and autonomy. Maintaining relational safety within the family is supported through the nervous system's most basic responses.

Polyvagal theory, developed by Dr. Stephen Porges, supports relational safety, giving rise to regulation and social engagement within families. Polyvagal theory provides a framework for conceptualizing an individual's adaptive survival behaviors (Dana, 2018; Delahooke, 2019; Porges, 2011, 2020a, 2020b).

If an individual does not feel safe, they automatically react with surface behaviors. If in *danger*, an active fight/flight response may be characterized in a child by aggression or running away or in an adult, strong anger. If in *life threat* or freeze/shut-down a child or adult may look stone-faced or fully withdrawn. However, if the child and family member/s feel safe in the environment and within the relationship, they will be prime to be well-regulated, attentive, and socially engaged (Dana, 2018; Delahooke, 2019; Porges, 2011, 2020a, 2020b).

These visible behaviors are adaptive, informative and communicative. They are adjusted within the autonomic nervous system. The autonomic nervous system balances

Table 21.1 Polyvagal theory.

Autonomic nervous system	Subconscious detection by the nervous system	Outward visible behavior
Sympathetic nervous system	Danger Fight/flight	Aggression, running away
Parasympathetic nervous system: ventral vagal	Safety Social engagement	Connected, warm, alert, attending, curious
Parasympathetic nervous system: dorsal vagal	Life threat Freeze/shut-down	Flat affect, disengaged, helpless

Source: Based on Porges (2011, 2020a, 2020b).

the interplay of its parts relative to stress and safety. The sympathetic branch is derived from the spinal cord and it mobilizes (fight/flight). The parasympathetic branch comprised of two portions of the cranial nerve X, the vagus nerve, links the body to the brain in both directions and triggers immobilization or connection (freeze/shutdown versus engagement). The neurophysiological responses are a result of the subconscious detection of the nervous system's *perception* of danger, life-threat or safety and they are the underpinnings for outward behaviors which provide information about internal regulatory states needed to support attention and readiness to engage (Dana, 2018; Delahooke, 2019; Porges, 2011, 2020a, 2020b; see Table 21.1).

Common for each person are these neurologically based responses to stress, but they are variable because of biological and environmental differences and relational experience. A response to a seemingly nonthreatening experience for one may lead another into a tailspin. Also, stress tolerance differs from person to person. Siegel delineates a "window of tolerance" that lies between fight/flight and shutdown (Siegel, 2011). Delahooke (2019) likens this area to Vgotsky's "zone of proximal development," (1978) a place prime for social engagement and managing stress (Lillas & Turbull, 2009).

It is within this window or zone, that families members connect or not, learning about each other and how to adjust or calibrate to one another's individual profiles. Together the family, led by caregivers, work to balance optimal arousal levels "to soothe and be soothed, to fluidly move in and out of connection" through a process called *coregulation* (Dana, 2018, p. 26). Families' members can build better adaptive capacity which improves the emotional environment. Tolerance increases and self-regulation grows. As practitioners support family members to attune to one another, family life becomes more cohesive and handles inevitable ups and downs more successfully.

Family members neurodiversity in the sensory and motor systems

While there are many elements to development, the authors chose to emphasize sensory and motor systems because they support or impede support to *integrate ALL areas* of development, based on severity of challenge (Ayres, 1989; Taylor & Trott, 1991).

Neurodiversity in families

Neurodiversity refers to brain differences which are a part of all human beings. Whether an individual has autism or not, all humans have neurological strengths and challenges (Silberman, 2015). When the differences are few, it is easier for families to balance between capacities and challenges. The attunement is easier. When there are greater challenges, the ability to make sensitive "just right" matches becomes more difficult. These variations are recognized as the child's ability to adapt to underlying neurophysiological development, rather than simply "traits" of a child with ASD (Delahooke, 2019; Torres & Whyatt, 2018).

Within families and within each of us, we are defined by our individual differences (Greenspan, & Wieder, 1998, 2006). There are inherent distinct characteristics which can be noted on neuroimaging based simply by how individuals approach tasks (Tavor et al., 2016). These differences form individuality, or as Robinson (2020) defines, a neurological "signature." Being human or having these individuated "signatures" is what makes our world interesting. When we are troubled by behaviors, we can make sense of the behaviors by tuning into individual neurodiversity or characteristics of how the person is within the world and with others, as we can learn to appreciate their meaning. Sensory and motor features are a part of this diversity.

The sensory system

Sensory Integration Theory, developed by Dr. A. Jean Ayres, can be simply conceptualized: incoming sensory information from the body and the world are continually processed in the brain. When the information is processed well, organized, and in sync, the resulting behavior is regulated, coordinated, and accurately experienced as sensation and emotion (1989).

There are eight senses that inform us about our world: taste, touch, smell, vision, hearing, body, movement, and emotional "feelings" associated with each (see Table 21.2). As sensations are processed simultaneously or integrated, this gives rise to perceptions (Ayres, 1989). When the brain makes a collective organized processing of sensations, there is meaning, dependent on developmental capacity.

Table 21.2 The eight senses.

The eight senses
Touch
Taste
Smell
Vision
Hearing
Body/muscles and joints
Movement/balance and motion
"Feelings"/ internal body senses and embodied affect

In utero, the sensory systems are developing and become more organized as a child grows. Rich developmental early life experiences of infancy, toddlerhood, preschool and beyond are fueled as the brain wires experiences within the sensory system. As a child interacts and learns about the world first through the sensory systems, motor development is driven. When a child is able to coordinate a look toward a caregiver with a smile and coo, we know that multisensory integration and affectual meaning are taking place. At the same time, emotionally laden sensations or "feelings" are emerging, inviting caregiver interest and connection. With synchronous sensory processing, robust relational exchanges occur and this developmental integration process occurs with relative ease.

However, with asynchronous processing of sensory information, outcoming behavior can be dysregulated, disorganized, or inefficiently modulated. When there are sensory processing challenges, information is like a "traffic jam" within the brain (Ayres, 1989). For example, a child may exhibit behaviors such as flapping hands, spinning, withdrawal from light touch or appearing uninterested in interaction. Because the processing is out of sync, the child reacts in an unexpected way that influences the relational and developmental process.

These behaviors can be confusing. Yet, they are a child's way of sharing their difficulties processing internal and external experiences or conveying their unique sensory preferences. If met with attentiveness and awareness, what appears foreign, actually begins to make sense. If unconventional responses are met by caregiver and practitioner with calm interest in making meaning together, *awareness of inherent developmental and neurological processes can occur so that the reciprocal response is matching the child*. For example, the child may be flapping in excitement, spinning because the body needs movement to regulate, withdrawing from touch and crying because of discomfort, or not responding to a social bid because their sensory system requires more input. Understanding the child's signals will support and respectfully define engagement, disengagement, or reciprocity. New opportunities and practice organize information, interaction, and meaning to connect the body and the mind within a relational lens, thus fostering developmental integration.

Over 90% of children on the autism spectrum have sensory processing differences (Chang et al., 2014). *Sensory Response Patterns* are part of those differences (Miller, 2007; Profectum, n.d.a, n.d.b, n.d.c). *Overresponsivity* often leads to a strong reaction to sensory information. A child may exhibit withdrawal, discomfort, caution, fearfulness, or body disorganization and restlessness. *Underresponsivity* is represented in a child who takes more effort to engage or tends to be "in his or her own world." A *sensory craving* child appears to have an insatiable desire for continual sensory input such as chewing, running, jumping, crashing, touching, spinning, visually exploring, or humming. A child with a *mixed profile*, which is often the case, exhibits any mixture of these response patterns. Practitioners support families when they can begin to make sense of the child's sensory response patterns and how they may be interpreted, and sensitively and meaningfully met as adaptations (see Table 21.3).

The motor system

From as early on as the prenatal period, there is evidence of differences in development within the sensorimotor parts of the nervous system related to timing,

Table 21.3 Sensory response patterns and outward visible behaviors.

Sensory response pattern	Outward visible behaviors linked to sensory differences
Overresponsivity is a stronger, often negative reaction than expected to sensory input	Seemingly benign sensation is perceived as noxious (e.g., tickles, shirt tags), strong food preferences, gags at smells, fearful or resistance to movement, places hand over ears; pulls away; anxious, fearful or easily irritated
Underresponsivity is a decreased response, than expected to sensory input; requires more sensory input for a acknowledged response	Slow to respond to sounds, decreased response to pain, visually unaware of others or environment, delayed reaction to movement, may not notice smells; sedentary, quiet, self-absorbed or withdrawn
Sensory craving is a seemingly unsatiated desire for sensation	Constant moving/incredibly active, crashing, spinning, chewing, smelling, touching, making noises/humming, visually captivated; intense presence and/or emotions; often lacks safety awareness
Mixed	Any combination of the above

Source: Based on Profectum (n.d.a, n.d.b, n.d.c), Miller (2007), Parham and Ecker (2007).

Table 21.4 Motor performance.

Expected motor performance	Outward visible behaviors linked to motor differences
Praxis includes generating ideas, planning, sequencing and putting novel plans into actions	Dyspraxia: clumsiness, challenges with rhythm and timing in interactions, uneven performance, uncertain how to use toys or go about multi-step tasks, repetitive patterns
Motor control is the cooperation within the central nervous system to direct and coordinate movements	Motor control challenges: uncoordinated use of hands, loss of balance, poor posture or muscle tone

Source: Based on Shumway-Cook and Woollacott (2007), Miller (2007), Kranowitz (2005).

sequencing, and motor control in autism, which then impact a child's motor affect signaling and ability to socially engage (Trevarthen & Delafield-Butt, 2013). A child develops the capacity to process the world and move intentionally within it as motor capacities are refined by sensory feedback and feedforward mechanisms. However, it is not atypical for a child on the autism spectrum to exhibit differences in motor control and delays in anticipating movement (Schmitz et al., 2003). These differences impact intentional movement, the rhythm and timing of interactions, and can effect synchrony among family members. Praxis, or creating ideas and generating plans and sequencing them into motor actions, as well as motor control such as balance, posture, and coordination, create a dynamic motor system and are interconnected with sensory processing. Linked together, praxis and motor control influence how, and if, and to what extent a child is able to participate in family activities and engage within relationships (see Table 21.4).

Motor development works hand in hand with sensory processing to propel the child's developmental integration. Most families place value on motor benchmarks such as rolling, crawling, and walking as notable developmental milestones. However, the practitioner partners with the family to value and navigate the interconnected motor and sensory systems for building rhythms in interactions and for purposeful and intentional movements as cornerstones for social emotional, communication/language, visual-spatial, and cognitive development to thrive.

Sensory-motor response pattern continuum within families

There is variety in the way sensory information is processed, and "none of us organizes sensations perfectly" (Ayres, 1989). Relationships in families are aligned or misaligned because of their individual differences. Within relationships "each [person] influences the other ... in a constantly evolving process of interaction" (Thomas & Chess, 1977, p. 67). Given the theorists' insights, taking the Sensory Response Patterns a step a further, these authors propose each are on a hypothetical Sensory-Motor Response Pattern Continuum (SMRPC).

The SMRPC provides knowledge of sensory and motor processing not only of the child, but also for the entire family. The SMRPC analyzes sensory response patterns in a graded manner for family members including outlying sensory response patterns in the child with ASD. It highlights variations within typical motor abilities; some are more agile and coordinated, while others may be middle of the road or even somewhat clumsy.

Knowing information about a child's patterns correlates with attachment (Whitcomb et al., 2015), but understanding one another's patterns can support interactions for *all* relationships and family life. Awareness of family member's differences or similarities—and how they fit or clash—affects sensitivity and responsivity within interactions on a small scale. These interactions support attunement and good matches which build and bind relationships. This awareness gives meaning to how and why a family may go about their daily living in ways that are uniquely theirs. The SMRPC has the potential to identify reasons for continued success or alleviating challenges in family life. (See Tables 21.5–21.8 which allow for the practitioner to begin to conceptualize family member's sensory and motor response patterns on the SMRPC.)

Putting foundations together for family: sensory-affective interactions

Sensory and motor signals are integrated and embedded within family social interactions. They are conveyed through affect such as facial expression, body posture and gestures. Sensory-affective interactions give emotional meaning to a family's actions, experiences, and have the potential to create synchrony and *togetherness* or disharmony

Table 21.5 Expanded example of family sensory and motor response pattern.

Sensory system response	Caregiver 1	Caregiver 2	Child 1	Child 2	Child 3
Overall response patterns to multiple senses	Overresponsive	Underresponsive	Overresponsive	Sensory craving	Mixed
Touch	Overresponsive	Underresponsive	Overresponsive	Sensory craving	Underresponsive
Muscle	Typical	Underresponsive	Underresponsive	Sensory craving	Underresponsive
Movement	Sensory craving	Underresponsive	Underresponsive	Sensory craving	Overresponsive
Hearing	Typical	Overresponsive	Overresponsive	Typical	Underresponsive
Vision	Typical	Typical	Typical	Typical	Sensory craving
Smell	Typical	Typical	Overresponsive	Typical	Typical
Taste	Typical	Typical	Overresponsive	Typical	Typical
"Feelings"	Overresponsive (quick to anger)	Underresponsive (slow to recognize anger)	Overresponsive (easily cries)	Sensory craving (boisterous emotions)	Underresponsive (limited facial expression)
Motor profile	Agile, enjoys athletics	Creative and pensive; prefers quiet activities	Clumsy, excels in fine motor/art	Exuberant and spirited and constantly moving	Stalls in repetitive motor patterns; fascinated with lining toys

Table 21.6 Simple example of family sensory and motor response patterns.

Sensory system response	Caregiver 1	Caregiver 2	Child 1	Child 2	Child 3
Overall response patterns to multiple senses	Overresponsive	Underresponsive	Overresponsive	Sensory craving	Mixed
Motor profile	Agile, enjoys athletics	Creative and pensive; prefers quiet activities	Clumsy, excels in fine motor/art	Exuberant and spirited and constantly moving	Stalls in repetitive motor patterns; fascinated with lining toys

Table 21.7 Blank expanded example of family sensory and motor response patterns.

Sensory system response	Caregiver 1	Caregiver 2	Child 1	Child 2	Child 3
Overall response patterns to multiple senses Touch Muscle Movement Hearing Vision Smell Taste "Feelings" Motor profile					

Table 21.8 Simple blank example of family sensory and motor response patterns.

Sensory system response	Caregiver 1	Caregiver 2	Child 1	Child 2	Child 3
Overall response patterns to multiple senses Motor profile					

if mismatched. Sensory-affective processing *is* the integration of emotional meaning and sensory and motor signaling within interactions (Tronick, 1989).

In her seminal work on sensory-affective processing in her dissertation evaluating the validity of an emerging measure, the Sensoriaffective Interactional Attunement Scale (unpublished), Alvarado states "the child's physiological responses to sensation and affective states are modulated by the caregiver's" (2017a, p. 6). Sensory-affective interactions are neuroscientifically, empirically, and theoretically supported and lay the framework for modulated matches between parent and child and within families to foster regulation, attention, and relational attunement via contingent in the moment responsivity (Alvarado, 2017a, 2017b). Learning to read the signals of a child with autism as well as one another's signals and match them through sensory-affective interactions leads to connecting socially and emotionally within families. Good signals can create balance in "optimizing their own interactive patterns with [each other]" (Alvarado, 2017a, 2017b) in daily life.

The central nervous system and sensory and motor system are highly influential for development and growth in a person's social and emotional interaction. Evidence-based neurological studies support sensory-affective interactions. In a groundbreaking neuroimaging study, interconnectivity differences within the brain in *both* sensory processing and social–emotional processing were evident in children with ASD. This finding *differed* from those with only Sensory Processing Disorder who showed inter-connectivity differences in *only* sensory connections (Chang et al., 2014). Alvarado further states that "differences in sensoriaffective integration in autism may better explain the significant corresponding relationship between sensory atypicalities and emotional atypicalities seen in this population" (2017, p. 15). In addition, the brain region of the insular cortex which is noted to have differences for the ASD population, is a multifunctional neurological structure that links social interactions and affect with multisensory processing and emotional states (Gogolla, 2017; Mahler, 2017).

Identifying the qualities within the sensory-affective interactions naturally shapes the milieu for using these modalities in relationship-based therapeutic intervention with a child and family.

> How we use our voices, breathing patterns; body language; body positioning; pace and rhythm of interactions; attention to our own [nervous system] patterns; and the use of playful non-judgmental, exploratory and empathetic interaction is quintessential to the therapeutic process.
>
> Paraphrased from A. Jean Ayres (1979) Sensory Integration and the Child.
>
> *Champagne (2011, p. CE-4)*

Champagne illustrates the process for the practitioner's therapeutic use of self. Furthermore, an understanding of sensory-affective interaction as described above supports the process of tailored matching, attuning, and connecting *within families to children and one another*. Also, self-awareness is as an integral part of the sensory-affective interaction process. MacCormack et al. (2019) finds awareness of self in the caregiver supports the child's social affective and emotional regulation, and Alvarado (2017a, 2017b) suggests this awareness leads to better sensory-affective capacity in the child.

The authors have identified 12 Modalities of Sensory-Affective Interactions that are found in the literature and practice (Alvarado, 2017a, 2017b, 2017c; Ayres, 1979; Bahrick & Todd, 2012; Champagne, 2011; Greenspan & Wieder, 1998; Haebig, McDuffie, & Ellis Weismer, 2013; Mahler, 2017; Rosello, 2018; Wieder & Wachs, 2012; Alvarado, 2017b; Gerber et al., 2012; Greenspan, 2002; Profectum, n.d.a; Profectum, n.d.b; Profectum, n.d.c; Salazar, 2012; White, 2011; White, n.d.). Table 21.9 outlines the sensory-affective modalities including language components. It also embeds experiences of rhythm, intensity, and pace which are perceived simultaneously across multiple senses (Bahrick & Todd, 2012) and can be used therapeutically to tailor sensory-affective interactions (Alvarado, 2017a, 2017b, 2017c; see Table 21.10).

By astutely spotting the sensory-affective signals of the child, in oneself and others, the caregiver and family can effectively use these signals as "ports of entry" (Alvarado, 2017a, 2017b; Stern, 2005). As they gain awareness, they *contingently match* the sensory affective state and bids of the child and other family members (Alvarado, 2017a, 2017b). Subtly calibrating rhythms, intensity, timing, and pairing of sensory-affective modalities while attending to emotional tags supports the regulation within interaction and creates patterns (Alvarado, 2017a, 2017b; Bahrick & Todd, 2012; see Table 21.10). These patterns of sensory-affective interactions

Table 21.9 12 Sensory affective interactions: types of sensory-affective signals and qualitative examples.

Sensory-affective interactions*Integrate sensory and motor signals and emotional meaning*	
Types of sensory-affective signals *Identified modalities*	**Qualitative examples *Impacted by rhythm, intensity, pace, and/or pairing inputs***
Facial expression	*Bright versus Muted*
Overall pace	*Fast versus Slow*
Overall rhythm and timing	*In rhythm together versus Out of sync*
Position	*Near versus Far*
Movements	*Complex versus Simple*
Touch	*Light Touch versus Deep Pressure*
Gesture	*Grand versus Subtle*
Intent	*Join child's ideas/actions versus Leading the child*
Use of language—playful and developmental	*Speaks at Child's Developmental Level versus Speaks above Child's Developmental Level*
Voice of the child/verbal commenting	*Mirroring child's actions and emotional textures versus Misaligned with child's actions and emotional textures*
Sound	*High Pitched versus Deep Tones*
"Feelings"/ internal body senses and embodied affect	*Fast breathing rate versus Slow breathing Rate*

Source: Based on Rosello (2018), Alvarado (2017a, 2017b, 2017c), Champagne (2011), Mahler, 2017, Bahrick and Todd (2012), Salazar (2012), Gerber et al. (2012), Haebig et al. (2013), Wieder and Wachs (2012), White (2011), Greenspan (2002), Greenspan and Wieder (1998, 2006), Ayres (1979), Profectum (n.d.a, n.d.b, n.d.c), White (n.d.).

Table 21.10 Tailoring sensory-affective interactions.

Tailoring sensory-affective interactions*The ways in which the sensory-affective signals are used and can be altered*
Rhythm: The sensory-affective modality is used in rhythmic or dysrhythmic manner
Intensity: The grading of the use of sensory-affective modality
Pacing: The amount of time between the use of each sensory-affective modality
Intersensory: The pairing and layering of sensory-affective modalities to create synchrony

Source: Based on Alvarado (2017a, 2017b, 2017c), Bahrick and Todd (2012).

become lived experiences and build attunement to establish emotional connections, and can be generalized within family activities and in the world.

A practitioner partners with a family to appreciate sensory-affective qualities within interactions as the framework to build synchrony and attunement. Identifying and using a child's strengths and capacities within sensory-affective interactions is the starting point to support social emotional growth. As families are responsive to the child's signals and optimize their own use of sensory-affective signaling, they move into synchrony. Together, when mindful of their own stress responses or "feelings" (e.g., breathing rate, muscle tension, heart rate) including the "window of tolerance," they are better able to create relational safety in family life. Highlighting individualities in the family members through the SMRPC will help family members to see strengths and identify challenges, thus being able to respond and support with the best fit. Practitioners have the responsibility to foster developmental growth and cohesiveness in the family life.

Vignette 3: Family Vacation: Working to "Fit" Together

This family tends to pair in dyads because of their individual differences. They have two children—Tommy, age 5 and *Penny*, age 3. Dad has some overresponsive tendencies. Mom can be underresponsive and Tommy is curious and sensory craving. Penny, diagnosed with ASD, has a mixed sensory profile with motor planning/praxis challenges. We will explore how they navigate their vacation at the shore. Take a close look at their experiences, feelings, and where they match and mismatch. Attempt to identify the qualities in the sensory-affective interactions used to support synchrony and attunement and to build family engagement.

Dad enjoys being at the side of the shore, yet guardedly watches his daughter. Penny searches intently for seashells under his gaze. Mom is in the ocean with Tommy, who is bobbing up and down in a large red inner tube, chuckling and splashing his mother. Naturally paired, the dyads have divided and settled into family activities. However, Tommy beckons his father and younger sibling to join to play in the ocean.

Penny looks out into the ocean with uncertainty, as does her father. The water makes her feel wobbly. She is content sitting, searching for shells, finding treasures, and lining them in the sand. Father appreciates his quiet time. However, recollecting from his daughter's therapy, he knows the importance of overcoming his own frustrations. He sits down directly beside her, puts one arm around her, and points toward Tommy and her mother who wave. "Hey—look!" Dad exclaims with wide eyes and a grin. Penny catches his eye, smiles, and stands. Dad takes her hand and slowly they walk part way through the cold and grainy, yet fresh sand. He checks in, bending close. Penny knows he is near. As the water reaches knee level, she whimpers. He swiftly carries her, instinctively, through the waves, and she clings tight. His heart pounds.

Upon arriving, Penny clings to Dad, but Mom keeps her cool and reminds Father to take a deep breath, to pat Penny's back slowly and rhythmically and to wait a little longer for Penny to feel comfortable. Penny hides her head in her father's shoulder as Tommy splashes. Mom tries to settle Tommy with a solid, yet gentle hand on his head and this slows the pace. Mom and Dad persist although not without considering that it may be better to go back to the hotel. "It's hard," Dad attunes to Penny's distress.

With time, Penny shows a budding curiosity as Tommy finally steadily holds up the bright red inner tube. It catches her eye. Mom's face brightens as she sees her little girl's interest. Dad delights, "Oh wow!" Mom looks into the inner circle. The "quiet" mother, laughing, deliberately moves farther into the tube, "Sweet Penny!" she chants as Tommy holds it and bounces in excitement alongside her. Dad sturdily leans Penny forward as she gazes and is captivated by her mother. Finally, after many moments, it happens. Brave Penny holds her arms out, giggling. Father cheers in deep low tones as he passes her into the center of the inner tube to her Mom.

Mom, Dad, and Tommy switch places and alternate holding the tube. Tommy joins and climbs through as well. Back and forth, back and forth, back and forth—they persist, molding and changing, mindfully recognizing their actions, their expressions and positions. They all move together in time and space, sometimes tumbling into synchrony, uniting, and reuniting merrily through a series of activities. Each has their own part. Different profiles and tendencies, all generate a profound family experience.

Discussion: Both father and mother recognized real struggles and differences, within themselves, within the children based on the neurobiopsychosocial profiles of each of the family members. Achieving synchrony took considerable willful effort to tailor their interactions to attune to one another, not always reaching success, but they persevered.

- Using the qualities of the sensory-affective interactions and understanding of individuality, builds the framework and offers greater possibilities for supporting the "fit" within families.
- Mismatches are likely to occur but can be viewed as learning opportunities.
- As the "fit" becomes more adaptive in families, developmental integration has greater potential to take place for the child and others.
- This process develops over time, often first with the practitioner present and then, it transfers and generalizes to other areas of family life so that self-awareness of and attunement with one another affects quality of togetherness.

Developmental, individual-differences, relationship-based model (DIR): a template for optimal relating and learning

We have been exploring the importance of identifying and using the individual differences that exist in a child with autism and in a family with all family members in order to better promote high quality synchrony, attunement, and healthy attachments. This is in the service of building a child's strong and autonomous sense of self as a competent person—to show that child that he or she is worthy of being loved and capable of loving. Across professional disciplines, DIR practitioners learn a detailed understanding of sensory and motor development and pragmatically utilize sensory-affective modalities as part of intervention. In identifying individual differences by understanding developmental details, we recognize that these differences take many forms. To further support social emotional development, DIR practitioners also delve into the intricacies and interplay of communication/speech and language, visual spatial, and cognition. They make meaning around this interplay and accompanying behaviors all which inform families to be even more sensitive to individual nuances and how they impact relationships and family life. Any combination of these developmental elements can impact relating and learning within relationships for caregivers and their children, especially their child with autism.

Consideration must also be given to language capacities including comprehension, attention, modulation, and self-regulation. Noticed behaviors such as anxiety, mood lability, impulsivity, overactivity, aggression, or excessive-withdrawal are the child's communications of the need for help. These behaviors are an important place for parents and practitioners to start and will need sensitive responses, so the child feels met and understood. However, the behaviors are the start of a deeper, more important set of developmental and relational factors which should be determined and used.

In such focused and detailed developmental formulations, the practitioner is directed to the DIR (Developmental, Individual-Differences, Relationship-based) model developed by Greenspan and Wieder (1998, 2001, 2006). Taking into consideration overt behaviors, this model offers a practical template for determining the individual neurobiopsychosocial profile of the child, children and caregivers within the family system and across other environments. Please see Fig. 21.1 to better understand the dynamic systems and how they influence each other.

An important part of being together and loving is engaging with sincere and deep interest in understanding another person's full self. Their intentions, preferences, and even passions, along with frustrations, avoidances, and failures all contribute to their individuality. DIR propagates this holistic, individualized approach and offers many valuable techniques to make use of relationships in the service of connecting with specifics and details about one another. Floortime, which is informed quality play, is one of these techniques. Often caregivers, loving their child, do not know how to play, relate, or make sense of their child's sometimes mysterious behaviors. Relating with shared meanings, practitioners can help parents and others to understand the details of how a child can function successfully and what derails that "feel good" integrated developmental functioning. As "I" individual characteristics are understood, parents can learn how to match, shift, recalibrate, and enjoin with their child.

In the DIR template the "D" provides a constant awareness of processes important in relational sequences for regulating, attending, engaging, sharing meanings, problem solving, and using ideas creatively and symbolically so as to think analytically and logically. Such processes are intensely and constantly affected by the "R" relationships. When relationships are fundamentally attuned, connected, and sensitive to micromoments of shared meanings, higher functioning will happen. Please see Fig. 21.2 that explains and illustrates the interplay and ongoing developmental processes.

The big picture: daily family living in action

The authors have emphasized, when the foundations of synchrony and attunement in the development of healthy "enough" attachment are in place, development integrates, functioning is stronger, and individuality is understood and valued. These processes are sometimes compromised and challenging due to many things, such as environment, life circumstances, or biological barriers. Yet, these realities of life can be supported through the therapeutic process and by putting necessary supports in place.

Each child is valued for his or her exceptionality and no matter the make-up, each family member offers unique contributions, as well as regrets and challenges to family life. Establishing opportunities for all to participate and fostering development in daily family living in both ordinary activities and those that deepen relationships is fundamental.

Participating in family life activities together

Through family activities, the family can grow their understanding of the child in both unconventional and conventional ways. With patience, a creative eye, and a developmentally and relationship-based focus, the child *can* be involved. With a strength-based focus, even unconventional ways *can* be considered contributions.

This contribution may be as simple as having the child *present*. Without pressure to fully engage, the stage is set for a child to see what the family is doing. Presence offers the periodic "check-in" with family members, giving a secure base for the child to feel appreciated and loved. Perhaps through this connection, there may be the chance to spark an interest for the child to be involved, even if unconventionally.

Another way to *include* the child more fully is by tailoring the activity to the child's sensory and motor response patterns including interests. Considering ways in which the child or family member, task, or environment can be adapted allows for better possibility of success (Dunn et al., 2003). There are a myriad of options, all dependent on many variables, but with the child's individual differences in mind, the likelihood of success increases.

The goal for some activities may be to *participate* in more conventional ways over time. Creating competence in simple actions will lead to more robust confidence (Osgood, 2020). This competence and confidence promotes participation, enhancing the child's autonomy and family life. Depending on the child and/or family members, participation within the activities will be determined by development and neurobiopsychosocial profiles, interests, preferences, and the nature of activity itself.

Table 21.11 identifies a reflective way for the practitioner to consider with the family ways that the child may be involved in family life.

Conclusion

When a family first comes for services, they usually come because the child is referred. A doctor, teacher, or the parents themselves have recognized that something is of concern about the child. The practitioner rightly begins by trying to understand the child.

The practical question, though, is how to understand the child without understanding their family. As we have shown, the quality of care improves dramatically when practitioners put the family relationships at the center of their approach.

To begin understanding the profile of the child, a practitioner starts by creating a setting where the child and caregiver (or caregivers) interact in a way that reveals something about their lives. A skilled practitioner looks for attunement between parent and child. They look for synchrony. This is possible through gathering information, conversation, activities, or play. By looking for capacities in the child AND

Table 21.11 Reflective analysis of everyday family living activities.

Activities for everyday family living	Given relational attunement and safety, how *can* a child take part through presence, inclusion, or participation and offer a contribution to family, based on his or her developmental level, strengths, interests, sensory response pattern/s, and motor profile?
Daily routines: morning Daily routines: bedtime Daily routines: entire daily schedule Mealtimes Self-care/self-help (e.g., dressing, bathing, grooming) School (e.g., homework, educational activities) Social opportunities Community activities (e.g., park, market, fair, music, theater, therapies, medical appointments, church, grocery store, amusement park, hike) Play (e.g., developmentally appropriate) Sleep and rest Holidays/celebrations (e.g., Christmas, Hanukkah, Birthdays) Child-rearing (e.g., values, spirituality, volunteering, discipline, sibling rivalry, growing autonomy)	

Source: Based on American Occupational Therapy Association (2020), Rosello et al. (2016), Honaker (2007), Honaker et al. (2006).

capacities in the caregiver, the practitioner can see connections. By seeing where they match or diverge, the practitioner is able to assess the authentic relationship of the child to caregiver. By adding piece to piece, the practitioner begins to see what the relationship really looks like.

Expectations matter a great deal.

More often than not, caregivers come for services with the idea that the child can somehow be fixed. The caregiver enters the situation with fantasies and preconceived notions of what a good life for the child should be. As soon as a parent knows they will become a parent, they begin to dream about the life of the child. The parents imagine their child one day matriculating at their own alma mater, taking over a family business, or volunteering in the family church. All of these ideas that the parents bring shape how they see succeed in the treatment and shape what they want for their child.

Practitioners must be sensitive to caregivers' dreams, but they must also shape the relationship in an authentic and realistic way. They must set an aspiration for the parent to meet their child where the child really is. The parent cannot simply drop off a child, head for a coffee, and return to a fixed child. Both caregiver and child must work together to improve the quality of their lives and to ensure that the child is on a path to independence.

Though the caregiver–child relationship is of primary importance, children also exist in a broader ecosystem. Too often we have seen families orient their lives around autism and the child in need. But other concerns also matter, families have to be able to have a range of motivations, sources of happiness, and feelings of purpose.

Consequently, the practitioner must probe to understand the broader context. Do the parents have a strong relationship? Are the siblings positively shaping the daily experience of the child? Does a family member struggle with mental illness? Is the family financially stable? Does an aunt's addiction create anxiety for the extended family? Is unrest in society upending the neighborhood? Should a sibling's or another family member's needs be prioritized? What are the rhythms of daily family life? What brings the child and family together or gives meaning to their days? Where do they find joy? How do upsets in routine daily life activities impact relationships and vice versa? These kinds of questions must be integrated into treatment.

Sociocultural context impacts parenting practices and should always be considered. Cultural context shapes parenting styles and may determine if the parent is predisposed to an authoritative or permissive approach. Societal inequities, like racism, religious discrimination, or sexism, may also be impacting the experiences of the dyad. Perhaps a child has visual sensitivities and would be more integrated in the suburbs than the city. Different cultures have different ideas about how a family can help a child be at his or her best.

Of the various models for treatment and engagement, the DIR model does the best job of integrating the child's ecosystem into the child's treatment. It maps the functioning and individuality of a child, while still recognizing the critical role of significant relationships. This model guides practitioners to spot the processes of regulation and shared attention, engaging and relating, two-way gesturing, problem solving, use of ideas and symbols and analytic/logical thinking. DIR trained professionals know how individual neurobiopsychosocial differences and affectual exchanges impact these processes.

Research of the DIR model by Casenhiser, Binns, McGill, Murderer, and Shanker (2014), Solomon et al. (2014) have further substantiated the approach, but building a broader evidence base would ensure DIR applies with equal efficacy to more diverse populations. Specifically, we see value in further research into its application to racial, ethnic, and cultural minorities.

In the end, the healthiest families stop trying to fix each other. They recognize each other's capabilities, passions, and propensities, while still acknowledging each family member may express their individuality in a way that grates on others or diminishes the family's sense of itself. A family becomes more synchronous through understanding, tolerance, and a shared commitment to grow together.

Life begins with family, and family is a process. It's unlikely that a magical moment of togetherness or perfection will be found, but through the realities of time and the complexities of life, families form the bonds that truly matter.

Vignette 4: Unexpected turn of events

This final vignette offers a gestalt illustrating how practitioners were able to support a family living with autism over time. By first building foundations of trust and security and capitalizing on strengths, the family provided for the needs of their child and family as a whole. Through their own valued process, they grew in understanding acceptance of themselves and their child, generating a profound deep love. With therapeutic support, their relationships became stronger as they navigated the realities of family life.

Five-year-old *Damien's* behaviors were confusing for his family. While highly verbal, he also exhibited frustration in daily family life. Morning routines were hectic and trying to get out of the home was nearly impossible. Mom and Dad, as responsible professionals, had to get to work on time and needed a more efficient morning routine. Damien preferred to wear a particular type of shorts and a soft shirt every day, and if the clothes were not available, he would cry. He insisted that the morning activities were the same each day and his parents complied. His mother often was indulgent to avoid aggression. Father distanced himself by making breakfast. In numerous daily life scenarios, Damien had a sequence, and the family followed suit to keep the peace.

The family began therapy with a DIR mental health professional who understood that Damien's behaviors communicated his needs to be comfortable and his feelings, and that the family's response promoted dysregulation rather than coregulation. She helped them understand that Damien's sensory sensitivities along with separation pangs underlaid the overt frustration behaviors. Damien was demonstrating a need to feel safe, loved, and secure, rather than exhibiting obstinance. With their practitioner's help, they realized Damien's communications expressed his needs to connect with his parents before separating for the day and that his sensitivity to clothing needed to be respected. Therefore, Dad and Damien, who both woke up early, used their time together by doing large motor activities such as kicking the soccer ball. Mom and Damien selected his clothes for the next day after tubby with Mom choosing the bottom and Damien selecting among three tops. When Mom realized that Damien preferred soft clothes, she was able to be more flexible.

Through the therapeutic process, the mental health clinician recognized that Damien appeared to have a mixed sensory profile, and while highly verbal, also seemed to have challenges creating shared meaning, even in context, and specifically around change. For this reason, she made referrals to an occupational therapist to help sort out his sensory response patterns as well as a speech language pathologist to better support his communication. In addition, she was in touch with his specialized preschool team to facilitate a better learning environment, as some of the aggressive behaviors were occurring there as well.

Overtime, Mom and Dad began to understand Damien, which improved family life and relationships. The occupational therapist helped them tailor their sensory-affective interactions to match Damien's individuality. The speech language pathologist provided an understanding that even though Damien was highly verbal, his comprehension challenges manifested as resistance. The professional team partnered with the parents to integrate these insights into the school program. While life still had upsets, Damien's caregiving at home and school became better attuned and developmental integration improved. Their relationships deepened, the rhythms of family and school life became more in sync and meaningful.

A year later they decided to try something they had been reluctant to do and go to a soccer game. Damien's mother excitedly recorded parts of this important event. Damien was sometimes sensitive to crowds, but they decided it was worth a try. In planning, they smartly arrived early and chose seats high in the stands to enjoy great views. Damien asked for spicy nachos with cheese! There he went in his new soccer shirt and ball.

Just before going through the gate, Damien ran down the long path leading to the riverfront. His father took this sign as an opportunity, recognizing he was excited. Rather than pushing Damien to go into the gate, his parents followed his lead and father and son began to play soccer. Mother videoed the unexpected turn of events, sharing in the fun as they carried on together for at least 15 minutes.

On their way to their seats, the concession line was long, crowded, and noisy. Because Damien really wanted his snack, he supported himself by holding his hands to his ears and then, with Mom, sang a favorite song. From his bleacher seat, he watched the boats on the river and ate his nachos. They relaxed before their team scored the first goal. This is when Dad could not contain himself, and in his enthusiasm, he lifted little Damien onto his shoulders. Damien cried at the unexpected movement. Mom noticed his distress, and brought Damien into her lap, snuggled him into her arms and they read a favorite soccer book. The family stayed a bit longer, but soon left in order for Damien to experience the positiveness of this event.

Sharing this experience and the video with their DIR team, together they assessed the outing. They reflected on their hopes for what the family experience may have been, including disappointments and what they might have done differently. The various team members were able to underscore their success by how Damien happily described the event. In reviewing their soccer game story they realized the great meaning in the shared "pregame" as well as the ability to have successful shared moments in the stadium. "One day we will stay for the whole game, but, for now we really enjoyed those moments more than we expected. For Damien and *our* family, *it was just right*."

References

Alvarado, C. (2017a). *The sensory affective interactional attunement scale: Development and preliminary validation of a measure geared toward interactional enhancement between-primary caregivers and their young children with autism spectrum disorder* (Unpublished Doctoral Dissertation). Santa Barbara, CA: Fielding Graduate University.

Alvarado, C. (2017b). *Promoting enhanced shared attention and shared positive affect in parent mediated autism intervention; preliminary validation of the sensory affective interactional attuenment scale. Relationships the key to progress*. Newark, NJ: Profectum.

Alvarado, C. (2017c). *The sensory affective interactional attunement scale manual.* [Unpublished Assessment].

American Occupational Therapy Association. (2020). Occupational therapy practice framework: Domain and process (4th ed.). *American Journal of Occupational Therapy, 74* (Suppl. 2). Advance online publication.

Ayres, A. J. (1979). *Sensory integration and the child*. Western Psychological Services.

Ayres, A. J. (1989). *Sensory integration and the child*. Western Psychological Services.

Bahrick, L. E., & Todd, J. T. (2012). Multisensory processing in autism spectrum disorders: Intersensory processing disturbance as a basis for atypical development. In B. E. Stein (Ed.), *The new handbook of multisensory processes* (pp. 657–674). Cambridge, MA: MIT Press.

Bebe, B., & Lachmann, F. M. (1988). The contribution of mother-infant mutual influence to the origins of self and object representations. *Psychoanalytic Psychology*, *5*(4), 305–337. Available from https://doi.org/10.1037/0736-9735.5.4.305.

Begum, R., & Mamin, F. A. (2019). Impact of autism spectrum disorder on family. *Open Access*, *9*, 244. Available from https://doi.org/10.35248/2165-7890.19.09.244.

Bornstein, M. H., Britto, P. R., & Nonoyama-Tarumi, Y. (2012). Visual habituation in human infants: Developmental and rearing circumstances. *Psychological Research*, *83*(1), 16–31.

Bornstein, M. H., Germaine, M., & Lecuyer, R. (1988). Visual habituation in human infants: Developmental and rearing circumstances. *Psychological Research*, *50*, 130–133.

Brazelton, T. B. (1981). *On becoming a family: The growth of attachment*. New York: A Merloyd Lawrence Book, Delta/Seymour Lawrence, Dell Publishing Co., Inc.

Casenhiser, D. M., Binns, A., McGill, F., Murderer, P., & Shanker, S. G. (2014). Measuring and supporting language function for children with autism: Evidence from a randomized control trial of a social-interaction-based therapy. *Journal of Autism and Developmental Disorders*, *43*(3), 846–857.

Champagne, T. (2011). Attachment, trauma and occupational therapy practice (CE article). *OT Practice*, *16*(5), CE-1–CE-8.

Chang, Y. S., Owen, J. P., Desai, S. S., Hill, S. S., Arnett, A. B., Harris, J., . . . Mukherjee, P. (2014). Autism and sensory processing disorders: Shared white matter disruption in sensory pathways but divergent connectivity in social-emotional pathways. *PLoS One*, *9*(7), e103038. Available from https://doi.org/10.1371/journal.pone.0103038.

Chen, F. (2017). Everyday family routine formation: A source of the development of emotional regulation in young children. In M. Fleer, F. Gonzalez Rey, & N. Versov (Eds.), *Perezhizvanie Emotions and Subjectivity* (p. 129). Singapore: Springer Nature. Retrieved September 10, 2017. <https://books.google.com/books?hl = en&lr = lang_en&id = t64sDwAAQBAJ&oi = fnd&pg = PA129&dq = families + reactions + to + child%27s + autism&ots = E1QklGi8Du&sig = OVNDfOCSgCStwDtUqJ8oQZf4R80#v = onepage&q = families%20reactions%20to%20child%20autism&f = false>.

Dana, D. (2018). *The polyvagal theory in therapy. Engaging the rhythm of regulation*. New York: W.W. Norton and Company.

DeGrace, B. (2003). Occupation-based and family centered care: A challenge for current practice. *American Journal of Occupational Therapy*, *57*(3), 347–350.

DeGrace, B. (2004). The everyday occupation of families with children with autism. *American Journal of Occupational Therapy*, *58*(5), 543–550.

Delahooke, M. (2019). *Beyond behaviors*. Eau Claire, WI: PESI.

Delaherche, E., Chetouani, M., Mahdhaoui, A., Saint George, C., Viaux, S., & Cohen, D. (2012). Interpersonal synchrony: A survey of evaluation methods across disciplines. *IEEE Transitions on Affective Computing*, *3*(3), 345–365.

Delobel-Ayoub, M., Ehlinger, V., Klapouszczak, D., Maffre, T., Raynaud, J. P., Delprerre, C., & Arnaud, C. (2015). Socioeconomic desparities and prevalence of autism spectrum disorder and intellectual disability. *PLoS One*, *10*(11), eO141064.

Dunn, W., Brown, C., & Youngstrom, M. J. (2003). Ecological model of occupation. In P. Kramer, J. Hinojosa, & C. Brasic Royeen (Eds.), *Perspectives of human occupation* (pp. 22–263). Baltimore, MD: Lippincott Williams & Wilkins.

Engel, G. L. (1977). The need for a new medical model. The challenge for biomedicine. *Science (New York, N.Y.)*, *196*(4286), 129–136.

Fiese, B., Tomocho, T., Douglas, M., Josephs, K., Poltrock, S., & Baker, T. (2002). A review of fifty years of research on naturally occurring routines and rituals: Cause for celebration. *Journal of Family Psychology*, *16*(4), 381–390.

Gerber, S., Cervenka, L., & Ricamato. (2012). *The language acquisition process in assessment as intervention.* DIR functional emotional developmental levels 1-3. [Videopodcast] retrieved from: <https://www.profectum.org>.

Gogolla, N. (2017). Primer the insular cortex. *Current Biology Magaizine*, *27*, R573–R591.

Greenspan, S. (2002, November 8). Autism and disorders of relating and communicating. Improving long term outcomes. The latest advances in psychological, biomedical, educational approaches and technology. In *Interdisciplinary council on development and learning 6th international conference*. Tysons Corner, VA.

Greenspan, S., & Wieder, S. (2006). *Engaging autism.* Cambridge, MA: De Capo Press.

Greenspan, S. I., & Wieder, S. (1998). *The child with special needs: Encouraging intellectual and emotional growth.* Reading, MA: Perseus Books. Addison-Wesley.

Haebig, E., McDuffie, A., & Ellis Weismer, S. (2013). The contribution of two categories of parent verbal responsiveness to later language for toddlers and preschoolers on the autism spectrum. *American Journal of Speech-Language Pathology*, *22*(1), 57–70. Available from https://doi.org/10.1044/1058-0360(2012/11-0004).

Honaker, D. (2007). *Family L.I.F.E. (Looking in Family Experiences).* [Unpublished Assessment].

Honaker, D., Santore, A., & Unger, I. (2006). Car pools, vacations, and holiday dinners: Defining family occupations. *Elizabethtown College Journal of Occupational Therapy*, 2–38.

Kranowitz, C. S. (2005). *The out-of-sync child: Recognizing and coping with sensory processing disorder.* New York: A Skylight Press Book/A Perigee Book.

Leclere, C., Viaux, S., Avril, M., Achard, C., Chetouani, M., Missonnier, S., & Cohen, D. (2014). *Why synchrony matters during mother-child interactions: A systematic review.* Paris, France: Institut des Systemes Intelligents et de Robotiques, CNRS, UMR 7222, Universite Pierre t Marie Curie.

Lillas, L., & Turbull, J. (2009). *Infant/child mental health. Early intervention and relationship-based therapies. A neurorelational framework for interdisciplinary practice.* New York: W.W. Norton Company, Inc..

MacCormack, J. K., Castro, V., Halberstadt, A. G., & Rogers, M. L. (2019). Mothers' interoceptive knowledgepredicts children's emotional regulation and social skills in middle childhood. *Social Development*. Available from https://doi.org/10.1111/sode.12418.

Mahler, K. (2017). *Interoception. The eighth sensory system.* Lenexa, KS: AAPC Publishing.

Miller, L. J. (2007). *Sensational kids. Hope and help for children with sensory processing disorder.* New York: Penguin Group.

Oppenheim, D. (2012). Emotional availability: Research advances and theoretical questions. *Developmental and Psychopathology*, *24*(11), 131–136.

Osgood, M. (2020, January 11). *Foundational capacities for development-FCD.* [Webcast]. Retrieved from: <https://profectum.org/Profectum/mod/lesson/view.php?id = 10>.

Parham, D., & Ecker, C. (2007). *Sensory processing measure manual and home form.* Western Psychological Services.

Piazza, E. A., Hasenfratz, L., Hasson, U., & Lew-Williams, C. (2019). Infant and adult brains are coupled to the dynamics of natural communication. *Psychological Science.* Available from https://doi.org/10.1177/0956797619878698, 095679761987869.

Porges, S. (2011). *Polyvagal theory.* New York: W.W. Norton and Company, Inc.

Porges, S. (2020a, June). *Autonomic state in the context of polyvagal theory.* Update safe & sound protocol (SSP). Integrated Listening Systems. [Videopodcast]. Retrieved from: <https://ils.docebosaas.com/learn>.

Porges, S. (2020b, June). *Polyvagal theory and social engagement.* Update safe & sound protocol (SSP). Integrated Listening Systems. [Videopodcast]. Retrieved from: <https://ils.docebosaas.com/learn>.

Profectum. (n.d.a). *Step 1. Profectum parent toolbox. Become your child's play partner.* Retrieved from: <https://profectum.org>.

Profectum. (n.d.b). *Step 2. Profectum parent toolbox. Discovering individual differences. Your child's individual profile.* Retrieved from: <https://profectum.org>.

Profectum. (n.d.c). *Step 3. Profectum parent toolbox. Build and extend circles of interaction moment to moment.* Retrieved from: <https://profectum.org>.

Provence, S. (1978). Application of psychoanalytic principles to treatment and prevention. In G. Glenn, & M. A. Scharfman (Eds.), *Child analysis and therapy.* New York: Jason Aronson, Inc.

Robinson, B. (2020, July 19). *Neuroscientists discover each of us has a distinct brain signature: Could it be used to project your job potential.* Forbes. <https://www.forbes.com/sites/bryanrobinson/2020/07/19/neuroscientists-discover-each-of-us-has-a-distinct-brain-signature-could-it-be-used-to-predict-your-job-potential/#97c0e9f72b4c>.

Rosello, S. S. (2018). *The 3R's program: Regulation, relationships and the right sensory inputs.* Waynesburg, PA: Intermediate Unit One.

Rosello, S. S. (2020) Family matters: Facilitating success in family occupations. Using a multi-faceted approach with children and families. In *American occupational therapy association national conference.* Aysnchronous Virtual Poster.

Rosello, S. S., Honaker, D., & Salazar, R. (2016). In A. Wagenfield, J. Kaldenbrer, & D. Honaker (Eds.), *Putting families first: Family occupations and family-centered therapy.* Slack.

Rutgers, A. H., Bakermans-Kranenburg, M. J., van IJzendoorn, M. H., & van Berckelaer-Onnes, I. A. (2004). Autism and attachment: A meta-analytic review. *Journal of Child Psychology and Psychiatry and Allied Disciplines*, *45*(6), 1123–1134.

Salazar, R. (2012). *The emotional voice of the child.* DIR Mentoring. Phone Meeting Notes. Pittsburgh, PA.

Salazar, R. (2019). Full circle autism care includes family relationships and dynamics. In D. Undurti, N. Papaneophytou, & T. El-Kour (Eds.), *Autism 360* (pp. 219–234). Elsevier Science, Academic Press.

Scharoun, S. M., & Bryden, P. J. (2016). Anticipatory planning in children with autism spectrum disorder: An assessment of independent and joint action tasks. *Frontiers in Integrative Neuroscience*, *10*, 29. Available from https://doi.org/10.3389/fnint.2016.00029.

Schmitz, C., Martineau, J., Barthélémy, C., & Assaiante, C. (2003). Motor control and children with autism: Deficit of anticipatory function? *Neuroscience Letters*, *348*(1), 17–20. Available from https://doi.org/10.1016/s0304-3940(03)00644-x.

Segal, R. (1999). Doing for others: Occupations within families with children who have special needs. *Journal of Occupational Science*, *6*(2), 53.

Segal, R. (2004). Family routines and rituals: A context for occupational therapy interventions. *American Journal of Occupational Therapy*, *58*(5), 499–508.

Shumway-Cook, A., & Woollacott, M. H. (2007). *Motor control: Translating research into clinical practice* (3rd ed.). Philadelphia, PA: Wolters Kluwer Health/Lippincott Williams & Wilkins.

Siegel, D. J. (2011). *Mindsight: The new science of personal transformation*. New York: Bantam Books.

Silberman, S. (2015). *Neurotribes: The legacy of autism and the future of neurodiversity*.

Solomon, R., Van Egeren, L. A., Mahoney, G., Quon Huber, M., & Zimmerman, P. (2014). Play Project home consultation intervention program for young children with autism spectrum disorders: A randomized controlled trial. *Journal of Developmental and Behavioral Pediatrics*, *35*(8), 475–485.

Stern, D. N. (1985). *The interpersonal world of the infant* (pp. 140–141). New York: Routledge.

Stern, D. N. (2005). Intersubjectivity. In E. S. Person, A. M. Cooper, & G. O. Gobbard (Eds.), *Textbook of psychoanalysis* (pp. 77–92). Washington, DC: American Psychiatric Association.

Tavor, I., Parker Jones, O., Mars, R. B., Smith, S. M., Behrens, T. E., & Jbabdi, S. (2016). Task-free MRI predicts individual differences in brain activity during task performance. *Science (New York, N.Y.)*, *352*(6282), 216–220. Available from https://doi.org/10.1126/science.aad8127.

Taylor, K., & Trott, M. (1991). Pyramid of development. In M. S. Willams, & S. Shellenberg (Eds.), *How does your engine run?* Albuquerque, NM: Therapyworks. (1996).

Thomas, A., & Chess, S. (1977). *Temperament and development*. Brunner/Mazel.

Torres, E., & Whyatt, C. (2018). *Autism: The movement sensing perspective*. Baca Raton, FL: CRC Press.

Trevarthen, C., & Delafield-Butt, J. T. (2013). Autism as a developmental disorder in intentional movement and affective engagement. *Frontiers in Integrative Neuroscience*, *7*, 49. Available from https://doi.org/10.3389/fnint.2013.00049.

Tronick, E. (1989). Emotions and emotional communication in infants. *American Pscychologist*, *44*(2), 112.

Vgotsky, L. S. (1978). *Mind in society: The development of higher psychological processes*. Cambridge, MA: Harvard University press.

Whitcomb, D. A., Carrasco, R. C., Neuman, A., & Kloos, H. (2015). Correlational research to examine the relationship between attachment and sensory modulation in young children. *American Journal of Occupational Therapy*, *69*, 06904220020. Available from http://doi.org/10.5014/ajot.2015.015503.

White, R. (2011). Sensory integration and individual differences. Synchrony of the sensory emotional social triad. In *Profectum inaugural conference*, New York.

White, R. (n.d.). *Your client's individual profile. Strategies to support the individual profile*. Profectum.

Wieder, S., & Wachs, H. (2012). *Visual/Spatial portals to thinking, feeling and movement: Advancing competencies and emotional development in children with learning and autism spectrum disorders*. Mendham, NJ: Profectum Foundation.

Further reading

Blacher, J., & Hatton, C. (2007). Families in context: Influences on coping and adaptation. In S. L. Odom, R. H. Homer, M. E. Sovell, & J. Blocher (Eds.), *Handbook of developmental disabilities* (pp. 531–551). New York: Guilford Press.

DePape, A. M., & Lindsay, S. (2014). *Parents' experiences of caring for a child with autism spectrum disorder* (pp. 1–14). Sage. Available from http://doi.org/10.1177/10497323/4552455.

McEvoy, M., Lee, C., O'Nell, A., Groisman, A., Roberts-Butler., Dinghra, K., & Porder, K. (2005). Are there universal parenting concepts among culturally diverse families in an inner-city population? *Journal of Pediatric Health Care: Official Publication of National Association of Pediatric Nurse Associates & Practitioners*, *19*(3), 142–150.

Osofsky, J., Wieder, S., Norona, C., Lowell, D., & Worthy, D. (2018). Effective mental health interventions and treatments for young children with diverse needs. *Zero To Three*, *33*(2), 13–22.

Sabatelli, R., & Mazor, A. (1985). Differentiation, individuation, and identity formation: The integration of family system and individual developmental perspectives. *Adolescence*, *20*(79), 619–633.

Semernov, A., & Zelazo, P. D. (2019). Mindful family routines and the cultivation of executive functioning skills in childhood. *Human Development*, *63*, 112–131.

Tremblay, R.E., Bolvin, M., Peters, R. De. V. (Eds.). (2015). *Parenting skills: Synthesis. Encyclopedia on early childhood development (online)*. <http://www.child-encyclopedia.com/parenting-skills/synthesis>.

Underwood PL. (2020). Are you overpraising your child? The New York Times, New York. <https://nyti.ms/3iAfXJW>.

Ventoia, P., Lei, J., Paisley, C., Lebowitz, E., & Silverman, W. (2017). Parenting a child with ASD: Comparison of parenting style between ASD, anxiety, and typical development. *Journal of Autism and Developmental Disorders*, *47*(9), 2873–2884. Available from https://doi.org/10.1007/s10803-017-3210.

Rhythm, rooting, range, and repetition: elements of play that promote regulation and engagement

22

Aditi Subramaniam[1] *and Kaitlin Mulcahy*[2]
[1]Massachusetts Society for the Prevention of Cruelty to Children, Boston, MA, United States, [2]Center for Autism and Early Childhood Mental Health, Montclair State University, Montclair, NJ, United States

In the first few sessions, I noticed the stillness and the patterned breath that Kyle presented, as he tried to make sense of his space around him. I mirrored Kyle's breath to attune to him as a way to introduce a "greeting" of play that held the intention; "I see you", "I hear you", "May we play"?. We breathed in and breathed out together. As the rhythm was repeated over sessions, it became a predictable game of embodied knowing and, eventually, a ritual greeting.

Introduction

In this chapter, we introduce an emerging method of regulation-informed interactive play which promotes arousal and affect regulation and engagement using the specific elements of rhythm, rooting, range, and repetition in playful interactions with children. Regulation-informed interactive play is grounded in theories of attunement, arousal and affect regulation, and the wisdom of the expressive arts. Regulation-informed interactive play includes activities that are repetitive and predictable, rhythmic and grounding, explore the full range of affect and arousal, and occur within a reciprocal, relational context. The elements of regulation-informed interactive play are an appropriate intervention for presentations of regulatory difficulties, including the arousal and affect dysregulation that is often manifest in the diagnosis of autism spectrum disorder (ASD). The elements are also appropriate to address other psychological and psychiatric presentations characterized by challenges to regulation, as well as systemic dysregulation found in family relationships or because of discriminatory or dangerous communities or contexts. Because of the prevalence of dysregulation in neurological, psychological, and systemic contexts, the use of the elements of regulation-informed interactive play has wide promotional and therapeutic application, and can be used by caregivers, classroom-based

Emerging Programs for Autism Spectrum Disorder. DOI: https://doi.org/10.1016/B978-0-323-85031-5.00026-8

staff, and clinicians. This chapter will review the foundational theories and techniques of this method of play, describe the four elements of regulation-informed interactive play, and provide examples of the use of the elements in clinical practice with families with children diagnosed with ASD.

Foundational theories of regulation-informed interactive play

Regulation-informed interactive play is a method of play influenced by multidisciplinary sources of knowledge, including literature on attachment and attunement, theories of arousal and affect regulation, and the wisdom from the expressive arts. These theories inform the foundational assumption of regulation-informed interactive play that suggests that synchronous attunement and mutual regulation are mutually reinforcing and complementary systems in the fostering of regulation and engagement in both adult and child, and this systematic process is promoted when enacted through body-based interactive play. The three theories that contribute to the foundational assumption of regulation-informed interactive play are reviewed below.

Attunement

Attunement is described in the literature as the kinesthetic, somatic, and emotional sensing of another (Stern, 1985), or the implicit process of nonverbal resonance (Devereaux, 2008; Sroufe, 1996). The process of attunement consists of accurately reflecting the experience of another through body movements, facial expressions, tone of voice, and/or vocabulary (Stern, 1985), which contributes to the ability to regulate arousal and affective states (Ostlund, Measelle, Laurent, Conradt, & Ablow, 2017). Attunement has also been described as mirroring (Tortora, 2006), kinesthetic empathy (Reynolds & Reason, 2012), and biobehavioral synchrony (Feldman, 2012), terms which well-describe the body-based nature of reflecting arousal and effect of another person, to and for that person. Yet, to feel "felt-with" (Furman, 1992) is not just to be mimicked (Stern, 1985), but instead to feel the quality of responsiveness of the attuning partner. To attune to another is not merely the bodily imitation of movement, but instead an embodied resonance of perceived intentionality and affect. Attunement allows for the development and regulation of the stress response (Porges, 2011), and is important for all future social, and emotional development (Kochanska, Aksan, Knaack, & Rhines, 2004).

Mutual regulation

Previous research has demonstrated that the development of the capacity for arousal and affect regulation is first developed through responsive, attuned, affective relationships between caregivers and infants (Bernier, Carlson, & Whipple, 2010;

Kopp, 1982; Siegel, 2001; Tronick, 2007). From infancy, the experience of regulation is obtained through an adult attuning to the organization of behaviors that are meant to establish and sustain connection with others (Ainsworth, Blehar, Waters, & Wall, 1978; Bowlby, 1969). These connections are preverbal, made through gesture, touch, voice tone, scent, and gaze (Schore, 2001). When behaviors of connection are attuned to by a sensitive adult caregiver, the infant's need is satisfied, and physiology is calmed. It is within the moment-to-moment relational context of attuned relationships that we learn to regulate emotions and affects, and to explore, access, modulate, and use emotions (Schore, 2001; Tronick, 2007). When these attuned interactions take place over time, the coregulatory benefits include an ability to self-regulate one's own body and emotions, build an early understanding of self and others, and, over time, build competency and a sense of resilience (Schore, 2010).

Expressive arts

The traditions of the expressive arts uphold the importance of body-based, nonverbal, playful encounters as a way of fostering relationship and regulation (Kossak, 2009; Levy, 1988; Malchiodi, 2016; McNiff, 1992). The expressive arts also offer avenues for attunement through rhythmic, kinesthetic, and multisensory interventions (Kossak, 2009; Malchiodi, 2016) that center nondominant ways of knowing (St. John, Thomas, & Noroña, 2012). Engaging in activities that involve movement, art, music and other rhythmic forms of nonverbal expression access neurological structures that potentiate regulation (Perry, 2006; Porges & Dana, 2018), and support attunement through the experience of kinesthetic empathy (Behrends, Müeller, & Dziobek, 2016; Tortora, 2006), embodied attunement (Lacson, 2020), and synchrony (Dvira, Lotanb, Vidermana, & Elefanta, 2020). Mirroring activities, which serve as a core component of the expressive arts, are used to support building of social communication (Bernstein, 1982) and enhancing empathy (McGarry & Russo, 2011). Play, or the interactive and dynamic space of embodied engagements (Krueger, 2011), can support and facilitate regulation and social connection (Axline, 1969; Lyons-Ruth et al., 1998). The techniques and enactments of expressive arts have been used to promote attunement and regulation in the human species over centuries (Albrecht, 1968; Blacking, 1977; Lévi-Strauss, Jacobson, & Schoepf, 1963), and are readily accessible and culturally congruent to all.

Regulation-informed interactive play and autism spectrum disorder

The diagnosis of ASD has been characterized by core deficits in communication and social engagement (American Psychiatric Association, 2013). Researchers have looked specifically at how these core deficits impact attunement and regulation, particularly in the areas of synchrony (Fitzpatrick et al., 2016), social engagement

(Baron-Cohen et al., 1996), and hyperarousal (Jahromi, Bryce, & Swanson, 2013; Kasari, Freeman, & Paparella, 2006; Laurent & Gorman, 2018). Previous research has also suggested that children diagnosed with ASD often have difficulty with self-regulation, which impacts social functioning (Uljarevic et al., 2018). Similarly, literature demonstrates that children with a diagnosis of ASD often present difficulties in the capacity to discern, and then organize, the sensorimotor information from the space around them (Lord & Spence, 2006), creating difficulties in social engagement (Samaritter & Payne, 2017).

The elements of regulation-informed interactive play are appropriate for addressing the documented deficits of the diagnosis of ASD, including synchrony, regulation, and engagement. Research has demonstrated that nonverbal, body-based activities are appropriate for increasing regulatory skills in children (Trevarthen & Delafield-Butt, 2013), and play-based interventions have shown improvements in regulation and interactions for children with ASD (Carden, 2009; Josefi & Ryan, 2004; Kasari et al., 2006; Mittledorf, Hendricks, & Landreth, 2001; Salter, Beamish, & Davies, 2016; Schottelkorb, Swan, & Ogawa, 2020; Solomon, 2020). Play-based models often used with children with a diagnosis of ASD, such as the work of Greenspan and Wieder (1999), suggest support of regulation and engagement as foundational to all subsequent capacities. Additionally, interactive, coregulatory activities with parents have been shown to bring about biobehavioral synchrony (Feldman, 2012) between parents and children (Althoff, Dammann, Hope, & Ausderau, 2019; Dawson, 2008; Dawson et al., 2010; Hirschler-Guttenberg, Golan, Ostfeld-Etzion, & Feldman, 2015; Kasari & Smith, 2013). Activities typically used by music therapists using rhythm and synchrony have demonstrated support to regulatory and engagement capacities for children with ASD (Sharda et al., 2019; Srinivasan & Bhat, 2013; Srinivasan, Park, Neelly, & Bhat, 2015), and the mirroring and rhythmic activities of dance movement therapy have similar findings (Devereaux, 2017; Scharoun, Reinders, Bryden, & Fletcher, 2014; Takahashi, Matsushima, & Kato, 2019; Tortora, 2006). Regulation-informed interactive play is guided by these previous findings to impact regulation and engagement. The elements are offered as ways of playing that are appropriate and supportive for children diagnosed with ASD.

The elements of regulation-informed interactive play

Regulation-informed interactive play suggests four elements of play—rhythm, rooting, range, and repetition—that can be used in play by caregivers, classroom-based staff, and clinicians to promote arousal and affect regulation and engagement. Regulation-informed interactive play upholds the importance of relational interaction and synchronous attunement in the promotion of regulation. Play activities are not given to a child to play alone, but instead done interactively, with caregiver and child playing together, encouraging reciprocation. Regulation-informed interactive play is not a manualized approach that is followed to fidelity, but instead a conceptual understanding of the qualities of play that promote a state of regulation. Regulation-informed interactive play is not constrained into procedural play activities, but instead affords caregivers, classroom-based staff, and clinicians the freedom to play in ways that are culturally responsive and developmentally relevant, using play materials that are available and preferred. Caregiving adults keep the elements in mind during play, and suggest playful activities using the elements that match the interests of the child and their perceived regulatory need. Additionally, the elements of play can be used within existing evidence-informed therapeutic models that utilize play.

In the section below, we describe the four elements of regulation-informed interactive play. Each of the descriptions suggest a few activities that may be considered during play to engage the element but are not meant to be prescriptive. Each element may be used in isolation in play, or more than one element can be incorporated in one playful activity to amplify the regulatory benefit. Ultimately, whatever play activities are chosen should be enjoyable to both child and adult, as play demonstrates maximized neurological benefits when it is experienced as fun and enjoyable to all players (Brown & Vaughan, 2009).

Rhythm

The expressive arts and body-based therapies integrate rhythm as a central medium to enhance regulation (Malchiodi, 2016) and synchrony (Venuti et al., 2017). Science and anthropological/cultural history (You, 1994) speak about regular rhythmic activities as regulatory, connecting even to our internal rhythms of heartbeat, breath, heart rate, and pulse. Rhythmic patterned activities are resonant with the neural patterns of our somatosensory networks (Berrol, 1992; Perry, 2006) and are soothing. The polyvagal theory (Porges, 2011) elucidates the importance of the regulation of the body's internal rhythms by understanding the ventral vagal network that is influenced by breathing patterns and social cues. Repetitive rhythmic activities of movement and music create opportunities for self-regulation and readiness to attune to another (Macy, Macy, Gross, & Brighton, 2003; Williams & Berthelsen, 2019). Studies in music therapy integrating beat synchrony and rhythmic entrainment afford an opportunity to better understand the integration of multiple systems to make sense of sensorimotor information (Thompson, White-Schwoch, Tierney, & Kraus, 2015). Synchrony supports the reciprocity or "serve and return" (Shonkoff, 2017) of mutual regulation (Tronick, 2007), and "moments of meeting" (Sander, 1995; Stern, 1985).

Rhythm can be incorporated into any kind of play when play actions are done in a rhythmic pattern (i.e., dump and fill play, drawing or painting, ball bouncing or tossing, swinging in a parachute or swing, or in object play). Additionally, playing with regular rhythms in actions like drumming, full body patting, and stamping or stomping will entrain the body to the regularity and regulation of the beat. These rhythmic activities offer ways to soothe, slow down, and bring individuals into the "here and now." Rhythmic activity need not always be whole body large and big movements. It can include mirroring and matching tempo to the child by assessing where they are in their energy level or breath. Engaging with rhythmic repetitive motions of breathing together or matching and attuning to the child's breathing patterns can initiate ways of joining in relationship with them. Rhythm can also be used to model a more optimal range of arousal, for example, speeding up the tempo of the rhythm of play for children who need upregulation, or slowing down the tempo of the rhythm for children who need downregulation. Rhythm can be played with by changing the tempo of movement to fast or slow, or light or heavy, thereby creating variation and expanding the range of embodied experience. The element of rhythm can also integrate vocal rhythms like singing songs which offer repetition and create a sense of predictability for the child.

Rooting

The element of rooting focuses on activities that engage the ground and help "root" the energy in our body downward, thus creating more stability and safety. Play activities that integrate rooting elements are a way to integrate the proprioceptive sense (Ayers, 2005), stimulating a process of downregulation (Pierce, 2014). Studies from the field of yoga and energy chakras (Maxwell, 2009; Nemri, 2004) have highlighted both the physiological, psychological, and spiritual aspects of "root" or ground centered activities. Grounding as a concept, coined by Lowen (2006), has been expanded by body-based and expressive arts psychotherapists (Levy, 2005; Meekums, 2002) to include the felt sense of connection to the "ground," as well as to the inner experiences of "self" with regard to control, safety, and autonomy (Anagnostopoulou, 2015). Rooting is developmentally foundational to the development of regulation through the sense of proprioception (Ayers, 2005). Young children, through their early developmental movement experiences of being held, laying, scooting, crawling, sitting, and walking, discover the relationship of weight of their body and the process of navigating and adaptation of that weight with the ground and space around them (Ayers, 2005). Rooting exercises and activities provide a means to be present in the "here and now" (Meekums, 2002) by bringing attention to the whole body and its relationship with the environment. Rooting activities in play can be used to bring kinesthetic awareness into the present for the child and caregiver, in service of the relationship between them.

Rooting can be integrated by caregiving adults and clinicians in play through activities that focus on sending energy into the ground through play like pounding games such as playing whack-a-mole or closing lids, or through pressing games, like kneading or creating shapes out of play dough. Play may also incorporate heavy work activities like pushing things on a small cart or carrying a few books or a weighted backpack. These activities engage the proprioceptive sense to feel more weighted and connected to the ground and offer opportunities for whole body integration and a sense of stability. Playing with materials or props to facilitate a sense of grounding can also be beneficial. Large elastic stretch bands that engage resistance of the body can foster the embodied sense of the self in relationship to the surrounding space. Everyday play that involves hanging from bars and wheelbarrow play are also ways to activate this relationship between body and ground. Materials like Play-Doh, Model Magic, or clay present with resistance and an intrinsic play scheme of pushing and prodding downwards. Play that includes kneading or pushing play dough can support the bodily sense of being in the here and now. Rooting activities that utilize the ground as support are also regulatory. Bringing play to the floor, rather than on a chair or at a table can serve to provide regulatory input (Greenspan & Wieder, 1999). Utilizing more of the ground, including laying down on the ground, can also provide a supportive coregulatory energy.

Range

The element of range plays with the capacity for modulation of arousal and affect. Modulation is a neurological process that serves to regulate physiological and emotional input to maintain balance of energy (Ayers, 2005; Schoen, Miller, & Sullivan, 2014). Modulation serves to manage inhibitory and excitatory influences to allow input that is needed by the body. This process is regulated by the central nervous system (CNS) (Porges, 2011). Many researchers have discussed modulation on a continuum from hypoactive (low CNS arousal) to optimal arousal to hyperactive (high CNS arousal) (Kinsbourne, 1987; Zentall & Zentall, 1983). Other researchers have identified the possibility of a neural imbalance in modulation which operates more like a seesaw than a continuum, resulting in extremes of behavioral presentation that teeters from hypoarousal to hyperarousal, rarely coming to balance in the optimal range (Schaaf et al., 2010). Siegel terms this optimal range as the "window of tolerance" (1999), which can be narrow or broad, depending on the capacity for modulation in the neurological system. Expressive and body-based therapeutic models (Blaustein & Kinniburgh, 2018; Kossak, 2009; Malchiodi, 2016; Ogden & Minton, 2000; Ogden, Minton, & Pain, 2006; Tortora, 2006), as well as the field of occupational therapy, include modulation in their treatment goals. Body-based expressive therapists use space in playing with modulation, allowing for both wide open spaces and contained spaces to mimic the internal window of tolerance (Devereaux, 2008; Laban, 1976; Tortora, 2006). The use of music has also been suggested to provide a neurological modulation function (Koelsch, 2009), and allow for preverbal or nonverbal connection and communication and social reciprocity (Geretsegger, Elefant, Mössler, & Gold, 2014). While modulation is a neurological process, it is mediated through positive caregiving (Callaghan & Tottenham, 2015; Gunnar & Donzella, 2002). In fact, the experience of coregulation allows for modulation of the nervous system. Both vagal tone, which is activated by detecting cues of safety from safe caregivers (Porges, 2011), and mirror neurons, which fire by watching others perform actions, including those of modulation (Pfeifer, Iacoboni, Mazziotta, & Dapretto, 2008), become involved because of coregulatory relationships (Ratcliffe, 2007), which can broaden the window of tolerance.

To use the element of range in play, clinicians and caregiving adults play with the full range of emotions and arousal by pushing the boundaries of high and low arousal to find the optimal arousal, or window of tolerance, for each person. By doing so, clinicians and caregiving adults assess movements, actions, and activities that increase and decrease a child's energy level, as well as identify the actions that are avoided. Play activities can mirror the modulation balance continuum by playing with opposites, such as big/little, loud/quiet, awake/sleep. This can be done by using full body play that travels the arousal continuum from low to high and back to low again by pretending to be an airplane that leaves the hanger, then races quickly in the sky, then returns for rest and relaxation. Examples of opposite play are found in traditional games played by children such as Red Light, Green Light or Freeze Tag, which play with the opposites of start/stop. The element of range can also be played by using a wide range of art materials across the textural spectrum. Dense textures like clay utilize more energy to manipulate, while fluid textures like water are more difficult to control. The element of range can use space as an example of range itself, playing with how wide or how contained a space is comfortable for the child, and whether the child needs a coregulatory partner to tolerate either of the extremes of space.

Repetition

The fourth element of repetition follows findings from early education research about the importance of repetition, consistency, and predictability in learning and healthy development (Lester, Allanson, & Notar, 2017; Watson & DiCarlo, 2015). This element also draws from research that has demonstrated the foundational neurological benefits of repetitive, patterned activity for regulatory growth (Dobson & Perry, 2010; Perry, 2006; Perry & Hambrick, 2008). Repetition also allows for automaticity, or the ability for a practiced skill to become procedurally automatic (Brabeck, Jeffrey, & Fry, 2010). Repetition is resonant with our most basic connection with nature, as repetition of pattern is inherent in the natural world (Ball, 2016). Similarly, repetition is inherently existent within rhythmic and movement activities, as regular rhythms repeat patterns and form.

To implement the element of repetition, a chosen regulation-informed interactive play activity is done repeatedly until the point of saturation (Warner, Finn, Wescott, & Cook, 2020) for the child. Many times, adults become saturated, or finished, with an activity well in advance of a child, and themselves suggest a change in the routine. However, children often need more repetition and practice to reach automaticity and to feel complete with an activity. The element of repetition also includes repetitive structure within a play activity. For example, when playing a game such as pretending to be animals, the element of repetition would not just be seen in playing the animal game many times, but also that play themes are repeated within the game, (i.e., each time the animal game is played, the animals wake up, then move out to explore, then head home to go to bed). Lastly, the element of repetition is done with reciprocation or turn-taking in mind. In regulation-informed interactive play, the adult repeats that which is offered by the child, and the child repeats that which is offered by the adult in play. This back-and-forth kinesthetic attunement serves to increase engagement.

The elements in practice with families

The authors have chosen three scenarios from our practice to demonstrate the application of regulation-informed interactive play to multiple systems of arousal and affect dysregulation, including neurological, relational, and systemic dysregulation. Each family has had their identifying information changed to protect and honor their confidentiality. However, the authors transparently share our positionality to highlight the importance of remaining aware of the systemic implications of interaction between clinician and family, particularly when considering attunement and regulation within the therapeutic relationship. The first author, Aditi, identifies as a South Asian of Indian descent, middle-class, heterosexual, cisgendered, clinician of color, informed by over 15 years of clinical practice in India and Boston, USA. The second author, Kaitlin, identifies as a third-generation, middle-class Irish, Catholic, cisgendered, heterosexual clinician, informed by over 20 years of clinical practice in New York City, Boston, and northern New Jersey, USA. Both Aditi and Kaitlin have been trained as licensed mental health counselors, with specialization in expressive therapies and Dance/Movement Therapy, play therapy, family therapy, and infant and early childhood mental health clinical practice. The stories of our work using regulation-informed interactive play with families are offered to highlight the method of play in action. The examples demonstrate the wide application of the four elements of regulation-informed interactive play to scenarios that all share the need for regulation, but in unique and family-specific ways. We have illuminated particular moments in our work with these families to highlight the "moments of meeting" (Sander, 1995, p. 589) during the play, using the four elements of regulation-informed interactive play—rhythm, rooting, range, and repetition.

Violet

The first example demonstrates the elements of regulation-informed interactive play with a child with significant neurological dysregulation. Kaitlin partnered with a family of 4-year-old Violet, diagnosed with ASD, to provide play-based family and developmental clinical support in a fee-for-service, outpatient setting. Violet's family identified as middle-class, first generation, Filipino, and consisted of her mother, father, older brother, and a supportive aunt that lived within close enough distance to share weekly contact. Sessions typically consisted of Violet, her mother, and her brother. Violet's father rarely participated in sessions due to his work schedule. During most of our time together, Violet entered session in significant distress, demonstrated by prolonged crying, screaming, and clinging to her mother. She was not able to use verbal language to communicate her wants and needs, so we were often challenged to decipher her core source of distress. Her mother was able to hold her and soothe her through calm tones and consistent physical containment, and instinctively sat on the floor with Violet on her lap. Kaitlin noticed that Violet was able to be coregulated through her mother's physical presence and use of the floor for grounding, but assessed Violet's window of tolerance (Siegel, 1999) to be quite narrow. Violet often moved out of the optimal range of arousal to hyperarousal or shutdown. If Violet's mother had to move her body position, if someone in the room used a voice that was too loud, if clinician attempted to make eye contact with Violet, or if anyone attempted what Violet perceived as intrusive attempts of connection, including face-to-face play, Violet would become hyperaroused and again begin expressing her significant distress. For the first sessions of treatment, Kaitlin struggled to know how best to help calm Violet's distress, so as to both assist Violet in increasing her window of tolerance, but also to provide her mother with support in her constant coregulatory relationship with Violet.

Over time, Kaitlin noticed that Violet appeared to calm more quickly when holding a bag of snacks or a "snuggle-lovey" clenched in her hand. The author noticed that the repetitive, rhythmic nature of eating her snack seemed to allow Violet to remain within her window of tolerance. The author noticed the rhythm and shape of Violet's eating of snack, noticing the steady arc of up and down motion, which harkened to a similar movement arc used in dump and fill play. Kaitlin then began to attune to this rhythmic repetition by slowly matching the movement through transferring soft but weighty bean bags from a bucket into another bucket that was placed slightly higher, thereby matching the movement trajectory from snack bag to mouth. This action used rhythm to attune to the movement that appeared calming to Violet, and, because of the weight of the bean bags causing the bean bag movement to ground when dropped, also incorporated the rooting needs that were already present by Violet's need to be supported by the floor and her mother's lap. Kaitlin did this action in parallel, with no eye contact, and no attempts at reciprocation, but repeated this action many times over. After noticing that the parallel kinesthetic attunement was tolerated by Violet, Kaitlin also increased the range of space between the bean bag and the bucket, expanding the boundaries of vertical and horizontal space in the play, thereby expanding the mirrored window of tolerance for Violet.

After some time of this rhythmic, repetitive attunement, Violet's mother was able to shift her body so that Violet would sit in between her mother's legs on the floor, allowing Violet to tolerate more of her own body posture, and positioning Violet with her body orientation out towards the room, rather than in and contained towards her mother. While this bodily shift might be considered inconsequential, this ability to demonstrate bodily autonomy and increased tolerance for expanded social interaction was perceived as significantly positive for the family. When Violet was able to expand her window of tolerance to sit on her own on the floor facing outwards from her mother, she was also able to engage in activities that continued to utilize the elements, including slowly rolling a rolling pin back and forth on the carpet together while softly singing songs with regular beats. Violet was also able to tolerate watching Kaitlin roll a car down a very slight ramp, and then was able to tolerate the increased height of the ramp, and the subsequent increased pace of the car, demonstrating her continually expanded tolerance for range expansion. She eventually became able to indicate her interest in repeating a play activity through body movements and eye contact with her mother.

This work with the expansion of Violet's range of regulatory tolerance and reciprocal interaction was fragile, delicate, and characterized by developmentally appropriate regressions and expansions (Brazelton, 1992). Most of the work was in assisting the family in determining the elements that could be done in their daily routines and supporting Violet's mother in her use of the elements at home. Over time, this way of being and playing together as a family allowed for continued progress toward the goals for an increased neurological regulatory capacity and expanded window of tolerance for Violet.

Kyle

The second example elucidates the integration of the regulation-informed interactive play method with a family and their 13-month-old son, Kyle, who was seen by Aditi in a home visiting setting. Aditi first met Kyle and his family, consisting of his mother, father, and older sibling, in their home after Kyle's eligibility for Part C services. The family identified themselves as a middle class, biracial family, with the mother identifying as Chinese and the father as German and they often spoke to the dynamics of multicultural raising of their children here in the United States. Kyle had a diagnosis of hydrocephalus, cortical visual impairment (CVI), and complex medical conditions. There were multiple therapists involved, including speech/feeding therapy, occupational therapy, physical therapy, and CVI therapy, to support various developmental areas for Kyle, along with a very cohesive and large medical team. The family expressed being committed to doing well by their child (Brazelton, 1992), and providing him with the best resources he needed to thrive.

However, over the course of observation with the family, Aditi noticed that Kyle's mother found "being-with" harder than "doing for" Kyle. In fact, the day Aditi met the family to partner with them, Kyle's mother named, "I don't know how to play with him." This became our developmental goal and began the sessions together. Though Kyle's mother was usually in the home for visits, she usually sat back at the stairs, reportedly waiting for Aditi to fix something about Kyle, or "do developmentally informed things" with Kyle. Kyle presented as still and curious about his environment as he heard a new voice in the room. Aditi noticed that whenever his sister or mother said something in a higher tone, Kyle would pout his lips and cry. Aditi assessed that his window of tolerance was narrow, and so began tentatively engaging with the element of rhythm. In the first few sessions, Aditi noticed the stillness and the patterned breath that Kyle presented, as he tried to make sense of his space around him. Aditi mirrored Kyle's breath to attune to him as a way to introduce a "greeting" of play that held the intention; "I see you," "I hear you," "May we play"? We breathed in and breathed out together. As the rhythm was repeated over sessions, it became a predictable game of embodied knowing and, eventually, a ritual greeting. After repeated breath play over many sessions, one day, Kyle initiated the breath game on his own. It was that day that his mother joined the session, and was henceforth always a part of the sessions, having physically moved in space from behind the stairs to face-to-face with Kyle.

The attuning to breathing in rhythmic patterns was a way that Kyle and his mother both came into the play of the here and now and being with one another. A new meaning and way of being with each other in mutual enjoyment was created (Tronick, 2007), helping to alleviate the relational dysregulation that was felt by Kyle's mother in not knowing how to connect with him. The moments of meeting (Sander, 1995) through the breath game expanded to a rhythmic greeting song that Kyle was able to tolerate. We then worked to expand his range of tolerance through tapping rhythms on his highchair. Over time, Kyle's mother noticed Kyle's rhythms and movements as expressions of connection and his selfhood and expanded or matched them with sounds, tapping, or playful back and forth games. They incorporated the play into their daily routines, like changing clothes, diaper, bath time. Playful games became central to their mutual enjoyment.

Kyle was eventually diagnosed with ASD at age 2 years. The author continued to see Kyle's family until he aged out of Part C services, and continued using the elements of rhythm, rooting, range, and consistent repetition, in play that involved the whole family. They would make music together, with his older sister on her violin, Kyle using a hollow mic to sing, his mother clapping and his father tapping. This became a ritual of mutual enjoyment in their home. The elements of regulation-informed interactive, specifically rhythm and repetition, in play, not only supported developmental goals of this child, but also supported ways of relationally regulating each member of the family to have more mutually enjoyable moments and tolerate moments of mismatch (Tronick, 2007) in their relationship over time.

Jenissa

The third example we share is the story of a 7-year old African American girl, Jenissa, diagnosed with ASD, and her mother, Alicia. Jenissa and her mother presented at Kaitlin's outpatient clinic with concerns related to social engagement and reciprocal play. Alicia and Jenissa recently moved from out of state after fleeing an unsafe relationship between Alicia and Jenissa's father. Alicia reported that the family did not have many social connections in the area, but as Jenissa had benefited from treatment for her autism diagnosis in the past, one of their first actions upon moving was to find a therapeutic relationship for Jenissa. During the first session, Kaitlin observed that Jenissa used scripted language including phrases from television shows to communicate her hopes and needs. Alicia reported that she did not find meaning in Jenissa's use of verbal language, and did not believe Jenissa could play, reporting that she preferred watching screens. Alicia expressed her core fear for Jenissa's safety, mentioning worry around Jenissa's inability to communicate with words, and that she would be more at risk because of the systemic racism that would not provide her empathy or permission for developmental delay. These concerns in mind, Alicia requested that services focus on functional play and communication.

Jenissa was assessed as being challenged to attend to initiated social interaction, and instead was perceived as interested in specific objects like the blinds on the window and her mother's keys. It appeared Jenissa used these preferred play schemes when she became overwhelmed and dysregulated by social engagement. After a short amount of play engagement, Jenissa would begin walking back and forth in front of the drawn blinds in the room in a particular rhythm, looking at the blinds out of the corners of her eyes. Kaitlin noticed this rhythm with Alicia and began walking in parallel along with Jenissa. Jenissa quickly noticed Kaitlin doing this attuned movement, so Kaitlin expanded the range of the attunement by adding a rooting element by stomping while walking. Jenissa quickly demonstrated enjoyment with this play by laughing and was able to follow Kaitlin's movement by attempting to stomp. After a few sessions of this play, Kaitlin initiated a rhythmic, rooting, repetitive play pattern by jumping on the small trampoline in the room. We used an uttered phrase used by Jenissa to make a rhythmic song and jumped up and down to the rhythm. We also practiced start and stop range play by jumping on the trampoline to the song of her words, and then saying "stop" to see if Jenissa could follow the pattern of the game, and engage in reciprocal start and stop directions. Over time, Jenissa was successful at this play, and appeared to enjoy the play very much, demonstrated through smiling, laughing, and increased initiation at starting play.

At first, Alicia reported that she did not want to join Jenissa during the play, and instead requested that Kaitlin reinforce language through repeated trials and drills without Alicia's participation. Kaitlin concurrently supported Alicia's regulatory capacity to coregulate and support Jenissa's needs through processing her own stress and trauma related to her relational history, her concerns with raising Jenissa on her own, and her justified concerns about the family's safety due to systemic oppression. After time in this concurrent work, Alicia was provided the regulatory space to be able to join in play with Jenissa. We worked together to notice Jenissa's increased cues of social engagement during the trampoline game and other rhythmic movement play. We also used videos that Alicia took of Jenissa at home to notice Jenissa's natural engagement with the elements, and to think of new ways to use the elements during play at home to increase engagement and functional communication. We also noticed that Jenissa could follow songs of words that were made of consonant-vowel combinations like "ba-na-na" while stomping in a circle, demonstrating the beginning of functional and reciprocal communication with social engagement. We continued to look for rhythm and repetition in Jenissa's use of scripts and began to try to follow the pattern of her script usage. The use of the elements of regulation-informed interactive play became the vehicle by which Alicia and Jenissa better came to engage with each other, while also concurrently calming Alicia's own stress about relevant systemic concerns that might add further dysregulation for Jenissa.

Conclusion

This chapter introduced an emerging method of regulation-informed interactive play which promotes arousal and affect regulation and engagement using the specific elements of rhythm, rooting, range, and repetition in playful interactions with children. The four elements serve as tools to expand attuned moments of "being-with" and enhance interactions of mutual regulation. The four elements of regulation-informed interactive play are available to all caregiving adults to help to promote arousal and affect regulation. The elements of rhythm, rooting, range, and repetition are particularly suited for working with children with a diagnosis of autism. Playing with the elements in mind can support challenges in regulation and engagement by expanding the window of tolerance (Siegel, 1999) for both caregiver and child, thereby encouraging mutual regulation and promoting engagement.

References

Ainsworth, M. D. S., Blehar, M., Waters, E., & Wall, S. (1978). *Patterns of attachment: A psychological study of the strange situation*. Erlbaum.

Albrecht, M. C. (1968). Art as an institution. *American Sociological Review*, *33*, 383–397.

Althoff, C. E., Dammann, C. P., Hope, S. J., & Ausderau, K. K. (2019). Parent-mediated interventions for children with autism spectrum disorder: A systematic review. *American Journal of Occupational Therapy*, *73*(3), 1–13.

American Psychiatric Association. (2013). *Diagnostic and statistical manual of mental disorders* (5th ed.). https://doi.org/10.1176/appi.books.9780890425596.

Anagnostopoulou, L. (2015). Vertical grounding: The body in the world and the self in the body. In G. Marlock, & H. Weiss (Eds.), *The handbook of body psychotherapy & somatic psychology* (pp. 684–691). North Atlantic Books.

Axline, V. (1969). *Play therapy* (Rev. ed.). Riverside Press.

Ayers, A. J. (2005). *Sensory integration and the child: Understanding hidden sensory challenges*. Western Psychological Services.

Ball, P. (2016). *Patterns in nature: Why the natural world looks the way it does*. Chicago Press.

Baron-Cohen, S., Cox, A., Baird, G., Swettenham, J., Nightingale, N., Morgan, K., ... Charman, T. (1996). Psychological markers in the detection of autism in infancy in a large population. *British Journal of Psychiatry*, *168*, 158–163.

Behrends, A., Müeller, S., & Dziobek, I. (2016). Dancing supports empathy: The potential of interactional movement and dance for psychotherapy. *Embodiment in Psychotherapy*, *13*, 99–131.

Bernier, A., Carlson, S. M., & Whipple, N. (2010). From external regulation to self-regulation: Early parenting precursors of young children's executive functioning. *Child Development*, *81*, 326–339.

Bernstein, P. (1982). *Eight theoretical approaches in dance-movement therapy*. Kendall/Hunt Publishing Company.

Berrol, C. F. (1992). The neurophysiologic basis of the mind-body connection in dance/movement therapy. *American Journal of Dance Therapy*, *14*, 19–29. Available from https://doi.org/10.1007/BF00844132.

Blacking, J. (1977). Towards an anthropology of the body. In J. Blacking (Ed.), *The anthropology of the body* (pp. 1–28). Academic Press.

Blaustein, M., & Kinniburgh, K. (2018). *Treating traumatic stress in children and adolescents: How to foster resilience through attachment, self-regulation, and competency* (2nd ed.). Guilford Press.

Bowlby, J. (1969). *Attachment and loss: Vol. I. Attachment*. Basic Books.
Brabeck, M., Jeffrey, J., & Fry, S. (2010). *Practice for knowledge acquisition (not drill and kill): Designing activities with the goal of transferring knowledge*. American Psychological Association. Retrieved on August 29, 2020 from: <https://www.apa.org/education/k12/practice-acquisition#:~:text=Practice%20is%20important%20for%20teaching,knowledge%20automatically%2C%20without%20reflection>.
Brazelton, T. B. (1992). *Touchpoints: Emotional and behavioral development*. Addison-Wesley.
Brown, S. L., & Vaughan, C. C. (2009). *Play: How it shapes the brain, opens the imagination, and invigorates the soul*. Avery.
Callaghan, B. L., & Tottenham, N. (2015). The neuro-environmental loop of plasticity: A cross-species analysis of parental effects on emotion circuitry development following typical and adverse caregiving. *Neuropsychopharmacology: Official Publication of the American College of Neuropsychopharmacology*, *41*, 163–176. Available from https://doi.org/10.1038/npp.2015.204.
Carden, M. (2009). Understanding Lisa: A play therapy intervention with a child diagnosed on the autistic spectrum who presents with self-harming behaviours. *British Journal of Play Therapy*, *5*, 54–62.
Dawson, G. (2008). Early behavioral intervention, brain plasticity, and the prevention of autism spectrum disorder. *Development and Psychopathology*, *20*, 775–803. Available from https://doi.org/10.1017/S0954579408000370.
Dawson, G., Rogers, S., Munson, J., Smith, M., Winter, J., Greenson, J., et al. (2010). Randomized, controlled trial of an intervention for toddlers with autism: The Early Start Denver Model. *Pediatrics*, *125*, 17–23. Available from https://doi.org/10.1542/peds.2009-0958.
Devereaux, C. (2008). Untying the knots: dance/movement therapy with a family exposed to domestic violence. *American Journal of Dance Therapy*, *30*, 58. Available from https://doi.org/10.1007/s10465-008-9055-x.
Devereaux, C. (2017). Neuroception and attunement in dance/movement therapy with autism. *American Journal of Dance Therapy*, *39*, 36–38.
Dobson, C., & Perry, B. D. (2010). The role of healthy relational interactions in buffering the impact of childhood trauma. In E. Gil (Ed.), *Working with children to heal interpersonal trauma: The power of play* (pp. 26–43). The Guilford Press.
Dvira, T., Lotanb, N., Vidermana, R., & Elefanta, C. (2020). The body communicates: Movement synchrony during music therapy with children diagnosed with ASD. *The Arts in Psychotherapy*, *69*, 1–9, DOI. Available from https://doi.org/10.1016/j.aip.2020.101658.
Feldman, R. (2012). Bio-behavioral synchrony: A model for integrating biological and micro-social behavioral processes in the study of parenting. *Parenting: Science and Practice*, *12*, 154–164. Available from https://doi.org/10.1080/15295192.2012.683342.
Fitzpatrick, P., Frazier, J. A., Cochran, D. M., Mitchell, T., Coleman, C., & Schmidt, R. C. (2016). Impairments of social motor synchrony evident in autism spectrum disorder. *Frontiers in Psychology*, *7*, 1323. Available from https://doi.org/10.3389/fpsyg.2016.01323.
Furman, E. (1992). On feeling and being felt with. *The Psychoanalytic Study of the Child*, *47* (1), 67–84. Available from https://doi.org/10.1080/00797308.1992.11822665.
Geretsegger, M., Elefant, C., Mössler, K. A., & Gold, C. (2014). Music therapy for people with autism spectrum disorder. *The Cochrane Database of Systematic Reviews*, *2014*(6), CD004381. Available from https://doi.org/10.1002/14651858.CD004381.pub3.

Greenspan, S. I., & Wieder, S. (1999). A functional developmental approach to autism spectrum disorders. *Journal of the Association for Persons with Severe Handicaps*, *24*, 147–161. Available from https://doi.org/10.2511/rpsd.24.3.147.

Gunnar, M. R., & Donzella, B. (2002). Social regulation of the cortisol levels in early human development. *Psychoneuroendocrinology*, *27*, 199–220.

Hirschler-Guttenberg, Y., Golan, O., Ostfeld-Etzion, S., & Feldman, R. (2015). Mothering, fathering, and the regulation of negative and positive emotions in high-functioning preschoolers with autism spectrum disorder. *Journal of Child Psychology and Psychiatry*, *56*(5), 530–539. Available from https://doi.org/10.1111/jcpp.12311.

Jahromi, L. B., Bryce, C. I., & Swanson, J. (2013). The importance of self-regulation for the school and peer engagement of children with high-functioning autism. *Research in Autism Spectrum Disorders*, *7*, 235–246.

Josefi, O., & Ryan, V. (2004). Non-directive play therapy for young children with autism: A case study. *Clinical Child Psychology and Psychiatry*, *9*, 533–551. Available from http://doi.org/10.1177/1359104504046158.

Kasari, C., Freeman, S., & Paparella, T. (2006). Joint attention and symbolic play in young children with autism: A randomized controlled intervention study. *Journal of Child Psychology and Psychiatry*, *47*, 611–620.

Kasari, C., & Smith, T. (2013). Interventions in schools for children with autism spectrum disorder: Methods and recommendations. *Autism: The International Journal of Research and Practice*, *17*, 254–267.

Kinsbourne, M. (1987). Specific learning disabilities and attention deficit with hyperactivity. In M. Gottlieb, J. Williams, & P. Zinkus (Eds.), *Textbook of developmental pediatrics*. Plenum Press.

Kochanska, G., Aksan, N., Knaack, A., & Rhines, H. M. (2004). Maternal parenting and children's conscience: Early security as moderator. *Child Development*, *75*, 1229–1242.

Koelsch, S. (2009). A neuroscientific perspective on music therapy. *The Neurosciences and Music Disorders and Plasticity*, *1169*(1), 374–384. Available from https://doi.org/10.1111/j.1749-6632.2009.04592.x.

Kopp, C. (1982). Antecedents of self-regulation: A developmental perspective. *Developmental Psychology*, *19*, 199–214.

Kossak, M. S. (2009). Therapeutic attunement: A transpersonal view of expressive arts therapy. *The Arts in Psychotherapy*, *36*(1), 13–18.

Krueger, J. (2011). Extended cognition and the space of social interaction. *Conscious Cognition*, *20*, 643–657. Available from https://doi.org/10.1016/j.concog.2010.09.022.

Laban, R. (1976). *Modern educational dance*. MacDonald and Evans Ltd.

Lacson, F. C. (2020). Embodied attunement: A dance/movement therapy approach to working with couples. *Body, Movement and Dance in Psychotherapy*, *15*(1), 4–19. Available from https://doi.org/10.1080/17432979.2019.1699859.

Laurent, A. C., & Gorman, K. (2018). Development of emotion self-regulation among young children with autism spectrum disorders: The role of parents. *Journal of Autism and Developmental Disorders*, *48*, 1249–1260.

Lévi-Strauss, C., Jacobson, C., & Schoepf, B. G. (1963). *Structural anthropology*. Basic Books.

Lester, R. R., Allanson, P. B., & Notar, C. E. (2017). Routines are the foundation of classroom management. *Education*, *137*(4), 398–412.

Levy, F. (1988). *Dance/movement therapy. A healing art*. Sage Publications.

Levy, F. (2005). *Dance movement therapy: A healing art* (Rev. ed.). National Dance Association.

Lord, C., & Spence, S. (2006). Autism spectrum disorders: Phenotype and diagnosis. In S. O. Moldin, & J. L. R. Rubenstein (Eds.), *Understanding autism: From basic neuroscience to treatment* (pp. 1–23). CRC Taylor and Francis.

Lowen, A. (2006). *The language of the body* (3rd ed.). Bioenergetics Press.

Lyons-Ruth, K., Bruschweiler-Stern, N., Harrison, A., Morgan, A. C., Nahum, J. P., Sander, L., … Tronick, E. Z. (1998). Implicit relational knowing: Its role in development and psychoanalytic treatment. *Infant Mental Health Journal, 19*(3), 282–289.

Macy, R. D., Macy, D. J., Gross, S. I., & Brighton, P. (2003). Healing in familiar settings: Support for children and youth in the classroom and community. In R. D. Macy, S. Barry, & G. G. Noam (Eds.), *New directions for youth development: Theory, practice, and research* (pp. 51–79). Jossey Bass.

Malchiodi, C. (2016). *Trauma and expressive arts therapy: Brain, body and imagination in the healing process*. The Guilford Press.

Maxwell, R. W. (2009). The physiological oundation of yoga chakra expression. *Journal of Religion and Science, 44*, 807–824.

McGarry, L. M., & Russo, F. A. (2011). Mirroring in dance/movement therapy: Potential mechanisms behind empathy enhancement. *The Arts in Psychotherapy, 38*(3), 178–184.

McNiff, S. (1992). *Art as medicine: Creating a therapy of the imagination*. Shambala Press.

Meekums, B. (2002). *Dance movement therapy. A creative psychotherapeutic approach.* Sage Publications.

Mittledorf, W., Hendricks, S., & Landreth, G. (2001). Play therapy with autistic children. In G. Landreth (Ed.), *Innovations in play therapy: Issues, process and special populations* (pp. 257–270). Brunner-Routledge.

Nemri, K. (2004). Aiijii healing and how the chakras relate to disease and healing. *Proceedings: Academy of Religion & Psychical Research*, 36–42.

Ogden, P., & Minton, K. (2000). Sensorimotor psychotherapy: One method for processing traumatic memory. *Traumatology, 6*(3), 149–173.

Ogden, P., Minton, K., & Pain, C. (2006). *Trauma and the body: A sensorimotor approach to psychotherapy*. W.W. Norton & Company.

Ostlund, B. D., Measelle, J. R., Laurent, H. K., Conradt, E., & Ablow, J. C. (2017). Shaping emotion regulation: Attunement, symptomatology, and stress recovery within mother-infant dyads. *Developmental Psychobiology, 59*(1), 15–25. Available from https://doi.org/10.1002/dev.21448.

Perry, B. D. (2006). The neurosequential model of therapeutics: Applying principles of neuroscience to clinical work with traumatized and maltreated children. In N. B. Webb (Ed.), *Working with traumatized youth in child welfare* (pp. 27–52). The Guilford Press.

Perry, B. D., & Hambrick, E. (2008). The neurosequential model of therapeutics (NMT). *Reclaiming Children and Youth, 17*(3), 38–43.

Pfeifer, J. H., Iacoboni, M., Mazziotta, J. C., & Dapretto, M. (2008). Mirroring others' emotions relates to empathy and interpersonal competence in children. *Neuroimage, 39*(4), 2076–2085. Available from https://doi.org/10.1016/j.neuroimage.2007.10.032.

Pierce, L. (2014). The integrative power of dance/movement therapy: Implications for the treatment of dissociation and developmental trauma. *The Arts in Psychotherapy, 41*, 7–15. Available from https://doi.org/10.1016/j.aip.2013.10.002.

Porges, S. W. (2011). *The polyvagal theory: Neurophysiological foundations of emotions, attachment, communication, and self-regulation*. New York: W.W. Norton & Company.

Porges, S. W., & Dana, D. (2018). *Clinical applications of the polyvagal theory: The emergence of polyvagal-informed therapies*. WW Norton.

Ratcliffe, M. (2007). *Rethinking commonsense psychology: A critique of folk psychology, theory of mind, and simulation*. Palgrave Macmillan.

Reynolds, D., & Reason, M. (2012). *Kinesthetic empathy in creative and cultural practice*. Intellect.

Salter, K., Beamish, W., & Davies, M. (2016). The effects of Child-Centered Play Therapy (CCPT) on the social and emotional growth of young Australian children with autism. *International Journal of Play Therapy*, *25*(2), 78–90.

Samaritter, R., & Payne, H. (2017). Through the kinesthetic lens: Observation of social attunement in autism spectrum disorders. *Behavioral Sciences*, *7*(1), 14. Available from https://doi.org/10.3390/bs7010014.

Sander, L. (1995). Identity and the experience of specificity in a process of recognition. *Psychoanalytic Dialogues*, *5*, 579–593.

Schaaf, R. C., Schoen, S. A., Roley, S. S., Lane, S. J., Koomar, J., & May-Benson, T. A. (2010). A frame of reference for sensory integration. In P. Kramer, & J. Hinojosa (Eds.), *Frames of reference for pediatric occupational therapy* (3rd ed., pp. 99–186). Lippincott Williams & Wilkins.

Scharoun, S. M., Reinders, N. J., Bryden, P. J., & Fletcher, P. C. (2014). Dance/movement therapy as an intervention for children with autism spectrum disorders. *American Journal of Dance Therapy*, *36*, 209–228. Available from https://doi.org/10.1007/s10465-014-9179-0.

Schoen, S. A., Miller, L. J., & Sullivan, J. C. (2014). Measurement in sensory modulation: The sensory processing scale assessment. *American Journal of Occupational Therapy*, *68*, 522–530. Available from http://doi.org/10.5014/ajot.2014.012377.

Schore, A. N. (2001). Effects of a secure attachment relationship on right brain development, affect regulation, and infant mental health. *Infant Mental Health Journal*, *22*, 7–66.

Schore, A. N. (2010). Relational trauma and the developing right brain: The neurobiology of broken attachment bonds. In T. Baradon (Ed.), *Relational trauma in infancy* (pp. 19–47). Routledge/Taylor & Francis Group.

Schottelkorb, A. A., Swan, K. L., & Ogawa, Y. (2020). Intensive child centered play therapy for children on the autism spectrum: A pilot study. *Journal of Counseling & Development*, *98*, 63–73.

Sharda, M., Silani, G., Specht, K., Tillmann, J., Nater, U., & Gold, C. (2019). Music therapy for children with autism: Investigating social behaviour through music. *The Lancet Child & Adolescent Health*, *3*(11), 759–761. Available from https://doi.org/10.1016/S2352-4642(19)30265-2.

Shonkoff, J. (2017). Breakthrough impacts: What science tells us about supporting early childhood development. *Young Children*, *72*(2), 8–16, Retrieved August 25, 2020, from. Available from https://www.jstor.org/stable/90004117.

Siegel, D. J. (1999). *The developing mind: Toward a neurobiology of interpersonal experience*. Guilford Press.

Siegel, D. J. (2001). Toward an interpersonal neurobiology of the developing mind: Attachment relationships, "mindsight", and neural integration. *Infant Mental Health Journal*, *22*, 67–94.

Srinivasan, S. M., & Bhat, A. N. (2013). A review of "music and movement" therapies for children with autism: Embodied interventions for multisystem development. *Frontiers in Integrative Neuroscience*, *7*, 22.

Solomon, R. (2020). The PLAY project autism intervention model. In F. Volkmar (Ed.), *Encyclopedia of autism spectrum disorders* (2nd ed.). Springer International Publishing.

Srinivasan, S. M., Park, I. K., Neelly, L. B., & Bhat, A. N. (2015). A comparison of the effects of rhythm and robotic interventions on repetitive behaviors and affective states of children with autism spectrum disorder (ASD). *Research in Autism Spectrum Disorders, 18*, 51–63. Available from https://doi.org/10.1016/j.rasd.2015.07.004.

Sroufe, L. A. (1996). *Emotional development: The organization of emotional life in the early years*. Cambridge University Press.

Stern, D. N. (1985). *The motherhood constellation: A unified view of parent–infant psychotherapy*. Basic Books.

St. John, M., Thomas, K., & Noroña, C. R. (2012). Infant mental health professional development: Together in the struggle for social justice. *Zero to Three Journal, 33*(2), 13–22.

Takahashi, H., Matsushima, K., & Kato, T. (2019). The effectiveness of dance/movement therapy interventions for autism spectrum disorder: A systematic review. *American Journal of Dance Therapy, 41*, 55–74. Available from https://doi.org/10.1007/s10465-019-09296-5.

Thompson, E. C., White-Schwoch, T., Tierney, A., & Kraus, N. (2015). Beat synchronization across the lifespan: Intersection of development and musical experience. *PLoS One, 10* (6), e0128839. Available from https://doi.org/10.1371/journal.pone.0128839.

Tortora, S. (2006). *The dancing dialogue: Using the communicative power of movement with young children*. Brookes Publishing.

Trevarthen, C., & Delafield-Butt, J. T. (2013). Autism as a developmental disorder in intentional movement and affective engagement. *Frontiers in Integrative Neuroscience, 7*, 49.

Tronick, E. Z. (2007). *The neurobehavioral and social-emotional development of infants and children*. Norton.

Uljarevic, M., Hedley, D., Nevill, R., Evans, D. W., Cai, R. Y., Butter, E., & Mulick, J. A. (2018). Brief report: Poor self-regulation as a predictor of individual differences in adaptive functioning in young children with ASD. *Autism Research, 11*, 1157–1165. Available from https://doi.org/10.1002/aur.1953.

Venuti, P., Bentenuto, A., Cainelli, S., Landi, I., Suvini, F., Tancredi, R., ... Muratori, F. (2017). A joint behavioral and emotive analysis of synchrony in music therapy of children with autism spectrum disorders. *Health Psychology Report, 5*(2), 162–172. Available from https://doi-org.ezproxy.montclair.edu/10.5114/hpr.2017.63985.

Warner, E., Finn, H., Wescott, A., & Cook, A. (2020). *Transforming trauma in children and adolescents: An embodied approach to somatic regulation, trauma processing, and attachment-building*. North Atlantic Books.

Watson, K. J., & DiCarlo, C. F. (2015). Increasing completion of classroom routines through the use of picture activity schedules. *Early Childhood Education Journal*, 1–8. Available from https://doi.org/10.1007/sl0643-015-0697-2.

Williams, K. E., & Berthelsen, D. (2019). Implementation of a rhythm and movement intervention to support self-regulation skills of preschool-aged children in disadvantaged communities. *Psychology of Music, 47*(6), 800–820. Available from https://doi.org/10.1177/0305735619861433.

You, H. (1994). Defining rhythm: Aspects of an anthropology of rhythm. *Culture, Medicine and Psychiatry, 18*, 361–384. Available from https://doi.org/10.1007/BF01379231.

Zentall, S., & Zentall, T. (1983). Optimal stimulation: A model of disordered activity and performance in normal and deviant children. *Psychological Bulletin, 94*, 466–471.

Asperger syndrome and adolescent girl: understanding the rhythm of emotions towards the struggle with social relationships—cognitive-behavioral and narrative therapy

23

Carla Vale Lucas[1], *Luísa Soares*[2,3] *and Filipa Oliveira*[1]
[1]Psychological Service, University of Madeira, Funchal, Portugal, [2]Faculty of Arts and Humanities, University of Madeira, Funchal, Portugal, [3]Larsys - ITI—Interactive Technologies Institute, Funchal, Portugal

Asperger syndrome and adolescent girl

Social skills represent a complex area within human behavior. Highly socially competent individuals are able to meet the demands of everyday life. They possess appropriate peer reinforcement behaviors, communications skills, problem solving skills, and social self-efficacy and can develop such adaptive behaviors as independent functioning, self-direction, personal responsibility, and functional academic skills (Elder, Caterino, Chao, Shacknai, & Simone, 2006).

Children and adolescents who have difficulties in social skills and who are poorly accepted by peers are at risk of developing some negative consequences. There is a high incidence of school maladjustment, delinquency, child psychopathology, and adult mental health difficulties, such as depression and anxiety (Elder et al., 2006). For people that have Asperger's syndrome (AS), social skills are the biggest life challenge.

This is a case study of a teenager named "Sandra" who was diagnosed with AS when she was 11 years old. Also she had to learn how to cope with absence seizures since the age of 9. Sandra struggled with the feeling of being different. She wanted to fit in social groups, but lacked the skills and social knowledge to do it.

Throughout individual therapy, framed in the grounds of cognitive behavioral and narrative therapy, we work toward helping her cope with these difficulties and become more independent. Additionally, we report the intervention with Sandra's parents, who struggle to learn how to cope with the diagnoses of epilepsy and AS and how to promote the development of their teenage daughter.

Emerging Programs for Autism Spectrum Disorder. DOI: https://doi.org/10.1016/B978-0-323-85031-5.00011-6

Sandra's case study

Sandra started attending the psychological sessions when she was 10 years old, on the transition for the 5th grade. She is now 12, and attends the 7th grade. She presented some immature behavior in the way she addressed her parents and also in the way she separated from them (with prolonged hugging and kissing). By the age of 9, she started having absence seizures. As she got older and since she got her menstruation at 11, they become more frequent. She is being medicated to prevent those seizures.

Sandra's parents looked for psychological counseling, due to difficulties in adjusting to the new school and getting along with colleagues. Through these difficulties, she maintained good grades.

In school, Sandra is a calm and shy girl, lacking confidence, as stated by one of her teachers. In some moments, she shows little control over emotions, crying in front of others out of the blue. At home, she presents a different behavior. She is extremely dependent on her parents (for instance, she isn't able to sleep and to take a bath alone). When stressed, she has aggressive behaviors toward her parents, calling them names. The problems about sleeping in her bedroom started after she was diagnosed with epilepsy. She gets more scared about the dark and her parents were afraid to leave her alone, due to the seizures.

During the psychological sessions, at the age of 11, she was diagnosed with Asperger's syndrome by a neuropsychiatrist, with expertise in Autism Spectrum Disorders.

Assessment and case conceptualization

Sandra's assessment included interviews with both parents for the purpose of obtaining a comprehensive developmental history, and also an interview with her to determine the level of communication, academic and social skills, and adaptive functioning. Also the assessment used some psychological tests and other activities.

Sandra presented a good level of intellectual maturity. The results of Child Behavior Checklist for ages 4–18 (Achenbach, 1991) showed high values on internalization scales, especially in the social problems scale, as well as in the syndrome scale of anxious/depressed. Although not entirely significant, some externalizations problems stood out. In the Family Drawing test, the characters were drawn as being very old, when compared to her real family. She showed strong fear of losing people and constantly talking about making birthdays. From the analysis of Roberts (Roberts & Gruder, 2005) it shows a vulnerable pattern of emotions and behaviors. She presented some features expected in a clinical profile of depression, with elevations in anxiety and rejection scales. Also she showed some difficulties in identifying problems, which seem anxiety related, when she have to acknowledge some emotions, such as fear. Likewise, she presented difficulties in finding age appropriate solutions to the problems presented. Moreover, she had difficulties in seeking help.

Observation was also an important component of the assessment. Sandra didn't want to come to the sessions. In the first session, she showed resistance and a disrespectful attitude towards her parents. Parents seem to be having difficulties in managing her behavior and establishing limits. In the interview, her father said, "probably we are protecting her too much." These difficulties were enhanced after Sandra's diagnosis with epilepsy.

Throughout the therapeutic process, Sandra struggled in separating from her mother. Also, she had difficulties in greeting and establishing eye contact. Despite the initial resistance in engaging with the sessions, we were able to establish a good therapeutic relationship. Nevertheless from time-to-time she presented some anxiety, expressed in nervous laughs, avoiding themes or tasks, or doing them very fast, and not confronting the results. She showed difficulties in understanding some abstracts concepts, like metaphors, and feeling somehow confused.

About herself she writes "I'm ugly," "I'm fat," "I'm an idiot." In sessions, these expressions are frequent. Also, she describes her epilepsy as "an evil in her head." She doesn't like to talk about that, as she states that she cannot understand what is happening with her. Her biggest wish is to not have epilepsy.

She talked about school in an aggressive way, "It sucks," "It's bad," "I want to change school." For her, the worse thing in school is the "breaks for lunch." During the therapeutic process and as she grew older, she became more worried and distressed about her lack of friends, showing her difficulties in understanding the social interactions. Also, older colleagues teased her, without her knowing that she was being deceived, and lacking the skill to self-defend.

Sandra has intense interests that guide all her conversations (i.e., age, a strong interest toward boys, more intense than typical teenage crushes), lacking the ability to understand and react in terms of the interest of the interlocutor.

Sandra's diagnosis

Throughout the assessment symptomatology of depression and anxiety stood out. Likewise, Sandra presented difficulties in the social domain, being self-centered and lacking social competencies. Also she presented struggles in managing emotions, like fear and anger, as well as having low self-esteem. Nevertheless, the struggle to adapt to school was not adequately and completely described by this symptomatology. Besides the difficulties presented in social relationships, she had also difficulties in using social language, and in understanding and using adequately facial expressions and gestures. With this in mind, we argue that Sandra's difficulties could be better explained by Asperger's syndrome, presenting also depressive and anxious symptoms.

Asperger's syndrome

The diagnosis of Asperger's disorder was first added to the American Psychiatric Association's Diagnostic and Statistical Manual of Mental Disorders, 4th edition as a pervasive developmental disorder belonging to the family of autism spectrum disorders (American Psychiatric Association (APA), 1994; Portway & Johnson, 2003).

Diagnosing individuals with AS is complex as there isn't any biological test to aid diagnosis (Portway & Johnson, 2005). Thus it is made solely on the basis of developmental and behavioral characteristics (National Autistic Society, 1999). Moreover individuals with AS present high rates of comorbid disorders (such as emotional disorders—anxiety and depression; as well as behavioral disorders—conduct disorder, oppositional defiant disorder; and attention-deficit/hyperactivity disorder), which might delay or obscure the diagnose of AS (Hoffmann et al., 2013; Park, Park, Kim, & Yoo, 2003; Portway & Johnson, 2005; Sotronoff, Attwood, & Hinton, 2005), leaving the child at risk of negative encounters, developing low self-esteem, anxiety, and depression (Portway & Johnson, 2003).

The mean age for a diagnosis of AS is approximately 8 years old (Elder et al., 2006). The difficulties presented are age-related, and need to be targeted in intervention. During elementary school, social skill deficits became more prominent. In middle school, children begin feeling their differences and express sadness, anxiety, and rejection. Teenagers faced increased anxiety, obsessive-compulsive, and ever-changing social skill deficiencies (Church, Alisanski, & Amanullah, 2000).

In DSM-5, an explicit diagnostic category "Asperger syndrome" will no longer exist. That doesn't mean that individuals with milder autistic symptoms, good cognitive and language abilities will disappear (Hoffmann et al., 2013).

People with AS are affected to different degrees in the way they think, communicate, relate to others, and understand the world around them (National Autistic Society, 1999). Individuals with AS have been identified as having difficulty with "theory of mind" tasks. That is, they lack an understanding and appreciation of the feelings, thoughts, needs, and intentions of others, how their behavior impacts others, and the meaning of reciprocity in relationships (Cumine, Leach, & Stevenson, 2006; Elder et al., 2006; Farrugia & Hudson, 2006). Due to these social deficits, the attempts made in social contexts are often clumsy and inappropriate. They can be fluent in verbal expression, but the content of conversations may be narrow and reflect circumscribed interests. The child may continue a conversation with little regard to the interest of the listener (Sotronoff et al., 2005), also having an inability to read social cues and to respond to those (Elder et al., 2006). There is likely to be a preference for fixed routines and structure, with significant distress at even minor changes. They have also a rigid thinking (Farrugia & Hudson, 2006). There can be signs of motor clumsiness, poor fine motor skills (Elder et al., 2006), hypersensitivity to specific auditory and tactile experiences, and problems with time/organization management (Sotronoff et al., 2005).

Genetic and environmental factors, like immunological factors, could be at the origin of AS. Still, no exogenous causes have been found that explain AS. According to Antunes (2009), the father sometimes has AS too. Also, the age of parents seems directly correlated with autism. These last two assumptions were found to be true in Sandra's case. Attwood (2010) states there is some evidence suggesting a dysfunction in the frontal or temporal lobe. Sandra's encephalogram to check the brain for electrical activity that can cause seizures, pointed out a lesion in the temporal lobe.

AS and epilepsy

Epilepsy is a neurological condition, which affects the nervous system. It is also known as a seizure disorder. Seizures seen in epilepsy are caused by disturbances in the brain's electrical activity. Over a third of people with autistic spectrum disorders develop epilepsy, the risk being linked to the degree of developmental delay and receptive language deficit. There is no specific study of epilepsy in AS, although the relatively normal ability and language suggest that the risk is lower, around 5%–10%, and that it is more likely to start later, in adolescence or early adulthood (Berney, 2004).

AS in girls

The proportion of boys and girls that are sent to a diagnostic evaluation is 10 boys to 1 girl. Nevertheless, the epidemiologic states a proportion of 4:1 (Ehlers & Gillberg, 1993). Although there aren't many studies, it has been found that in general, boys showed a higher expression of social deficits, very irregular profiles of social skills, and a tendency toward disturbing or aggressive behavior, especially when they feel frustrated or under tension. In contrast, girls tend to be relatively more skilled in social play and reveal a more balanced profile of social skills. Often, they have the ability to post imitate social behaviors. They watch other kids and copy them, but their actions, unlike the other children do not occur at the right time and are not spontaneous (Attwood, 2010).

Girls with AS are considered more immature than unusual. They may still be "invisible" children, socially isolated, concerned about their imaginary world, but do not constitute a disruptive influence in the classroom. According to the author's experience, the prognosis of girls is better in the long term. They appear to be better able to learn to integrate socially, although they may appear aloof, awkward, shy, or otherwise overly friendly and intrusively talkative (Attwood, 2010; Wing, 1996).

Understanding the diagnosis in Sandra's adolescence

Transition times are very difficult, as they break the routine. In a study made by Portway and Johnson (2003) the school years were seen as being particularly and progressively problematic, due to the increase of social expectations from the child as well from peers, teachers, parents, and society in general (Berney, 2004; Portway & Johnson, 2003). In Sandra this seems particularly true. She coped well in her primary school. However, when she moved to a bigger school, her true degree of disability became apparent.

The transition from childhood to adolescent is seen as stressful for both family and child. Adolescents with AS experience difficulties arising from the core symptoms presented but also in coping with the need to become less dependent, more responsible, and the need to make decisions (Portway & Johnson, 2003). They often struggle to separate from primary caregivers because they have no peer group to whom they can turn or with whom they can fit in (McKinsey, 2009). Also the syndrome distorts relationships with family and peers. Sometimes they can feel angry by the person's self-centered insensitivity, obsessiveness, and rigid inflexibility.

Between the ages of 9 and 13, friendships are based on similarities, sharing adventures, and giving each other emotional support. Teenagers with AS are often eager to understand and experience the social and relationship world of their peers, including relationships and sexual experiences (Moreno, Wheeler, & Parkinson, 2012), which seems to be Sandra's case. Adolescents with AS also struggle with the feeling of being different from others on many occasions (Portway & Johnson, 2003). Likewise, there is the stress that grows from the limited achievement and sense of failure, when compared with more autonomous and successful siblings or peers (Berney, 2004). Sandra struggles with this and with self-esteem problems, common within this developmental stage, being more vulnerable to anxiety and/or depression.

Adolescents with AS may express their distress in different ways. They may have a strong awareness of their need for contact with others or a desire for closeness (Sandra's case), or they may cope with environmental stress by withdrawing or isolating themselves. Nonetheless, children with AS often learn strategies to cope, that can mask the true extent of their difficulties.

Prognostic and treatment

As with other developmental disorders, autistic spectrum disorders improve with age. Nevertheless there isn't any cure or medicine that might significantly alter the ability of socialization or empathy, or cognitive rigidity (Antunes, 2009). Symptoms such as stereotypies may resurface with arousal, whether from anxiety, boredom, anger, or excitement (Berney, 2004). The problems of people who have AS and the associated risks cannot be completely ameliorated by appropriate educational interventions and greater understanding by others, but can be greatly exacerbated by their absence (Portway & Johnson, 2005).

When diagnosed, treatment involves a multimodal approach, thus being complex and multifaceted (McKinsey, 2009). It can include individual and family psychotherapy, psychopharmacology, special education, occupational therapy, speech and language therapy, and social skills training (Elder et al, 2006).

Therapeutic intervention

Therapeutic intervention in AS cases is usually long term. We started the sessions on a regular basis (weekly). After some time, they became fortnightly, in order to monitor the achievements and continue working with her social skills. The intervention process was based on the theoretical framework of Cognitive Behavioral

Therapy (CBT), the principles of narrative therapy of White and Epston (1990), and also integrated some systemic principles, as it was very important to intervene with family, supporting parents and improving the relationship between family members.

CBT only recently has been applied to children and adults with AS. Although few empirical studies have been reported, outcomes have been positive (Sotronoff et al., 2005). The use of narrative therapy aimed at helping Sandra to deconstruct narratives about school, about herself and epilepsy, and elaborate other narratives that are more adaptive and flexible.

The therapeutic intervention had the following aims: establish a satisfactory therapeutic relationship; help the adaptation process to school and colleagues; psych educate about AS and epilepsy; psych educate about emotions; develop strategies to cope with stress, anxiety, and aggression; develop social competences; improve self-esteem and self-confidence; enhance her autonomy and help parents to accept the diagnosis; decrease the tension felt; and promote Sandra's development.

Intervention process

In order to facilitate the understanding of the intervention process, we systematized the therapeutic goals into six moments.

First moment: establishing a satisfactory therapeutic relationship

Although the initial resistance engaging in the sessions, we started working as a coach and a trainee. Sandra also had in the therapist a coping model for careful reasoning, nonanxious behavior, and other social competencies, which was a key element in the therapeutic process. One important thing that helped in establishing the therapeutic relationship was the flexibility shown to adjust the sessions to the emotional state of Sandra. We used writing exercises, art exercises, reading materials carefully selected, games and videos, that were age and interests appropriate.

Second moment: psych educating about the problem (AS and epilepsy)

Sandra and her family had to cope with two diagnoses: epilepsy and AS. Both diagnostics caused anxiety. It was important to give accurate information about them. Some books and other materials were provided to the family (Antunes, 2009; Cumine et al., 2006; Welton, 2004). After receiving this information, we were better able to work together as a team.

Sandra's parents showed some resistance to revealing the AS diagnosis to Sandra, feeling that she was not prepared. In fact, as cited by McKinsey (2009), children tend to accept more readily the "label," while adolescents tend to struggle more, especially when issues of self-identity are prominent, which was Sandra's case. Nevertheless, it was important to educate Sandra regarding her diagnosis and what it meant for her. Together we elaborated a list of abilities and difficulties of each member of the family, as suggested by Attwood (2010). Afterwards, it was explained that doctors had given a name to the main characteristics presented in her list: Asperger syndrome. Also, we searched for famous people with AS. As stated by McKinsey (2009), Sandra's understanding of how her brain may work differently was essential, as a way to help to improve self-esteem.

Third moment: developing social competences

It was essential to develop Sandra's social competences, through social skills training. This training was aimed at increasing her self-awareness, to develop strategies to compensate for social deficits, to improve conversational skills, and to encourage independent living skills. Social skills treatment is a well-documented and important intervention for children with AS, although little empirical evidence exists to support this premise (Attwood, 2000, Elder et al., 2006).

We helped her to learn how to initiate a conversation; to acknowledge signs that point at the time to answer, interrupt, or change subject; to use eye contact; to ask for clarifications or for help (...). Also it was important to explain and clarify why certain behaviors are expected in specific contexts.

For these purposes we use techniques as modeling, role-playing, and feedback. We analyzed videos with social behaviors as well as reading materials and social stories (Attwood, 2000; Elder et al., 2006; Gray, 2000). Also we constructed some comic strip conversations that allowed her to analyze and understand the range of messages and meanings that are part of natural conversation, an activity suggested by Attwood (2000). Likewise we used structured games like card and board games to teach pragmatic language. Body language, facial cues, gestures, and voice tone were then practiced using these tools. We also trained problem-solving skills. We shared experiences inside and outside the therapy office, as suggested by Kendal (1992). Those were an opportunity for modeling, to discuss interpersonal interactions and to give feedback to her (experiences like to great the therapist or other person, to start a conversation, besides others).

Also we suggested that Sandra participate in social group activities, as an opportunity to know people with similar capacities and interests, to learn how to self-reveal and listen to others, as well as acknowledging her and the thoughts and feelings of others.

Fourth moment: psych educating about emotions and developing coping strategies

Attwood (2000) suggested that social skills training might target the identification of specific emotions, the contexts in which they might be appropriate, and modulation skills to help manage the intensity of the emotions. Hence, we explore individually each emotion. We questioned, for instance, "How can you know that a person is sad? What could you say or do to help? What makes you feel sad?" We have done exercises like mimics to help her read and express body signs and facial expressions. Furthermore, to describe and explore events and comments that drive toward a feeling, we try to recall some of her own events and explain that others could experience similar feelings, as a way to promote empathy development.

We encourage her to write the events, impressions, thoughts, and feelings. Stress, anxiety, and aggression were symptoms strongly presented in Sandra, thus it was important to teach how to cope with them. One of the exercises done was the fears hierarchy. She had fears like "being different," "being teased," "getting alone," "death," "dark." Thus to better learn ways to cope with fear we applied the benefits of bibliotherapy (Lucas & Soares, 2013), using for instance the book of Gonçalves (2000). Afterwards, we trained anxiety management techniques, such as diaphragmatic breathing, progressive muscle relaxation and visualization imagery. At some point, after facing some fears, she wrote: "it is worth facing and overcoming fear."

We have done exercises to help her anticipate the consequences, and others to remind her what to do when angry. Although there were some difficulties in self-control, as time passed she become more capable to hold/wait and to manage better the feeling of frustration.

Fifth moment: promoting the development of autonomy and self-esteem

As she presents negative speech about herself, to increase self-esteem and self-confidence we suggested some activities that she could do, focusing on what she is doing right, and complimenting the child and teaching her to compliment herself, as suggested by Elder et al. (2006).

To achieve these purposes, we use books as a tool (i.e., Welton, 2004). Through reading about others that experienced similar feelings and behaviors, she gained increased understanding of her social awkwardness. Also we registered all her conquests during sessions as she wrote the "Adventures of Sandra," reporting some of her accomplishments.

During the therapeutic process, progressively, she changed her negative speech about herself (i.e., "I'm ugly," "I'm fat"). She brought to the session a letter that she wrote for the therapist:

> *I am writing to tell you what I think about me. I think I have a sense of humour; I like my friends and my family, especially my parents, but sometimes I'm not tolerant with the rules; I'm sweet with animals, especially with my kitty; I like to work out to be a good student; I'm smart and pretty (...). This is Me! Kisses and hugs.*

Enhancing her autonomy was a very important goal to be achieved in therapy, as a means to increase her self-esteem and self-efficacy. Note she faced difficulties in sleeping alone, doing homework tasks by herself, taking baths, and taking the epilepsy medication, etc. Now, she is more responsible about these things, being able to accomplish them. We have done some therapeutic contracts like "I, Sandra, will sleep alone in my bed. I know sometimes it will be hard but I'll try... I WILL ACHIEVE!," writing down every time she could do it, monitoring the process. These agreements had witnesses, the therapist and her parents, as a way to better work together to achieve our goals. Another accomplishment was the fact she started coming to sessions alone. She wrote, "Before, when I couldn't do something, I asked my mother to do it. Now, first I try. That is like gold!"

Since she faced so many changes in her body, which led to anxiety and stress, we addressed these questions. After some time, she felt more comfortable, accepting her body changes, taking more care about herself, and becoming more vain. Another question that still is very important to address in sessions is sexuality and boyfriends. For several times, she asked "How can I get a boyfriend?" Boys themes were constant in school, at home, and in sessions. So it was very important to give accurate information on attraction, the dating game, and sexuality, as she has difficulties in correctly interpreting someone's intentions (Moreno et al., 2012).

Sixth moment: parents intervention

The parents' involvement was a very important part of the therapeutic process. They struggle with doubts and guilty feelings, questioning if they could prevent it. It was important to work toward these anxieties that were enhancing Sandra's handicaps, by confronting some thoughts and developing their coping mechanisms.

We had to work especially with the mother, who showed some high levels of anxiety, worrying that Sandra could not have a normal life. Also, she worried about others not being able to understand what Sandra had, and so judging her ability as a mother. Wishing to protect the daughter, she struggled in establishing limits, saying no, and assigning tasks, which was increasing Sandra's difficulties in getting more responsible and independent. So Sandra's mother was a key factor through the intervention. As she became more confident she was able to better encourage Sandra's autonomy, responsibility, to set limits, help her understand social situations, and develop social competences.

Conclusions

> *Once upon a time there was a girl named Sandra. She had brown hair, blue eyes and freckles (...). What made her happy was being with friends. When Sandra was younger she had some fears, as to do a somersault. But in the 6th grade she learned how to do it and was very good at it. Also, she was afraid to sleep in her bed and of the dark. Nevertheless, she was able to face those fears. She decided to tell other people how she had overcome the fears. When Sandra went to the new school she felt ashamed and afraid because she didn't knew anything or anyone. Now she already knows colleagues and gets along with them. She now says to other kids who face this fear: "Make friends!," "It takes courage to make friends and I was brave!"*
>
> *Sandra's adventures: 1st chapter*

This is one of the many chapters of Sandra's history. She wrote this chapter during sessions, when facing some fears and after struggling to adapt to school. She has achieved many conquests but the most important one was making friends.

In adolescence, there is the desire of intimacy, love, and the wish to develop friendships. However, Sandra faced some difficulties in knowing how to do it, that was explained by the AS diagnosis. Antunes (2009) states that people with AS are bad dancers in the emotions dance, and like a bad dancer they try to imitate others, but they cannot understand the rhythm of emotions. So Sandra's individual therapy was aimed at helping her to better cope with the daily challenges and to develop social skills.

To better sum up the therapeutic process, we can divide it in two big periods: Sandra during 5th grade and Sandra during 6/7nd grade. During 5th grade the goals were to adjust to the new school, develop her autonomy, and help face the intense fears presented. After a couple months of therapy she faced some fears, and changed the way she spoke about school, being more adjusted to it. Nevertheless, she still felt like an outlier from classmates. During the 6th and 7nd grade, we saw her flourish. Teenage worries, such as friends and boyfriends, were the main topics of sessions. She faced social difficulties in getting along, as well as the big desire to be with them. She also had to face the feeling of being different, but also to cope with all her body changes, and with the seizures that were intensifying. As she made more friends, she felt more comfortable, and capable of developing the strategies for managing stress, anxiety, and aggression. However, as the social relationships got better, the school grades got a little worse. Nevertheless, she is more able to find things that she feels good at it. She is more independent and responsible.

One important part of the therapeutic process was the intervention with the parents. Sandra's family were scared about her diagnosis. The tension was big, and was getting in the way of her autonomy, responsibility, and other core aspects of her development. It was urgent to address and to work in collaboration with her parents to better help Sandra.

The therapeutic intervention still is onset to better help understand daily situations and to train social skills, that are important for the development of a positive sense of identity and competence, and to prevent the symptoms of anxiety and depression that she already had. There are also some aspects that need to be further addressed, namely the way she sometimes expressed affection, excessively/overfriendly, and questions of sexuality and boyfriends.

This is Sandra's history. Probably throughout her development Sandra will continue facing challenges. The transition to a new school could be one of those. Peer relationship difficulties will continue to be a source of frustration, anxiety, and confusion. To better help children and adults fit in society more effectively and achieve their full potential it is essential to make an earlier detection of AS and improve our knowledge about AS (Portway & Johnson, 2003).

AS has no cure. A child/adolescent with AS "is like a Ferrari. The problem is that the road of life is not smooth. For the Ferrari to go on as fast as their potential, we must put tires more suited and to repair at least some holes of the road" (adapted from Antunes, 2009, p. 122). Therefore, treating people with AS implies firstly educating the family, then the school, and whenever possible the society about the challenges they face. So, changing the tires of the Ferrari means giving the child tools to deal with life's obstacles.

Acknowledgment

The parents signed a consent form allowing this publication. This study received no external funding.

The authors have declared that they have no competing or potential conflicts of interest.

References

Achenbach, T. (1991). *Manual for the child behaviour checklist/4-18 and 1991 profile*. Burlington, VT: University of Vermont, Department of Psychiatry.

American Psychiatric Association (APA). (1994). *Diagnostic and statistical manual for mental disorders*. Washington, DC: APA.

Antunes, N. L. (2009). *Mal-entendidos*. Lisboa: Verso de Kapa.

Attwood, T. (2000). Strategies for improving the social integration of children with Asperger syndrome. *Autism*, *4*(1), 85–100.

Attwood, T. (2010). *A Síndrome de Asperger*. Lisboa: Verbo.

Berney, T. (2004). Asperger syndrome from childhood into adulthood. *Advances in Psychiatric Treatment*, *10*, 341–351.

Church, C., Alisanski, S., & Amanullah, S. (2000). The social, behavioral, and academic experiences of children with Asperger syndrome. *Focus on Autism and Other Developmental Disabilities*, *15*(1), 12–20.

Cumine, V., Leach, J., & Stevenson, G. (2006). *Compreender a Síndrome de Asperger. Guia Prático para Educadores*. Porto: Porto Editora.

Ehlers, S., & Gillberg, C. (1993). The epidemiology of Asperger syndrome. A total population study. *Journal of Child Psychology and Psychiatry*, *34*, 1327.

Elder, L. M., Caterino, L. C., Chao, J., Shacknai, D., & Simone, G. (2006). The efficacy of social skills treatment for children with Asperger syndrome. *Education and Treatment of Children*, *29*(4), 635–663.

Farrugia, S., & Hudson, J. (2006). Anxiety in adolescents with Asperger syndrome: Negative thoughts, behavioral problems, and life interference. *Focus on Autism and Other Developmental Disabilities*, *21*(1), 25–35.

Gonçalves, M. (2000). *Pôr o medo a fugir: As aventuras de Joana contra o medo*. Porto: Campo de Letras.

Gray, G. (2000). *New social stories: Illustrated edition*. Arlington, TX: Future Horizons.

Hoffmann, W., Konig, U., Heinzel-Gutenbrunner, M., Mattejat, F., Becker, K., & Kamp-Becker, I. (2013). Early identification of Asperger syndrome in young children. *Research in Developmental Disabilities*, *34*, 640–649.

Kendall, P., Chansky, T., Kane, M., Kim, R., Kortlander, E., Ronan, K., ... Siqueland, L. (1992). *Anxiety disorders in youth: Cognitive-behavioral interventions*. Massachusetts: Allyn and Bacon.

Lucas, C. V., & Soares, L. (2013). Bibliotherapy: A tool to promote children's psychological well-being. *Journal of Poetry Therapy: The Interdisciplinary Journal of Practice. Theory, Research and Education*, *26*(3), 137–147.
McKinsey, L. L. (2009). An Asperger's diagnosis and success in individual therapy. *CABL, The Brown University Child and Adolescent Behavior Letter*, *25*(6), 6–7.
Moreno, S., Wheeler, M., & Parkinson, K. (2012). *The partner's guide to Asperger syndrome*. London and Philadelphia, PA: Jessica Kingsley Publishers.
National Autistic Society. (1999). *The autistic spectrum – A handbook*. London: The National Autistic Society.
Park, S., Park, M.-H., Kim, H. J., & Yoo, H. J. (2003). Anxiety and depression symptoms in children with Asperger syndrome compared with attention-deficit/hiperactivity disorder and depressive disorder. *Journal Child Family Studies*, *22*, 559–568.
Portway, S. M., & Johnson, B. (2005). Do you know I have Asperger's syndrome? Risks of a non-obvious disability. *Health, Risk & Society*, *7*(1), 73–83.
Portway, S., & Johnson, B. (2003). Asperger syndrome and the children who "don't quite fit in". *Early Child Development and Care*, *173*(4), 435–443.
Roberts, G. E., & Gruder, C. (2005). *Roberts-2 manual*. WPS.
Sotronoff, K., Attwood, T., & Hinton, S. (2005). A randomised controlled trial of a CBT intervention for anxiety in children with Asperger syndrome. *Journal of Child Psychology and Psychiatry*, *46*(11), 1152–1160.
Welton, J. (2004). *Posso explicar-te o que é a Síndrome de Asperger? Um guia para amigos e familiares*. Porto: Verbo.
White, M., & Epson, D. (1990). *Narrative Means to Therapeutic Ends*. New York: Norton.
Wing, L. (1996). *The autistic spectrum: A guide for parents and professionals*. London: Constable.

Emotion regulation: a target for improving mental health in autism 24

Ru Ying Cai[1,2] *and Mirko Uljarević*[3]
[1]Aspect Research Centre for Autism Practice, Autism Spectrum Australia, Melbourne, Vic, Australia, [2]Faculty of Medicine, Nursing and Health Sciences, School of Psychological Sciences, Monash University, Melbourne, Vic, Australia, [3]Faculty of Medicine, Dentistry and Health Sciences, Melbourne School of Psychological Sciences, University of Melbourne, Melbourne, Vic, Australia

Emotion regulation

Emotions were traditionally thought to be irrational and to cause problems in adaptive functioning (for a critical overview, see Damasio, 1994). Subsequent research has demonstrated that emotions allow us to adapt to our environmental demands via activation of attentional, behavioral, and physiological resources (Levenson, 1994). Emotions can be classified as positive, negative, or neutral (emotional valence). Positive emotions include "pleasant or desirable situational responses, ranging from interest and contentment to love and joy, but are distinct from pleasurable sensation and undifferentiated positive affect" (Cohn & Fredrickson, 2009, p. 13). In contrast, negative emotions such as anger, sadness, or fear involve "unpleasant, often disruptive, emotional reactions" (American Psychological Association, 2020). Neutral emotions are expressed as feelings of indifference, "nothing in particular, and a lack of preference one way or the other" (Gasper, Spencer, & Hu, 2019, p. 3).

Researchers have demonstrated that both positive and negative emotions have adaptive functions. Positive emotions can help us to broaden our cognitive and behavioral repertoires (Fredrickson, 2004), assist in the recovery from daily stresses (Ong, Bergeman, Bisconti, & Wallace, 2006), and enhance our self-efficacy, relationship satisfaction, mental health, and work satisfaction (Schutte, 2014). Negative emotions and moods have been shown to reduce judgment bias (Fiedler, Asbeck, & Nickel, 1991; Forgas, 2011) and improve memory accuracy (Bäuml & Kuhbandner, 2007; Forgas, Laham, & Vargas, 2005; Storbeck & Clore, 2011). Although the majority of emotion regulation research focus on negative emotions, there is an increasing interest in understanding the mechanisms and impact of positive emotions (Carl, Soskin, Kerns, & Barlow, 2013).

We are intrinsically motivated to feel good, hence we tend to approach or avoid stimuli that make us feel good or bad, respectively (Larsen, 2000). For this reason, we tend to reduce the intensity or frequency of our negative emotions

Emerging Programs for Autism Spectrum Disorder. DOI: https://doi.org/10.1016/B978-0-323-85031-5.00016-5

(downregulation) and more readily accept our positive emotions (Gross, Richards, & John, 2006). Imagine a scenario where you are stuck in traffic and running very late for an important business meeting. With every minute that passes, the frustration that you feel increases. When you realize how you are feeling and that there is nothing you can do to change your situation, you decide to reduce your frustration by calling your colleagues to notify them of your lateness, apologize for it, and then drive as calmly as you can to the office. This complex process of monitoring and modifying our emotional responses is called emotion regulation (Eisenberg & Spinrad, 2004). Emotion regulation can modify the intensity, duration, and types of emotions experienced (Thompson, 1991). Emotion regulation can be goal-directed or be automatic and outside of one's consciousness (Gyurak, Gross, & Etkin, 2011). The first step of emotion regulation is to identify the emotions that require regulating (Gross, 2015), which then triggers the implementation of emotion regulation strategies to either increase or decrease these emotions.

Long-term emotion dysregulation is a trans-diagnostic risk factor for experiencing mental health conditions in the general and autistic populations (Aldao, Gee, De Los Reyes, & Seager, 2016; Cai, Richdale, Uljarević, Dissanayake, & Samson, 2018; Gross & John, 2003). Some people experience difficulties identifying their own or other people's emotions (alexithymia). Since the critical and initial step of emotion regulation is identifying emotions that require modification, experiencing alexithymia is not helpful for emotion regulation. Indeed, people with alexithymia show great emotion regulation difficulties (Pandey, Saxena, & Dubey, 2011) and tend to experience more mental health symptoms such as anxiety and depression (Honkalampi, Hintikka, Tanskanen, Lehtonen, & Viinamäki, 2000; Karukivi et al., 2010).

People are capable of using a variety of different strategies within and across situations to regulate emotions (Aldao & Dixon-Gordon, 2014; Aldao & Nolen-Hoeksema, 2013). Research findings in the general population indicate that the habitual use of certain strategies (e.g., rumination, expressive suppression) is associated with an increase in negative emotions and internalizing symptoms such as anxiety and depression (Aldao, Nolen-Hoeksema, & Schweizer, 2010). These strategies are known to be maladaptive. Conversely, the use of other strategies (e.g., emotional acceptance and savoring positive experiences) is related to reduced negative emotions and better psychological well-being. Hence, these strategies are seen as adaptive. It is important to note that consistent use of adaptive strategies across all situations may not be healthy. Matching the appropriate emotion regulation strategy to the situation and being able to regulate flexibly is very important for well-being (Gross & John, 2003; Quoidbach, Berry, Hansenne, & Mikolajczak, 2010). For example, although cognitive reappraisal is generally thought to be an adaptive emotion regulation strategy due to its association with better mental health (Aldao et al., 2010; Gross & John, 2003), it is only adaptive in situations where stress is uncontrollable (Troy, Shallcross, & Mauss, 2013). In situations where stress is controllable, problem-solving (i.e., taking actions to improve one's circumstances) may be more suitable and adaptive.

Emotion regulation in autistic individuals

Researchers have suggested that poor emotion regulation may be inherent in autistic individuals (Mazefsky & White, 2014; Mazefsky et al., 2013). All autistic traits are associated with emotion dysregulation (Berkovits, Eisenhower, & Blacher, 2017), with restricted and repetitive pattern of behaviors, activities, and interests showing the strongest association (Samson et al., 2014). In addition to these core autistic traits, cognitive factors such as lower executive functioning have also been shown to be associated with poorer emotion regulation in autistic children (Cibralic, Kohlhoff, Wallance, McMahon, & Eapen, 2019).

Emotion regulation research in autistic individuals to date has largely focused on group differences (autistic and nonautistic groups) in alexithymia and emotion regulation, relationships between emotion regulation and outcome variables, and effectiveness of interventions targeting emotion regulation. A systematic review showed that there is a higher prevalence of alexithymia in autistic individuals than nonautistic individuals (49.93% vs 4.89%; Kinnaird, Stewart, & Tchanturia, 2019). As a group, autistic individuals experience more emotion regulation difficulties when compared to nonautistic individuals. A recent systematic review of emotion regulation in autistic children found that they have poorer emotion regulation abilities and used simpler and less effective emotion regulation strategies during times of distress compared to typically developing children (Cibralic et al., 2019). Research evidence also indicates autistic individuals show a maladaptive pattern of strategy use (e.g., using more frequently strategies that are associated with poorer mental health). Our recent commentary has shown that most studies reported autistic individuals using less adaptive patterns of emotion regulation than nonautistic individuals (Cai et al., 2018). We also noted that strategies may have differing effects on autistic individuals. For example, inconsistent findings thus far preclude firm conclusions in terms of the long-term impact of avoidance for autistic individuals. Avoidant strategies are generally thought to be maladaptive due to their association with more depressive symptoms in nonautistic youth (Seiffge-Krenke & Klessinger, 2000). However, the use of avoidant strategies is associated with reduced symptoms of depression in autistic youth (Pouw, Rieffe, Stockmann, & Gadow, 2013).

Apart from mental health, emotion regulation is shown to be associated with various other health and life outcomes such as social skills (Berkovits et al., 2017), peer social engagement (Jahromi, Bryce, & Swanson, 2013), social adjustment (Nader-Grosbois & Mazzone, 2014), and academic performance (Konstantareas & Stewart, 2006). Furthermore, we recently found a positive association between emotion regulation and heart rate variability, an index of cardiac vagal control and autonomic flexibility (Cai, Richdale, Dissanayake, & Uljarević, 2019). Autistic adults who can reappraise a situation to help themselves feel better had higher resting heart rate variability.

Coregulation of emotions in autistic children

Not only is the ability to manage one's emotional response important for well-being across the lifespan, the child development literature has shown that coregulation of emotions is also highly relevant. Coregulation has been defined as "a bidirectional linkage of oscillating emotional channels (subjective experience, expressive behavior, and autonomic physiology) between partners, which contributes to emotional and physiological stability for both partners in a close relationship" (Butler & Randall, 2013, p. 203). Extensive research evidence suggests that a bidirectional dependence exists in parent-infant interactions and infants depend on their caregivers for emotional homeostasis (Feldman, 2003; Kopp, 1982). During typical development of emotion regulation from infancy through to preschooler age, children move from caregiver-driven coregulation to self-driven regulation (Grolnick, Bridges, & Connell, 1996).

Researchers have studied coregulation of emotions in autistic children. Nuske et al. (2017) found that autistic children tend to rely on others for comfort more than themselves, whereas nonautistic children were more self-reliant. The researchers suggested that autistic children have delayed emotion regulation strategy development, specifically, a delay in the shift from coregulation to self-regulation. Parents of autistic children engage in a similar range of emotion coregulation behaviors (Gulsrud, Jahromi, & Kasari, 2010; Hirschler-Guttenberg, Feldman, Ostfeld-Etzion, Laor, & Golan, 2015) and are as responsive and sensitive to children's cues as parents of nonautistic children (Hirschler-Guttenberg et al., 2015; Siller & Sigman, 2002). Guo, Garfin, Ly, and Goldberg (2017) videotaped mother–child play interactions in a home setting to study patterns of emotion coregulation. They found that although mother–child dyads in the autism group exhibited greater flexibility (wider range of emotional-engagement states, more frequent changes in states), they spent more time in mismatched emotion-engagement states (e.g., child negative and mother positive) and less time in mutual positive engagement states than dyads in the nonautistic group. These findings indicate that mothers and their autistic children do not sustain dyadic positive engagement patterns in a low-stress, home environment.

Researchers have also investigated the impact of coregulation of emotions by parents on their autistic children's outcomes. Greater parental scaffolding (i.e., sensitive responses to child), higher levels of parental emotion coaching behaviors, and child's knowledge of emotion regulation strategies were associated with fewer externalizing behaviors in autistic children (Ting & Weiss, 2017; Wilson, Berg, Zurawski, & King, 2013). Greater dyadic flexibility and more mutual positive engagements also predict lower levels of maladaptive outcomes for autistic children (Valentovich, Goldberg, Garfin, & Guo, 2018).

Emotion regulation supports for autistic children

Treatment research focusing on emotion regulation in autistic individuals is in its infancy, with the majority of research being conducted in the last decade (Beck et al., 2020). Emotion regulation supports and treatments have used various techniques including cognitive behavioral therapy (CBT), behavioral principles, school-based approaches, and mindfulness (see Table 24.1 for list of emotion regulation interventions).

Table 24.1 List of emotion regulation interventions for autistic individuals.

Intervention	Age group	Treatment type	Intervention components	Covers emotional awareness	Covers emotion regulation strategies
Exploring FeelingsCognitive Behavior Therapy to Manage Anxiety/Anger (Attwood, 2004a, 2004b, 2004c)	ChildrenParents	CBT	*Children*: 6 group sessions (pairs) that cover exploring pleasant and unpleasant emotions, emotional awareness, relaxation and emotion regulation tools, social tools, thinking tools, social stories, group discussions, and home-based projects. *Parents*: 6 group sessions (pairs) focusing on the same content covered in the children's sessions. Parents were encouraged to help children with their home-based projects.	Yes	Yes
Stress and Anger Management Program (Scarpa et al., 2013)	Young childrenParents	CBT	*Children*: 9 group sessions (2–3 children) focusing on understanding positive (happiness and relaxation) and negative emotions (anger and anxiety) as well as teaching various emotion regulation tools (relaxation, cognitive restructuring, social support, appropriate vs inappropriate). All sessions have the following components: welcome time, singing, story time, activity/lesson time, snack, and goodbyes.*Parents*: 9 psychoeducational group sessions to review the children's educational material and discuss/troubleshoot strategy use outside of the clinical setting. Include watching children's sessions. Parents were also given homework assignments to practice with their children.	Yes	Yes

(*Continued*)

Table 24.1 (Continued)

Intervention	Age group	Treatment type	Intervention components	Covers emotional awareness	Covers emotion regulation strategies
Secret Agent Society: Operation Regulation (Beaumont, 2013)	Children and youth	CBT	Ten individual sessions targeting emotional awareness as well as implementation of relaxation strategies, and tools to cope with difficult emotions like anger and anxiety. Sessions involve progress checks, multimedia activities, modeling and role-playing to practice skills, relaxation and mindfulness activities, generalization strategies, and a token reinforcement system to maintain attention and motivation. Each session consisted of the child, parent(s), and one therapist.	Yes	Yes
Resilience Builder Program (Auden et al., 2014)	Children	CBT	Twelve group sessions targeting behavioral (problematic social behaviors), cognitive (accurate vs inaccurate thoughts), and affective deficits (aggressive and destructive behaviors when feeling frustrated) in social contexts. RBP implements common CBT techniques such as role-playing and CBT relaxation techniques. The program also focuses on resilience skills such as adapting to stressors and social challenges. Each session consists of 3 components: an interactive didactic component, a free play/behavioral rehearsal component, and a relaxation/self-regulation component.	Yes	Yes

Westmead Feeling Program (Wong et al., 2010)	ChildrenParentsTeachers	CBT	*Children*: 16 group sessions broken down into 3 modules (including a booster session) focusing on identifying emotions, emotional problem solving, understanding other people's emotions, and managing emotions (covers various emotion regulation strategies).*Parents*: 5–7 group sessions consisting of psychoeducation, CBT as well as training in emotion coaching, self-monitoring and evaluation.*Teachers*: 5–7 group sessions consisting of psychoeducation, CBT as well as training in emotion coaching, self-monitoring and evaluation.All sessions are run by school counselors with assistance from a member of school staff, most typically a teacher or teacher's aide.	Yes	Yes
CBT and behavior analytic techniques program (Parent et al., 2016)	Children	CBTBehavior analytic	There were no predetermined session numbers. Tailored programs were developed for each of the two autistic individuals based on interviews with teachers and parents. Intervention consisted of three phases: (1) Assessment (individual's ability to identify emotions and understand social situations, assess challenging behaviors etc.); (2) Skills acquisition (CBT used to help participants identify triggers, feelings, actions, and thoughts, and acquire emotion regulation skills, such as relaxation, distraction, reappraisal); (3) Skills generalization (CBT + generalization procedures to ensure skills developed can be shifted from classroom environment to a variety of other contexts).	Yes	Yes

(*Continued*)

Table 24.1 (Continued)

Intervention	Age group	Treatment type	Intervention components	Covers emotional awareness	Covers emotion regulation strategies
Emotion recognition and emotion regulation intervention (Walker, 2017)	Young children	Discrete trial training Video modeling	The 8-week intervention included two weekly sessions of emotion recognition training using discrete trial training method (focused on identifying happiness, sadness, anger, and fear) and video modeling of emotion regulation (taught 3 adaptive emotion regulation strategies: squeezing a stress ball, blowing a pinwheel, and using a handheld fan). Calm down coaching was provided by the researcher and behavioral assists to help children use the adaptive emotion regulation strategies during emotional episodes throughout the intervention period.	Yes	Yes
Regulation of Emotional Lability in Autism Spectrum Disorder through Caregiver Supports (Rispoli et al., 2019)	Young children	Behavioral approach	Eight sessions with mother and child in home settings. Sessions involve setting up the home, identifying children's emotions, psychoeducation on parent emotion regulation, training on emotion regulation strategies with visual tools, review of behavioral data to understand dysregulation, and generalization of strategies to other situations.	Yes	Yes

Emotion regulation app (Fage et al., 2019)	Children and youth	Technology	The intervention period was 3 months. The application consisted of two steps: (1) emotion identification (participant is invited to identify their emotions by clicking on emoticons; emotions were anger, sadness, joy and fear); and (2) coregulation strategies (relaxation methods, coregulation strategies, and taking a break).	Yes	Yes
EmotionAwareness and Skills Enhancement Program (Conner et al., 2019)	Adolescents	CBTMBSRMBCT	Sixteen individual weekly sessions with a therapist. An initial needs assessment is conducted with parent and autistic individual. Sessions included two introductory sessions and fourteen intervention session covering four modules (ABCD): Awareness (mindful awareness of emotion, goals, and practicing mindful awareness outside of clinic), Breathing (mindful breathing and practicing mindful breathing outside of clinic), Change (emotions and thoughts, distancing and reframing, consolidation of skills, and practicing distancing and reframing outside of the clinic), and Distract (distraction, practicing all skills outside of the clinic).	Yes	Yes
MYmind (de Bruin et al., 2015)	Youth and young adultsParents	Mindfulness	*Youth:* 9 group sessions focusing on bodily awareness and self-control via mindfulness exercises (e.g., breathing meditation and sensory awareness exercises, yoga).*Parents:* 9 group sessions focusing on meditation practices and mindful parenting issues (e.g., parental reactivity, unbiased attention to child, understanding boundaries).	No	Yes

(*Continued*)

Table 24.1 (Continued)

Intervention	Age group	Treatment type	Intervention components	Covers emotional awareness	Covers emotion regulation strategies
Mindfulness-based individual therapy (Conner & White, 2018)	Young adults	Mindfulness	Six individual sessions covering psychoeducation on mindfulness, meditation practices, emotions, emotion regulation, and coping strategies. Six emotion regulation modules were used: acceptance, reappraisal, problem solving, rumination, avoidance, and blowing up/shutting down. Specific emotion regulation modules were selected for each participant depending on their habitual emotion regulation strategy use.	Yes	Yes
Emotion regulation intervention (Hartmann et al., 2019)	Young adults	CBTDBT	Twelve group sessions and two follow-up sessions facilitated by clinicians. Each session includes a mindfulness introduction, a didactic portion (20–30 min), a short break, and a longer practice portion (45–60 min) with a final cool-down period at the end of the session. The intervention included demonstration exercises, practice of specific DBT and CBT skills and concepts (e.g., role plays, modeling), and homework to practice skills between sessions.	Yes	Yes

Cognitive behavioral therapy

One of the earliest CBT programs developed for improving emotional well-being is Attwood's (2004a, 2004b, 2004c) Exploring Feelings: Cognitive Behavior Therapy to Manage Anxiety/Anger. This program was designed to be highly structured and informative to help autistic individuals manage two unpleasant emotions (anxiety and anger). Sofronoff, Attwood, and Hinton (2005) and Sofronoff, Attwood, Hinton, and Levin (2007) evaluated this CBT program in children diagnosed with Asperger syndrome age between 10 and 14 years using randomized controlled trials. In the study focusing on anger (Sofronoff et al., 2005), the researchers found that children postintervention were able to generate more effective strategies to manage anger and parents reported that the number of anger episodes decreased at 6-week follow-up. Parents also felt more confident in managing anger in their children. In the study focusing on anxiety (Sofronoff et al., 2007), parents reported that the CBT program effectively reduced anxiety symptomatology in children. Parents also reported fewer social worries of their children. Similar to the anger study, the children developed more strategies to cope with unpleasant situations (anxiety-provoking ones).

Recognizing the effectiveness of CBT programs for improving emotion regulation in autistic children, Scarpa and Reyes (2011) modified Attwood's programs to target younger autistic children without intellectual disability (ID) aged between 5 and 7 years in a pilot study, which later became the Stress and Anger Management Program (STAMP; Scarpa, Wells, & Attwood, 2013). Notable modifications included greater use of play activities, stories and songs, shorter sessions, and more active parent-training that involved evaluating their children's sessions. Scarpa and Reyes (2011) conducted a pilot of STAMP. After participating in the intervention, parents reported that the children experienced less negative lability, better emotion regulation skills, and shorter outbursts. Parents also reported greater confidence in their ability and their children's ability to manage anxiety and anger. STAMP was further evaluated by Factor et al. (2019) in 4- to 7-year-old autistic children through a randomized controlled trial and found that compared to the waitlist group, children showed significant decreases in parent-reported negativity and emotional lability, and parent perceptions of children's ability to regulate anger and anxiety increased in the treatment group. However, parent-reported emotion regulation did not improve significantly.

The Secret Agent Society: Operation Regulation (Beaumont, 2013) is a game-based, CBT program that aims to improve emotion regulation of autistic children and youth. This program is a modified version of the Junior Detective Program (Beaumont & Sofronoff, 2008; also named as the Secret Agent Society), a group-based program for autistic children to develop social skills. Thomson, Riosa, and Weiss (2015) examined the feasibility of Secret Agent Society: Operation Regulation and found high satisfaction levels among parents, children, and therapists. Attendance (100%) and retention were also high and treatment fidelity was strong. More recently, Weiss et al. (2018) conducted a randomized waitlist-controlled trial of the program and demonstrated that autistic children in the treatment group showed improvements in emotionality, ability to regulate emotions, and reductions in internalizing and externalizing symptoms (using composite score), and overall psychiatric symptom severity, as reported by parents.

The Resilience Builder Program (Aduen, Rich, Sanchez, O'Brien, & Alvord, 2014) is a comprehensive CBT-based manualized program developed to address social skills and resilience, in addition to emotional competence. Unlike the CBT-based interventions described above, emotion regulation strategies are not explicitly taught as part of the Resilience Builder Program. Instead, training sessions focus mostly on developing social skills, self-regulation, and resilience. Aduen et al. (2014) evaluated the effectiveness of the program by assessing the social, emotional, and behavioral domains of participants. The researchers found that parent-reports of children's social skills and responsibility improved, however, children's internalizing problems also increased. Child-reports indicated better emotional control and less negative emotions. Although the researchers specified that Resilience Builder Program covers emotion regulation, it is not possible to conclude whether or not participating in the program improves emotion regulation when no emotion regulation outcome measure was used. They used *How I feel* (Walden, Harris, & Catron, 2003) to measure emotional arousal and emotional control of positive and negative emotions (e.g., "I was in control of how often I felt mad"). It is questionable if *How I feel* adequately covers emotion regulation. Widely used emotion regulation measures such as Emotion Regulation Questionnaire (Gross & John, 2003) and Difficulties in Emotion Regulation Scale (Gratz & Roemer, 2004) assess one or more relevant emotion regulation aspects such as emotion regulation strategy use, emotional awareness and understanding, emotional acceptance, and ability to appropriately use emotion regulation strategies in a flexible manner. Another notable limitation of the research on the Resilience Builder Program is the lack of control group.

School-based programs

The Westmead Feelings Program (or formerly known as the Emotion-Based Social Skills Training; Wong, Lopes, & Heriot, 2010) is based on emotional intelligence and emotional competence theories that aim to teach autistic children emotional competence skills. It was initially developed for use in a clinical setting and subsequently adapted for use in schools. The participants of the training include autistic children as well as their parents and teachers. There are two versions of Westmead Feelings Program. Westmead Feelings Program 1 is aimed at supporting autistic children with mild ID. Ratcliffe, Wong, Dossetor, and Hayes (2014) examined the effectiveness of Program 1. The Emotions Development Questionnaire (EDQ; Wong, Heriot, & Lopes, 2009) was used to measure emotional competence and it covered four aspects: emotional understanding, empathy/theory of mind, emotion regulation, and parent emotion coaching skills. The researchers found that autistic children in the treatment group had significantly better emotional competence than children in the control group after treatment, as reported by teachers. Parents did not note any difference in emotional competence. Additionally, teachers and parents did not report any significant differences between groups on social skills and mental health difficulties. Ratcliffe et al. suggested various reasons why parents did not report improvements in emotional competence, which included children's difficulties with generalizing emotional skills across environment, differences in parents' and teachers' abilities to report observations, and family factors such as psychopathology in parents.

Wong and Costley (2016) also conducted a project to pilot Westmead Feelings Program 1 at Aspect Vern Barnett School. Six children, 12 parents, and two teachers participated in the pilot. The project found that the program was feasible for Aspect schools and recommended conducting a large pilot project. No outcome measures were used in this pilot. Westmead Feelings Program 2 was developed for autistic children with higher cognitive functioning. Ratcliffe, Wong, Dossetor, and Hayes (2019) investigated the effectiveness of this program and found that children from the treatment and control groups did not significantly differ on emotional competence, mental health difficulties, and social skills, as reported by parents and children. Even though the emotional competence results were not significant, they trended in the expected direction. Limitations of the research studies included not being able to randomly assign participants and low response rate for the outcome measures. For example, data for outcome measures were collected for 92 children pretreatment in the study by Ratcliffe et al. (2014), however, at 6-months follow-up, data was collected from only 13 children.

Another school-based intervention is one developed by Parent, Birtwell, Lambright, and Dubard (2016) which leveraged both CBT and behavior analytic techniques. The researchers conducted a pilot program consisting of two adolescent males with ID (verbal) in a special school setting. The authors reported a reduction in frequency and intensity of students' severe aggressive behavior and increase in students' use of coping skills, self-advocacy and social participation. The efficacy of the program is currently unknown, given that only two individuals participated in the pilot program without a control group. More research using larger sample sizes is needed to determine the actual efficacy of the program using statistical analyses.

Walker (2017) developed an emotion recognition and emotion regulation intervention for young autistic children in a preschool setting as part of her PhD. Walker conducted a pilot study with two preschool autistic children and another main study with three preschool autistic children and found that children improved in identifying four basic emotions and increased their adaptive emotion regulation behaviors when coaching was provided. Unfortunately, similar to Parent et al.'s (2016) research, it is not possible to determine the efficacy of the intervention due to the very small sample size and lack of a control group.

Other interventions

Several other interventions have been designed and researched to improve autistic children's emotion regulation. The Regulation of Emotional Lability in Autism Spectrum Disorder through Caregiver Supports (RELACS) is a parent-mediated intervention, grounded in behavioral principles for supporting preschool children, and implemented in the family home (Rispoli, Malcolm, Nathanson, & Mathes, 2019). Rispoli et al. (2019) conducted a feasibility study of RELACS involving five children (aged 3–6 years) and their parents. The study found that the intervention was acceptable to parents, fidelity was high, and emotion dysregulation postintervention was significantly lower for three of the five children.

Another emotion regulation support that leveraged coregulation with the use of mobile technology is the app developed by Fage et al. (2019) for school-aged autistic children within a mainstream school setting. A participatory design approach was used involving 30 families, 10 teachers, 3 special-education teachers, 5 school aids, and 3 psychotherapists. Results indicate high usability of the application, better self-regulation, and improved emotional self-awareness and emotional fluency (individual's ability to express emotions via language).

The Emotion Awareness and Skills Enhancement Program (EASE) was developed to reduce the emotion dysregulation of autistic adolescents using a combination of CBT, Mindfulness-Based Stress Reduction (MBSR), and Mindfulness-Based Cognitive Therapy (MBCT; Conner et al., 2019). EASE teaches participants to develop nonjudgmental awareness of emotions and incorporates some cognitive behavioral exercises without focusing on problem-solving. The ultimate goal of EASE is to help participants remain in situations eliciting strong negative emotions without avoiding negative thoughts or emotions. Conner et al. (2019) conducted a pilot study to examine the feasibility and acceptability of EASE as well as to evaluate the effectiveness of EASE to reduce emotion dysregulation and improve mental health outcomes. Findings suggest that EASE is feasible and acceptable by participants. Parent-reported emotion regulation and mental health improved postintervention and child-reported depression symptoms reduced postintervention. Overall, findings indicate EASE is a promising intervention for improving emotion regulation in autistic adolescents.

An intervention that does not specifically focus on emotion regulation, but overall self-regulation, is The Zones of Regulation (or Zones). It is a cognitive behavioral approach that teaches children self-regulation by categorizing feels and states of alertness into four concrete colored zones: red (extremely heightened states and intense emotions), yellow (heightened state of alertness and elevated emotions), green (calm state of alertness), and blue (low state of alertness and feeling down). There is currently no research examining the efficacy of the Zones for supporting autistic children. An unpublished study from 2015 of 46 US preschool children found no significant benefits of participating in a modified Zones of Regulation curriculum (Kuypers, 2020). In Australia, the Zones has been embedded into a school practice model (REWIRE) at an NSW Department of Education school. The REWIRE practice model aims to facilitate a school environment that can adequately support the needs of maltreated and traumatized children within the NSW public education school. Although the school counselor reported positive outcomes, no outcome measures were used (Costa, 2017).

Interventions for autistic youth and adults

Unlike the extensive amount of work on emotion regulation interventions for autistic children, very little research has been conducted to design and evaluate emotion regulation interventions for adults. The majority of existing research studies in the adult space have targeted autistic youth and young adults (below 26 years of age). A CBT-based intervention for emotion regulation has been designed for autistic adults, however, only the study protocol has been published (see Kuroda et al., 2013) and not the feasibility or effectiveness of the program. Given that all interventions were developed in the last few years, it is unlikely that these interventions are used widely.

One research group designed MYmind, a mindfulness-based, group training for parents and their autistic children (adolescents and youth; de Bruin, Blom, Smit, van Steensel, & Bögels, 2015). Two studies have shown that MYmind improved quality of life and mindfulness, and decreased rumination of autistic youth (de Bruin et al., 2015; Ridderinkhof, de Bruin, Blom, & Bögels, 2018). Parent-reported decreases in their children's autism symptoms as well as internalizing and externalizing symptoms. Parent's social communication, emotional and behavioral functioning, parenting-related stress, parenting style and quality of life also improved. A more recent study of MYmind found that emotion regulation skills of autistic youth improved (Salem-Guirgis et al., 2019).

Another mindfulness-based intervention that more actively targets emotion regulation difficulties is an individual-based therapy designed by Conner and White (2018). This intervention drew heavily from MBCT (Segal et al., 2004) and was tailored to support young autistic adults in individual therapy sessions. Nine participants participated in the intervention study and seven individuals demonstrated improvement in at least one of the following areas: impulse control, access to emotion regulation strategies, and emotional acceptance.

Finally, an intervention for young autistic adults that targets both emotion regulation and social communication is one developed by Hartmann et al. (2019), which used CBT and dialectical behavior therapy (DBT) approaches. Hartmann et al. (2019) evaluated the intervention using a single-case design to study the effectiveness of the intervention for seven autistic youth aged between 18 and 24 years and found that although social communication, social cognition and social awareness improved, improvements in emotion regulation were not significant.

Common features of emotion regulation support

The key features of good practice in providing emotion regulation supports for people on the autism spectrum are:

- *Help individuals understand their own emotions.* The first step of emotion regulation is to identify one's emotional states and determining whether or not emotion regulation is required. Given that people tend to regulate negative emotions (unpleasant) more often than positive emotions (pleasant), it is important to first determine if emotion regulation is required for the situation. Therefore almost all of the interventions summarized above helped autistic individuals identify their emotions.
- *Teach various strategies to regulate and manage emotions.* Once emotions have been identified and the goal to regulate emotions set, individuals must have a repertoire of

regulation strategies to choose from. Since research has shown that autistic individuals tend to use maladaptive strategies, it is important to teach individuals more adaptive strategies to regulate emotions and apply these strategies in their own lives as difficult situations arise. All of the interventions summarized above have modules that teach individuals how to better regulate emotions via strategies such as relaxation, cognitive reappraisal, problem-solving.

- *Understand the importance of coregulation and build it into interventions.* Apart from autistic children's emotion regulation abilities, research has shown that parent's sensitive responses to the child and emotion coaching influences children's externalizing behaviors. Some of the researchers recognized the importance of coregulation by parents and build parental training into their emotion regulation interventions for autistic children.

Conclusions

The ability to regulate emotions is crucial for ensuring good mental health. Overall, autistic individuals tend to have emotion dysregulation. Given the high prevalence of mental health conditions including anxiety and depression in autistic children and adults, it is crucial to design and develop interventions to improve autistic people's emotion regulation capacities. Emotion regulation interventions have focused mostly on autistic children and adolescents, and these include CBT-based, behavioral, mindfulness, and technology-based approaches. Currently, only three interventions focused on young autistic adults have been developed and evaluated, and no research exists on emotion regulation supports for older adults. Key features of emotion regulation support programs include helping individuals understand their own emotions, teaching various strategies to regulate and manage emotions, and building coregulation aspects into interventions. Although there are some encouraging preliminary findings, the quality of the majority of studies is weak and randomized controlled trials are lacking. Given the key role of emotion regulation in mental health and its viability as a treatment target, the relative lack of dedicated interventions and stringent research evaluations is surprising. Therefore further research utilizing randomized controlled trials, larger samples, and more stringent assessments of emotion regulation and mental health outcomes are needed.

References

Aduen, P. A., Rich, B. A., Sanchez, L., O'Brien, K., & Alvord, M. K. (2014). Resilience builder program therapy addresses core social deficits and emotion dysregulation in youth with high-functioning autism spectrum disorder. *Journal of Psychological Abnormalities in Children*, *3*(2). Available from https://doi.org/10.4172/2329-9525.1000118.

Aldao, A., & Dixon-Gordon, K. L. (2014). Broadening the scope of research on emotion regulation strategies and psychopathology. *Cognitive Behavior Therapy*, *43*(1), 22–33. Available from https://doi.org/10.1080/16506073.2013.816769.

Aldao, A., Gee, D. G., De Los Reyes, A., & Seager, I. (2016). Emotion regulation as a transdiagnostic factor in the development of internalizing and externalizing psychopathology:

Current and future directions. *Development and Psychopathology*, *28*(4pt1), 927–946. Available from https://doi.org/10.1017/S0954579416000638.

Aldao, A., & Nolen-Hoeksema, S. (2013). One versus many: Capturing the use of multiple emotion regulation strategies in response to an emotion-eliciting stimulus. *Cognition and Emotion*, *27*(4), 753–760. Available from https://doi.org/10.1080/02699931.2012.739998.

Aldao, A., Nolen-Hoeksema, S., & Schweizer, S. (2010). Emotion-regulation strategies across psychopathology: A meta-analytic review. *Clinical Psychology Review*, *30*(2), 217–237. Available from https://doi.org/10.1016/j.cpr.2009.11.004.

American Psychological Association. (2020). *APA dictionary of psychology: Negative emotion*. Retrieved from <https://dictionary.apa.org/negative-emotion>.

Attwood, T. (2004a). Cognitive behavior therapy for children and adults with Asperger's syndrome. *Behavior Change*, *21*(3), 147–161. Available from https://doi.org/10.1375/bech.21.3.147.55995.

Attwood, T. (2004b). *Exploring feelings (Anger)*. Arlington, TX: Future Horizons.

Attwood, T. (2004c). *Exploring feelings: Cognitive behavior therapy to manage anxiety*. Arlington, TX: Future Horizons.

Bäuml, K. H., & Kuhbandner, C. (2007). Remembering can cause forgetting—But not in negative moods. *Psychological Science*, *18*(2), 111–115. Available from https://doi.org/10.1111/j.1467-9280.2007.01857.x.

Beaumont, R. (2013). *Secret agent society: Operation regulation anual*. Milton, Australia: Social Skills Training Institute.

Beaumont, R., & Sofronoff, K. (2008). A multi-component social skills intervention for children with Asperger syndrome: The Junior Detective Training Program. *Journal of Child Psychology and Psychiatry*, *49*(7), 743–753. Available from https://doi.org/10.1111/j.1469-7610.2008.01920.x.

Beck, K. B., Conner, C. M., Breitenfeldt, K. E., Northrup, J. B., White, S. W., & Mazefsky, C. A. (2020). Assessment and treatment of emotion regulation impairment in autism spectrum disorder across the life span: Current state of the science and future directions. *Child and Adolescent Psychiatric Clinics of North America*, *29*(3), 527–542. Available from https://doi.org/10.1016/j.chc.2020.02.003.

Berkovits, L., Eisenhower, A., & Blacher, J. (2017). Emotion regulation in young children with autism spectrum disorders. *Journal of Autism and Developmental Disorders*, *47*(1), 68–79. Available from https://doi.org/10.1007/s10803-016-2922-2.

Butler, E. A., & Randall, A. K. (2013). Emotional coregulation in close relationships. *Emotion Review*, *5*(2), 202–210. Available from https://doi.org/10.1177/1754073912451630.

Cai, R. Y., Richdale, A. L., Uljarević, M., Dissanayake, C., & Samson, A. C. (2018). Emotion regulation in autism spectrum disorder: Where we are and where we need to go. *Autism Research*, *11*(7), 962–978. Available from https://doi.org/10.1002/aur.1968.

Cai, R. Y., Richdale, A. L., Dissanayake, C., & Uljarević, M. (2019). Resting heart rate variability, emotion regulation, psychological well-being T and autism symptomatology in adults with and without autism. *International Journal of Psychophysiology*, *137*, 54–62. Available from https://doi.org/10.1016/j.ijpsycho.2018.12.010.

Carl, J. R., Soskin, C. P., Kerns, C., & Barlow, D. H. (2013). Positive emotion regulation in emotional disorders: A theoretical review. *Clinical Psychology Review*, *33*(3), 343–360. Available from https://doi.org/10.1016/j.cpr.2013.01.003.

Cibralic, S., Kohlhoff, J., Wallance, N., McMahon, C., & Eapen, V. (2019). A systematic review of emotion regulation in children with autism spectrum disorder. *Research in Autism Spectrum Disorders*, *68*. Available from https://doi.org/10.1016/j.rasd.2019.101422.

Cohn, M. A., & Fredrickson, B. L. (2009). Positive emotions. In S. J. Lopez, & C. R. Snyder (Eds.), *Oxford handbook of positive psychology* (pp. 13–24). New York: Oxford University Press.

Conner, C. M., & White, S. W. (2018). Brief report: Feasibility and preliminary efficacy of individual mindfulness therapy for adults with autism spectrum disorder. *Journal of Autism and Developmental Disorders, 48*(1), 290–300. Available from https://doi.org/10.1007/s10803-017-3312-0.

Conner, C. M., White, S. W., Beck, K. B., Golt, J., Smith, I. C., & Mazefsky, C. A. (2019). Improving emotion regulation ability in autism: The Emotional Awareness and Skills Enhancement (EASE) program. *Autism: The International Journal of Research and Practice, 23*(5), 1273–1287. Available from https://doi.org/10.1177/1362361318810709.

Costa, D. A. (2017). Transforming traumatized children within NSW department of education schools: One school counsellor's model for practice – REWIRE. *Children Australia, 42* (2), 113–126. Available from https://doi.org/10.1017/cha.2017.14.

Damasio, A. R. (1994). *Descartes' error: Emotion, reason, and the human brain*. New York: Avon Books.

de Bruin, E. I., Blom, R., Smit, F. M., van Steensel, F. J., & Bögels, S. M. (2015). MYmind: Mindfulness training for youngsters with autism spectrum disorders and their parents. *Autism: The International Journal of Research and Practice, 19*(8), 906–914. Available from https://doi.org/10.1177/1362361314553279.

Eisenberg, N., & Spinrad, T. L. (2004). Emotion-related regulation: Sharpening the definition. *Child Development, 75*(2), 334–339. Available from https://doi.org/10.1111/j.1467-8624.2004.00674.x.

Factor, R. S., Swain, D. M., Antezana, L., Muskett, A., Gatto, A. J., Radtke, S. R., & Scarpa, A. (2019). Teaching emotion regulation to children with autism spectrum disorder: Outcomes of the Stress and Anger Management Program (STAMP). *Bulletin of the Menninger Clinic, 83*(3), 235–258. Available from https://doi.org/10.1521/bumc.2019.83.3.235.

Fage, C., Consel, C., Etchegoyhen, K., Amestoy, A., Bouvard, M., Mazon, C., & Sauzéon, H. (2019). An emotion regulation app for school inclusion of children with ASD: Design principles and evaluation. *Computers & Education, 131*, 1–21. Available from https://doi.org/10.1016/j.compedu.2018.12.003.

Feldman, R. (2003). Infant–mother and infant–father synchrony: The coregulation of positive arousal. *Infant Mental Health Journal, 24*(1), 1–23. Available from https://doi.org/10.1002/imhj.10041.

Fiedler, K., Asbeck, J., & Nickel, S. (1991). Mood and constructive memory effects on social judgement. *Cognition and Emotion, 5*(5-6), 363–378. Available from https://doi.org/10.1080/02699939108411048.

Forgas, J. P. (2011). Can negative affect eliminate the power of first impressions? Affective influences on primacy and recency effects in impression formation. *Journal of Experimental Social Psychology, 47*(2), 425–429. Available from https://doi.org/10.1016/j.jesp.2010.11.005.

Forgas, J. P., Laham, S. M., & Vargas, P. T. (2005). Mood effects on eyewitness memory: Affective influences on susceptibility to misinformation. *Journal of Experimental Social Psychology, 41*(6), 574–588. Available from https://doi.org/10.1016/j.jesp.2004.11.005.

Fredrickson, B. L. (2004). The broaden-and-build theory of positive emotions. *Philosophical Transactions of the Royal Society of London, 359*(1449), 1367–1378. Available from https://doi.org/10.1098/rstb.2004.1512.

Gasper, K., Spencer, L. A., & Hu, D. (2019). Does neutral affect exist? How challenging three beliefs about neutral affect can advance affective research. *Frontiers in Psychology*, *10*, 2476. Available from https://doi.org/10.3389/fpsyg.2019.02476.

Grolnick, W. S., Bridges, L. J., & Connell, J. P. (1996). Emotion regulation in two-year-olds: Strategies and emotional expression in four contexts. *Child Development*, *67*(3), 928–941. Available from https://www.jstor.org/stable/1131871.

Gulsrud, A. C., Jahromi, L. B., & Kasari, C. (2010). The co-regulation of emotions between mothers and their children with autism. *Journal of Autism and Developmental Disorders*, *40*(2), 227–237. Available from https://doi.org/10.1007/s10803-009-0861-x.

Guo, Y., Garfin, D. R., Ly, A., & Goldberg, W. A. (2017). Emotion coregulation in mother-child dyads: A dynamic systems analysis of children with and without autism spectrum disorder. *Journal of Abnormal Child Psychology*, *45*, 1369–1383. Available from https://doi.org/10.1007/s10802-016-0234-9.

Gratz, K. L., & Roemer, L. (2004). Multidimensional assessment of emotion regulation and dysregulation: Development, factor structure, and initial validation of the difficulties in emotion regulation scale. *Journal of Psychopathology and Behavioral Assessment*, *26*, 41–54. Available from https://doi.org/10.1023/B:JOBA.0000007455.08539.94.

Gross, J. J. (2015). Emotion regulation: Current status and future prospects. *Psychological Inquiry*, *26*(1), 1–26. Available from https://doi.org/10.1080/1047840X.2014.940781.

Gross, J. J., & John, O. P. (2003). Individual differences in two emotion regulation processes: Implications for affect, relationships, and well-being. *Journal of Personality and Social Psychology*, *85*(2), 348–362. Available from https://doi.org/10.1037/0022-3514.85.2.348.

Gross, J. J., Richards, J. M., & John, O. P. (2006). Emotion regulation in everyday life. In D. K. Snyder, J. Simpson, & J. N. Hughes (Eds.), *Emotion regulation in couples and families: Pathways to dysfunction and health* (pp. 13–35). Washington, DC: American Psychological Association.

Gyurak, A., Gross, J. J., & Etkin, A. (2011). Explicit and implicit emotion regulation: A dual-process framework. *Cognition and Emotion*, *25*(3), 400–412. Available from https://doi.org/10.1080/02699931.2010.544160.

Hartmann, K., Urbano, M. R., Raffaele, C. T., Kreiser, N. L., Williams, T. V., Qualls, L. R., & Elkins, D. E. (2019). Outcomes of an emotion regulation intervention group in young adults with autism spectrum disorder. *Bulletin of the Menninger Clinic*, *83*(3), 259–277. Available from https://doi.org/10.1521/bumc.2019.83.3.259.

Hirschler-Guttenberg, Y., Feldman, R., Ostfeld-Etzion, S., Laor, N., & Golan, O. (2015). Self- and co-regulation of anger and fear in preschoolers with autism spectrum disorders: The role of maternal parenting style and temperament. *Journal of Autism and Developmental Disorders*, *45*(9), 3004–3014. Available from https://doi.org/10.1007/s10803-015-2464-z.

Honkalampi, K., Hintikka, J., Tanskanen, A., Lehtonen, J., & Viinamäki, H. (2000). Depression is strongly associated with alexithymia in the general population. *Journal of Psychosomatic Research*, *48*(1), 99–104. Available from https://doi.org/10.1016/S0022-3999(99)00083-5.

Jahromi, L. B., Bryce, C. I., & Swanson, J. (2013). The importance of self-regulation for the school and peer engagement of children with high-functioning autism. *Research in Autism Spectrum Disorders*, *7*, 235–246. Available from https://doi.org/10.1016/j.rasd.2012.08.012.

Karukivi, M., Hautala, L., Kaleva, O., Haapasalo-Pesu, K., Liuksila, P., Joukamaa, M., & Saarijärvi, S. (2010). Alexithymia is associated with anxiety among adolescents. *Journal of Affective Disorders*, *125*(1–3), 383–387. Available from https://doi.org/10.1016/j.jad.2010.02.126.

Kinnaird, E., Stewart, C., & Tchanturia, K. (2019). Investigating alexithymia in autism: A systematic review and meta-analysis. *European Psychiatry*, *55*, 80–89. Available from https://doi.org/10.1016/j.eurpsy.2018.09.004.

Konstantareas, M. M., & Stewart, K. (2006). Affect regulation and temperament in children with autism spectrum disorder. *Journal of Autism and Developmental Disorders*, *36*, 143–154. Available from https://doi.org/10.1007/s10803-005-0051-4.

Kopp, C. B. (1982). Antecedents of self-regulation: A developmental perspective. *Developmental Psychology*, *18*(2), 199–214. Available from https://doi.org/10.1037/0012-1649.18.2.199.

Kuroda, M., Kawakubo, Y., Kuwabara, H., Yokoyama, K., Kano, Y., & Kamio, Y. (2013). A cognitive-behavioral intervention for emotion regulation in adults with high-functioning autism spectrum disorders: Study protocol for a randomized controlled trial. *Trials*, *14* (231). Available from https://doi.org/10.1186/1745-6215-14-231.

Kuypers, L. (2020). *Research around the zones of regulation*. Retrieved from <https://www.zonesofregulation.com/research-studies.html>.

Larsen, R. J. (2000). Toward a science of mood regulation. *Psychological Inquiry*, *11*(3), 129–141. Available from https://doi.org/10.1207/S15327965PLI1103_01.

Levenson, R. W. (1994). Human emotion: A functional view. In P. Ekman, & R. J. Davidson (Eds.), *The nature of emotion: Fundamental questions* (pp. 123–126). New York: Oxford University Press.

Mazefsky, C. A., Herrington, J., Siegel, M., Scarpa, A., Maddox, B. B., Scahill, L., & White, S. W. (2013). The role of emotion regulation in autism spectrum disorder. *Journal of the American Academy of Child and Adolescent Psychiatry*, *52*(7), 679–688. Available from https://doi.org/10.1016/j.jaac.2013.05.006.

Mazefsky, C. A., & White, S. W. (2014). Emotion regulation: Concepts and practice in autism spectrum disorder. *Child and Adolescent Psychiatric Clinics of North America*, *23*(2), 15–24. Available from https://doi.org/10.1016/j.chc.2013.07.002.

Nader-Grosbois, N., & Mazzone, S. (2014). Emotion regulation, personality and social adjustment in children with autism spectrum disorders. *Psychology (Savannah, Ga.)*, *5*, 1750–1767. Available from https://doi.org/10.4236/psych.2014.515182.

Nuske, H. J., Hedley, D., Woollacott, A., Thomson, P., Macari, S., & Dissanayake, C. (2017). Developmental delays in emotion regulation strategies in preschoolers with autism. *Autism Research*, *10*(11), 1808–1822. Available from https://doi.org/10.1002/aur.1827.

Ong, A. D., Bergeman, C. S., Bisconti, T. L., & Wallace, K. A. (2006). Psychological resilience, positive emotions, and successful adaptation to stress in later life. *Journal of Personality and Social Psychology*, *91*(4), 730–749. Available from https://doi.org/10.1037/0022-3514.91.4.730.

Pandey, R., Saxena, P., & Dubey, A. (2011). Emotion regulation difficulties in alexithymia and mental health. *Europe's Journal of Psychology*, *7*(4). Available from https://doi.org/10.5964/ejop.v7i4.155.

Parent, V., Birtwell, K. B., Lambright, N., & Dubard, M. (2016). Combining CBT and behavior-analytic approaches to target severe emotion dysregulation in verbal youth with ASD and ID. *Journal of Mental Health Research in Intellectual Disabilities*, *9*(1-2), 60–82. Available from https://doi.org/10.1080/19315864.2016.1166301.

Pouw, L. B. C., Rieffe, C., Stockmann, L., & Gadow, K. D. (2013). The link between emotion regulation, social functioning, and depression in boys with ASD. *Research in Autism Spectrum Disorders*, *7*, 549–556. Available from https://doi.org/10.1016/j.rasd.2013.01.002.

Quoidbach, J., Berry, E. V., Hansenne, M., & Mikolajczak, M. (2010). Positive emotion regulation and well-being: Comparing the impact of eight savoring and dampening strategies. *Personality and Individual Differences*, *49*(5), 368–373. Available from https://doi.org/10.1016/j.paid.2010.03.048.

Ratcliffe, B., Wong, M., Dossetor, D., & Hayes, S. (2014). Teaching social–emotional skills to school-aged children with autism spectrum disorder: A treatment versus control trial in 41 mainstream schools. *Research in Autism Spectrum Disorders*, *8*(12), 1722–1733. Available from https://doi.org/10.1016/j.rasd.2014.09.010.

Ratcliffe, B., Wong, M., Dossetor, D., & Hayes, S. (2019). Improving emotional competence in children with autism spectrum disorder and mild intellectual disability in schools: A preliminary treatment versus waitlist study. *Behavior Change*, *36*(4), 216–232. Available from https://doi.org/10.1017/bec.2019.13.

Ridderinkhof, A., de Bruin, E. I., Blom, R., & Bögels, S. M. (2018). Mindfulness-based program for children with autism spectrum disorder and their parents: direct and long-term improvements. *Mindfulness*, *9*(3), 773–779. Available from https://doi.org/10.1007/s12671-017-0815-x.

Rispoli, K. M., Malcolm, A. L., Nathanson, E. W., & Mathes, N. E. (2019). Feasibility of an emotion regulation intervention for young children with autism spectrum disorder: A brief report. *Research in Autism Spectrum Disorders*, *67*, 101420. Available from https://doi.org/10.1016/j.rasd.2019.101420.

Salem-Guirgis, S., Albaum, C., Tablon, P., Riosa, P. B., Nicholas, D. B., Drmic, I. E., & Weiss, J. A. (2019). MYmind: A concurrent group-based mindfulness intervention for youth with autism and their parents. *Mindfulness*, *10*, 1730–1743. Available from https://doi.org/10.1007/s12671-019-01107-9.

Samson, A. C., Phillips, J. M., Parker, K. J., Shah, S., Gross, J. J., & Hardan, A. Y. (2014). Emotion dysregulation and the core features of autism spectrum disorder. *Journal of Autism and Developmental Disorders*, *44*, 1766–1772. Available from https://doi.org/10.1007/s10803-013-2022-5.

Scarpa, A., & Reyes, N. M. (2011). Improving emotion regulation with CBT in young children with high functioning autism spectrum disorders: A pilot study. *Behavioral and Cognitive Psychotherapy*, *39*(4), 495–500. Available from https://doi.org/10.1017/S1352465811000063.

Scarpa, A., Wells, A., & Attwood, T. (2013). *Exploring feelings for young children with high-functioning autism or Asperger's disorder: The STAMP treatment manual*. London: Jessica Kingsley Publishers.

Schutte, N. S. (2014). The broaden and build process: Positive affect, ratio of positive to negative affect and general self-efficacy. *The Journal of Positive Psychology*, *9*(1), 66–74. Available from https://doi.org/10.1080/17439760.2013.841280.

Segal, Z. V., Teasdale, J. D., & Williams, M. G. (2004). Mindfulness based cognitive therapy: Theoretical rationale and empirical status. In S. C. Hayes, V. M. Follette, & M. M. Linehan (Eds.), *Mindfulness and acceptance: Expanding the cognitive-behavioral traditions* (pp. 45–65). New York: Guilford Press.

Seiffge-Krenke, I., & Klessinger, N. (2000). Long-term effects of avoidant coping on adolescents' depressive symptoms. *Journal of Youth and Adolescence*, *29*(6), 617–630. Available from https://doi.org/10.1023/A:1026440304695.

Siller, M., & Sigman, M. (2002). The behaviors of parents of children with autism predict the subsequent development of their children's communication. *Journal of Autism and Developmental Disorders*, *32*(2), 77–89. Available from https://doi.org/10.1023/a:1014884404276.

Sofronoff, K., Attwood, T., & Hinton, S. (2005). A randomized controlled trial of a CBT intervention for anxiety in children with Asperger syndrome. *Journal of Child Psychology and Psychiatry*, *46*(11), 1152–1160. Available from https://doi.org/10.1111/j.1469-7610.2005.00411.x.

Sofronoff, K., Attwood, T., Hinton, S., & Levin, I. (2007). A randomized controlled trial of a cognitive behavioral intervention for anger management in children diagnosed with Asperger syndrome. *Journal of Autism and Developmental Disorders*, *37*(7), 1203–1214. Available from https://doi.org/10.1007/s10803-006-0262-3.

Storbeck, J., & Clore, G. L. (2011). Affect influences false memories at encoding: Evidence from recognition data. *Emotion (Washington, D.C.)*, *11*(4), 981–989. Available from https://doi.org/10.1037/a0022754.

Thompson, R. A. (1991). Emotional regulation and emotional development. *Educational Psychology Review*, *3*(4), 269–307. Available from https://doi.org/10.1007/BF01319934.

Thomson, K., Riosa, P. B., & Weiss, J. A. (2015). Brief report of preliminary outcomes of an emotion regulation intervention for children with autism spectrum disorder. *Journal of Autism and Developmental Disorders*, *45*(11), 3487–3495. Available from https://doi.org/10.1007/s10803-015-2446-1.

Ting, V., & Weiss, J. A. (2017). Emotion regulation and parent co-regulation in children with autism spectrum disorder. *Journal of Autism and Developmental Disorders*, *47*(3), 680–689. Available from https://doi.org/10.1007/s10803-016-3009-9.

Troy, A. S., Shallcross, A. J., & Mauss, I. B. (2013). A person-by-situation approach to emotion regulation: Cognitive reappraisal can either help or hurt, depending on the context. *Psychological Science*, *24*(12), 2505–2514. Available from 10.1177/0956797613496434.

Valentovich, V., Goldberg, W. A., Garfin, D. R., & Guo, Y. (2018). Emotion coregulation processes between mothers and their children with and without autism spectrum disorder: Associations with children's maladaptive behaviors. *Journal of Autism and Developmental Disorders*, *48*(4), 1235–1248. Available from https://doi.org/10.1007/s10803-017-3375-y.

Walden, T. A., Harris, V. S., & Catron, T. F. (2003). How I feel: A self-report measure of emotional arousal and regulation for children. *Psychological Assessment*, *15*(3), 399–412. Available from https://doi.org/10.1037/1040-3590.15.3.399.

Walker, B. L. (2017). *Evaluating the effectiveness of a combined emotion recognition and emotion regulation intervention for preschool children with autisms spectrum disorder* (Doctoral dissertation). Available from OhioLINK (miami1498150504281695).

Weiss, J. A., Thomson, K., Riosa, P. B., Albaum, C., Chan, V., Maughan, A., & Black, K. (2018). A randomized waitlist-controlled trial of cognitive behavior therapy to improve emotion regulation in children with autism. *Journal of Child Psychology and Psychiatry*, *59*(11), 1180–1191. Available from https://doi.org/10.1111/jcpp.12915.

Wilson, B. J., Berg, J. L., Zurawski, M. E., & King, K. A. (2013). Autism and externalizing behaviors: Buffering effects of parental emotion coaching. *Research in Autism Spectrum Disorders*, *7*(6), 767–776. Available from https://doi.org/10.1016/j.rasd.2013.02.005.

Wong, M., Heriot, S., & Lopes, A. (2009). *The emotions development questionnaire*. Sydney, Australia: The Children's Hospital at Westmead.

Wong, M., Lopes, A., & Heriot, S. (2010). *Emotion-based social skills training (EBSST) for children with high functioning autism and Asperger's disorder*. Sydney, Australia: The Children's Hospital at Westmead.

Wong, M. G., & Costley, D. (2016). *Emotion-based social skills training at aspect: A pilot project*. Sydney: Final report. The Children's Hospital at Westmead.

Autism Spectrum Disorder and child maltreatment: forensic considerations

25

Kirsten Byrnes[1,2]
[1]Audrey Hepburn Children's House, Hackensack University Medical Center, Hackensack, NJ, United States, [2]Psychiatry and Behavioral Health, Hackensack Meridian School of Medicine, Nutley, NJ, United States

According to current statistics on child maltreatment in the United States, 4.3 million referrals were received by child protection agencies, concerning 7.8 million children, with approximately 678,000 children having been confirmed to have experienced abuse (U.S. Department of Health and Human Services, 2020). Approximately 85% of these youth (used throughout to signify minors) have experienced one form of maltreatment, while 15.5% of youth have experienced two or more forms, with physical abuse and neglect being the most common combination. Just over 60% of these youth experienced neglect. In examining those youth who have experienced such abusive behaviors, almost 92% of the maltreatment was at the hands of a parent. While this is obviously not a thorough discussion of the scope of child maltreatment across the United States and elsewhere, it does highlight the degree of vulnerability youth experience as related to those in their environment. These vulnerabilities may be heightened when youth experience symptomology and deficits associated with autism spectrum disorder (ASD). ASD is a neurodevelopmental disorder characterized by difficulties in communication, social interactions, and behavioral challenges in the form of restricted interests and repetitive behaviors (American Psychiatric Association, 2013). These symptoms and behaviors, while occurring along a wide spectrum and varying in presentation between youth, contribute to a range of impairment in several domains of functioning (e.g., social, occupational). The following chapter will review research suggesting that those diagnosed with ASD may be more vulnerable to experience maltreatment at higher rates and the issues related to accurate tracking of the prevalence of maltreatment, how presentations associated with ASD may complicate investigation and contribute to certain outcomes, and relevant forensic considerations pertaining to both criminal investigation and child protective services (CPS) involvement.

Emerging Programs for Autism Spectrum Disorder. DOI: https://doi.org/10.1016/B978-0-323-85031-5.00029-3

Challenges in assessing the scope of the issue

General definitions and monitoring

Though there is a degree of variability by state, definitions of various types of maltreatment at a minimum had been set forth originally by Child Abuse Prevention and Treatment Act (U.S. Congress, 1974), which has been amended (1988; CAPTA Reauthorization Act of 2010) and adjusted throughout the years to include varying types of maltreatment (e.g., Justice for the Victims of Trafficking Act of 2015, Comprehensive Addiction and Recovery Act of 2016) and increased sensitivity to the needs of children and families (Child Welfare Information Gateway, 2019). Broadly speaking, child abuse, as defined by CAPTA (U.S. Committee on Health, Education, Labor and Pensions, 2010), is:

> *any recent act or failure to act on the part of a* parent *or* caretaker *which results in death, serious physical or emotional harm, sexual abuse or exploitation; or an act or failure to act, which presents an imminent risk of serious harm.*

Emphasis was added in the above quote to highlight that the individual engaging in the abusive act must be in a caretaking role during the course of the abuse to be considered child abuse from a CPS perspective. Physical abuse, sexual abuse, and neglect have historically been considered as abusive acts, while more recently, states have begun to consider other experiences, such as psychological maltreatment, exposure to intimate partner violence, and exposure to substance abuse to be considered due to the propensity for pervasive negative impacts upon children. Relatedly, the National Child Abuse and Neglect Data System (NCANDS) assists with the tracking and analysis of child maltreatment data.

There is a general recognition that youths' emotional, behavioral, interpersonal, and intellectual/cognitive functioning may impact the level of risk as related to the experience of maltreatment. With this in mind, National Child Abuse and Neglect Data System (2019) data collection includes nine child risk factors to assist in research pertaining to prevention and intervention. Of these risk factors, several pertain to assessing the presence or absence of deficits or symptoms related to ASD, including intellectual disability (ID), emotional disturbance, visual and/or hearing impairment, learning disability, physical disability, behavior problem, and/or other relevant medical problem. Of note, workers and agencies have the option of omitting this information because individuals documenting data can default to blank spaces or coding indicating "unknown or missing," and thus findings are not aggregated and specifically reported in annual *Child Maltreatment* reports. Moreover, it has been noted that these risk factors are difficult to assess, as some symptoms might go undetected or unrecognized by families, some families do not openly discuss diagnoses or symptom presentation with CPS investigators, and many of these risk factors require diagnosis by a professional, which may not occur prior to the close of the investigation (U.S. Department of Health and Human Services, 2020). Additionally, CAPTA requirements instituted in 2010 and 2012 require agencies to document the number of children referred to or eligible for referral to early intervention services. However, if victims are older than 3 years old, it is up to the states' discretion as to whether to report this information (U.S. Department of Health and Human Services, 2020). While these changes are clearly a step in the right direction in understanding maltreatment, especially as related to those with difficulties in these various areas of functioning, there is likely a significant degree of underreporting. Moreover, it could be argued that separating out each of these separate risk factors may both fail to recognize the interactive effects of deficits in multiple domains commonly found with ASD and underappreciate the possibility of increased risk as related to ASD youth in general.

Difficulties in establishing prevalence rates of maltreatment and ASD

Several decades ago, it was recognized that children with developmental and/or intellectual disabilities may be at increased risk of experiencing maltreatment (Gil, 1970; Jaudes & Diamond, 1985; Ratnofsky, 1994; Sandgrund, Gaines, & Green, 1974; Soeffing, 1975). These authors reasoned that physical abuse and/or neglect was partially precipitated by parents' disappointments secondary to having children that were different, or by youth engaging in challenging, provocative, or aggressive behavior. With this understanding, legislation was enacted to track child maltreatment perpetrated against those diagnosed with a disability (The Child Abuse and Prevention, Adoption, and Family Services Act of 1988), though it was rare until CAPTA's reauthorization in 2010. Since that point, studies have suggested that those with intellectual or developmental disabilities are at an elevated risk (1.5–3.4 times) for experiencing maltreatment when compared to neurotypical individuals (Dinkler et al., 2017; Hibbard & Desch, 2007; Sullivan & Knutson, 2000). Relatedly, some studies sought to examine the type of deficit or symptomology associated with risk of maltreatment. Sullivan and Knutson (2000) found that children with communication disorders experienced rates of physical abuse and neglect at five times the rates of their peers and were three times more likely to be sexually abused. Youth with developmental disabilities and behavioral issues were at the greatest risk for maltreatment (Govindshenoy & Spencer, 2007; Helton & Cross, 2011; Jaudes & Mackey-Bilaver, 2008; Sullivan & Knutson, 2000), with one study in particular finding these youth were seven times more likely to experience physical or emotional abuse, or neglect (Sullivan & Knutson, 2000).

These early studies established a much-needed foundation for an understanding of the risk associated with various symptom presentations and deficits. However, until recently, many of the existing studies focused broadly on disabilities or symptom presentations rather than specifically on the risk related to those diagnosed with ASD (Kildahl, Bakken, Iversen, & Helverschou, 2019). Moreover, many of the existing studies pertain to adults experiencing abuses later in life or adults disclosing previous abuse earlier in life. In their research on children with ASD and maltreatment, Fisher et al. (2018) argued that "in order to develop systems of care that include maltreatment prevention, response, assessment, and intervention strategies, it is extremely important for states to know the proportion of children who interact with their child protection systems who have specific forms of disabilities" (p. 1335). As such, Fisher and colleagues conducted a study utilizing Tennessee's CPS database, cross-referencing it with the records from the Autism and Developmental Disabilities Monitoring network (ADDM) to examine a large population study including 387 youth diagnosed with ASD. The study revealed that of the 24,306 children considered, 17.3% of those diagnosed with ASD were referred to CPS versus 7.4% of children without a diagnosis of ASD. The authors were also interested in what happened to these referrals after coming to the attention of CPS, whether they were dismissed as not worthy of further investigation, or referred for further action. Those without ASD were considered in need of additional action (91.6%), while just over 60% of youth with ASD were referred. Substantiation rates for both groups (determinations that abuse occurred) were similar.

McDonnell et al. (2019) used a similar strategy to assess differences in maltreatment related to presence of ASD and ID. In this study, odds ratios for risk of child maltreatment were calculated pertaining to youth with ID alone, ASD alone, ASD with ID (ASD + ID), and youth without either. A particular strength of this study was that the authors also controlled for gender, ethnicity, socioeconomic status, and parental education. Youth diagnosed with ASD were more likely to experience physical abuse compared to all other groups. However, in general, those in the ASD + ID and the ID groups were two to three times more likely to have experienced any form of maltreatment. Youth in the ASD and ID groups experienced more instances of both physical abuse and neglect and tended to be victimized by more people, including an emphasis on the immediate family, than others in the study.

Both studies (Fisher et al., 2018; McDonnell et al., 2019) address various factors contributing to the vulnerability of experiencing maltreatment in youth with ASD. McDonnell et al. (2019) anchored largely in a transactional-ecological model of maltreatment and risk as set forth by Cicchetti and Valentino (2015). As such, it is understood that there are varying developmental needs at each age. Characteristics of the youth interact with characteristics of caretakers, which are also influenced by processes or experiences in other levels of their ecology. In an optimal situation, youth have an easy temperament, are socially engaging, and do not demonstrate challenging behaviors associated with poor affect regulation. These attributes, combined with adequate parental skills and support on other levels (e.g., familial supports, stable finances and housing, community supports, embedded within a chronology, and culture/political situation supportive of the family and their situation), provide the foundation for optimal development throughout childhood. However, for children with ASD, deficits in social relatedness and affect regulation have the propensity to alter the attachment bonds in the child–caretaker dyad. Relatedly, both studies noted challenging behaviors and complex cognitive and language deficits commonly exhibited by youth diagnosed with ASD. Parents of children with ASD often experience significant stress related to parenting in this context, which may be further exacerbated by limited family support and isolation (Mandell et al., 2005) and complex, systems-related factors. There are also factors independent of child maltreatment that may contribute to higher levels of referral for youth with ASD to CPS. Fisher et al. (2018) reasoned that perhaps since these youth are involved with numerous professionals providing various services, most of whom are mandated reporters, more concerns are noted and reported. There is also the possibility that a misinterpretation of complex behaviors, self-injurious behaviors, or injuries obtained from nonabusive experiences lead to referral, which was later recognized as such.

The above highlights the opportunity for various points of intervention related to prevention of child maltreatment for families with children on the spectrum, including additional parenting classes, psychoeducation pertaining to child maltreatment and its prevention, behavior modification and applied behavior analysis (ABA) interventions. Interventions can also include additional tailored supports for parents to assist in mitigating the stresses of parenting in challenging contexts and provide additional support. By extension, there are also lessons to be learned for the CPS system. Given the differences in referrals for more intensive investigation for children without ASD, there are some concerns pertaining to the investigative process and caseworker or investigator education. For example, were referrals not made due to youths' inability to verbalize or otherwise communicate actual abusive experiences? After observing youths' problematic or aggressive behaviors or hearing parents' accounts of having to restrain or otherwise physically react to these behaviors, were caseworkers and/or investigators more apt to ascribe injuries or bruises received in an abusive situation to challenging but more benign interactions viewed as "justified" (Manders & Stoneman, 2009) forms of restraint? Moreover, as pertains to caseworker and/or investigator documentation, disability status is generally conveyed through overly simplistic assessments of *present* or *absent*, which inevitably fails to separate out the vast and different types of disabilities, impairments and presentations (Fisher et al., 2018). These issues speak directly to the need of caseworker and investigator training in the area of developmental disabilities and more specifically in youth with ASD (Fisher et al., 2018). Training should include information pertaining to a greater understanding of ASD and its possible presentations, and how such information and observations could meaningfully contribute to CPS investigations. Relatedly, there should be an emphasis on the *spectrum* aspect, reiterating the wide range of presentations with youth with ASD. The simple presence of ASD does not mean youth are nonverbal or do not have functional language, are significantly cognitively impaired, and that a meaningful interview cannot be conducted. Child protection and law enforcement agencies would benefit from a greater understanding of the ecological factors contributing to abuse in general and more specific to ASD presentations, which would both contribute to enhanced empathy for families, while also facilitating an approach to more accurately appraise risk and presence of abuse. Additional considerations revolve around understanding the unique communication impairments of children with ASD and issues related to obtaining disclosures.

Forensic interviews and evaluation of child maltreatment

When concerns of maltreatment arise, both the criminal and child protective (civil) systems may become involved, conducting their own investigations in attempts to both ascertain the presence or absence of child maltreatment and the assess possible harm or impact as a result (Blair & Steinberg, 2011; Budd, Connell, & Clark, 2011; Condie, 2014; Faller, 2015). Interviews are conducted by a range of professionals, consisting of but not limited to CPS caseworkers, detectives and law enforcement investigators, medical professionals, and various mental health professionals. Interviews at various stages seek to inform the process in different ways through gathering evidence for prosecution, assisting CPS in making their determinations, assessing the impact of maltreatment and, ultimately, providing recommendation for treatment or other safety related interventions. While each of these interviews conducted in civil, legal, and mental health agencies may be used differently or garner slightly different information, many of the same foundations and structure serve as guidance for conducting an appropriate and clinically and forensically defensible interview. There are high stakes involved in this process, as results may have a direct impact on the health and safety of youth, or greatly impinge on the civil liberties of parents as related to their children. There is a tenuous balance between attempting to enact safeguards against false disclosure while at the same time enabling or empowering disclosures of actual abuse. As such, out of respect for the interests and need for protection of the rights of all involved, a growing understanding of developmental level and how question types (e.g., suggestive, closed vs open-ended) impact interviews, the field of forensic interviewing has become more structured and nuanced (Faller, 2015). For the purpose of the current discussion, the term *forensic interview* will apply to those interviews conducted by CPS or law enforcement, and *forensic psychosocial evaluations* will be used to apply to not only an assessment of the disclosure of abuse, but the possible impact of such abuse and recommendations pertaining to treatment and safety issues stemming from such evaluations. General expectations pertaining to these types of interviews will be reviewed, followed by a discussion of relevant considerations and areas for further research related to the ASD population.

Early guidance was provided by the Kempe National Center for the Prevention and Treatment of Child Abuse and Neglect in 1985 (see Faller, 2015), suggesting interviewers thoroughly review the record prior, reassure the child that the nonoffending parent(s) is close and supportive, conduct one interview, and encourage the videotaping or audio recording of forensic interviews. It was recommended that interviewers establish rapport prior to an abuse inquiry, that the abuse inquiry largely rely upon open-ended questioning, and that the interviewer obtain as many specific details as possible. A closure phase is also usually included to focus on the needs of youth, allow for questions, and discuss safety or other relevant educational issues. Since these early years, significant concerns have arisen regarding suggestive or leading questions, the need to account for context or alternative hypotheses, the recognition that props (e.g., anatomical diagrams or dolls) may elicit false information in the absence of interviewer training, management of interviewer biases, and the impact of development upon participation and presentation in an interview (Faller, 2015).

Over the years, several protocols for forensic interviews of youth suspected of experiencing maltreatment have been developed (e.g., guidance or protocols developed by American Professional Society on the Abuse of Children, Corner House, the Gundersen National Child Protection Training Center, the National Children's Advocacy Center, and the National Institute of Child Health and Human Development). While each have slightly different nuances to them, the underlying structure and focus are generally the same (Faller, 2015; Newlin et al., 2015). There is a general consensus that children who experience abuse are likely to present differently in their ability to recall and communicate their experience and in reflecting upon their thoughts, feelings, and reactions. It is expected that interviews will rely upon open-ended questions as much as possible through eliciting free recall and spontaneous narrative of experience. Prompts are used to encourage greater detail (e.g., "and then what happened?," "Tell me about..."). Interviewers are expected to allow for silence and to adjust pacing depending on the communication style of youth. Depending on the developmental level of youth, more focused questions are used later in the interview to clarify information provided. The idea is that interviewers will be well-versed and knowledgeable in culture, development, the impact of trauma, the impact of disabilities, and the general process of disclosure.

Interviews typically begin with a rapport-building phase in which general ground rules and instructions are provided. At this early stage in the interview, youth are provided with an opportunity to discuss an innocuous, free-narrative, personal experience (e.g., narrative practice/episodic memory training), as well as a discussion of youths' understanding of truth and lie, with a promise to discuss things that only happened in reality (Faller, 2015, 2020; Newlin et al., 2015). The substantive phase focuses on obtaining as many details as possible regarding the reason for referral to assist in determinations of whether abuse occurred. Rather than progressing immediately to potentially emotionally evocative topics (e.g., the reason for referral), initial questions in this phase of the interview typically begin with topics such as family and peer relationships. However, information gathered as related to these relationships and interpersonal functioning is much more superficial than in a forensic psychosocial evaluation. Open-ended questions are utilized to elicit narrative accounts of youths' experiences, combined with prompts to elaborate, though without specific questioning, making sure not to introduce information into the discussion. Once these narratives have been fully explored, including other possible instances or types of abuse other than the specific referral, the interviewer, in a nonleading fashion, elicits information regarding the reason for referral through more focused questions to obtain sensory details, greater clarification about previously made statements or depictions, and/or other salient details relevant to prosecution or litigation. Some interview protocols allow for the use of other tools or media to assist in information gathering (e.g., anatomic diagrams or anatomical dolls; see Gunderson National Child Protection Training Center, 2020). Great attention is paid to monitoring for leading questions and being mindful of asking similar questions repeatedly, as they may contaminate the interview through suggestion or the influence of social demand characteristics (Ceci & Bruck, 1995; Malloy & Quas, 2009). At times, it is appropriate to introduce information garnered outside of the interview that youth have not openly discussed in the interview, though caution is warranted in these instances. In addition, during this segment of the interview, interviewers must attempt to rule out possible alternative hypotheses (e.g., misattribution, coaching) or consider contexts in which the contact or detail would make sense in a nonabusive fashion (e.g., genital touch in the context of toileting or application of medication to a rash). The interview then enters a formal closure phase in which youth are asked if the interviewer missed any relevant information and the youth is provided with the opportunity to ask questions. The interview concludes with the relevant psychoeducation when appropriate and the youth are thanked for their participation (American Professional Society on the Abuse of Children (APSAC), 2012; Faller, 2015; Newlin et al., 2015).

Forensic psychosocial evaluations, or psychological evaluations of youth suspected of experiencing maltreatment, incorporate many of the same principles noted above in terms of information gathering and examining details associated with possible maltreatment. In assessing for the presence of maltreatment, Condie (2014) specifies considering the following information: developmental context of the disclosure (e.g., hygiene ritual versus sexual touch; consideration of age and ADL development), explicit details, details that exceed developmental knowledge (e.g., advanced sexual knowledge in the case of sexual abuse), idiosyncratic details or phrases (e.g., sensation or phrases likely used during the commission of that abuse, etc.), inclusion of peripheral or unnecessary information, consistency of account and details, information relayed from youths' perspective rather than appearing rehearsed (e.g., coaching or other influence), descriptions of the "grooming" process or means to maintain youths' silence (seduction, isolation, coercion, bribes/enticements, escalation of threats and aggression), youths' depictions of ways to avoid the abuse, affective responses and presentation of youth (pp. 267–268). While obviously evaluators are not present at the time of the referral incident(s) and thus cannot definitively remark upon whether the abuse occurred (in the absence video evidence), this information assists in assessing the credibility or veracity of disclosures or descriptions, while also weighing them against possible alternative hypotheses. Forensic evaluators memorialize their findings in reports to the court, documenting (ideally) transparent and logical lines of thinking that contributed to clinically-informed opinions as to whether abuse likely occurred, there was not enough evidence in the interview to suggest it occurred, or there was an absence of information to opine in either direction (Otto, DeMeir, & Boccaccini, 2014).

Forensic psychosocial evaluations also seek to address the psycholegal question of not only did an abusive action occur, but did this abusive action cause harm and what treatment, services or accommodations would be warranted (American Psychological Association, 2011; Blair & Steinberg, 2011; Budd et al., 2011; Condie, 2014; Faller, 2015; Kroncke, Willard, & Huckabee, 2016). Such assessments must consider whether there were underlying conditions that should be considered as related to functioning and harm (e.g., underlying vulnerabilities often referred to as "thin skulls," "crumbling skulls," and "eggshell psyches"), the extent of the harm, a causal link between current presentation (harm) and the abusive act and that the actor is responsible for the harm, and relevant recommendations for intervention (Budd et al., 2011; Condie, 2014; Koch, Douglas, Nicholls, & O'Neill, 2006; Kroncke et al., 2016).

ASD and forensic interviews and evaluations

Often times, and especially as related to concerns of sexual abuse, disclosures obtained in forensic interviews and evaluations are the primary source of evidence (Faller, 2015), as there is a general absence of clear physical evidence. These demands require that interviewers and evaluators be highly skilled in interviewing children of differing developmental levels and abilities and understand the impact of trauma upon youths' presentation. This is especially relevant as there have been concerns noted that allegations of child maltreatment against youth with intellectual disabilities may not receive appropriate attention from the CPS and justice system due to investigators', prosecutors', and judges/juries' skepticism over such youths' ability to provide credible, meaningful, and robust information that would hold up to the adversarial process (Aarons & Powell, 2003; Aarons, Powell, & Browne, 2004; Brown & Lewis, 2013; Henry, Ridley, Perry, & Crane, 2011). In light of the possibly complicated and differing presentations of youth with ASD, including disruptions in attention, memory, language, and other aspects of functioning, evaluators must consider several factors both prior and during the interview or evaluation process. Kroncke et al. (2016) highlighted the following areas as relevant to the functional impairments of ASD and the potential impact of these impairments during the interview process: "concrete, literal processing, linear, sequential thinking, selective attention, weaknesses in processing speed, anxiety, repetitive thinking and behaviors, difficulty recalling events, weaknesses or deficits in social skills, impairments in perspective taking" (pp. 362–364). Of particular relevance to the current discussion, Faller (2020) recently noted that despite all of the progress made in our understanding in interviewing youth regarding possible experiences of maltreatment, and the development of various interview protocols, there are still several areas of concern that directly impact interviews of those with ASD. More specifically, Faller acknowledged the field is still uncertain as to how to meet the needs of those who require more than one interview to disclose, how to determine which youth are most suggestible, and how to best make decisions based on information provided in forensic interviews.

Early on, due to possible taint and the impact of leading or suggestive questioning, it was determined that a single, focused forensic interview was the desired method and became standard practice. However, more recently, the field has developed an understanding that more than one interview might be required to establish rapport or trust, accommodate youths' communication styles or limitations, and to assist in facilitating "reminiscence" (Faller, 2020; La Rooy, Katz, Malloy, & Lamb, 2010). Interviewers and evaluators trained in an extended evaluation process may want to consider, based on information provided in the referral materials, whether to meet with youth for more than one session (Williams, Nelson-Gardell, Faller, Tishelman, & Cordisco-Steele, 2016; Wyman, Lavoie, & Talwar, 2019). Such a format would enable youth more than one opportunity to disclose, as well as a slower pacing that may be more conducive to disclosure in light of attentional, memory, communication or other concerns. Of course, it is imperative that these decisions are based upon well trained interviewers who are knowledgeable about development and acutely aware of the impact of leading or suggestive questions.

While of course not an exhaustive list, youth diagnosed with ASD may evidence difficulties in their verbal abilities, rigidity in shifting attention, perseveration, relevantly responding to open-ended tasks, inhibiting responses and overall impairments in metacognition and metamemory, which is the capacity to reflect upon one's own thinking or memory processes (e.g., where they learned particular information; see White, Burgess, & Hill, 2009). Considering the importance of youths' descriptions of their experiences, significant impairments in language abilities has the potential to significantly compromise the investigative process. Moreover, instances of disclosure of abuse through the use of "facilitated communication" have proven not only extremely controversial but have also resulted in numerous false allegations with significant ramifications (Elliot, 2016; Regal, Rooney, & Wandas, 1994). As such, gathering information through such means is highly contraindicated, especially as the origin of the information or disclosure (youth or facilitator) cannot be confirmed or validated (International Society for Augmentative & Alternative Communication, 2014). There is limited, if any, research related to obtaining credible and legally defensible disclosures from those without the capacity to verbally communicate. By extension, while the use of sign language may assist in communicating abuse experiences, drawbacks and limitations have been noted in the literature (Neave-DiToro, Fuse, & Bergen, 2018). This highlights the great need for additional research to help protect and obtain justice for those with significant communication issues.

Previous studies support the notion that those interviewing youth about possible experiences of abuse feel unprepared when interviewing youth with ASD (Aarons & Powell, 2003; Aarons et al., 2004). By extension, it would not be unrealistic to expect that a large number of interviewers would be unfamiliar with some of the following when interviewing youth with ASD: heightened reactivity; sensory issues; stereotyped or repetitive behaviors; monotone voice or communications lacking emotional intonation; concrete, literal thinking; issues with pragmatic aspects of language (e.g., turn-taking); difficulty dealing with open-ended tasks with limited rules; heightened focused on precise or specific details while not appreciating the whole or the greater context; deficits in episodic memory; impairments in theory of mind; being less likely to reference their own mental states; poor frustration tolerance (McVey et al., 2018). Emergence of these difficulties during the course of a forensic interview conducted by someone naïve to these presentations could lead to the employment of ineffective interviewing strategies that fail to garner important information. More specifically, potentially problematic interview strategies employed by an evaluator include (but are not limited to) closed ended and forced choice questions that are apt to taint the interview (Brown, Lewis, Stephens, & Lamb, 2017), interviewer frustration that leads to premature ending of the interview (thereby preventing implementation of safety measures or obtaining justice), and a misinterpretation of the presentation (possibly interpreting behavior as dissimulation or attempts to lie or obstruct the process).

As noted above, open-ended questions/invitations are imperative in obtaining information related to abusive experiences to control for leading questions, suggestion or other interviewer influence that may taint the interview. In order to respond appropriately to open-ended questions, individuals generally need to demonstrate the capacity for implicit understanding of social contingencies, expectations, and an understanding of what the interviewer is asking for (Kenworthy, Yerys, Anthony, & Wallace, 2008; White et al., 2009). Youth with ASD may approach these open-ended questions in a more egocentric fashion, providing seemingly unrelated or irrelevant information to the task at hand. Interviewers must be aware of this possibility so as not to become exasperated during the interview process and/or misinterpret such responses as being deceitful, dissimulation, or representative of an overall inability to provide relevant information pertaining to possible abuse experiences. Relatedly, those with ASD often evidence difficulties with maintaining attention, may generally experience heightened anxiety, be prone to engaging in impulsive behaviors, and otherwise demonstrate challenging behaviors throughout the interview. It is imperative that interviewers and evaluators are familiar with such presentations to help buffer against potentially misinterpreting these behaviors as related to the referral and disclosure. Another relevant consideration is that of echolalia. Throughout the interview, youth may appear to perseverate on particular facts or interactions, especially if emotionally relevant, thus possibly appearing echolalic. However, interviewers and evaluators must conduct appropriate collaterals, as echolalia may not be present in some youths' history, contributing to a misinterpretation of this behavior as meaningless. Furthermore, interviewers must be appropriately trained in order to recognize that behaviors typically experienced as evasive or indicative of lying (e.g., avoidance of eye contact, avoidance of answering questions directly or relevantly) may be more a reflection of the youth's ASD presentation, rather than of deliberately evasive behaviors.

Interviews pertaining to child maltreatment rely heavily upon language and associated processing abilities, attentional capacities, and episodic or autobiographical memory. However, it is recognized that youth with ASD may experience significant deficits in these domains (Mattison, Dando, & Ormerod, 2015; McVey et al., 2018), which is evidenced in impaired free-recall in the absence of further scaffolding or support for memory retrieval (Hershkowitz, Lamb, Orbach, Katz, & Horowitz, 2012). Moreover, due to attentional or other memory-related deficits, information that would be considered forensically relevant and important (e.g., time periods, frequency, intent, penetration), may not have been attended to or subsequently encoded (Condie, 2014). Elaborating further on the forensic interview process during the substantive stage, interviews begin with open-ended invitations (e.g., "tell me everything you can remember") focusing on free-recall and minimal scaffolding. To gather additional information, "wh-" questions (e.g., who, what, where, when, and how) are employed, starting with relatively broad questions and progressing to more specific questions to assist in information gathering (Brown et al., 2017; Child Welfare Information Gateway, 2017). Research has suggested that these "wh-" questions may provide appropriate and productive support for memory retrieval (Ahern, Andrews, Stolzenberg, & Lyon, 2015; Hershkowitz, et al., 2012). Recognition prompts are also utilized through the use of option posing (e.g., "were your clothes on, off or something else?") to clarify information further, but it is strongly recommended that interviewers delay employing recognition prompts or options for as long as possible (American

Professional Society on the Abuse of Children (APSAC), 2012; Brown et al., 2017). In consideration of the developmental difficulties (e.g., communication, comprehension, attention) experienced by youth with ASD, there is a tenuous balance between spending adequate time in the interview attempting to gather information using open-ended invitations and appropriately progressing to more specific questioning. However, ultimately, interviewers must be mindful not to employ more specific questions at the early stages of the interview process in order to mitigate the possibility of suggestive questions in response to perceived or actual disability (Brown et al., 2017). Related to the issue of suggestibility and false memories, one recent study suggests that those with ASD are less susceptible to the impact of these concerns as compared to their nonclinical peers (Griego, Datzman, Estrada, & Middlebrook, 2019). The authors posited that the results may partially stem from individuals with ASD relying less upon "gist" memory, thus making them less susceptible to influence. However, the same study found increased vulnerability for both suggestibility and false memories in regard to individuals with intellectual disabilities. Clearly this area requires greater understanding and research, which in turn would inform the interview and evaluative process, as well as interpretations of information provided by ASD youth.

Another relevant issue pertains to source monitoring. Often, during the course of a forensic interview or evaluation, youth are asked to reflect upon how they *know what they know*, which helps investigators and the trier of fact (e.g., judge or jury) make judgments related to credibility. Through the use of open-ended questions, the interviewer attempts to account for misattribution, external influences such as coaching, or other sources from whence information relayed in the interview (e.g., pornography) may have originated. Impairments in metacognition and metamemory may meaningfully impact these responses. Moreover, youth with ASD and significant intellectual disabilities may have impairments in discerning reality from fantasy or rely upon and relay information obtained from others in speaking of past experiences (Wyman et al., 2019).

Clearly this discussion is not an exhaustive address of all the relevant issues, but rather highlights some key areas of concern related to interviewing youth with ASD suspected of having experienced child maltreatment. Greater dissemination of this information to forensic interviewers and evaluators will not only assist in obtaining better information, which in turn would help protect and obtain justice for abused youth, but would also enable these professionals to explain to the triers of fact why possibly confusing presentations emerged and how they are not incompatible with credible disclosures. Moreover, given the heightened risk for youth diagnosed with ASD, it is imperative that we continue to research forensic interviewing and evaluation techniques (Faller, 2020; Wyman et al., 2019).

Psycholegal issues of harm or trauma

All of the above information is relevant to information gathering during the course of a forensic psychosocial evaluation. However, one of the hallmark differences is that the forensic psychosocial evaluation not only examines issues pertaining to the disclosure itself (e.g., the degree of detail, consistency, idiosyncratic information not otherwise accounted for, reliability, considering alternative hypotheses), but it also seeks to address the issue of whether the abusive act created measurable harm and what recommendations would derive from the results (Budd et al., 2011; Condie, 2014; Kroncke et al., 2016; Melton et al., 2018). Pervasive and significant harm to the child perpetrated by a caretaker or known to a caretaker and not appropriately addressed can lead to limitations on caretakers' natural rights to their children. This section will speak more specifically to issues or emotional or psychological harm. Several considerations must be weighed in making these determinations, including high comorbidity of anxiety, PTSD and lifetime exposures to Adverse Childhood Experiences (ACEs; Kerns, Newschaffer, Berkowitz, & Lee, 2017) in youth with ASD that may not be due solely to child maltreatment (Haruvi-Lamdan, Horesh, Zohar, Kraus, & Golan, 2020); challenges in assessing presence, absence, or severity of symptoms (e.g., reliance upon caretakers for observational data, limitations in ASD youth conveying their internal emotional experiences, comorbid conditions); and the need for corroboration, a thorough history, and a clear link between the abuse and the harm (e.g., decline, traumatic reaction).

According to the National Institute of Mental Health (2017), 3.6% of adults experience PTSD in a given year, with a lifetime prevalence rate of 6.8%. The U.S. Department of Veterans Affairs (2019) estimates that between 5% and 8% of youth have experienced PTSD but current research on youth and PTSD lack definitive studies to determine prevalence rates. In comparison to neurotypical youth, some studies have reported much higher prevalence rates in the ASD population (Haruvi-Lamdan et al., 2020). These traumatic reactions in youth (regardless of ASD diagnosis) are not solely in reaction to child maltreatment but could also be in response to any of the ACEs (Felitti et al., 1998), including divorce, bullying, racism, aggression or abuse by another outside of the household, and/or neighborhood violence. This is important to note, as the presence of PTSD does not necessarily indicate that child maltreatment by a caretaker occurred, or that the clinical presentation *must* be related to child maltreatment. Moreover, it is similarly important to note that a diagnosis of PTSD is not necessary to highlight harm and that there is no "typical" traumatic presentation (Kisiel et al., 2014a, 2014b; van der Kolk, Roth, Pelcovitz, Sunday, & Spinazzola, 2005). Additionally, youth with ASD may also experience high rates of comorbidity of anxiety, which may stem from experiences including social confusion, rejection or bullying, sensitivity to sensory stimuli, and other sources of stress (Wood & Gadow, 2010). A contrasting concern is that due to "diagnostic overshadowing" (Helverschou, Bakken, & Martinsen, 2011) trauma responses may be misunderstood as or misattributed to preexisting comorbid disorders such as anxiety or depression (Kildahl et al., 2019).

One significant concern is an overreliance upon parental/caregiver report of changes in behavior, affective expression, and interpersonal functioning (Haruvi-Lamdan et al., 2020; Howlin & Clements, 1995; Kildahl et al., 2019; Kroncke et al., 2016). Firstly, assuming the parent providing the collateral information is not suspected of being the offending parent, they may inadvertently amplify the impact of the alleged abuse. Conversely, if parents are not aware of various alterations related to traumatic reactions, they may not recognize changes in youths' presentation, or by extension, realize this information is important to relay to evaluators. While these concerns highlight the need for corroboration and independent observation (e.g., evaluator) they are not significant enough to discount parental input altogether. In response to these concerns regarding ASD, trauma, and psycholegal issues related to abuse and harm, Howlin and Clements (1995) developed an interview schedule focusing on functioning in five domains: social-communication skills, behavior problems associated with stressful experiences, problems related more specifically to ASD (e.g., rituals), self-help skills, and general health. In the development of this interview approach, the researchers collected information on functioning in these areas, including behavioral ratings of frequency and degree of disturbance, from three time periods (e.g., prior to the abuse, during the abuse, and current functioning) to serve as a basis of comparison. Moreover, the authors made attempts to then corroborate descriptions through independent records from multiple sources (e.g., various therapies and assessments, medical records, school records). While admittedly an extremely small sample size, this study demonstrated that it was indeed possible to assess for traumatic impact or harm, even when youth with ASD were nonverbal. In response to the maltreatment experienced by the participants, the authors noted increases in dependent behaviors, deterioration in behavior (e.g., school refusal, changes in eating, tantrums, aggression), mood swings, and an increase in fear, though other skills, such as self-help and language skills remained mostly intact.

While also considering studies on adults, Kildahl et al. (2019) conducted a review of 18 studies examining experiences of trauma in those diagnosed with ASD and ID. The authors highlighted the above concerns and advocated for additional research to better understand trauma symptomology in those diagnosed with ASD and ID. However, their review revealed many studies noted alterations in arousal and an exacerbation in negative thoughts and emotions, which could be easily observed in an increase in dysregulated behaviors. Echoing some of these results, McDonnell et al. (2019), not included in the review, found maltreatment in youth with ASD was associated with higher levels of aggression, tantrums, self-harm, fears, and hyperactivity as compared to their nonabused peers. In their review, Kildahl et al. found that individuals exhibited an exacerbation of restriction in interests, stereotypic movement, and motor mannerisms, which they posited were likely to help alleviate altered arousal or facilitate avoidance. Further, they suggested that avoidance may instead be misinterpreted as challenging behaviors associated with ASD or general noncompliance. Kildahl et al. (2019) also reasoned that due to the tendency of traumatic memory to be stored in perceptual memory and an overreliance on sensory-based processing, youth with ASD experience "formation of poorly contextualized and disjointed memories, resulting in the development of intrusive trauma memories and symptoms of reexperiencing" (p. 16). Thus while youth with ASD may experience the flashbacks and intrusive ideation that are hallmarks of a PTSD diagnosis, they may not be able to report on these experiences.

An important consideration in the assessment of changes in functioning is examining whether youths' presentation is consistent with general skills deficit, a decline in functioning (versus some of the decalage associated with ASD) or is a complete regression. Through understanding the varying functional impairments and presentations of trauma experienced by youth with ASD, professionals in the field can better understand whether the presentation may be suggestive of a traumatic reaction (Kroncke et al., 2016). Additionally, Kerns, Newschaffer, and Berkowitz (2015) provide a useful review of the impact of traumatic events upon those with ASD, as well as a through discussion of issues relevant to notions of "thin skulls," "crumbling skulls," and "eggshell psyches." These legal doctrines pertain to assessing the relationship between previously existing vulnerabilities and the impact of abuse.

Conclusion

Clearly youth with ASD represent a particularly vulnerable population as related to child maltreatment. The above review highlights how youth with ASD are at increased risk for experiencing maltreatment and are referred at greater rates to the authorities and CPS. Yet many of these youth may not receive the intervention necessary due to a lack of caseworker or investigator training, perceptions of utility or credibility of the information that could be gathered in interviews, lack of specialized training in forensic interviewing of youth with ASD and intellectual disabilities, symptoms and skills deficits that complicate cognitively demanding and verbally based interviews, and a body of research that is generally in its infancy. It is imperative that there is a shift toward educating professionals that interact with youth suspected to have been maltreated at the earlier stages of professional training so that biases and lack of knowledge do not cripple investigations before they really start. Interviewers and evaluators must become well versed in the various presentations and possible complications posed by associated symptoms and deficits, to avoid some of the pitfalls that lead to a spoiled or prematurely ended interview. Moreover, legal, civil, and psychological professionals are in a unique position to explain to others within the system (e.g., prosecutors, triers of fact) why such confusing presentations do not render disclosure meaningless, fully prevent an assessment of impact, or mean the case unable to be prosecuted.

References

Aarons, N. M., & Powell, M. B. (2003). Issues related to the interviewer's ability to elicit reports of abuse from children with an intellectual disability: A review. *Current Issues in Criminal Justice*, *14*, 257–268.

Aarons, N. M., Powell, M. B., & Browne, J. (2004). Police perceptions of interviews involving children with intellectual disabilities: A qualitative inquiry. *Policing and Society*, *14*, 269–278. Available from https://doi.org/10.1080/1043946042000241848.

Ahern, E. C., Andrews, S. J., Stolzenberg, S. N., & Lyon, T. D. (2015). The productivity of wh- prompts in child forensic interviews. *Journal of Interpersonal Violence*, *33*(13), 2007–2015. Available from https://doi.org/10.1177/0886260515621084.

American Psychiatric Association. (2013). *Diagnostic and statistical manual of mental disorders (5th ed.)*. Arlington, VA: Author.

American Psychological Association. (2011). *Guidelines for psychological evaluations in child protection matters*. <www.apa.org/pus/journals/features/child-protection.pdf>.

American Professional Society on the Abuse of Children (APSAC). (2012). *Practice guidelines: Forensic interviewing in cases of suspected child abuse*. <https://www.apsac.org/guidelines>.

Blair, G., & Steinberg, A. G. (2011). Child abuse and neglect. In E. Y. Drogin, F. M. Dattilio, R. L. Sadoff, & T. G. Guthiel (Eds.), *Handbook of forensic assessment: Psychological and psychiatric perspectives* (pp. 391–415). John Wiley & Sons, Inc.

Brown, D., Lewis, C., Stephens, E., & Lamb, M. (2017). Interviewers' approaches to questioning vulnerable child witnesses: The influences of developmental level versus intellectual disability status. *Legal and Criminological Psychology*, *22*(2), 332–349. Available from https://doi.org/10.1111/lcrp.12104.

Brown, D. A., & Lewis, C. (2013). Competence is in the eye of the beholder: Perceptions of intellectually disabled child witnesses. *International Journal of Developmental Disabilities and Education*, *60*, 3–17. Available from https://doi.org/10.1080/1034912X.2013.757132.

Budd, K. S., Connell, M., & Clark, J. R. (2011). *Evaluation of parenting capacity in child protection*. Oxford University Press.

Ceci, S., & Bruck, M. (1995). *Jeopardy in the courtroom: A scientific analysis of children's testimony*. American Psychological Association.

Child Welfare Information Gateway. (2019). *About CAPTA: A legislative history*. <https://www.childwelfare.gov/pubPDFs/about.pdf>.

Child Welfare Information Gateway. (2017). *Forensic interviewing: A primer for child welfare professionals*. <https://www.childwelfare.gov/pubPDFs/forensicinterviewing.pdf>.

Cicchetti, D., & Valentino, K. (2015). An ecological-transactional perspective on child maltreatment: Failure of the average expectable environment and its influence on child development. In D. Cicchetti, & D. J. Cohen (Eds.), Developmental psychopathology: Risk, disorder and adaptation (pp. 129–201). John Wiley & Sons, Inc.

Condie, L. O. (2014). Conducting child abuse and neglect evaluations. In I. B. Weiner, & R. K. Otto (Eds.), *The handbook of forensic psychology* (4th ed., pp. 237–278). John Wiley & Sons, Inc, ol.3456789.

Dinkler, L., Lundström, S., Galwani, R., Lichtenstein, P., Gillberg, C., & Minnis, H. (2017). Maltreatment-associated neurodevelopmental disorders: A co-twin control analysis. *Journal of Child Psychology and Psychiatry*, *58*(6), 691–701. Available from https://doi.org/10.1111/jcpp.12682.

Elliot, J. (2016). *The battle over a controversial method for Autism communication*. The Atlantic. <https://www.theatlantic.com/education/archive/2016/07/a-controversial-method-for-autism-communication/491810/>.

Faller, K. C. (2015). Forty years of forensic interviewing of children suspected of sexual abuse, 1974–2014: Historical benchmarks. *Social Sciences*, *4*, 34–65. Available from https://doi.org/10.3390/socsci4010034.

Faller, K. C. (2020). The cutting edge of forensic interviewing. *Journal of Child Sexual Abuse*, *29*(2), 129–137. Available from https://doi: 10.1080/10538712.2020.1718819.

Felitti, V. J., Anda, R. F., Nordernberg, D., Williamson, D. F., Spitz, A. M., Edwards, V., ... Marks, J. S. (1998). Relationship of childhood abuse and household dysfunction to many of the leading causes of death in adults: The Adverse Childhood Experiences (ACE) study. *American Journal of Preventive Medicine*, *14*(4), 245–258. Available from https://doi.org/10.1016/S0749-3797(98)00017-8.

Fisher, M. H., Epstein, R. A., Urbano, R. C., Vehorn, A., Cull, M., & Warren, Z. (2018). A population-based examination of maltreatment referrals and substantiation for children with autism spectrum disorder. *Autism: The International Journal of Research and Practice*, *23*(5), 1335–1340. Available from https://doi.org/10.1177/1362361318813998.

Gil, D. G. (1970). *Violence against children: Physical child abuse in the United States*. Harvard University Press.

Govindshenoy, M., & Spencer, N. (2007). Abuse of the disabled child: A systematic review of population-based studies. *Child: Care, Health & Development*, *33*(5), 552–558. Available from https://doi.org/10.1111/j.1365-2214.2006.00693.x.

Griego, A. W., Datzman, J. N., Estrada, S. M., & Middlebrook, S. S. (2019). Suggestibility and false memories in relation to intellectual disability and autism spectrum disorder: A meta-analytic review. *Journal of Intellectual Disability Research*, *63*(12), 1464–1474. Available from https://doi-org.proxy.library.nyu.edu/10.1111/jir.12668.

Gunderson National Child Protection Training Center. (2020). *Child first/finding words*. Winona, MN: Gunderson National Child Protection Training Center.

Haruvi-Lamdan, N., Horesh, D., Zohar, S., Kraus, M., & Golan, O. (2020). Autism spectrum disorder and post-traumatic stress disorder: An unexplored cooccurrence of conditions. *Mental Health Across the Lifespan*, *24*(4), 884–989. Available from https://doi.org/10.1177/1362361320912143.

Helton, J. J., & Cross, T. P. (2011). The relationship of child functioning to parental physical assault: Linear and curvilinear models. *Child Maltreatment*, *16*(2), 126–136. Available from https://doi.org/10.1177/1077559511401742.

Helverschou, S. B., Bakken, T. L., & Martinsen, H. (2011). Psychiatric disorders in people with autism spectrum disorders: Phenomenology and recognition. In J. L. Matson, & P. Sturmey (Eds.), *International handbook of autism and pervasive developmental disorders* (pp. 53–74). Springer.

Henry, L. A., Ridley, A., Perry, J., & Crane, L. (2011). Perceived credibility and eyewitness testimony of children with intellectual disabilities. *Journal of Intellectual Disability Research*, *55*, 385–391. Available from https://doi.org/10.1111/j.1365-2788.2011.01383.x.

Hershkowitz, I., Lamb, M. E., Orbach, Y., Katz, C., & Horowitz, D. (2012). The development of communicative and narrative skills among preschoolers: Lessons from forensic interviews about child abuse. *Child Development*, *83*, 611–622. Available from https://doi.org/10.1111/j.1467-8624.2011.01704.x.

Hibbard, R. A., & Desch, L. W. (2007). Maltreatment of children with disabilities. *Pediatrics*, *119*(5), 1018–1025. Available from https://doi.org/10.1542/peds.2007-0565.

Howlin, P., & Clements, J. (1995). Is it possible to assess the impact of abuse on children with pervasive developmental disorders? *Journal of Autism and Developmental Disorders*, *25*(4), 337–354. Available from https://doi-org.proxy.library.nyu.edu/10.1007/BF02179372.

International Society for Augmentative and Alternative Communication. (2014). ISAA position statement on facilitated communication. *Augmentative and Alternative Communication*, *30*(4), 357–358. Available from https://doi.org/10.3109/07434618.2014.971492.

Jaudes, P. K., & Diamond, L. J. (1985). The handicapped child and child abuse. *Child Abuse & Neglect*, *9*, 341–347. Available from https://doi.org/10.1016/0145-2134(85)90030-4.

Jaudes, P. K., & Mackey-Bilaver, L. (2008). Do chronic conditions increase young children's risk of being maltreated? *Child Abuse & Neglect*, *32*(7), 671–681. Available from https://doi.org/10.1016/j.chiabu.2007.08.007.

Kenworthy, L., Yerys, B. E., Anthony, L. G., & Wallace, G. L. (2008). Understanding executive control in autism spectrum disorders in the lab and in the real world. *Neuropsychology Review*, *18*, 320–338.

Kerns, C. M., Newschaffer, C., & Berkowitz, S. (2015). Traumatic childhood events and autism spectrum disorder. *Journal of Autism and Developmental Disorders, 45*, 3475–3486. Available from https://doi.org/10.1007/s10803-015-2392-y.

Kerns, C. M., Newschaffer, C., Berkowitz, S., & Lee, B. K. (2017). Examining the association of autism and adverse childhood experiences in the National Survey of Children's Health: The important role of income and co-occurring mental health conditions. *Journal of Autism and Developmental Disorders, 47*(7), 2275–2281. Available from https://doi.org/10.1007/s10803-017-3111-7.

Kildahl, A. N., Bakken, T. L., Iversen, T. E., & Helverschou, S. B. (2019). Identification of post-traumatic stress disorder in individuals with autism disorder and intellectual disability: A systematic review. *Journal of Mental Health Research in Intellectual Disabilities, 12*(1–2), 1–25. Available from http://dx.doi.10.1080/19315864.2019.1595233.

Kisiel, C., Fehrenback, T., Torgersen, E., Stolbach, B., McClelland, G., Griffin, G., & Burkman, K. (2014a). Constellations of interpersonal trauma and symptoms in child welfare: Implications for a developmental trauma framework. *Journal of Family Violence, 29*, 1–14.

Kisiel, C., Fehrenbach, T., Liang, L., Stohlbach, B., McClelland, G., Griffin, G., ... Spinazzola, J. (2014b). Examining child sexual abuse in relation to complex patterns of trauma exposure: Findings from the National Traumatic Stress Network. *Psychological Trauma: Theory, Research, Practice and Policy, 6*(1), S29–S39. Available from https://doi.org/10.1037/a0037812.

Koch, W. J., Douglas, K. S., Nicholls, T. L., & O'Neill, M. L. (2006). *Psychological injuries: Forensic assessment, treatment, and law*. Oxford University Press.

Kroncke, A. P., Willard, M., & Huckabee, H. (2016). *Assessment of autism spectrum disorder: Critical issues in clinical, forensic, and school settings*. Springer International Publishing.

La Rooy, D., Katz, C., Malloy, L. C., & Lamb, M. E. (2010). Do we need to rethink guidance on repeated interviews? *Psychology, Public Policy, and Law, 16*(4), 373–392. Available from https://doi.org/10.1037/a0019909.

Malloy, L. C., & Quas, J. A. (2009). Children's suggestibility: Areas of consensus and controversy. In K. Kuehnle, & M. Connell (Eds.), *The evaluation of child sexual abuse allegations: A comprehensive guide to assessment and testimony* (pp. 267–297). John Wiley & Sons, Inc.

Mandell, D. S., Novak, M. M., & Zubritsky, C. D. (2005). Factors associated with age of diagnosis among children with autism spectrum disorders. *Pediatrics, 116*(6), 1480–1486. Available from https://doi.org/10.1542/peds.2005-0185.

Manders, J. E., & Stoneman, Z. (2009). Children with disabilities in the child protective services system: An analog study of investigation and case management. *Child Abuse & Neglect, 33*(4), 229–237. Available from https://doi.org/10.1016/j.chiabu.2008.10.001.

Mattison, M. L. A., Dando, C. J., & Ormerod, T. C. (2015). Sketching to remember: Episodic free recall task support for child witnesses and victims with autism spectrum disorder. *Journal of Autism and Developmental Disorders, 45*, 1751–1765. Available from https://doi.org/10.1007/s10803-014-2335-z.

McDonnell, C. G., Boan, A. D., Bradley, C. C., Seay, K. D., Charles, J. M., & Carpenter, L. A. (2019). Child maltreatment in autism spectrum disorder and intellectual disability: Results from a sample population. *Journal of Child Psychology and Psychiatry, 60*(5), 576–584. Available from https://doi.org/10.1111/jcpp.12993.

McVey, A. J., Schiltz, H. K., Haendel, A. D., Dolan, B. K., Willar, K. S., Pleiss, S. S., ... Van Hecke, A. V. (2018). Social difficulties in youth with autism with and without anxiety and ADHD symptoms. *Autism Research, 11*(12), 1679–1689. Available from https://doi.org/10.1002/aur.2039.

Melton, G., Petrila, J., Poythress, N. G., Slobogin, C., Otto, R. K., Mossman, D., & Condie, L. O. (2018). *Psychological evaluations for the courts: A handbook for mental health professionals and lawyers*. The Guilford Press.

National Child Abuse and Neglect Data System. (2019). *Child file codebook*. <https://www.acf.hhs.gov/sites/default/files/cb/ncands_child_file_codebook.pdf>.

National Institute of Mental Health. (2017). *Post-traumatic stress disorder (PTSD)*. <https://www.nimh.nih.gov/health/statistics/post-traumatic-stress-disorder-ptsd.shtml>.

Neave-DiToro, D., Fuse, A., & Bergen, M. (2018). Law enforcement interactions: The role of communication sciences and disorders professionals. *Communication Disorders Quarterly*, *40*(4), 250−256. Available from https://doi.org/10.1177/1525740118810898.

Newlin, C., Steele, L.C., Chamberlin, A., Anderson, J., Kenniston, J., Russel, A., . . . Vaughan-Eden, V. (2015). *Child forensic interviewing: Best practices*. Office of Juvenile Justice and Delinquency Prevention. <https://ojjdp.ojp.gov/sites/g/files/xyckuh176/files/pubs/248749.pdf>.

Otto, R. K., DeMeir, R. L., & Boccaccini, M. T. (2014). *Forensic reports & testimony: A guide to effective communication for psychologists & psychiatrists*. John Wiley & Sons, Inc.

Ratnofsky, A. C. (1994). *A report on the maltreatment of children with disabilities*. National Center on Child Abuse and Neglect.

Regal, R. A., Rooney, J. R., & Wandas, T. (1994). Facilitated communication: An experimental evaluation. *Journal of Autism and Developmental Disorders*, *24*(3), 345−355. Available from https://doi.org/10.1007/BF02172232.

Sandgrund, A., Gaines, R. W., & Green, A. H. (1974). Child abuse and mental retardation: A problem of cause and effect. *American Journal of Mental Deficiency*, *79*(3), 327−330.

Soeffing, M. (1975). Abused children are exceptional children. *Exceptional Children*, *42*, 116−133. Available from https://doi.org/10.1177/001440297504200302.

Sullivan, P. M., & Knutson, J. F. (2000). Maltreatment and disabilities: A population-based epidemiological study. *Child Abuse and Neglect*, *24*, 1257−1273. Available from https://doi.org/10.1016/S0145-2134(00)00190-3.

U.S. Committee on Health, Education, Labor and Pensions (2010). *CAPTA Reauthorization Act of 2010: Report (to accompany* S. 3817). U.s. G. P. O. U.S. Congress. *(1974). S. 1191 (93rd) Congress: Child Abuse Prevention and Treatment Act.* https://www.govtrack.ur/congress/bills/93/s1191.

U.S. Congress. (1974). Child Abuse Prevention and Treatment Act (CAPTA). P.L. 93–247.

U.S. Department of Health & Human Services, Administration for Children and Families, Administration on Children, Youth and Families, Children's Bureau. (2020). *Child maltreatment 2018*. <https://www.acf.hhs.gov/cb/research-data-technology/statistics-research/child-maltreatment>.

U.S. Department of Veterans Affairs. (2019). *PTSD: National center for PTSD, PTSD in children and adolescents*. <https://www.ptsd.va.gov/professional/treat/specific/ptsd_child_teens.asp>.

van der Kolk, B., Roth, S., Pelcovitz, D., Sunday, S., & Spinazzola, J. (2005). Disorders of extreme stress: The empirical foundation of a complex adaptation to trauma. *Journal of Traumatic Stress*, *18*, 389−399. Available from https://doi.org/10.1002/jts.20047.

White, S. J., Burgess, P. W., & Hill, E. L. (2009). Impairments on "open-ended" executive function tests in autism. *Autism Research*, *2*(3), 138−147. Available from https://doi.org/10.1002/aur.78.

Williams, J., Nelson-Gardell, D., Faller, K. C., Tishelman, A., & Cordisco-Steele, L. (2016). Perceptions of the value of extended assessments to resolve allegations of sexual abuse: It's the performance that counts. *Journal of Social Service Research*, *42*(1), 57−69. Available from https://doi.org/10.1080/01488376.2015.1077493.

Wood, J. J., & Gadow, K. D. (2010). Exploring the nature and function of anxiety in youth with autism spectrum disorders. *Clinical Psychology: Science and Practice*, *17*, 281–292. Available from https://doi.org/10.1111/j.1468-2850.2010.01220.x.

Wyman, J. D., Lavoie, J., & Talwar, V. (2019). Best practices in interviewing children with intellectual disabilities in maltreatment cases. *Exceptionality: A Special Education Journal*, *27*(3), 167–184. Available from https://doi.org/10.1080/09362835.2018.1425623.

The use of scripts by children with autism spectrum disorder: a puzzle and an opportunity

26

Sima Gerber
Queens College, City University of New York, Queens, NY, United States

What is scripting?

The speech, language, and communication patterns of children on the autism spectrum are often thought of as deviating from the language acquisition processes of both typically developing children and other populations of children with challenges in these areas. The use of echolalia and scripting are two of the most often cited examples of this departure. From one perspective, these language forms are dismissed relative to their place in the process of acquiring language and their function during communication exchanges. This despite the fact that research from 40 years ago (Prizant & Duchan, 1981; Prizant & Rydell, 1984) described immediate and delayed echolalia as forms of gestalt language learning, which were used to express communicative functions similar to those noted in typical development. More recently, the conversational analysis of echolalia has led to positive interpretations of the use of echolalia by children with autism spectrum disorder (ASD) during interpersonal interactions (Sterponi, de Kirby, & Shankey, 2015). While research on echolalia, both historic and recent (Stiegler, 2015), set the stage for a "new" appreciation of its communicative power, scripting is still often considered an inappropriate behavior.

Sterponi et al. (2015) suggest that the analysis of the language of individuals with autism is colored by the researcher's view of language. This is certainly the case in clinical interactions as well. These authors argue that adopting a *multidimensional view of language* has wide ranging implications, deepening our understanding of autism's core features and developmental trajectory. Two paradigms, one developmental and the other linguistic, will be used in this discussion to represent a "multidimensional view of language" and serve as the basis of the discussion of gestalt forms. Issues such as how scripts can be understood from a developmental lens and the role of gestalt forms in conversational exchanges will be explored. From here, we can move seamlessly to an intervention approach which both values the child's use of scripting and sees it as an opportunity to facilitate a more conventional language and communication system. Case material will be presented to support the perspective presented.

Emerging Programs for Autism Spectrum Disorder. DOI: https://doi.org/10.1016/B978-0-323-85031-5.00025-6

The question of where scripting fits vis-a-vis traditional definitions of language is a fair one to begin with. Language is typically defined as a code whereby ideas about the world are expressed through a conventional system of arbitrary signals for communication (Lahey, 1988). Scripting, like echolalia, departs from several hallmarks of this definition, specifically relative to the notion of a "conventional system" of language. Since the use of scripts is not a *shared* convention and since scripts are more imitative than self-generated, the reasons scripting might be considered "less than" are apparent.

However, if we assume that echolalia and scripting are being used to communicate the child's thoughts and feelings and to participate in conversational interactions, the fact that the forms are unconventional rather than conventional becomes less significant. Our most productive attempts to help children who struggle with language will come from using well-established stages of typical development and insights from conversational analysis, as a starting point for understanding what the child might be trying to accomplish given his limitations in the comprehension and production of language.

Before continuing, two clarifications should be made. In terms of definitions, the line between echolalia and scripting is not always clear and at times, these terms are used interchangeably. While echolalia and scripting share common features, such as the imitative nature of the forms, in this discussion, scripting will be considered a subset of gestalt forms used by children with autism (and other children as well) where the forms are exact or close approximations of lines from movies, books, and songs rather than the immediate repetitions of other speakers' utterances. In some ways, the distinction between echolalia and scripting is less important than the hallmark characteristics of gestalt language which they share. These include:

- Imitative versus self-generated forms of language
- Unconventional forms used to communicate meaning and feelings
- Adherence to the semantic-syntactic structure of the "borrowed" language forms
- Continuum of exact repetitions to modified ones

Another, quite different use of the term scripting, refers to an intervention strategy. In this context, the child is introduced to a verbal and/or written description about a specific skill or situation that provides a model for how to interact in a certain context. The thinking here is that the "script" will help the child anticipate the dimensions of the situation and give him guidelines for participating in that activity. After scripts are practiced, the child is expected to use the scripts in real life and their use is then faded. This use of the term scripting will not be dealt with in this chapter.

Language and communication challenges of children with ASD

The speech, language, and communication challenges of children on the autism spectrum are typically described as impairments in social communication, and language and related cognitive skills. According to the American Speech-Language-Hearing Association (ASHA) (asha.org), deficits in *social communication* include problems in joint attention, social reciprocity, and social cognition. Among the many manifestations of these problems, the following communicative behaviors might be observed:

- restricted range of communicative functions to seek engagement and comfort from others;
- difficulty initiating bids for interaction;
- problems responding to bids for interaction initiated by others;
- limitations with maintaining turn-taking in interactions;
- difficulty recognizing and repairing breakdowns in communication; and
- understanding and regulating emotions.

In terms of impairments in *language and related cognitive skills*, the following patterns are noted:

- delayed acquisition of words, word combinations, and syntax;
- more delayed receptive language than expressive language;
- use of echolalia;
- limitations in understanding and applying social norms of conversation (e.g., balanced turn-taking, vocal volume, proximity, prosody, and conversational timing);
- provision of inappropriate and unnecessary information in conversation;
- provision of too little detail in conversation;
- preference for topics of special interest; and
- lack of or limited question asking in conversation.

Many of the communicative challenges mentioned above are considered part of the component of language referred to as pragmatics or *use*, in the form-content-use model introduced by Lahey (1988). In fact, deficits in pragmatics are often considered a defining feature of the language and communication patterns of children on the autism spectrum. Early research suggested that the pragmatic profiles of children with ASD were distinguished not only from typically developing children but also from other groups of children with language disorders. For example, when the discourse abilities of children with autism were compared to children with Down's syndrome, it was found that the conversational patterns were quite different (Tager-Flusberg & Anderson, 1991). Specifically, the children with autism who were matched on age and language level, produced fewer adjacent, contingent, and relevant utterances. Differences in pragmatic abilities have also been noted between children with autism and children with specific language impairment. Surian, Baron-Cohen, and Van der Lely (1996) found that children with ASD had more violations of the conversational maxims, such as be informative but not redundant.

Over the last 40 years, studies have documented the particular challenges in the pragmatics of language that are typically seen in children with autism, including children who are nonverbal as well as those who are highly verbal (Parsons, Cordier, Munro, Joosten, & Speyer, 2017). It is beyond the scope of this chapter to review this literature, but taken together, there is clear evidence to support the particular vulnerability that children on the autism spectrum experience with the pragmatic aspects of language. These challenges are seen in the fundamental areas of pragmatics, including discourse management, communicative functions, conversational repair, and presupposition. Difficulties in early developing pragmatic skills such as joint attention, joint engagement, initiating communication, and range of communication acts, as well as later developing skills such as cohesion, referencing, adequate responsiveness, and adapting to different conversation partners are noted. Differences in nonlinguistic communication such as unusual prosody and eye gaze often are seen throughout the person's lifetime.

Although integrally tied, when the form and function of language are thought of somewhat separately, research suggests that the use of gestalt forms are often attempts at accomplishing some of the pragmatic functions mentioned above, such as expressing communicative intent, initiating conversations, and responding to the bids of others (Prizant & Duchan, 1981). In fact, one of the most welcome shifts in the analysis of the language of children on the spectrum came with the pragmatic revolution. For the first time, taxonomies were available which did not focus on syntax alone and therefore could be used to analyze more holistically the communication challenges that children with autism faced. On the positive side, pragmatic analysis provided the researcher and the clinician with paradigms that prioritized the interactional aspects of language rather than only the structural forms and thus potentially led to the realization of the universality in the functions of language regardless of the semantic-syntactic structures being used to express them.

How can we view scripting from a developmental language perspective?

Gerber (2003) recommended that speech-language pathologists use developmental language acquisition principles as the foundation for language-communication assessment and intervention for children on the autism spectrum.

> *Those clinicians who embrace a developmental approach to language intervention do so with the understanding that the universal and unique features of the language acquisition process of children with autism, as with all children, can best be understood, explained, and responded to with a keen awareness of the forms and functions of typical language acquisition.*
>
> *Gerber (2003, p. 75)*

This position may be challenged by speech-language pathologists and educators who approach the unconventional patterns of children on the autism spectrum with deficit explanations of their use. This in turn leads to approaches in intervention which may in fact negatively impact the child's potential source of a developmental language pathway, especially, when parents are counseled to ignore or discourage the use of scripts. Suskind (2014a) notes that when he first reported that he might be able to connect to his son through scripting, the speech-language therapist did not embrace his enthusiasm.

In terms of the developmental language perspective, scripting will be framed relative to language acquisition principles to achieve two goals: (1) to place scripting in the larger framework of typical language acquisition, and (2) to direct our intervention priorities and strategies for children who script. The science of language acquisition has provided a map of how children move from preintentional sounds to using language to participate in conversations and narratives. The developmentalist views these theories, models, paradigms, and facts of language acquisition as the science on which to base her understanding of atypical language acquisition and as the starting point for understanding the complexities of the intervention process. Three principles will be reviewed:

> Language Acquisition Principle 1—Language is learned in the context of spontaneous, natural social interactions between the caregiver and the child.

Some interventionists believe that if language is not learned naturally, there is less concern with using the "typical" science as a reference point to guide a therapeutic approach. This departure raises important questions about which alternatives are best to adopt when the goal is to facilitate the generative use of language and the potential to communicate thoughts and feelings.

The relational context of language learning between child and caregiver is unique and formative. Regardless of the child's disability, most would agree that the attachment between the child and the caregiver is the strongest one the child has. The attachment might be manifested differently or unconventionally, but relative to that child and his capacity for relationships, there is little question, that the relationship with the mother or father or grandmother is primary. This is true despite the conflict and anxiety that parents may experience when they have a child with a disability.

In 2020 we know so much about the unmistakable place of the caregiver–child relationship in each child's healthy development of both mind and body (National Scientific Council on the Developing Child, 2020). The recent work by Singletary (2015) supports the idea that the altered patterns of parent–child interactions experienced by children with ASD reduces their experience of growth-promoting interactions. Clearly, the primary work of the clinician or educator supporting a family with a child with ASD is to help the caregiver create and magnify moments of togetherness. First and foremost, we hope to engineer qualitative and quantitative improvements in interpersonal engagement between parent and child. Not to take advantage of this natural learning context seems to be a clear misstep.

In my work with a child who scripted when I met him at 4 years of age and to some degree, uses scripts now, at 19 years of age (Gerber, in press), the most significant and positive aspects of his development of language, can be traced to his mother's acceptance and response to his scripts. This mother delighted in Mark's talking and wanted to encourage dialogue rather than monologue. In joining the scripts, she listened attentively and let Mark take the lead on the topic of conversation. She did this when she knew the reference and when she did not.

The difference between communication being heard and "read" by your loved ones versus not being responded to is the difference between being acknowledged as a person and being marginalized. Surely, this response from your love object would make a difference in how you viewed yourself as a communicator and as a person.

In some ways, this response to gestalt forms is reminiscent of the perlocutionary stage of language (Bates, Benigni, Bretherton, Camaioni, & Volterra, 1979) where caregivers imbue their infant's vocalizations and gurgles with meaning in order to engage in a communicative interaction. There is no question that experiences of being read, affectively and communicatively, contribute significantly to the child's emerging sense of the power and the joys of communicating.

Each language acquisition principle leads directly to an intervention principle, which will set the stage for how the parent, clinician, and educator can think about their response to the child's scripting.

Intervention Principle 1

Scripting provides an opportunity for the parent or caregiver to be an integral part of the therapeutic process.

> Language Acquisition Principle 2—The development of language begins with the child's thoughts and feelings.

Bloom and Tinker (2001) proposed a model of language acquisition referred to as the Intentionality Model. This model embraced the well-known Form–Content–Use paradigm of language (Lahey, 1988) and expanded it to include broader developmental areas, referred to as *effort* (cognitive development) and *engagement* (social-emotional development). Among the most helpful constructs introduced in this work was the idea of "contents of mind." This simple but elegant construct underscores that children talk about what they are thinking or feeling. For children who use more conventional systems of nonlinguistic communication, language, and play, determining what the child is thinking or feeling can be somewhat transparent. However, for a child whose comprehension and production of language is compromised and possibly seriously so, scripts can be an alternative window into the child's thoughts and emotions. With this in mind, the issue isn't whether the content is relevant to the moment or even if we can precisely decipher what the child is trying to communicate. By using the scripts, the child has offered us access to his world. And the child's thoughts take precedence over the listener's judgment of the content.

In terms of intervention, rather than introducing more arbitrary material for the child to talk about, taken from the clinician's agenda, this developmental language principle dictates that we begin our therapeutic interactions where language begins—with the contents of the child's mind. Again, even if the forms of communication are unconventional and somewhat opaque, the role of the speaker's intentions and meanings take precedence as they reflect the origins of all human language (Gerber, 2003).

Beyond this, clinicians who join the child's scripts, much like Suskind (2014b) did with his son Owen, find that the child who was minimally verbal or conversational will participate with a gleam in his eye when the adult joins the dialogue and takes on roles in the scripts.

Intervention Principle 2

Scripting may be unconventional but it does reflect the contents of the child's mind, that is, what the child is thinking and what the child is feeling. This is where language begins.

Language Acquisition Principle 3—The child's stage of comprehension and production can be determined by referring to developmental information.

Children with delays in the acquisition of language can be placed on the developmental trajectory of language to better understand what they can and cannot comprehend, what they can and cannot produce, and what would be next in the process. Blanc (2012) has proposed a developmental sequence observed in children who use gestalt forms, which supports the template of linguistic stages as a foundation for determining therapeutic goals and strategies. Another possibility is to use a map of typical developmental language stages, such as the one proposed by Gerber and Prizant (2001).

Stage 1—Preintentional (0–8 months)
(*The communicative partner infers the child's messages, feelings, and intentions*)

Stage 2—Prelinguistic Intentional (8–12 months)
(*Emergence of intentional communication*)

Stage 3—First Words (12–18 months)
(*Emerging symbolic communication, that is, meaningful words and phrases*)

Stage 4—Two-Word Utterances (18–24 months)
(*Vocabulary explosion and early multiword combinations*)

Stage 5—Early Pragmatic-Semantic-Syntactic Development (24–36 months)
(*Later multiword, beginning complex sentences*)

Stage 6—Later Pragmatic–Semantic–Syntactic Development (36 months +)
(*The child uses more complex language to talk about events and engages in various kinds of discourse*)

*Adapted from Gerber and Prizant (2001).

Despite deviations, it is possible to place every child somewhere on this map. The use of developmental language stages provides the adult with two advantages:

1. The parent, clinician, or educator can begin to understand what expectations might be appropriate for this particular child. For example, if the child is approximately at Stage 2, the adults would not yet model or expect more complex utterances.

2. The parent, clinician, or educator can begin to target goals at the next level. For example, if the child is at Stage 2, addressing the comprehension of early-occurring phrases (*give Mommy a kiss*) would be prioritized.

Intervention Principle 3

Scripting is a reflection of challenges with the comprehension and/or production of language. We can approximate the child's stage of comprehension and production and begin intervention there.

The overarching thinking in using principles of language acquisition to generate intervention principles is consistent with contemporary views about developmental approaches across disciplines.

> *Regardless of the specific discipline, developmental approaches begin with the assumption that all strategies of intervention, regardless of the target group or desired outcome, can be derived from normative theories of development. That is to say, the general principles of development apply to all children independent of their biological variability or the range of environments in which they live.*
>
> *(National Research Council and Institute of Medicine, 2000)*

Finally, it should be noted that these intervention principles place the parent center stage in the therapeutic process. Although the clinician or educator will guide, coach, and/or counsel the parent, the view that the parent becomes the primary interactant during intervention is foundational to this thinking. Parents will naturally wonder why their child is using atypical forms and understandably be uncomfortable with the idiosyncrasy of these utterances. In order for the language acquisition process to maintain the joyfulness that typically developing children and their caregivers experience, the parents of children who use gestalt forms will need support to understand why we are honoring and valuing the scripts despite their unconventionality. In this regard, intervention with children who use alternative forms of language must embrace the child's caregivers robustly and sensitively during therapeutic interactions.

How can we view scripting from a conversational analysis perspective?

The second paradigm considered here is a conversational analysis perspective, which leads to a rich and complex understanding of how children with autism use language to communicate, interact, and experience others (Sterponi et al., 2015).

> *Conversation Analysis examines language in the natural communicative context of social interaction, showing how sentences are never isolated, self-contained entities that merely describe states of affairs in the world.*
>
> *Sterponi et al. (2015, p. 517)*

In this view, all conversational turns are seen as the coconstruction of an interaction between speakers. Researchers coming from this perspective have examined the effect of communicative context and the contribution of the partner's language on the communicative performance of children with autism. As with the developmental language perspective presented above, when scripting is thought of from the viewpoint of conversation, interaction, and communicative partners, clinicians are provided with a much more positive starting point for addressing the use of gestalt forms, a welcomed alternative to the view that these forms are automatic and noncommunicative. As Sterponi et al. (2015) suggest,

> *This view urges us to consider even those utterances that appear most self-directed, or free from content relevant to the immediate interaction, as potentially having social or affective import for the child. Such utterances, therefore, may be potentially important resources upon which the child can draw to facilitate her being-in-the-world and with others (p. 524).*

In this same vein, Hobson, Hobson, and García-Pérez's (2012) analysis of verbal exchanges between individuals with autism and adult conversational partners, led the authors to introduce the concept of *dialogic resonance*. Dialogic resonance refers to conversation patterns where one of the participants in the interaction selectively reproduces segments of language structure of another participant in a previous discourse. In this, we have a description of a discourse pattern and strategy, which is often seen in children on the autism spectrum and shifts the lens from disorder to difference.

The link to intervention is again a direct one and can be put into practice in two ways. First, ignoring or suppressing the child's attempt to be in the world with others would be counterproductive to all we are trying to encourage in children who are less interpersonally engaged. Contrast the child who is nonverbal with the child who primarily uses gestalt forms and we can immediately appreciate the portal that echolalia and scripts provide the child and the adult. Secondly, if the conversational partner not only acknowledges the child's linguistic contributions but also provides the child with language that is more easily understood and responded to (following analysis of the discourse patterns of the particular child), the nature of the interaction can be more balanced and authentic. The very act of participating in conversational exchanges may be one of the most important experiences for the child relative to his social, emotional, cognitive, language, and communicative development.

To review, the previous discussion has been grounded in the idea of how researchers and clinicians evaluate children's use of gestalt forms, specifically scripting. A developmental language perspective and conversational analysis provide frameworks for positive views of unconventional forms of language. Taking this one step further, children whose language development is atypical should have the same affective opportunity to learn language in the context of loving, primary relationships, as do children who are typically developing. Their thoughts and feelings should be "heard" and responded to in an attempt to create an interaction between the caregiver and the child. Secondly, conversational analysis allows us to appreciate the integration of language, communication, and context at a much deeper level and to bring the analysis of language to the level of what is happening between speakers, even if one of the speakers is imitating part of the other's utterances, or using language heard in another context. When the parent is brought into the treatment in a vital way, many of the child's scripts can be traced back to their origins and disambiguated and understood. Thus, within the caregiver–child relationship, the connection between what the child means when he uses scripts can be made and the child's world can be entered. Finally, analysis of the child's comprehension and production of language allows us to determine an approximate stage of language development and tailor communicative interactions to that stage.

Case illustration

As mentioned above, the author, a speech-language therapist, has worked with a child who used scripts extensively when she met him at 4 years old. He is now a young man of 19. The longitudinal experience of following this child, who initially scripted more than he produced spontaneous novel language, has provided an opportunity to understand the role of scripts in a child's language acquisition. The following comments about Mark are anecdotal and qualitative, more of a story than a research report and are a brief summary of 15 years of intervention with the child (young man) and collaboration with his mother.

When I met Mark, he had been diagnosed on the autism spectrum. Mark's prelinguistic communication, including reciprocal interactions and interpersonal communication were at a pre-12-month level, suggesting significant socioemotional and early pragmatic challenges. Table 26.1 illustrates Mark's constrictions in nonlinguistic and linguistic forms of communication. Both his understanding of gestures, facial expressions, and body language and his use of these forms were restricted. His language production was at about a 24-month level, although a great deal of what he said included the use of scripts from movies, books, and songs. Production exceeded comprehension, which is not unusual for children on the spectrum (primarily because of their use of gestalt forms), but quite unusual for typically developing children. Mark's speech, specifically articulation, was age appropriate.

In terms of communicative intentions, Mark expressed requests for actions and objects as well as protests, often with conventional forms. Other functions of

Table 26.1 Mark's language and communication profile (4–6 years).

Communicative intentions	Comprehension	Production
1. **Nonlinguistic communication** • Gesture/ • Facial expression/ • Body language	Constricted	Constricted
2. **Linguistic communication** • Novel word combinations • "Scripted" utterances[a]	Constricted	Frequent[a]

[a]Scripted utterances account for the frequent linguistic communication.

language such as labels, comments, and requests for information were either infrequent or expressed with unconventional forms.

Based on the strengths and challenges of Mark's language and communication, it was clear that Mark's challenges in joint attention were significantly impacting his growth in many areas of development. The capacity for joint attention has been associated with social relationships, symbolic play abilities, and language development (Kasari, Freeman, & Paparella, 2006). Therefore facilitating joint attention was considered the first and most important intervention goal during the first phase of Mark's intervention.

Joint attention is often described relative to initiating and responding. When initiating joint attention, a baby uses gestures and eye contact to direct the adult's attention to objects, events, and themselves. Responding to joint attention refers to infants' ability to follow the direction of the gaze and gestures of the caregivers in order to share a common point of reference. Joint attention is a hallmark capacity which emerges early in life and leads to interpersonal interactions, intersubjectivity, and eventually proto-conversations between caregiver and child. From this capacity, the ability to understand and produce language is spawned.

From an intervention perspective, following into the scripts that Mark used was the key to promoting joint attention. Many studies have shown that responsive parental behaviors, for example, where the adult follows the child's focus of attention and activity, lead to positive results relative to language as well as other areas of development (Green et al., 2017; Pickles et al., 2016; Siller, Hutman, & Sigman, 2013). The question of how to facilitate joint attention for children who seem self-absorbed and repetitive in their use of scripts is often a dilemma. When Mark produced scripts from the *Finding Nemo* movie, for example, his mother and/or the clinician repeated lines that he was saying with exaggerated affect and eventually, took roles in the "story." Within this context, Mark looked at the clinician or his mother and began to talk *to* them rather than to no one in particular. In reference to the language acquisition principles mentioned above, Mom and the clinician followed the *contents of Mark's mind*, joining his play theme or script contingently. Intermittently, the communication partners modeled early language forms and meanings for the scripts that Mark was using, but that he may not have understood. For example, when Mark said, "take a deep breath … don't be scared," during the dentist scene, the clinician might say, "uh oh this is going to hurt." Tracking Mark's progression in engagement, interaction, communication, and language reinforced the benefits of joining his scripts relative to promoting the essential ability of joint attention including:

- Creating opportunities for moments of shared attention, affective engagement, reciprocity, shared intentions, shared meanings and more extended moments of interaction, that is, the capacities that set the stage for the comprehension and production of language.
- Creating opportunities for expanding schemas and symbolic representation—"where's the tree?" "who's the monster?"—that is, the nature of language capacity.
- Creating opportunities for the awareness of and expansion of affective themes—"we're scared," that is, the origins of interpersonal dimensions of language.
- Providing "meaningful" contexts for the comprehension and production of language, that is, the milieu for language acquisition.
- Providing opportunities for the child to experience another person's attention to his interests.

At the same time that Mark was receiving therapy oriented in this way, his mother was given advice about his scripting from other professionals with other perspectives. This advice, which she rejected, included explanations such as, scripting was Mark's way of regulating himself, it was a self-stimulatory behavior, and it was meaningless. Based on these interpretations, the recommendation was to discourage and ignore Mark's use of these forms of language. This perspective did not resonate with Mark's mom. She felt more comfortable honoring and enjoying Mark's "talking," rather than ignoring or discouraging it. Interestingly, Mark's father agreed that ignoring and even reprimanding Mark might be the best response to his scripting, as he worried that joining the scripts would increase the frequency with which they were used.

It should be noted that there were times when Mark's scripting did increase. This was interpreted positively as his attempt to be more communicative and join the world of language users. Due to his very significant challenges in language, our understanding was that scripts were his lifeline, especially as increased scripting led to increased interpersonal communication. One could even say that Mark had found a very promising compensating strategy to participate in conversation.

When Mark was between 7 and 9 years of age, important signs of progress could be noted (see Table 26.2). For example, Mark began to both understand and frequently use nonlinguistic communication. His comprehension and production of early stages of language had evolved. His continuing use of scripts signaled his continuing challenges in the comprehension of language and the importance of targeting this area in intervention rather than the production of language. His ability to participate in conversation, either as a listener or a speaker, was constricted.

In terms of language intervention goals, joining and honoring the scripts continued to be a priority. More focused language goals were added such as introducing early vocabulary, typical of preschool development and modeling simple sentences coding early semantic relations such as action (*open this*), location (*it's in the box*), and state (*I want two*). By doing this, the therapist narrowed the world of language input and looked for opportunities to model a small core of words and utterances. This was done in natural play contexts to assure comprehension. Finally, the comprehension of early-occurring

Table 26.2 Mark's language and communication profile (7–9 years).

file	Comprehension	Production
1. **Nonlinguistic communication** • Gesture/ • Facial expression/ • Body language	Emerging	Frequent
2. **Linguistic communication** • Sentences • "Scripted" utterances	Frequent	Frequent
3. **Conversation**	Constricted	Constricted

Wh- question words—who, what, where—was addressed in therapy at salient moments in the play context. For example, when Mark was playing with a butterfly cage, the clinician would ask, "Where's the yellow one?" to which Mom would model/respond with language and a gesture, "there it is!"

As Mark's therapy progressed, it became clear that there were developmental benefits to responding to his use of scripts in a positive and productive way. In order to move semantic-syntactic language learning ahead at the same time that the scripts were supported, the following strategies were used to facilitate the comprehension and production of language:

- Reduce the complexity of the language input—maintain the "grammar" of the language, the melody, and the interactive flow of communication.
- Embed comprehension work in contexts that are familiar to the child relative to schemas and that are affectively potent.
- Pair language with the child's actions, providing contextual support, that is, where these phrases naturally occur in a play context.
- Present targeted language in many familiar contexts to promote the generativity of learning language forms

As noted above, the opportunity to follow Mark's development of language in the context of supporting his use of scripts led to insights about the place of scripts (and echolalia) in a child's long-term language acquisition. Many of the hypotheses that we began with, such as the developmental value of joining scripts, were confirmed. To conclude this section on Mark, we offer the foundational principles about scripting that a parent, speech-language therapist, or educator might consider when working with children whose use of these forms is frequent or minimal. These include:

- Scripting is a reflection of a significant language disorder and therefore is best approached from the perspective of language challenges, rather than as inappropriate behavior.
- Scripting may be unconventional but it does reflect the contents of the child's mind, that is, the foundations of language.
- Scripts have meaning and intention, although without an informant it is difficult to make these connections.
- Increases in the amount of scripting may actually represent the child's expansion of ideas, representation, and/or communicative attempts.
- Even when the child develops the capacity to generate novel language, scripting may continue to be used.
- The form of scripting changes over time, as do the interpersonal functions.
- The first goal for the clinician is to make the child's use of scripts interpersonal—assuring joint attention, reciprocity, and protoconversation.
- Joining the scripts is a way to promote the child's sense of himself as a communicator, as a person who is making meaning, and as a partner in an interaction.
- All of the child's communicative partners should come to a consensus about how to address the child's use of scripts as it often represents the child's best available entrée into language.

Behavioral and emotional challenges

Often, children on the autism spectrum are described as having a range of behavioral and/or emotional problems. The list below from the ASHA (asha.org) website is typical:

- anxiety and social withdrawal
- using early-developing and/or idiosyncratic strategies for self-regulation (e.g., chewing on clothing, rocking, hand flapping, vocal play)
- using unconventional behavioral strategies and emotional expressions (e.g., aggression, tantrums, bolting from situations)
- restricted, repetitive patterns of behavior, interests, or activities
- problems with self-management
- problems dealing with changes in routine and/or changing from one activity to the next

These behavioral or emotional problems are typically attributed to sensory and regulatory challenges. From the perspective presented here, the impact of language and communication challenges on the emotional life and growth of the child, on his very personhood, is seen as foundational. There seems to be no question that challenges in understanding and producing language affect the inner life of the child, which is obviously a part of every human child's make-up regardless of developmental differences.

Reviewing the list above with an eye to how these behaviors (self-regulation, anxiety, changes in routines) are typically processed and managed with the use of language makes a strong case for the connection between language disorders and behavioral and emotional restrictions. More specifically, it has been found that children with pragmatic impairments, which as noted above is a common challenge for children with ASD, are more likely to have behavioral problems than children with other types of language disorders (Ketelaars, Cuperus, Jansonius, & Verhoveven, 2010).

As Foley (2006) suggests, language along with other symbolic developments underlie many key aspects of developmental progression. For example, advancements in symbolic ability allow children to solve problems through mental combinations, to gain access to peer relationships, to gain greater independence and connectedness, to form relationships with caregivers, and to access imagination and pretend play. In discussing the powerful role of symbolic ability in the child's life, Foley (2006) suggests that the child's ability to problem solve, communicate affectively, and engage in pretend play provides him with the means to process his inner life and the external world of relationships and reality. When symbolic capacities are compromised, emotional and behavioral problems may be inevitable.

The enormous role of language in all of the domains of child development, leads us to wonder what the behavioral and emotional outcomes would be if there were greater acceptance of the child's unconventional language patterns. If all of the child's nonlinguistic and linguistic communication was first and foremost seen as a reflection of his mind and heart, the child's expression of his needs, struggles, concerns, and worries would be acknowledged and responded to. Alternatively, if these unconventional channels of expression are ignored, the emergence of emotional and behavioral problems seems inevitable.

Conclusion

The previous discussion is in sync with the contemporary science of language and communication development. The mandate derived from these theories and paradigms is to reconsider the communication deficits of children on the autism spectrum through a new lens (Kliffer & Salt, 2014). Although studies from a number of disciplines have moved in this direction, the intervention provided by educators and clinicians often reflects outdated ways of thinking about the unconventional forms used by children on the autism spectrum. It is the author's hope that future discussions and interventions will embrace the thinking presented here, and elsewhere, turning toward a positive interpretation of a child's use of scripts. We can then look forward to both research and clinical studies that explore the impact of using developmental language models and conversational analysis on the child's progress in language, communication, and personhood.

References

American Speech-Language-Hearing Association (ASHA). ASHA.org. Autism.

Bates, E., Benigni, L., Bretherton, I., Camaioni, L., & Volterra, V. (1979). *The emergence of symbols: Cognition and communication in infancy*. New York: Academic Press.

Blanc, M. (2012). *Natural language acquisition on the autism spectrum: The journey from echolalia to self-generated language*. Communication Development Center.

Bloom, L., & Tinker, E. (2001). The intentionality model and language acquisition. *Monographs of the Society for Research in Child Development*, *66*(4), Serial No. 267.

Foley, G. (2006). Self and social-emotional development in infancy: A descriptive synthesis. In G. M. Foley, & J. D. Hochman (Eds.), *Mental health in early intervention* (pp. 139–173). Baltimore, MD: Brookes Publishing.

Gerber, S. (2003). A developmental perspective on language assessment and intervention for children on the autistic spectrum. *Topics in Language Disorders*, *23*, 74–95.

Gerber, S. (in press). An introduction to the DIR® model (developmental individual-difference relationship based) and its application to children with autism spectrum. In P. Prelock & R. Mac McCauley (Eds.), *Treatment of autism spectrum disorders: Evidence-based intervention strategies for communication and social interaction*. Baltimore, MD: Brookes Publishing.

Gerber, S., & Prizant, B. (2001). *A developmental approach to assessment and intervention with speech and language challenges. Clinical practice guidelines: Redefining the standards of care for infants, children and families with special needs* (pp. 85–122). Bethesda, MD: ICDL Press.

Green, A., Pickles, A., Paco, R., Bedford, R., Wan, M., Elsabbagh, M., ... Johnson, M. (2017). Randomised trial of a parent- mediated intervention for infants at high risk for autism: longitudinal outcomes to age 3 years. *Journal of Child Psychology and Psychiatry*, *8*(12), 1330–1340.

Hobson, P. R., Hobson, J. A., García-Pérez, R., et al. (2012). Dialogic linkage and resonance in autism. *Journal of Autism and Developmental Disorders*, *42*, 2718–2728.

Kasari, C., Freeman, S., & Paparella, T. (2006). Joint attention and symbolic play in young children with autism: A randomized controlled intervention study. *Journal of Child Psychology and Psychiatry*, *47*(6), 611–620.

Ketelaars, M., Cuperus, J., Jansonius, K., & Verhoveven, L. (2010). Pragmatic language impairment and associated behavioural problems. *International Journal of Language & Communication Disorders*, *45*, 203–214.

Kliffer, M., & Salt, M. (2014). *Pragmatics and autism spectrum disorders: A preliminary review*. <www.lacus.org/volumes/39>.

Lahey, M. (1988). *Language disorders and language development*. Wiley.

National Research Council and Institute of Medicine. (2000). *From neurons to neighborhoods: The science of early childhood development*. Washington, DC: National Academy Press.

National Scientific Council on the Developing Child. (2020). *Connecting the brain to the rest of the body: Early child-hood development and lifelong health are deeply intertwined*. Working Paper No. 15. Retrieved from <www.developingchild.harvard.edu>.

Parsons, L., Cordier, R., Munro, N., Joosten, A., & Speyer, R. (2017). A systematic review of pragmatic language interventions for children with autism spectrum disorder. *PLoS One*, *12*(4), e0172242. Available from https://doi.org/10.1371/journal.pone.0172242.

Pickles, A., Couteur, A., Leadbitter, K., Salomone, E., Cole-Fletcher, R., Tobin, H., ... Green, J. (2016). Parent-mediated social communication therapy for young children with autism (PACT): Long-term follow-up of a randomised controlled trial. *Lancet*, *388*, 2501–2509.

Prizant, B. M., & Duchan, J. F. (1981). The functions of immediate echolalia in autistic children. *Journal of Speech and Hearing Disorders*, *46*, 241–249.

Prizant, B. M., & Rydell, P. J. (1984). An analysis of the functions of delayed echolalia in autistic children. *Journal of Speech and Hearing Research*, *27*, 183–192.

Siller, M., Hutman, T., & Sigman, M. (2013). A parent-mediated intervention to increase responsive parental behaviors and child communication in children with ASD: A randomized clinical trial. *Journal of Autism and Developmental Disorders*, *43*(3), 540–555.

Singletary, W. M. (2015). An integrative model of autism spectrum disorder: ASD as a neurobiological disorder of experienced environmental deprivation, early life stress and allostatic overload. *Neuropsychoanalysis*, *7*(2), 1–101.

Sterponi, S., de Kirby, K., & Shankey, J. (2015). Rethinking language in autism. *Autism*, *10* (5), 517–526.

Stiegler, L. N. (2015). Examining the echolalia literature: Where do speech-language pathologists stand? *American Journal of Speech-Language Pathology*, *24*(4), 750–762.

Surian, L., Baron-Cohen, S., & Van der Lely, H. (1996). Are children with autism deaf to Gricean maxims? *Cognitive Neuropsychiatry*, *1*(1), 55–71.

Suskind, R. (2014a). *Reaching my autistic child through Disney*. New York Times. <http://www.nytimes.com/2014/03/09/magazine/reaching-my-autistic-sonthroughdisney.htm>.

Suskind, R. (2014b). *Life, animated: A story of sidekicks, heroes, and autism*. Glendale, CA: Kingswell.

Tager-Flusberg, H., & Anderson, M. (1991). The development of contingent discourse ability in autistic children. *Journal of Child Psychology and Psychiatry*, *32*, 1123–1134.

Further reading

Bates, E. (1976). *Language and context: The acquisition of pragmatics*. San Diego, CA: Academic Press.

Prizant, B. (1982). Gestalt language and gestalt processing in autism. *Topics in Language Disorders*, *3*, 16–23.

Transformed by the journey: building community with diverse fathers of people with autism

27

Michael D. Hannon[1] *and Robert A. Naseef*[2]
[1]Department of Counseling, Montclair State University, Montclair, NJ, United States,
[2]Alternative Choices, Philadelphia, PA, United States

Group counseling in all forms has been found to be effective in supporting peoples' mental health and wellness (Edwards & Ray, 2010; Perusse, Goodnough, & Lee, 2009). Corey, Corey, and Corey (2014) identified three general types of counseling groups: psychoeducational groups, counseling groups, and psychotherapy groups, each with its own purpose and usually distinguished by the level of support provided by the people facilitating the groups. Psychoeducational groups function primarily to assist group members in learning about a particular topic or further developing a skill, and can present in ways that are largely instructional (e.g., parenting skills). Counseling groups function to help members address normative challenges (e.g., grief) but also have a distinct focus on interpersonal processes of the group experience. That is, the group facilitators leverage their knowledge of a particular topic and use members' experiences in the group as a learning and/or therapeutic tool. Psychotherapy groups are those created to treat or remediate members' mental health challenges. People might join psychotherapy groups for treatment for addiction, depressive, or eating disorders. Additionally, psychotherapy group facilitators often draw on the tenets of other types of groups (i.e., counseling, psychoeducational) in ways to support members.

Yalom (1995) offered 12 therapeutic factors that influence positive outcomes for group counseling participants. They are: (1) universality, (2) instillation of hope, (3) facilitating interpersonal learning, (4) fostering group cohesion, (5) impartation of information, (6) helping through altruism, (7) corrective recapitulation (i.e., family reenactment), (8) socializing techniques, (9) imitative behavior, (10) catharsis, (11) self-understanding, and (12) existential factors. These factors can function to assist members in a variety of groups and have been documented to be useful in groups for parents of people with autism, which includes fathers (Ananpatiwet & Blauw, 2016; Dudziak, 1986; Lodder, Papadopoulos, & Randhawa, 2019). What follows is a brief review of literature about the effectiveness of group counseling for parents of people with autism, with special attention given to groups for fathers. We will also provide an account of our experiences and insights starting and facilitating an open, counseling (i.e., process) diverse group for fathers of people with autism. Finally, we will offer considerations for agencies and professionals seeking to facilitate groups for fathers of people with autism.

Emerging Programs for Autism Spectrum Disorder. DOI: https://doi.org/10.1016/B978-0-323-85031-5.00027-X

Groups for parents of individuals with autism

The experiences of parents of individuals with autism has been and continues to be widely reported in a variety of outlets including refereed journals, magazine articles, newsletters, and books. A large share of portion of this content, particularly in refereed journals, documents the parents' reports of daily stressors of parenting children with autism (Gong et al., 2015; Haya & Haris, 2018; Hartley & Schultz, 2015; Reed, Sejunaite, & Osborne, 2016; Rivard, Terroux, Parent-boursier, & Mercier, 2014; Yusuf et al., 2019), stress from being stigmatized (Gray, 2002, 2003; Lodder et al., 2019), and the consequential stress on couple/marital relationship between the parents (Allen, Bowles, & Weber, 2013; Aylaz, Yilmaz, & Polat, 2012; Fisman, Wolf, & Noh, 1989; Lavee, Sharlin, & Katz, 1996).

Given the documented challenges for parents of individuals with autism in a variety of contexts (e.g., community, school, family), group counseling has been one intervention used to connect with and provide support to parents of individuals with autism. Dudziak (1982) suggested psychiatric nurses could provide counseling support—via psychoeducational and process groups—to support mothers of children with autism. Ananpatiwet and Blauw (2016) found that a parent training program based on positive psychology to promote parent happiness among parents of individuals with autism in Thai was effective in supporting those parents experiencing hardships based on their children's diagnoses. Acknowledging parents of individuals with autism can internalize stigmatizing experiences, Lodder et al. (2019) are testing the feasibility and influence of a stigma support intervention, Stigma of Living as an Autism Carer (SOLACE), for parents and caregivers in the hope of reducing the internalized stigma among parents of individuals with autism. Finally, Lilly and Tungol (2015) tested the effectiveness of mindfulness-based psychoeducational program for mothers of individuals with autism, which were found to significantly reduce their stress compared to the study's control group.

These aforementioned studies are a fraction of the important research being done to understand how group counseling in all of its forms can help parents of individuals with autism. However, there is scant information about how group counseling can specifically support fathers of individuals with autism. What follows is an overview of how research informs the utility of groups for such fathers.

Groups for fathers of individuals with autism

Unfortunately, the experiences of fathers of individuals with autism are understudied and underrepresented in refereed journals, resulting in their needs frequently being misunderstood.

Some research that does exist informs that these fathers respond to their children's needs differently than mothers (Davis & Carter, 2008; Gray, 2003; Pottie & Ingram, 2008) and have concerns about their children's social and developmental trajectory (Seligman & Darling, 2007). Also, some research suggests that these fathers experience a unique orientation and adjustment phase to their children's needs (Hannon & Hannon, 2017; Hannon, Blanchard, & Storlie, 2019; Naseef, 2001, 2013). Past research also informs that securing effective and comprehensive therapeutic services for their children can be a predictor of their parents' healthy adjustment to their unique needs (Garcia-Lopez, Sarria, Pozo, & Recio, 2016). These considerations—among many others—help illustrate fathers' sources of concern for themselves and their children. They also illustrate focal points for potential group counseling support.

Elfert and Mirenda (2015) reported the impact of a support group for fathers of children with autism to compare pre- and postintervention measures of depression, marital adjustment, parenting stress, optimism, among others. While the results indicated no significant changes on most measures, the fathers strongly endorsed the utility of the support group. Others have also advocated for the use of groups for fathers of individuals with autism. Black and Latinx fathers of students with autism in Hannon, Johnson, Christian, and Hannon's (2017) study recommended schools finding ways to connect fathers of children of varying special educational needs as a way to support each other and engage with the school community. Hannon (2017) also advocated for the value of school-based family counseling support for Black fathers of students with autism.

Acknowledging the general value of group counseling for racially, ethnically, and spiritually diverse fathers of individuals with autism, we have been fortunate to cofacilitate an open, process/personal growth group for this population in our region. What follows is an account of the formation and facilitator reflections of our time running the group beginning fall 2019 through summer 2020.

A.J. Drexel Autism Institute dads' group

At a social get-together attended by Robert Naseef, the idea of a fathers' support group came up, and the possibility that it could be hosted by the A.J. Drexel Autism Institute was proposed. This affiliation seemed ideal according to its mission statement. It reads,

The A.J. Drexel Autism Institute is the first research organization built around a public health science approach to understanding and addressing the challenges of autism spectrum disorders. The Autism Institute's mission is to *discover*, *develop*, *promote*, and *disseminate* population-level and community-based approaches that will prevent autism-associated morbidity and disability and improve the quality of life for individuals with autism of all ages (A.J. Drexel Autism Institute, n.d.).

We are both mental health professionals (i.e., professional counselor, clinical psychologist) and fathers of individuals with autism and have been acquainted for several years. We participated together at conferences and webinars focused on fatherhood. So after speaking together, we decided to pursue the opportunity. With the Drexel sponsorship, it would be possible to engage the interracial and interfaith diversity of the autism community in the Philadelphia metropolitan region, minimally including portions of Pennsylvania, New Jersey, Delaware, and perhaps beyond. After meeting with the Center's social worker and social media director, a flyer was developed to publicize the group. The flyer included head shots of the facilitators, brief biographies of their professional and personal experiences, as well as monthly meeting dates on Saturdays, from 10:00 to 11:30 a.m. beginning in September 2019.

The flyer announcing the group was posted on the Center's social media as well as our social media accounts. Over 40 men registered for the first meeting fulfilling —and perhaps exceeding—our expectations. A tentative agenda with structured activities was prepared to accommodate those who would attend. Sixteen men, including us (cofacilitators), showed up. Our structured plan was not what the guys wanted or needed. After our brief opening including our lived experience as fathers raising children on the spectrum, the group spent the rest of our time together sharing our respective stories. When the meeting concluded, we met and concluded that this group would not be primarily psychoeducational. Instead, what had just unfolded reflected more of a personal growth group where the members intentionally seek support from one another to be better men and fathers and have a willingness to openly process what is happening in the room and with themselves in real time. We were truly excited to have begun this group's journey.

Our October meeting was smaller, but very engaging. Using an icebreaker, connections formed while we shared photos of ourselves and our families on our cell phones. The first man who shared brought up anger regarding his son's educational program. This opened a broad discussion about anger and strategies to deal with it as men raising children with autism (e.g., challenges of autism symptoms, living an experience that wasn't expected, wanting to hear expressions of love from their children, etc.). A more nuanced vocabulary was developed using descriptors such as frustrated, hurt, or slighted with more specificity. Guys were also encouraged to share the victories they or their children are experiencing, and this moved the group from focusing on deficits to focusing on strengths.

News of our group reached the national organization, Autism Speaks, headquartered in New York City and on October 24, we spoke to Felipe Maya of Autism Speaks about their experiences as fathers and our role—and privilege—of supporting other fathers raising autistic children. The podcast is available at: http://bit.ly/AutismSpeaksDadsPodcast. Our November meeting included 10 men, several of whom were unable to attend the October meeting. Mixed feelings of loving but not always liking our children on the spectrum emerged and this acknowledged lived experiences that were deeper and more nuanced. Much of the day's content was about reconciling not liking our children at times. The guys were encouraged to realize that we can both love and not like our kids. We also acknowledged the need to "learn our kids' language" and to appreciate how our children's senses are different and sometimes better than our own. This comes out when they can sense anger, tension, and conflict. We frequently used the terms, "good" and "bad" energy. There was a lot of hope expressed in the session along with a deep sense of relief in not being alone with uncomfortable mixed feelings. We began the practice of asking each man to share a brief "take away" from our time together.

In December, we met as facilitators with the Drexel team to begin planning for the spring. We agreed to start using GroupMe, a mobile group messaging app, for the fathers' group members to exchange texts, photos, and videos between our meetings to share experiences and resources. We also began thinking about a special event for Autism Awareness and Acceptance Month in April. When we met on December 21, our session explored our children's holiday challenges and how it can be frustrating for family members and friends who don't understand that children on the autism spectrum may not respond to gift giving and exchanges in ways that neurotypical people expect. As a coping strategy, preparation was suggested for what may feel like rejection or just a minimal or muted reaction. There was conversation about how we are always learning about ourselves and our children. As facilitators, we led by sharing personal examples. Many of the guys—with kids of various ages—shared similar sentiments. We ended our last meeting of the year by reflecting on what we've learned as a result of being in the group. Many talked about learning about themselves and the value of connecting with each other.

We've learned we have a shared experience and identity and this experience has made us better men, fathers, partners, and people.

In January, our Drexel planning team met prior to the group to discuss ideas for our program in April for Autism Awareness and Acceptance. We settled on a theme for the program "Transformed by the journey: Fathering individuals on the autism spectrum." This theme represented our lived experiences and the group's development. Our plan was to offer the men in the group the opportunity to weigh in on the theme and give them a sense of the overall vision of the program. Family members and professionals in the autism community would be invited to a panel discussion that would include food and childcare. Several new guys came to the meeting which occurred on Martin Luther King, Jr. weekend. A pattern has emerged of four to five fathers who attend regularly, and others come for the first time, which is typical for a drop-in group. The new guys were vocal and immediately engaged. There was an awkward moment when one dad was introducing himself and being really long-winded; everyone there noticed. At one point, one of us simply asked, "So what are you looking forward to while you're here?" The man clearly said, "To see what I don't normally see."

Notions of racial justice were an integral part of the meeting. Guys talked about being even more sensitized to injustice based on their children's ability status. The added layer of vulnerability for children of color on the autism spectrum was acknowledged in terms of the difficulty getting an accurate diagnosis and access to the appropriate services. This discussion really enriched our group's time together and having it in the container of our multiracial, multiracial group was extremely encouraging.

In our February meeting, about 16 men attended, returning and new, who engaged readily with the process that had become typical for the group focusing on ourselves as men, fathers, and partners. Overall, the group has evolved into a life and process of its own, with guys coming and leaving in small groups. New guys were invited to briefly introduce themselves, and then returning guys would do so when they shared for the first time. A father, from a previous group who is on the spectrum himself, came for the first time. When he shared his perspective of fathering twins on the spectrum, two more fathers identified as being on the spectrum. This was a welcome new aspect of diversity; we were running a group for fathers of people with autism that included fathers with autism. It was exciting and bittersweet simultaneously. We were a bit discouraged that there were only three men of color including one of us. We talked about shame and pride and how ashamed we are to admit that we are sometimes embarrassed in public when people stare at our children.

There was a memorable moment when some of the dads were talking about the value of their children using contextually appropriate but profane language, citing the example of one of the children saying, "Fuck off!" While we want our children to be happy and fulfilled, their safety has to be realized first. Some Black and Brown people with autism aren't safe when they use profanity toward authority figures. In retrospect, as facilitators we agreed that we should have stayed with this moment a bit longer than we did. In addition, the intersectionality that we are aspiring to for the group will continue to need intentional effort to keep fathers of color engaged. We acknowledged that white fathers and fathers of color are not used to sharing space. The classic book, *Why Are All the Black Kids Sitting Together in the Cafeteria*?: *And Other Conversations About Race*, was mentioned in the context of this issue.

By the time our March 21 meeting arrived, we were essentially in a lockdown due to the COVID-19 virus. We made the decision to meet as scheduled via Zoom. Only five guys were there including us. The session was rich with access to more context from the guys who were all participating from their homes. Guys were seen and heard responding to their children and other home dynamics. We spoke more than usual about the importance of acknowledging the limited control we have in general, and especially in times like these along with issues such as family stability, control, and health. The value of increased time with loved ones was contrasted with the challenges of balancing work and family in home locations with supporting their school-age children with online learning. The privilege of being able to work from home was also acknowledged for those able to do so. One man, an essential worker who repairs heating, ventilation, and air conditioning (HVAC) systems, shared how he has to go into homes with gloves and a mask while risking others and his family. Using faith as a springboard, one father discussed how his Islamic faith was an anchoring force for him in these times. Observing the other men appreciating this sentiment, the facilitators used this moment to weave their own spiritual traditions into the session as a tool to care for ourselves and others. Another man shared how many of his relatives think the pandemic is a hoax and how frustrating that is for his immediate family. We also considered more frequent meetings during the crisis for the rest of the academic year along with the possibility of meeting over the summer which was not in our original plan.

During our April meeting, six of us attended. We agreed to host the meeting for 1 hour versus 90 minutes in response to the demand of being online for an extended period of time.

Their general mood and disposition, appearance, and general comradery between them continued to be very positive. All men participated equally sharing reflections on their own mental health/wellness, their families' level of functioning, reports of good and challenging news, and other accounts of being primarily homebound with their families for the past month. One man shared how life in his house was becoming more tense, especially for him. Another father talked about the pandemic as a "life changing experience" and wanting to be an example to others.

There was a deep sense of loss over the life we had regarded as normal. There were feelings of being cheated of experiences because of the pandemic (e.g., children's promotion activities, graduations, etc.), and expressions of grief due to the loss of some freedoms and privileges. In terms of acceptance, it was now described as a moving target. We discussed trying to pay attention to what is going right in our lives, adjusting expectations, and doing everything we can to make a difference while balancing perspectives. We agreed that we feel the safest when we are home with our families, and we resolved to take it easy and be kind to ourselves, especially when feeling inadequate to the enormous challenges of living through the pandemic. We also agreed to meet in two weeks.

Our May 2 meeting included five of us in the third virtual meeting which continued to be smaller but no less profound in terms of the support expressed and offered to each other. The men shared reflections on topics about their self-care strategies and how they wanted to honor the mothers in their lives as we looked forward to Mothers' Day. Reflecting the open nature of the group, it should be mentioned that all of the participants were first-time Zoom attendees, although two of the three have attended in person groups. The men shared their own plans for Mothers' Day which included typical gifts (e.g., flowers) and more elaborate gifts developed by the fathers and their children (e.g., videos/iMovies). Another father described great rewarding moments while doing schoolwork with his son because he had no idea his son could do so much.

At the tenth group meeting on May 16, 2020, a total of 12 fathers attended virtually.

Three men were first-time attendees. The men reintroduced themselves and their children to each other in order to be inclusive of the first-time participants. The group further discussed some of the unique challenges their children are having as a result of the pandemic, particularly restricted diets/palates and sensory issues with masks. Discussion about these two topics generated open and honest responses from the men. Several group members used the chat feature of the Zoom platform to exchange personal emails with the intention of communicating outside of the meeting times. There was a discussion of the stereotypical males' urge to fix that is especially counterproductive during the pandemic. One father, employed in a healthcare facility that includes patients with COVID-19, shared his fear for himself and his family. A man who had immigrated from the Middle East shared that he had experienced war, his parents' divorce, and two sons with autism. We shared openly about the group experience of hearing about the challenges and victories of coping through these especially challenging times. There was a sense expressed that it has been encouraging to have a sense of common struggle as opposed to the "Why me?" reaction. "The dialogue eases your heart," according to one man.

To promote our May 30 meeting, we sent this update to the email list and posted it on social media:

> *Our neurodiverse fathers' support group was going strong and meeting monthly until COVID-19 struck in March. While it would have been easy to stop meeting, we upped our commitment to supporting ourselves and each other. We have switched to virtual meetings using the Zoom platform and we are now meeting bi-weekly. We're happy to share that our reach now extends beyond the Philadelphia area for any fathers who want to connect.*
>
> *On Saturday, May 16th, we spent our time talking about challenges and victories brought on during the shutdown. Topics included helping our kids through sleep issues, managing meltdowns, and creative food ideas. It was encouraging to hear about common struggles and offer each other support.*

This meeting brought 13 of us together; four of whom were first-time attendees. The emotions expressed increased with honesty and raw intensity. The safety of the group allowed men to admit to anger, irritability, anxiety, depression, and increased alcohol consumption. One father shared that his resources for coping seemed spent. The men also talked briefly about the ongoing protests in cities across the world in response to lethal police violence against Black people. The stress of being locked in place, racialized violence, ensuing protests, and diverse family needs are intersecting for these men as they are for people and families across the world. These terrible times were reframed as an opportunity to be better men. We also had an international visitor from Toronto who remarked that "It never gets old to find that I'm not alone." We started to end each meeting with a minute of quiet reflection on what we are taking away for ourselves.

As we contemplated the times we are living in, we issued another special update giving context to our group inviting fathers to participate. On June 10, we shared via email and social media along with a screenshot of the most recent Zoom meeting:

> *Being part of the change, we want to see. Brought together by our love for children growing up on the autism spectrum, a diverse group of fathers has been meeting since September 2019 with the support of the A.J. Drexel Autism Center. Drs. Michael Hannon and Robert Naseef have facilitated drawing from a depth of lived and professional experience. It's generally rare, but so welcome and vital, to see people of color and white people sharing the same space for support. Our group has often discussed the disparities that children of color and their families face getting the ASD diagnosis as well as the vital intensive services necessary. Our last meeting via Zoom aired our honest, pent-up frustrations after over 10 weeks of quarantine. There was anger at the world, anxiety, depression, shorter responses to loved ones, more alcohol consumption, and all this as cities across the country burned with the flames of protest against racial injustice. Our virtual meetings are open to fathers everywhere to join in to listen and participate. Mark your calendars for Saturday, June 13 at 10:00 a.m. We are living through some horrible moments as "I can't breathe" echoes deep in our collective souls. Nonetheless in these moments, there are opportunities to be better men, fathers, partners,*

brothers, and friends. As we continue to be transformed by the journey of raising children on the spectrum, as a diverse group we have an opportunity to be a part of the change we want to see in the world.

Stay Safe and Peace brothers, Michael & Robert

On June 13, attendance maxed out at 14 fathers. It was a really diverse group with another international attendee from Kuwait. We also had attendees from South Florida and Chicago, as well. Again, we shared an update with our email and social media followers reminding them that our virtual meetings are growing and open to fathers everywhere to participate for our June 27 meeting. Participation was invited in the form of solely listening or actively contributing to our conversations. As we reported:

We stand at the intersection of celebration and sorrow. On one hand, summer has arrived. Summer represents—for many of us—an opportunity for reprieve and more engaged family time. We just celebrated Fathers' Day and we are so grateful! Many of our families and partners celebrated our contributions and support we provide our families. At the same time, the pandemic and systemic racism are not taking a vacation, so we invite you to join us to talk about how to support each other facing these realities. In the midst of these moments, as we ponder the dangers in sending our children back to school, there exist countless opportunities to step up and become better men, fathers, partners, brothers, and friends. We continue to be transformed by the journey of raising children on the spectrum, as we support each other in a multiracial, multiethnic, and multifaith group of fathers.

Our group has broached and acknowledged the disparities that children of color and their families face getting an ASD diagnosis as well as the vital intensive services necessary for our children's success and quality of life. In our last meeting via Zoom, we talked about how to explain the protests against systemic racism to our children. One father shared the difficulty in explaining the curfew in Philadelphia to his son. It's difficult. Another father, who is an immigrant, shared how his son with autism was told to go back where he came from even though he has only lived in the United States. This was clear evidence that racism is alive and well in our most intimate communities. As a group we shared our deeply seated fears about the added vulnerability dealing with the police and the criminal justice system that our children, especially children of color, live with every day. Our meetings give us time, space, and safety to help make sense of our world. We honor the men who have engaged with us so far, and we invite you (if applicable) and your father friends to engage with us in this historic time.

Stay Safe and Peace brothers, Michael & Robert

On June 27, our dads' group included 15 total attendees; two men were first-time attendees, and the group included men from our region and also Florida and Chicago. The session was spent sharing how the group has been valuable to them, given this was scheduled to be our last meeting. The men shared the value of universality, accountability, and how beneficial it is to be in a community. There was an expressed sense of being of service to each other, and some men reported being in touch with each other outside of the meetings. There was predictable discourse about challenges in their fathering experiences and also successes and funny anecdotes shared as well. We processed at points what it was like to seek help in this way even when the men were encouraged to participate in the group and found out about it through their wives or partners.

On July 11, our dads' group included 16 men. Five men were first-time attendees. This session focused on two main themes—relationship challenges with our children's mothers and return to school concerns. The men discussed, in several ways, how the pandemic has illuminated and/or caused relationship strain between parents. Some men who are already separated or divorced talked about the increased challenge of better communication. The men who had intact romantic partnerships discussed more frequent conflict and communication barriers. One father revealed a recent in-home separation and the ongoing commitment of both for their child. Several men also discussed their concerns about returning to school, citing safety fears. Some reported already taking steps to enroll in full-time cyber schools, and one father who is a teacher discussed considering taking leave time for the entire year given the spike in cases where he lives in Florida. It was significant and valuable for the men to experience enough safety to be vulnerable, especially about their relationships. The pandemic is inflicting different forms of pain and strain for individuals and families living with autism, causing the kind of serious symptoms that were shared today. One father, recently separated, reported how he was finding his way in the relationship with his 16-year-old by following his son's lead. While expressing gratitude is very important, it was noted that it doesn't always refill the emotional tank that is often empty during the pandemic.

On July 25, our group met with 17 men total. The men opened with reflections about the personal value of the group, given this would be the last meeting until August 29. Frequently occurring sentiments about universality and shared experience were expressed. The idea was expressed that there was great value in the range in age of the fathers' children on the spectrum. For fathers with school aged children, it was encouraging to hear to hear from fathers whose children were in their 30s and 40s. Since our conversation seemed very practical, the session wrapped up with encouragement for dads to share something vulnerable. In response, fathers expressed feelings of fear, disappointment, frustration with a range of things related to COVID, home instruction, and fear for their kids possibly going back to school. The men are especially grateful for a designated time and place where they can honestly share and demonstrate some vulnerability. The scars of racialized trauma which have become more widely open since the summer of police violence against Black people was also acknowledged. The White fathers of children of color have added their perspective to the conversation in recent meetings. There is also a building need for more directive and specific resources in addition to the now established space where they are processing their feelings and experiences. Some men commented on how their partners seemed to get resources quickly through the online communities they were a part of. This led to increased activity on the GroupMe app around toilet training and eating issues. Our Drexel team will be considering a more comprehensive set of resources for the men in the coming months.

Are you thinking about starting a fathers' group?: Our lessons learned

At the close of every group meeting, we encourage the fathers to share one take-away from the time we have spent together. The men respond to this prompt verbally, and in the case of our virtual meetings, some use the Zoom chat feature if they are not as inclined to raise their voices. In that spirit, we offer seven lessons we have learned—or been reminded—for individuals and agencies who might consider developing a group for fathers of individuals with autism.

First, prepare for the likelihood of a small group. There is a Biblical scripture that translated into English says, "Despise not small beginnings." We were excited to know that over 40 fathers registered for our group's first in-person meeting in September 2019. As with many groups, only a fraction of them actually attended. Further, attendance fluctuated greatly during the 10 months we ran the group. Sometimes only five people—including us—were there. We encourage you to be prepared for whoever attends; it is an acknowledgment from those who show up a desire to find community and seek support. Persist in your efforts and keep meeting with regularity.

Second, we are continually reminded that diversity in all of its forms is incredibly valuable. Racially, our group is primarily attended by white fathers. However, there is a critical mass of Black fathers who attend with some frequency, which helps. Ethnically, we are proud that we have fathers attending from Kuwait and Canada, attempts from a father in China and first- and second-generation American immigrant fathers of individuals with autism. We pride ourselves on sharing that our group is multiracial and multifaith, representing fathers who do not subscribe to a particular spiritual or religious tradition, those who identify as Christian, and those who identify as Muslim. And we are grateful to have fathers who are men living on the spectrum. This kind of diversity continues to inform us, challenge us, and deepen our empathy for each other and the world around us. We are sharing spaces that have not been well lit and attempting to shine a light for growth towards a just society where all are included.

Third, we want to remind facilitators to be prepared for engagement by the fathers to be very solution-focused. Novice and experienced mental and behavioral health professionals know that people—particularly men—seeking support are often driven by a desire to solve problems; this was very present in our fathers' group. Our fathers were very willing and eager to tell each other how to address and solve issues in ways that worked for them. Be prepared for this.

Fourth, and relatedly, we encourage facilitators to resist the impulse to be entirely solution-focused and stress the importance of processing the fathers' experiences and feelings in an effort to support their intrapersonal and interpersonal development. We were and will continue to be intentional about this aspect of our group. Modeling, when needed, and providing opportunities to express feelings like pride, guilt, despair, frustration, grief, victory, elation has been incredibly valuable. Our fifth recommendation is related to the third and fourth. It is to provide a mechanism for the fathers to connect outside of group meetings to give the kind solution-focused support they often seek. Using the GroupMe app has provided the fathers in our group the chance to share resources, recommendations, referrals, and celebrations beyond our monthly or biweekly meetings. We genuinely believe relationships have developed and deepened as a consequence of this step.

Our final two recommendations may seem intuitive but are worth explicitly sharing. We want to remind facilitators to regularly and intentionally monitor group dynamics while in session. Do your best to notice and acknowledge body language, fathers who are overly verbal and those who are not. And, with gentleness and confidence, acknowledge what is happening in the room in order to affirm to the fathers you are entirely engaged with them.

Finally, our seventh recommendation is to be courageous. Developing and running a group for fathers of individuals with autism is an endeavor wrought with risk and doubt from others. But, we know—based on what research says and our own experiences—that this kind of intervention for fathers is valuable, helpful, energizing, and most importantly, needed in the autism community.

References

Allen, K. A., Bowles, T. V., & Weber, L. L. (2013). Mothers' and fathers' stress associated with parenting a child with autism spectrum disorder. *Autism Insights*, *5*, 1–11. Available from https://doi.org/10.4137/AUI.S11094.

Ananpatiwet, S., & Blauw, J. N. (2016). The development and testing of a positive psychology-based program for increasing happiness among parents of children with autism spectrum disorder in Thailand. *Au Graduate School of Education Journal*, *8*(2), 106–121.

Aylaz, R., Yilmaz, U., & Polat, S. (2012). Effect of difficulties experienced by parents of autistic children on their sexual life: A qualitative study. *Sexuality and Disability*, *30*(4), 395–406. Available from https://doi.org/10.1007/s11195-011-9251-3.

Corey, M. S., Corey, G., & Corey, C. (2014). *Groups: Process and practice*. Belmont, CA: Brooks/Cole.

Davis, N. O., & Carter, A. S. (2008). Parenting stress in mothers and fathers of toddlers with autism spectrum disorders: Associations with child characteristics. *Journal of Autism and Developmental Disorders*, *38*(7), 1278–1291. Available from https://doi.org/10.1007/s10803-007-0512-z.

Dudziak, D. (1986). *Parenting the autistic child. Journal of Psychosocial Nursing and Mental Health Services*, *20*(1), 11–16.

Edwards, O. W., & Ray, S. L. (2010). Value of family and group counseling models where grandparents function as parents to their grandchildren. *International Journal for the Advancement of Counselling*, *32*, 178–190. Available from https://doi.org/10.1007/s10447-010-9098-9.

Elfert, M., & Mirenda, P. (2015). Evaluation of a support group for fathers of children with autism spectrum disorder. *Canadian Journal of Counselling and Psychotherapy*, *49*(2), 115–138. Available from https://cjc-rcc.ucalgary.ca/article/view/61054.

Fisman, S. N., Wolf, L. C., & Noh, S. (1989). Marital intimacy in parents of exceptional children. *Canadian Journal of Psychiatry*, *34*(6), 519–525. Available from https://doi.org/10.1177/070674378903400607.

Garcia-Lopez, C., Sarria, E., Pozo, P., & Recio, P. (2016). Supportive dyadic coping and psychological adaptaion in couples parenting children with autism spectrum disorder: The role of relationship satisfaction. *Journal of Autism and Developmental Disorders*, *46*, 3434–3447. Available from https://doi.org/10.1007/s10803-016-2883-5.

Gong, Y., Du, Y., Li, H., Zhang, X., An, U., & Wu, B. (2015). Parenting stress and affective symptoms in parents of autistic children. *Science China Life Sciences*, *58*, 1036–1043. Available from https://doi.org/10.1007/s11427-012-4293-z.

Gray, D. E. (2002). Everybody just freezes. Everybody is just embarrassed": Felt and enacted stigma among parents of children with high functioning autism. *Sociology of Health & Illness*, *24*(6), 734–749. Available from https://doi.org/10.1111/1467-9566.00316.

Gray, D. E. (2003). Gender and coping: The parents of children with high functioning autism. *Social Science and Medicine*, *56*(3), 631–642. Available from https://doi.org/10.1016/S0277-9536(02)00059-X.

Hannon, M. D. (2017). Black American fathers, their children with autism, and the utility of school-based family counseling: A narrative inquiry. *International Journal of School-Based Family Counseling*, *8*, 1–16. Retrieved from: <http://bit.ly/Hannon2017IJSBFC>.

Hannon, M. D., Blanchard, R., & Storlie, C. (2019). Microaggression experiences of fathers with children with autism spectrum disorder. *The Family Journal: Counseling and Therapy for Couples and Families*, *27*(2), 199–208. Available from https://doi.org/10.1177/1066480719832512.

Hannon, M. D., & Hannon, L. V. (2017). Father' orientation to their children's autism diagnosis: A grounded theory study. *Journal of Autism and Developmental Disorders*. Available from https://doi.org/10.1007/s10803-017-3149-6.

Hannon, M. D., Johnson, K. F., Christian, N. A., & Hannon, L. V. (2017). Black and Latino fathers of students with autism: Culturally responsive support. *Journal of School Counseling*, *15*(10). Retrieved from: <http://www.jsc.montana.edu/articles/v15n10.pdf>.

Hartley, S. L., & Schultz, H. M. (2015). Support needs of fathers and mothers of children and adolescents with autism spectrum disorder. *Journal of Autism and Developmental Disorders*, *45*(6), 1636–1648. Available from https://doi.org/10.1007/s10803-014-2318-0.

Haya, A. P. V., & Haris, F. (2018). Parental stress and coping strategies among parents of autistic children. *Indian Journal of Health and Wellbeing*, *9*(6), 841–844.

Lavee, Y., Sharlin, S., & Katz, R. (1996). The effect of parenting stress on marital quality: An integrated mother-father model. *Journal of Family Issues*, *17*(1), 114–124. Available from https://doi.org/10.1177/019251396017001007.

Lilly, J., & Tungol, J. R. (2015). Effectiveness of mindfulness based psycho-educational program on parental stress of selected mothers of children with autism. *Indian Journal of Positive Psychology*, *6*(1), 52–56.

Lodder, A., Papadopoulos, C., & Randhawa, G. (2019). Stigma of living as an autism carer: A brief psycho-social support intervention (SOLACE). study protocol for a randomised controlled feasibility study. *Pilot and Feasibility Studies*, *5*(34), 1–8. Available from https://doi.org/10.1186/s40814-019-0406-9.

Naseef, R. A. (2001). *Special children, challenged parents: The struggles and rewards of raising a child with a disability*. Baltimore, MD: Brookes Publishing.

Naseef, R. A. (2013). *Autism in the family: Caring and coping together*. Baltimore, MD: Brookes Publishing.

Perusse, R., Goodnough, G. E., & Lee, V. V. (2009). Group counseling in the schools. *Psychology in the Schools*, *46*(3), 225–231. Available from https://doi.org/10.1002/pits.20369.

Pottie, C. G., & Ingram, K. M. (2008). Daily stress, coping, and well-being in parents of children with autism: A multilevel modeling approach. *Journal of Family Psychology*, *22* (6), 855−864. Available from https://doi.org/10.1037/a0013604.

Reed, P., Sejunaite, K., & Osborne, L. A. (2016). Relationship between self-reported health and stress in mothers of children with autism spectrum disorders. *Journal of Autism and Developmental Disorders*, *46*(3), 934−941. Available from https://doi.org/10.1007/s10803-015-2638-8.

Rivard, M., Terroux, A., Parent-boursier, C., & Mercier, C. (2014). Determinants of stress in parents of children with autism spectrum disorders. *Journal of Autism and Developmental Disorders*, *44*(7), 1609−1620. Available from https://doi.org/10.1007/s10803-013-2028-z.

Seligman, M., & Darling, R. B. (2007). *Ordinary families, special children: A systems approach to childhood disability* (3rd ed.). New York: Guilford Press.

Yalom, I. D. (1995). *The theory and practice of group psychotherapy* (4th ed.). New York: Basic Books.

Yusuf, A., Peltekova, I., Savion-Lemieux, T., Frei, J., Bruno, R., Joober, R., ... Elsabbagh, M. (2019). Association between distress and knowledge among parents of autistic children. *PLoS One*, *14*(9), 1−12. Available from https://doi.org/10.1371/journal.pone.0223119.

A relationship-based integrative model of intervention for autism spectrum disorders

28

Barbara Kalmanson[1] *and Stephen Seligman*[2,3]
[1]KidsAttuned.org, Fielding Graduate University, Santa Barbara, CA, United States,
[2]Clinical Professor of Psychiatry, University of California, San Francisco, United States,
[3]Training and Supervising Analyst, San Francisco Center for Psychoanalysis, CA, United States

In this chapter the authors illustrate the application of the relationship-based principles of infant mental health for use in multidisciplinary early intervention practice for children with autism spectrum disorders (ASD) and their families. They compare the more traditional practice with an integrated model of relationship-based intervention. The focus of the chapter is on the current conceptions of whom we serve, the nature of the work, the phases of intervention, the use of ourselves as practitioners, and the scope of mental health in the treatment of ASD.

Relationships are central to the effectiveness of interventions offered by professionals from any discipline and any theoretical orientation toward intervention. Parents are most apt to ally with professionals they trust and experience as attuned to their inner thoughts and feelings as parents. The focus on relationships is in itself a curative factor in the intervention and a necessary component of any successful treatment. The quality of the relationship influences how the interventionist can ameliorate the stress on the family and on the emotional availability of the family members to engage in the therapeutic work. This is especially true in the treatment of ASD where the primary developmental issues are located in the interpersonal world of reciprocal social communication and interaction. Recognition of early signs of Autism Spectrum symptoms is an uncertain and perplexing process for parents. These children are confusing social partners who tend to elicit more worries in parents about their own parenting capacities than about which developmental functions are constricting their child's capacities to relate, engage, communicate, or process and regulate sensory, motor, or social stimulation. Parents need the nonjudgmental partnership of the professional informed by mental health practices to navigate the complex feelings and reactions that will ultimately allow them to become well attuned coregulators of their child's experience and development. In this chapter, we unpack the therapeutic elements of building and sustaining the therapeutic working alliance with parents that enables them to identify their child's developmental challenges, and to understand and sustain empathy for their child's struggles to engage in relationships.

Emerging Programs for Autism Spectrum Disorder. DOI: https://doi.org/10.1016/B978-0-323-85031-5.00007-4

Our own orientation to intervention with children with ASD emphasizes the caregiving relationships in the child's family, along with the specific developmental difficulties and "symptoms" that the child presents. We regard parent–child relationships as the most powerful potential sources of progress, as the parents have the most intimate relationships with the children and are the ones who spend the greatest amount of time with them. Therefore, we make every effort to include the parents (and where appropriate, other caregivers) at the center of the intervention, working to enhance the parents' emotional range, awareness of their own feelings (including negative feelings), along with the various responses and behaviors that are so tied up with those feelings. We are interested in how the parents' experience their child, including but not restricted to their "ASD"; this might involve the parents' own childhood experiences, their relationships to one another, and the feelings about the therapist(s) and the intervention(s).

Thus we are advocates of a relationship-oriented approach here, as in infant and child therapies in general. We are, of course, aware of the significant influence of behaviorally oriented interventions in our field, and have learned from these in a variety of ways. Our interest in relationships may seem, at first glance, to be at odds with the behavioral approaches, however, we believe that a relational orientation that includes attention to emotional, interpersonal, and intrapersonal factors will enhance whatever intervention is proposed. As we have said, the effect of any intervention will be influenced by the emotional climate within which it is offered and unfolds. Patients of whatever kind of health professional are more likely to make positive use of their interventions when they feel confident and collaborative about what is happening, rather than anxious or otherwise resistant.

The relationship as the client

Traditionally, practitioners in all fields of health and development have conceptualized their treatment efforts in terms of individuals. The person, of whatever age, was the unit of intervention. In traditional autism intervention programs, parents are taught specific therapeutic techniques by professionals and are shown how to implement these interventions with their children on their own time (Dawson et al., 2010; Rogers et al., 2019).

In the last decades, recognition of the importance of relationships, especially the infant–caregiver relationship, has transformed our understanding of development. A general consensus has emerged, that relationships are the central organizing focus of early development (see, e.g., Sameroff & Emde, 1989; Stern, 1985). From the beginning, babies and their parents are immersed in dynamic, interactive, relational systems that integrate all domains of development. Positive emotional development is a requirement for healthy physical development; cognitive, linguistic, and motor development, all depend upon early experiences of caregivers' loving responsiveness. These lead the infant to feel vital, confident, and effective, so as to support the exploration and motivation that are essential to growth in all spheres. Similarly, infant researchers are amassing substantial evidence that the quality of infant–parent relationships predict subsequent development (see, e.g., Main, 2000). Overall, this new perspective has begun to influence a commitment to integrated early intervention programs for children with autism spectrum diagnoses, and attempts to shift the focus of intervention from the individual to the relationship (Davlantis, Estes, Dawson, & Rogers, 2019; Kalmanson, 1998, 2009; Kalmanson & Seligman, 1992; Schreibman et al., 2015; Zeanah, 2000).

As the client focus shifts to the relationship, so does the nature of the work. Traditionally, autism interventions focus either on direct intervention with the child, with a parent observing on the sidelines or directed to the waiting room, or on direct instructions to the parent regarding specific interventions the parent is expected to carry out with the child during the intervals between intervention sessions. In a traditional early intervention center, for example, one might see stations set up for parents and their infants to move around a room in a kind of "assembly line" of services. Perhaps some time is reserved for parents to separate from their children and meet as a group with a counselor. During these sessions, parents receive intervention advice and possibly some help advocating for the services their children need now or in the future.

In the home-based variant of this individual model, the practitioner comes to the family, often bringing materials or equipment. The practitioner either uses the visit to demonstrate intervention techniques with the child to the parent or applies interventions directly with the child. In either scenario, the parent's role is to observe the provider and possibly carry out specific, task-oriented exercises with the child as demonstrated by the practitioner. In either scenario, the nature of the practitioner's work is didactic.

In contrast, in an integrated, relationship-oriented early intervention setting, the nature of the work is interpersonal. The power of the didactic or developmental instruction is dependent upon the quality of the relationship between providers and parents. Practitioners and parents enter into a collaborative process to describe the child and clarify the meaning of the child's behavior in the context of the relationship.

Assessment and intervention planning

In a traditional intervention program, the child is referred for standardized assessments by several professionals in the field, yielding a diagnosis of the child's developmental challenges, and leading to specified intervention goals and objectives, often determined by the child's performance on the tests. In some settings a mental health practitioner, often a social worker, may also assess the parents, usually along the lines of suitability to parent the child, either related to patterns of abuse, neglect, or substance abuse, or to rule out or to diagnose parental psychopathology. If the parent(s) are assessed as in need of intervention, those treatments are typically carried out separately from the interventions for the child. More frequently, parents are assumed to possess the faculties and stamina to follow professional didactic direction and are never asked about their personal experience of caring for their child.

Practitioners using an integrated relationship-based model begin by developing the working relationship with the family. They assess how best to serve each family based on its unique needs; setting a cooperative tone for the assessment is regarded as essential. Questions that set the tone for the relationship are considered. "Should a single or primary practitioner initiate the relationship rather than multiple practitioners?" "How will we develop a shared understanding of the family's perceptions of the child and family relationships, and develop a shared language for talking about the child, the family, and the work they are about to embark on with the practitioner(s)?" Before going forward, parents and practitioners should agree on the usefulness of formal assessments under consideration, and on how they will be used, either by the practitioner or by the service system, and the plan for using them will be developed collaboratively. The description of the child's needs and goals is developed in the context of the family processes. For example, a single mother raising four children may be more focused on developing her child's independent functioning than an extended adoptive family with one child, who may be more focused on the child's recognition of the mother as a primary attachment figure. Overall, primary caregivers are seen in terms of their relationships with the child, and vice versa. For example, in families with children with severe developmental disabilities that require exceptional attention, parents whose relationships tend toward overprotectiveness and dependence may find these qualities regarded as strengths in terms of the child's needs and their capacity to work well with practitioners, who will have to provide extensive guidance about handling the child.

The individual differences in the child's development are mutually described by sorting through the parents' perceptions and misperceptions about the child, while the practitioner consistently seeks to understand the subjective experiences of the parents in relation to the child. Intervention goals are derived from the collaborative work between parents and providers and are written as statements of dyadic interaction. The focus is not on the diagnosis of the child's condition, nor is it on the limitations of the parent. Instead, the strengths of each member are emphasized in the everyday events that build the ongoing relationships between family members. This work is steeped in the real-life interactions among family members. The practitioner is the witness to child–parent interaction, with all of the heightened emotions of the moment. As Fraiberg (1980) described, we are not discussing the napping baby in the other room with the distance of reporting on the past. Our interventions address feelings before they turn to memories and can be changed by the passage of time in the perception of the parent.

In a relationship-oriented approach, the nature of the work shifts from discrete interventions aimed at a deficit model of development and functioning to a focus on the microevents of interaction in everyday life that support development across domains by supporting the affective connection between caregivers and children. For example, a child who has not developed a reciprocal social smile would not be "taught" to smile by pairing central nervous system stimulation with a prompt for smiling. Rather, observations of child and parent, and discussion about the nature of their interactions and the parents' feelings regarding the absence of the smile are discussed. In one family, this process with the practitioner revealed a pattern in which mother was hurt and disappointed when her smiles were not reciprocated, and she withdrew from the child. The practitioner was able to observe a generally slow response time in the child and wondered what would happen if the mother stayed with the contact and waited for her daughter to process the communication. The mother needed the support of the practitioner to wait quietly, without confusing the child with more talking, movement, or requests. When the mother waited, the child's delayed smile brought tears to her eyes and recognition that processing speed and not interpersonal rejection was at the root of the child's challenge.

The initial contact with the family: building the working alliance

It takes emotional courage and an open heart for parents to begin an intervention process with professionals focused on their child. Practitioners should respect parents' struggles throughout the evaluation process, asking themselves what they can offer to parents, what the parent is ready to hear from them, and what will be the most supportive and useful way to give assistance. From this perspective, the interpersonal quality of the initial contact is crucial because it sets the stage for how the family will feel about all future contact with helping professionals. The primary purpose of the initial session is to build a working alliance with the family. This is the opportunity to give parents confirmation of their central importance to the child, a fact that may have become clouded in the emotional and bureaucratic process of sorting out an emerging awareness of a child's developmental neurodiversity. Practitioners should give parents a feeling of being understood, and invited into a truly collaborative process.

In traditional early intervention settings, family contact often begins with an intake worker who does not plan to develop an ongoing relationship with the family. Frequently, this unknown person requests tender and personal information from the family during an initial contact, without making emotional contact, sometimes in a questionnaire format and sometimes over the telephone. Running through a checklist of developmental milestones cannot create the empathic connection with parents that will facilitate their trusting professional guidance or experiencing themselves and their children as supported and nurtured. As practitioners request developmental information they may consider neutral, they should not overlook the possible emotional meaning of such dismaying events as their child not smiling, talking, or taking comfort in their arms within the typical window for acquisition of such milestones.

The initial interview needs time and open-ended inquiry. It can be quite useful to make explicit to the family that the goal of the first visits is to form a team on the child's behalf, including using the assessment process to get to the point where parents and team members "see the same child" (Seligman, 2000, p. 213). Practitioners are more successful in gaining a perception of the family's felt experience when they ask facilitative and elaborative questions, rather than yes/no or ages and stages questions. The feeling tones of the family interactions emerge when parents are asked for concrete examples about the developmental information. For example, a father, concerned about his son's social connection with him, reports, in the abstract, that his child is very friendly. On exploration, he clarifies the concern with an example of his child being idiosyncratically friendly toward a neighbor he smiles to, but can only see through the windows of a light-well in their apartment. This same child never greets his dad upon his return home from work nor looks for a parent when he has fallen or hurt himself. In this situation, the father's feelings of disappointment and rejection will affect his stances toward his son *and* toward the intervention, and they must be taken into account in communicating and planning work with him and his child.

Rather than relying on developmental questionnaires eliciting memories often distorted by anxiety and time, practitioners should encourage parents to let their stories unfold with all of the heightened emotion attached to revisiting difficult or traumatic events. In this way, practitioners come to know the internal experience of the family members, which can guide them in building relationships with the family and enable the work together to proceed. When parents experience themselves as collaborative partners with practitioners, they are less likely to feel helpless or intruded upon, and more likely to feel that the working relationship will be flexible and responsive to their needs.

For example, the initial contact with a child development assessment unit at a major teaching hospital left Sarah, a young mother, feeling unheard. She later told the relationship-based therapist she had been concerned about her son for several months, and after bothering the pediatrician about her concern, he sent her to the university assessment unit to get her "out of his hair." In making the referral for infant–parent therapy, the social worker at the assessment unit described Sarah to the therapist as extremely anxious, and the baby's physical development as "on target." She speculated that this baby was avoidant in order to protect himself from the mother's anxiety. During the initial session with the family Sarah told the therapist she thought she was going crazy. "My baby can do all the normal things, but he acts like he doesn't know I exist. He doesn't look at me even if I hold him or call his name. When I feed him he looks the other way." Sarah further revealed her concern about medicines she'd taken for the flu during her first trimester of pregnancy. She thought these were the cause of her baby's problems. When the therapist spoke to the acuity of the mother's observations, and the reasonableness of her feelings, Sarah was able to tell the therapist, "It feels so good to finally meet someone who doesn't treat me like I'm out of my mind."

In certain more traditional medical models, the mother in this case would have been referred for treatment for her anxiety, and the baby would be placed in a "wait and see" category, to be followed up at a later time. Meanwhile, the mother would continue to feel unheard, the dynamic of misalignment between parent and child would become exacerbated, and the child's developmental challenges would become more acute and set in his developmental trajectory. By connecting with the mother's concerns as real, and reasonable, and worthy of investigation, the therapist creates an alliance with the parent to learn about the child together. This sets the stage for a trusting, caring therapeutic relationship that will make room for the mother's developing further insight about her child.

Case formulation as a relational process

Citing Shevrin and Shechtman (1973), Hirshberg (1993) has described the goal of the clinical interviews as

> *not to gather objective data, but to form a personal relationship through which the assessor can elicit and observe in the family a range of... functioning on the basis of which the problem can be understood and a plan made cooperatively to solve it...what is learned about the infant and family is a picture or account that is constructed in the course of an active, dynamic exchange between family members and evaluator (pp. 174–175).*

It can be quite useful to make this aspect of the assessment process explicit to the family: We often tell the parents that a central goal of the assessment phase of our work is to form a sense of being a team, on behalf of the child with a crucial part of this being getting to the point where we see the same child; in order to emphasize this, as well as to gather information, we ask explicitly about these aims as the process unfolds. For similar reasons, it is essential that these discussions be conducted in ordinary language.

Indeed, such accounts are especially compelling because they are rooted in the direct, evolving experiences of the evaluation, and they are often supported by their positive effects, both on the child's and parents' emotional state and on the observable details of the intervention and the overall child–parent interaction. Progress in the intervention formulation and the evolving therapeutic relationship can be mutually reinforcing: to the extent that the parents feel that they have been collaborative partners in the assessment, they will be more able to embrace the treatment process. Rather than feeling blamed, intruded upon, or helpless, so as to recapitulate some of the difficulties that brought them to the assessment in the first place, the parents are more likely to feel optimistic that the therapeutic relationship will be responsive and flexible when their thinking about both the child and the evaluation process are given a central role. Although such effects vary with the parents' personalities, an overall sense of effectiveness is more likely to ensue, which may contribute to overall progress in the intervention.

Therapeutic effects of the evaluation process

Under such congenial conditions, the assessment effort will be one of the cornerstones of the unfolding intervention process. The interventionists' capacity to think through the problems of the family offers a new vantage point from which the difficulties can be reviewed so as to yield new understandings, along with new solutions. This is especially important in work with children and parents where things have begun to go badly, since such situations are often characterized by absorption in powerful and often painful emotions. The calm, but engaged reflective interest of the intervention team can often serve to interrupt, or at least dampen, such "firestorms," so as to create space for at least a bit of reflective thinking. This can sometimes lead to some immediate reduction in distress and at times, to new and more progressive solutions. Along related lines, the hopeful presence of the intervention can offer some hope, both in the promise of a solution based on the interventionist's expertise and experience as well as through the evocation and amplification of whatever residues of helpful relationships lie within the parents' inner worlds.

An example from a multimodal intervention with a mother and her infant, who had a neurologically based hypersensitivity to novel stimuli potentially related to an autism spectrum disorder, can illustrate the complex effects of such processes. Although early interventionists may not always have access to all aspects of the parents' pasts, such factors are always in the implicit background, and often do come up explicitly.

Natalie had become overwhelmed as her daughter became inconsolable whenever she left her with a babysitter. During infant–parent psychotherapy, this mother realized that she had been left to cry herself to sleep as an infant, although she did not remember this at the beginning of the assessment. Clarifying the role of the daughter's neuropsychologically determined hypersensitivity freed the mother to think more emotionally about her early memories of abandonment, especially as she was beginning to trust the intervention team. Once these synergistic processes were in process, the therapist and mother were able to add a behavioral strategy of slowly increasing the girl's time with new caretakers, in very gradual increments. An effective intervention process ensued.

Forming a working relationship through the evaluation process: establishing the matrix of care

The initial meetings, then, provide the basis from which the essential working relationship can proceed; the success of all interventions will rest on the quality of parent–provider relationships, even when the relationship itself is not the focus of the intervention. Establishing a basic background of empathy, reciprocity, and support, to whatever extent possible, will enhance the quality of both the initial interviews and whatever subsequent therapies are offered. Parents are more likely to collaborate and offer information about themselves and their infants when they feel safe and accepted. At the same time, the family's strengths are more likely to emerge in a sympathetic atmosphere, which will allow for a more complete evaluation as well as providing a basis upon which subsequent intervention can draw.

Forming and maintaining the working relationship can have direct therapeutic effects. Intervention referrals can be especially trying for families who are already in distress sorting out their child's unusual behavior and reactions, leaving them feeling even more set apart and alienated from others. Without attention to such issues, parents are susceptible to a heightened sense of guilt, humiliation, and helplessness; this is a special pitfall in work with the parents of young children, whose identity is intertwined with their parental roles so as to leave them especially vulnerable to such feelings.

Alternatively, setting an acceptant and tolerant tone in the initial interviews can offer some relief from such haunting emotions; the direct effects of the positive working relationship are more pervasive than is often recognized. Effective and sympathetic working relationships enhance parents' all too often neglected recognition that it is their efforts that are ultimately most important to their children. When professionals communicate their understanding of this central clinical fact in the earliest sessions, immediate gains can often be observed, including an enhancement of the parents' forthrightness and reflectiveness and at times, a reduction in emotional distress and behavioral symptoms. Overall, the prospect of a good therapeutic relationship with a professional can enhance the sense of being understood and supported, which can, in turn, lead to more effective interventions (Kalmanson & Seligman, 1992, 2006; Seligman & Pawl, 1984).

Assessment as a collaborative process

In an integrated intervention, how the assessment takes place is as important as what is to be assessed. In contrast, most traditional assessments take place in a clinical setting, using an arena multiple assessment model, often separating the parents from the child and administering standardized instruments of infant development, usually normed on a typically developing population. The data from such an assessment leads to a deficit model for describing the infant's developmental needs and intervention goals. Parents tend to feel left out of the assessment process and especially when early medical interventions were necessary, the parents feel, once again, relatively unimportant to the well-being of their baby in light of all the health and education professionals' expertise.

The integrated point of view implies that evaluators should always consider how to discuss the assessment process with the family and mutually arrive at decisions about observations, interviews and testing. Parents experience the process as more supportive and informative when practitioners assess for strengths and emerging capacities rather than simply highlighting deficits. Issues regarding where the assessment sessions take place, which and how many practitioners will be present and observe or interact directly with the family, whether audio, video recording, or note taking will be comfortable for parents, and how information will be shared, should all be addressed. Parents who are encouraged to collaborate with practitioners in these decisions enter the assessment process fully informed and invested in the work together.

For example, Mr. and Mrs. Greene, followed through on a referral to see a highly respected mental health professional because they were concerned about behaviors in their younger son that resembled descriptions they were reading about autism on the internet. They had spoken with the doctor who seemed knowledgeable and professional on the phone and arranged a meeting with him. When they arrived for their appointment they were ushered into the therapist's office by a man carrying a laptop. He sat across from them and identified himself as Dr. Williams. He opened his laptop and began asking questions about their child, typing as they answered him. The parents ended the interview quickly and politely, but never returned for further treatment. Mrs. Greene later reported to the relationship-based therapist they eventually saw, that she and her husband were appalled by Dr. Williams' arrogance and assumption that he had their permission to record their answers to his intrusive questions without inquiring whether they were comfortable with his typing while they spoke. Further, Mr. Greene mentioned how he felt devalued as a person when Dr. Williams remained focused on his questionnaire and his screen, and not on Mr. Greene as a person.

When to include the infant or child

Another area of decision-making influencing parents' comfort is the handling of inclusion or exclusion of the child in the interview sessions. In general, infants who are still "in arms" and nonverbal, can be brought even to sessions designed to primarily learn about the parents needs and expectations. The advantage of the infant's presence is the opportunity to observe the spontaneous caregiving patterns and contact with the baby. The practitioner can learn about the demands on the family system. Whether the baby sits passively in an infant seat or cries despite Mom's best efforts to soothe, begins to inform the practitioner about the baby's individual constitutional patterns and the effects on the care giving system. Similarly, if Mom does the childcare while Dad does all the talking, the practitioner may have an early insight into the importance of Dad's role as family spokesperson and decision-maker.

As infants and young children become increasingly mobile and comprehend language, the practitioner's suggestion to meet without the baby may be an instructive intervention regarding early development and confirm for parents the provider's consideration of their privacy as well as protection of the toddler or child from potentially complex and difficult feelings, including some about the child or the parents' relationship. Whenever parents are going to want to discuss information they prefer the child not overhear, the practitioner should divide assessment sessions focused on parent interview from those focused on interacting with the child.

Recording and communicating information to other professionals

The role of the practitioner in taking written information and the process of sharing information is often taken for granted by the provider but may arouse distrust or suspicion in the parent. Even when providers are well accustomed to their routines for sharing information, parents may feel sensitive about one professional telling others what has been offered in an atmosphere of emotional risk and confidence. It is essential to remember that practitioners' assumptions of our own goodwill in providing services may seem to be novel and even frightening experiences for families. Parents and practitioners should come to explicit agreement about whether and how information will be shared and how the coordination will work. Inattention to this often overlooked detail can leave parents feeling isolated on the outside of their child's life and abandoned by a process we have suggested would be collaborative.

History taking in context

Historical and developmental information gathered in the process of building the working alliance with the family yields the affectively richer story of the parents' past in relationship to their reflections on the present situation with the child. An expectation that the developmental history will unfold over the course of several assessment sessions, will counteract the urge to gather the data from questionnaires, in the name of "efficiency," which too often yields emotionally flat information.

Specifically, in an assessment informed by infant mental health approaches, the practitioner will try to understand whom the child represents to each of the parents. Children often evoke particular memories and feelings from the parents' childhoods. These memories affect parents' feelings about the child as well as the dynamics of the family system.

Overall, then, flexibility, openness, and concern for process are imperative in work with the special situations of distressed or developmentally perplexing children and families, both in broad planning and in the moment-to-moment flux of responsiveness within the sessions. Families will be relieved and vitalized when the therapist can embody a sense of confidence in their dialogue as the central vehicle for the treatment process: Outcome will flow from the interpersonal process. This parallels what is now widely thought to be one of the most essential elements of progressive development in all areas of child development—the mutual regulation process between child and parents. Children with ASD are known to have difficulty with both sensory-motor and emotional regulation, creating a particular challenge for parents to provide the much needed mutual regulation or coregulation for their child. The interventionist who models mutual regulation at every stage of the intervention, creates a parallel process to increase the likelihood that positive outcomes of intervention will be enhanced.

For example, Joanna, the mother of a 3-year-old boy with an Autism Spectrum diagnosis, complained bitterly to the child's therapist about her effort to have a nice day at the beach with her son. She was discouraged by his obsessive interest in moving rocks in his bucket from one side of a puddle to another. Her attempts to join his play only aggravated her sense of unimportance to her son. Joanna and the therapist explored the boy's motivation to organize himself in space and time on the sandy beach that challenged his tactile sensitivity accompanied by the loud sound of the wind and the ocean's waves that challenged his auditory sensitivity.

About a week later, Joanna reported to the therapist how she had failed in her attempts to have time for herself for exercise. She had obsessively chosen to rearrange kitchen cabinets when she was hoping to use her free time to take a walk. This revelation allowed the therapist to provide a parallel regulatory exploration with Joanna, as she had around her son's beach experience. Nonjudgmental recognition of the similarity between the mother and child helped build Joanna's empathy for her son, recognizing their similarity in regulating through obsessional activity when they were experiencing stress. Joanna's insight about the similarity of her own and her son's regulatory strategies opened a pathway to increased empathy and more attuned coregulation.

The advantages of home visiting

When possible, a family should be seen in relevant contexts, including at home where the child is apt to be at her best and family members are most likely to engage in typical patterns of care and interaction. Home visiting offers many advantages in both assessments and treatment, although it presents a number of logistical and technical challenges. In many cases, there is no other way to reach the families that are most in need of treatment, and even in less challenging cases, the gains are quite substantial. Home visiting provides access to otherwise unavailable information about families lives' and reassures parents that the demands that come with the birth and development of a young child with a disability are being understood on a practical level. Parents of children with disabling conditions often find themselves uncharacteristically isolated at home, and welcome a new "friend" visiting them and taking interest in their child. In some cases, parents are so overwhelmed that getting to a clinic appointment is itself a source of strain. At other times, it will only be through concrete action that the therapist can demonstrate appreciation of how difficult the family's psychological and practical situation really feels to them; this is especially true in cases with histories of profound interpersonal insecurity and disappointment, and where actions, rather than words, have been the most important carriers of meaning.

Home visits have the distinct advantage of allowing the practitioner to experience life as the child lives it. For example, if the stereo and the TV are on simultaneously in a household with a child who is hypersensitive to sound, we are painfully aware of the issue before us in providing optimal intervention for the child. If a practitioner observes a father who is briefly present in the child's life, sweeping him up in a momentary whirlwind of interaction and disappearing as quickly as he appeared, our initial disapproval may turn to compassion once we observe that father come and go in three different uniforms to three different jobs in his efforts to provide for his son.

With these benefits, however, come a number of particular challenges. Home visits can be unpredictable and oversaturating. Home visitors will struggle to find a comfortable mode for maintaining their professional status while fitting in to the rhythm of the household. For even the most flexible and gifted practitioners, it can be a challenge, to remain nonjudgmental and open-minded, upon entry into a home with heavy metal music blasting, the soaps on TV, the overwhelming smell of old kitty litter, or a serious weapons display cabinet. Practitioners assume the task of adjustment, allowing the family the comfort of their natural surroundings. This reverses the position parents often find themselves in when they feel trapped in a clinic setting, on alien turf and negotiating a foreign culture: The usual office routines are not available to structure the practitioner's actions and the physical set up of an office is not available to communicate the practitioner–client relationship. Roles are reversed, too, with regard to cultural issues, since the practitioner is on the family's home turf.

When the practitioner leaves the office or clinic to become the practitioner in the family room or kitchen, he or she must define the role for herself as well as for the family. The practitioner becomes a professional guest, differentiated from a friend because the practitioner doesn't talk freely about his or her own life, but maintains focus on the family and the child (Hochman & D'Emery, 2006). This is not to suggest a traditional psychotherapeutic model in which the practitioner maintains a distant or remote stance that could be interpreted by parents as indifference. The voice of the practitioner is the voice of compassion, caring, and professional wisdom (Fraiberg, 1980).

When it is not possible to arrange regular home visits, it will be worth considering including one or two visits in the assessment plan. Even when home visits are entirely precluded, because of agency constraints, the family's sensitivity about housing conditions, or geographic distance from the clinical center, naturalistic observation should not be abandoned. The center's environments can be set up with some of the ambience of a homelike environment, with the therapist following the family's lead to a greater extent than is typical in the usual clinical interview.

A final note on home visiting: when home visiting has been integrated into the assessment procedure, the clinic visit should always be offered as an alternative, both for the initial interviews and throughout the treatment. Even when parents do not agree to a home visit, they are likely to appreciate the offer to come to their home.

The practitioner's role in building and maintaining the working relationship

When the work of the practitioner is didactic, as in traditional intervention models, the burden of the emotional work that sustains the motivation to maintain the intervention lies with the parents. All too commonly, practitioners in these settings complain about how little parents comply with their recommendations between intervention sessions, or how poorly a child is progressing due to lack of full participation on the part of the parents (Leiter, 2004). Practitioners from every discipline will be more successful in their interventions if they conceptualize their own role in developing the working alliance with the family as central to their work (Kalmanson & Seligman, 1992; Seligman & Pawl, 1984).

The working alliance is built on the practitioners' empathy, self-reflection, and thoughtful action. A sincere interest in the ideas, feelings, and experiences of the family members in relation to the infant is essential to developing a sturdy collaboration. This often entails open-mindedness about a family's values, feelings, and cultural identity. In building the alliance, practitioners also need to become aware of their own feelings and reactions, and learn to use them to inform the work and support the relationships with family members. From the outset, parents are making meaning from their infant's behavior. It is from these subjective experiences of the child that the provider can work with the family to formulate effective intervention goals. If they are uninformed by the parents' subjective interpretations, providers' systematic intervention objectives may lack meaning for the family. Seemingly sound advice and instructions may be met with polite interest and surface agreement, but without follow-through. Parents are not going to understand even the best intentions of the practitioner, until providers attune themselves with the realities of family life with this child. The practitioner should encourage parents to tell their stories, listening attentively to an array of feelings as parents revisit their prior experiences, whether with a bossy nurse in the NICU, an impatient grandparent, or a physician who represented a future of doom and gloom. Similarly, practitioners need to empathize with the feelings associated with severe sleep deprivation since the baby was born, or the feelings of helplessness that arise when one is unable to soothe one's own child after hours of listening to a crying baby.

Acceptance of the widest range of feelings as a core aspect of intervention

In addition, practitioners' capacity for empathy and acceptance, no matter what their profession, enables them to use the parents' negative reactions, along with their positive regard for our work, so as to best meet their hopes or expectations. When practitioners are prepared to tolerate the wide range of parents' negative reactions and feelings toward them as holding the same value to the work as the parents' positive feelings toward them, providers will be in the best position to form a relationship that can weather the inevitable wariness and disappointments parents experience in the course of the demanding collaboration with interventionists.

In a paper entitled "Why how you feel matters," referring to infant mental health therapists, one of us wrote that

> *.... It is almost impossible to stay detached when working with babies and their families, and those workers who do are often the least effective... But our strong reactions can also impede the progress of our most well-intentioned and technically sophisticated efforts. Whether these responses become exhausting obstacles or sources of insight and vitality will depend on how we handle our reactive thoughts and feelings.... We can become aware of our reactions and tolerate and use them as informative data, even when they initially seem negative or inappropriate.*
>
> *Seligman (1993, p. 2)*

Although this was written for psychotherapists, the same applies for interventionists in all fields: Practitioners must be ready to hear possible distrust and to respond without defensiveness. Parents legitimately wonder how interventionists can help when no one else has the answers, or when they have to make sense out of conflicting answers, or the wrong answers. Open to heartfelt sadness and loss, practitioners can invite parents to tell them when they are asking questions, in the name of helping, that parents don't feel they can answer, or have already answered too many times before. If the practitioner responds without need for self-defense or criticism of the parent, he or she will be in the best position to untangle the perceptions that are creating obstacles to the emerging nurturing relationship with the child.

In other words, self-reflective capacity in the practitioner is not reserved for the mental health field. In every discipline, practitioners experience reactions or responses outside one's expectations. Learning not to act on one's personal feelings, but to use those reactions as useful information and insight into the internal experience of the parent, supports the provider's capacity to sustain empathy for the family. This benefits the child–parent relationship through the parallel process engendered by the parents' experience of feeling understood, and not punished or criticized in their vulnerable moments.

Karen, a young mother of a toddler engaged in the process of diagnosis for an Autism Spectrum Disorder, told the diagnostician that she had been in a car accident during the second trimester of her pregnancy. She was convinced that this trauma had caused her child to behave so differently from other children she knew, adding that the doctors she had spoken with so far reassured her that the accident had no relation to her child's development. Karen told the diagnostician in a theatrical aside, that the doctors don't know everything and when they try to help, what they offer is too little and too late. Rather than become defensive, or protective of the other professionals involved, the diagnostician understood Karen's story as a plea to take her seriously, and to appreciate the vulnerability involved in harboring such strong and fearful emotions.

Parallels between the child–parent relationship and the parent–provider relationship

Parents' relationships with the practitioners have uncanny parallels to their relationships with their child. The success of the working alliance is often a reflection of how well the practitioner observes the complex interplay of past and present in the evolving relationship. Although this phenomenon is well-documented (Fraiberg, 1980; Lieberman, Silverman, & Pawl, 2000; Seligman, 1994), the enactment of such repetitions from the past can surprise practitioners. Tracking the ebb and flow of the influence of internal states on external reality can prove an essential tool in guiding the practitioner's interventions in all fields.

The therapeutic attitude: reflection and self-reflection at the core of all interventions

In an integrated early intervention setting, then, our attention must extend beyond one's area of professional training in communication, cognition, sensory regulation, or motor development, to a steady interest in feelings, including one's own reactions, in supporting the quality of the intervention relationship. In order to maintain a therapeutic attitude toward families who are frequently in great distress and whose behavior is often not transparent or comprehensible, it is useful to all practitioners to be informed about several concepts from the theories supporting mental health intervention. Providers' best work with families happens when they are reflectively aware of their own reactions, tolerant of them, whether positive or negative, and able to use their reactions to inform their intervention processes (Seligman & Pawl, 1984).

The psychoanalytic concepts of transference and countertransference are perhaps the most valuable in clarifying the complexities of all intervention relationships. Freud proposed the concept of transference to give meaning to the ever-present influence of past experience, feelings, memories, and fantasies (especially those with primary caregivers) on current interactions and experiences. Greenson's (1967) description of transference works well for practitioners in all fields,

> *Transference is the experiencing of feelings, attitudes, fantasies, expectations, etc. toward a person in the present which do not befit that person but are a repetition of reactions originating in regard to significant persons of early childhood, unconsciously displaced onto figures in the present (p. 171).*

Why how you feel matters: the therapist's reactions as data source

Clinical work with young preverbal children and parents is among the most evocative of all mental health interventions. The most basic psychological issues are at play, and affective and other nonverbal communications predominate, such that therapists will often respond with more raw and unmediated emotions than in other situations. In addition, the vulnerable and dependent state of the child, combined with the sense of urgency that often accompanies referrals of children with ASD is especially evocative.

Sometimes, a parent's reaction to a comment or a suggestion made by a practitioner takes that practitioner by surprise. This surprise reaction is often a clue that the parent is unconsciously bringing something reexperienced from his or her past into the current moment in the work together. Transference reactions are mysteriously both self-protective and revelatory of inner worries. Often, family members are not able to articulate how they feel, but they are able to make the practitioner feel how they feel. In this way, the practitioner may feel trapped between the invitation to become involved in the worry and the message to keep one's distance, and may experience a distortion of the very same feeling one is expected to understand. Thus practitioners find themselves confronting their own inner feelings toward their clients' efforts at self-protection. If the practitioner responds by withdrawing or acting without reflection in these inexplicable moments, regressions in the progress of the intervention may ensue.

The psychodynamic concept of countertransference is helpful here in maximizing the effectiveness of interventions when faced with these challenges. Countertransference is sometimes taken to refer to all the feelings that arise in a practitioner in the course of the relationship with the family, and at other times to those reactions that arise specifically in response to the transference. Either way, these feelings become part of the data that practitioners can use to understand our impact on the family and their experience of the intervention.

Rather than withdraw from these difficult feelings, or react to them, practitioners can gain insight from them by learning to monitor their personal internal responses and reflect on them. Tolerating and reflecting on our reactions will generally prove more useful than succumbing to the pressures to suppress and censor them or to prematurely act on them. Optimally, psychologically oriented, reflective consultation should be made available on a regular basis to practitioners in every field, as a resource and so as to enhance learning about the use of the self to enhance the working alliance, especially at difficult moments in the intervention process (Shahmoon-Shanok, 2006).

Interventionists are as vulnerable as parents to the feelings children on the autism spectrum can elicit. As a young special education teacher, Vicki was excited and determined to change the rigid routines of her student, Sam. She was convinced she could create novel experiences for him that would stretch his capacity to incorporate something new into his day. One day she decided she would take Sam to the donut shop down the street from the school. She carefully prepared Sam for the outing including expectations for ordering and eating his donut. Sam had many rituals, but the one that made Vicki most uncomfortable was Sam's oration of a Maxipad commercial. When the pair arrived at the counter, Vicki nodded toward Sam to encourage him to place his order. In the loudest possible voice, Sam recited the Maxipad commercial to the cashier and of course, to the entire café. Vicki turned bright red and hastily ushered Sam out of the donut shop, pulling on his coat sleeve to get him to move as quickly as possible down the street and back inside the school. Sam could not understand his teacher's reaction and began to scream and pull away from her. Vicki was ready to quit her job, feeling like a complete failure and drowning in embarrassment. Fortunately, she and her supervisor were able to gain insight into the events and feelings from Vicki's past that made such a public moment so unmanageable for her. Vicki came to understand her reaction to Sam's behavior and began learning how to use reflective process in her work.

Integrating mental health concepts: when the inner world gets in the way

Mental health interventions are indicated when issues for the parents, in the child, or in the relationship between the parent and child, have become obstacles to the experiences of pleasure and mutuality that are the foundation for healthy emotional development. These range from serious parental psychopathology to emotional conflicts specific to being a parent of a child with special needs in an otherwise "healthy" personality. Careful attention to such concerns is especially important in work with children with ASD because such issues can be especially emotionally painful, and the child's difficulties may become exacerbated by stresses in the child–parent relationships. A child with ASD is a confusing social partner for any parent. Within the range of children on the spectrum, a child may be exceptionally fussy, fearful, active, sleepless or passive, avoidant, and self-absorbed. Parents need an ally in discerning which behaviors and reactions are related to constrictions caused by the disability, such as sensory sensitivities causing flight responses or receptive language issues relating to physical outbursts.

One specific form of "infant–parent psychopathology" involves the repetition of parents' traumatic past as it is reevoked by the baby. Fraiberg, Adelson, and Shapiro's (1975) much cited metaphor of "ghosts in the nursery" brought the constructs of infant mental health into the professional and public arena. She coined this phrase, the ghosts in the nursery, to refer to the child's engulfment in the parents' unresolved psychological conflicts. The ghost of the parent's past lays the groundwork for the intergenerational transmission of disorders of attachment and emotional health. The image of the ghosts in the nursery captured the imaginations of many practitioners, and this phrase has become shorthand for the baby's role in the family as the unconscious representative of ominous figures from the parent's past. Uninvited by the baby, the parent transfers unacknowledged and unexorcised pain, anger or disappointment experienced in his or her own early relationships onto the relationship with the baby (Lieberman, 1991). The parents' internal representations—their fantasies about the baby and their perceptions of the baby's behavior become distorted by disturbing and unresolved experiences from their own childhood.

For example, a baby's cry is usually perceived as a call for help. But what happens to the unfolding relationship when this cry is perceived as an accusation that the parent can't do anything right, and deserves nothing but criticism and rejection for her ineptness? A parent who perceives her baby's cries this way is unlikely to be able to sensitively attend to her baby's distress no matter how much we try to persuade her or educate her to do so. The original infant parent psychotherapy was developed to free infants from the distortions and displaced affects engulfing them in parental conflict through a process of helping a parent explore and understand his or her own internal experiences which are repressed or denied. Infant–parent psychotherapists are the infancy fields' modern ghostbusters—freeing the infant–parent relationship from the haunting parental past and from the parents' distortions in their current worldview. Revisiting and understanding the past enables the parent to diminish its power to invade the present.

New parents are both most accessible and most likely to find themselves at the mercy of their ghosts. The emotional demands of the baby create openings one might not see in individual adult psychotherapy where suppressed early memories may remain undercover. Sometimes insight-oriented work can only begin after months of contact with other practitioners to establish a strong enough treatment alliance for parents to allow themselves to be vulnerable in a therapist's presence.

In some situations, the parental contribution to the impediments in the relationship arises as a specific reaction to a particularly perplexing or difficult infant. This situation needs sensitive understanding of a complex issue. For example, the infant who is unable to elicit caregiving or signal clear preferential interest in the parent can set in motion an array of feelings in the parent. When parents' natural expectations are violated, they feel confused, unimportant to their child, and even rejected. In these situations, direct education of the parent about the infant's developmental issues rarely ameliorates the relational problems without keen therapeutic attention to the parents' subjective experiences of themselves in relation to the child. Careful observation of the real life, repeated moment to moment interactions between the parent and the child can buffer the feelings of rejection and help parents learn to read the child's frequently confusing signs of recognition and interest. Often, when parents feel rejected and helpless they withdraw from opportunities for interaction. Similarly, these babies can withdraw easily due to hyper- or hyporeactivity to stimulation, seemingly signaling their parents to cut off interaction. The following vignette illustrates the integration of mental health concepts with the understanding of the infant's unique developmental profile.

Henry's parents were distraught about their failure to recognize early signs of withdrawal from interpersonal contact. Mother felt guilty and full of self-blame for the difficulties that occurred during Henry's delivery and her subsequent postpartum depression. He was already 20 months old when they first sought out intervention. They described him as alternately content and aloof, or very irritable if one of his parents attempted to compete with or disrupt his attention to his current obsessive object of interest. In the playroom, Henry showed an interest in music. He alerted when a parent sang a song or clapped a regular beat. Henry found a large box of tinker toys that had a metal lid and bottom. Following his natural interest in music and rhythm, the therapist suggested they use the container as a drum and the sticks inside as drumsticks. Henry was already banging the sticks as the therapist noticed his limited motor repertoire. Henry picks up on the idea of the "drum" as soon as the therapist shows him he could bang on the lid to make a big noise. The therapist offers sticks to his mother and suggests she join him in his activity, and pause to attune to his rhythm, creating a full joint stop action complete with big gestures and anticipatory facial expression. Henry is engaged, as Mom and therapist join his activity. This shared experience turns Henry into the conductor of the band and opens a door for mutual shared pleasure and shared regulation. Amidst the liveliness of this activity, Mom notices with a sinking look on her face and fallen body posture, that Henry's gaze is directed toward the therapist for the moment of mutual pleasure and a signal to return to the banging of the drum. The therapist perceives Mom's emotional state and understands her likely interpretation that Henry is enjoying the therapist rather than his mother. The therapist however, notices that Henry orients his gaze toward the right in general, and wonders about the possibility that constrictions in his early motor development have affected his visual search. The therapist helps the parents understand that perhaps Henry is hoping to see his mom when he stops drumming but is constricted in how he can use his neck and shoulders to turn and look. She switches places with Mom on the floor, which results in Henry looking animatedly toward his mother as he pauses the drumming, and beams up at her as he begins to drum again. The mother's affect brightens. She becomes available to enjoy the game with Henry and experience her primary importance to her son.

Practitioners in all fields can help parents empathize with their child's unique endowment and special sensitivities; and rather than withdraw and suffer disappointment, parents can gain resilience and sustain interaction, bringing the child increasingly into the social world. When innate endowment inhibits expression of emotional connections, it is often difficult for parents to perceive the cues for the affective messages appropriate to the child's stage of development. All too often, social and emotional development is overlooked, or facilitation of social development is neglected because of other glaring developmental challenges or health needs. In these cases, it is always rewarding to recognize that relationships provide the central organizing function from which all domains of development unfold.

This vignette also illustrates how the ordinary experience of a mother interacting with her child can lead to a parent's misperceptions about how and why her child is not responding to her nor eliciting social interaction. When these misperceptions derail the parents' capacities to sustain an empathic connection with the child, an infant mental health intervention can help to set the relationship back on track.

Monitoring the working relationship: infant mental health practice clarifying an early intervention

Although professionals in other fields may not be in a position to take up all of the psychological issues evoked here, they are often influential in many interventions, as a parent may experience herself most allied with any member of an intervention team. The team collaboration and mental health consultation is crucial in supporting the integrated treatment of the child and family. As the working relationship is the crucial locus for intervention, it also provides essential data: Since parents' relationships with providers often parallel their relationships with their children, observing the evolving intervention relationship can provide important information about parents and experiences of one another. As has been noted, these relationship patterns often reflect the parents' childhood experiences of their own parents; although this is well acknowledged (see, e.g., Fraiberg, 1980; Stern, 1995, among others), the actuality of such striking repetitions can still be quite startling to clinicians. From the infant mental health perspective, remembering that the evolving therapeutic relationship is always a reflection of a complex interplay of past and present and internal and external realities is an essential part of both assessment and treatment, as well as providing a formidable guide for formulation and moment-to-moment intervention decisions. Such attention can be especially fruitful when the developments in a therapeutic relationship are monitored in tandem with other information emerging in the ongoing assessment and treatment process.

These themes were well illustrated in an infant mental health intervention with the family of a toddler with Autism, Jackson, whose primary caretaker was his grandmother, Harriet. Increasingly, Harriet's daughter, Jennifer, had left Jackson's care to Harriet; this was consistent with her general pattern of unreliability and disappointing responses to her parents. In the face of Jennifer's absences, Harriet would make ever more strenuous efforts to gain her own daughter's loyalty by giving her gifts and extending other, self-sacrificing offers of support. Harriet had recently reported that her own mother had left her in the care of her grandaunt when Harriet's father died when she was 3 years old, in order to return to work in another city; although Harriet had always known this fact, she felt little emotion about how it must have been. Dr. A.'s suggestion that Harriet's relationship with her daughter Jennifer had evoked similar feelings was similarly met with assent, but little emotion.

The therapist, Dr. A., had announced that he would miss an upcoming session because of a commitment to speak in a distant city. Harriet began the meeting immediately preceding the cancelation by inquiring about the details of the talk, wishing him well, and saying how Dr. A.'s mother, who lived nearby Dr. A.'s destination, must be proud of him. After thanking Harriet for her kind words, Dr. A. wondered whether Harriet might be also preparing herself for his absence, since their work together had been growing quite important to her. Harriet agreed that this might be true, since she would indeed miss him. Dr. A. then wondered whether her kindness, too, might reflect a pattern of responding to inner disappointment with solicitousness, as with her daughter, and wondered whether that might distance her from the painful anticipation of his absence; he also added that he did not mean to devalue her good wishes about the talk.

Tearfully, Harriet said that this seemed true, and that she saw how she sometimes really worked hard, without realizing it, to avoid those feelings. She wondered whether something similar was at work with her efforts to think about what she felt when her father died. This led to a further elaboration of the feelings surrounding those early years, and more broadly, a more emotional elaboration of the themes of abandonment, disappointment, and the efforts to compensate for such distressing emotions by excessive attention to others' needs.

Another, apparently paradoxical aspect of this situation is worth mentioning. As Harriet became increasingly committed to caring for Jackson, she became an exceptionally dedicated caregiver. In consultation with colleagues, Dr. A. imagined that Harriet's dedication was partly a repetition of the self-sacrificing style that had served as a compensation for her feelings of disappointment and abandonment with both her father and her daughter. With Jackson, this style might turn out to be especially adaptive, since Jackson's difficulties meant that he could make use of whatever attention she could offer. This situation illustrates how different relationship configurations influence how individual characteristics come to be expressed, and which effects they have, within those specific configurations.

In this interview, Dr. A. used Harriet's way of relating to him as a central source of data, drawing on its correspondence with Harriet's history and her current extra-therapeutic relationships. As he inquired about Harriet's way of handling the canceled session, he was developing a sense of an "internal working model" (Bretherton, 1990) theme that seemed common in all three situations, and used it to guide his empathic inquiry. As Harriet's reactions both confirmed and broadened his own working formulation, his growing understanding deepened Harriet's self-awareness and her sense that the therapy was helpful to her. Thus the mutual and reciprocal nature of the assessment-intervention process synergistically served both diagnostic and therapeutic purposes.

Correlating the infant–parent and therapist–parent relationships

Such processes can be even more dynamically augmented, as well as taking on greater subtlety, when observations about the child–parent relationship are integrated into the emerging evaluation–intervention process. The child–parent relationship and therapist–parent relationships often contain similar themes, although they may be managed and articulated in different ways.

This can be further illustrated with reference to the observation of Harriet and Jackson's emerging relationship: as Harriet became more involved as Jackson's primary caretaker, she began to feel that something was "not right" about him. Indeed, Dr. A. shared this sense, and a neurological assessment was initiated. As troubling findings did indeed begin to emerge, Harriet zealously devoted herself to finding the best array of special intervention resources for her grandson. Dr. A. began to feel that Jackson's difficulties had provided an occasion for Harriet to become activated in her characterological pattern of self-sacrifice as a way to sidestep feelings of distress (here, over the possibility that Jackson's prognosis was quite poor), but did not comment on this, feeling both that this might be too upsetting for her and also, that this particular mode might prove actually to be an adaptive strength if Jackson's special needs proved to be very great. Instead, he took a generally supportive stance, both in gently exploring her feelings and in helping her negotiate the complex maze of medical and developmental services in which she was becoming involved. Along these lines, he functioned as an information coordinator/case manager with regard to the various professionals (cf. Greenspan & Wieder, 1998), which also augmented his own assessment process.

However, his understanding of the underlying psychological dynamics in this complex "internal–external relationship system" (Rebecca Shahmoon-Shanok, personal communication) became especially useful when Harriet began to feel quite disappointed in the pediatric neurologist, Dr. D. Amidst a growing sense of grievance, she felt unable to speak directly with Dr. D., and instead began to miss appointments. As the evaluation became stalled, Dr. A. now spoke more explicitly with Harriet about the themes about abandonment that they had discussed earlier, saying, "It must be so difficult when someone from whom you had so much hoped for help appears not to care, nor to understand how crucial that care could be to you and your grandson" Harriet was moved to tears by this, and feeling understood by Dr. A., was able to now think more explicitly about whether to talk with Dr. D. or to seek another neurologist, and eventually chose the latter path, with very positive results.

Summary

In importing insights from the infant mental health field, practitioners can augment their relationships with the families in several ways. They can create a parallel process so that their working alliance with the family creates a positive emotional experience for the parents, and the quality of that relationship can be transferred or passed on in their relationship with the child. In addition, they can become more aware of how the past links to the present, so as to highlight how everyday experiences can either get people stuck or under the right conditions, transform repetitive patterns of interaction so as to enhance parents' more flexible and adaptive senses of themselves.

References

Bretherton, I. (1990). Communication patterns, internal working models, and the intergenerational transmission of attachment relationships. *Infant Mental Health Journal, 11*(3), 237–252.

Davlantis, K. S., Estes, A., Dawson, G., & Rogers, S. J. (2019). A novel method for measuring learning opportunities provided by parents to young children with autism spectrum disorder. *Autism: The International Journal of Research and Practice, 23*(6), 1563–1574.

Dawson, G., Rogers, S., Munson, J., Smith, M., Winter, J., & Greenson, J. (2010). Randomized, controlled trial of an intervention for toddlers with autism: The Early Start Denver Model. *Pediatrics, 125*(1), e17–e23.

Fraiberg, S. (Ed.), (1980). *Clinical studies in infant mental health: The first year of life*. New York: Basic Books.

Fraiberg, S., Adelson, E., & Shapiro, V. (1975). Ghosts in the nursery: A psychoanalytic approach to the problem of impaired infant-mother relationships. *Journal of American Academy of Child Psychiatry*, 387–422.

Greenspan, S. I., & Wieder, S. (1998). *The child with special needs*. Reading, MA: Addison-Wesley.

Hirshberg, L. M. (1993). Clinical interviews with infants and their families. In C. J. Zeanah, Jr. (Ed.), *Handbook of infant mental health*. New York: Guilford Press.

Hochman, J. D., & D'Emery, C. (2006). An integrated model of infant mental health and early intervention: The practitioner perspective. In G. Foley, & J. D. Hochman (Eds.), *Mental health in early intervention*. Baltimore, London, Sydney: Paul H. Brookes Publishing.

Kalmanson, B. (1998). Missteps in mutual engagement and regulation: The effects of developmental vulnerabilities in an infant on emerging family relationships. *The Journal of Developmental and Learning Disorders, 2*, 199–215.

Kalmanson, B. (2009). Echoes in the nursery: Insights for treatment of early signs of autism in a baby sibling. *Journal of Infant, Child, and Adolescent Psychotherapy, 8*, 40–48.

Kalmanson, B., & Seligman, S. (1992). Family-provider relationships: The basis of all interventions. *Infants and Young Children, 4*, 46–52.

Kalmanson, B., & Seligman, S. (2006). Process in an integrated model of infant mental health and early intervention practice. In G. Foley, & J. D. Hochman (Eds.), *Mental health in early intervention*. Baltimore, London, Sydney: Paul H. Brookes Publishing.

Leiter, V. (2004). Dilemmas in sharing care: Maternal provision of professionally driven therapy for children with disabilities. *Social Science & Medicine*, *58*(4), 837–849.

Lieberman, A. F., Silverman, R., & Pawl, J. (2000). Infant-parent psychotherapy: Core concepts and current approaches. In C. J. Zeanah, Jr. (Ed.), *Handbook of infant mental health* (2nd ed.). New York: Guilford Press.

Main, M. (2000). The organized categories of infant, child, and adult attachment: Flexible vs. inflexible attention under attachment related stress. *Journal of the American Psychoanalytic Association*, *48*(4), 1055–1097.

Rogers, S. J., Estes, A., Vismara, L., Munson, J., Zierhut, C., Greenson, J., ... Talbott, M. (2019). Enhancing low-intensity coaching in parent implemented early start denver model intervention for early autism: A randomized comparison treatment trial. *Journal of Autism and Developmental Disorders*, *49*(2), 632–646.

Sameroff, A. J., & Emde, R. N. (1989). *Relationship disturbances in early childhood: A developmental approach*. New York: Basic Books.

Schreibman, L., Dawson, G., Stahmer, A. C., Landa, R., Rogers, S. J., McGee, G., ... Halladay, A. (2015). Naturalistic developmental behavioral interventions: Empirically validated treatments for autism spectrum disorder. *Journal of Autism and Developmental Disorders*, *45*, 2411–2428.

Seligman, S. (1993). Why how you feel matters: Countertransference reactions in intervention relationships. *WAIMH News*, *1*(2), 1–6.

Seligman, S. (1994). Applying psychoanalysis in an unconventional context. *Psychoanalytic Study of the Child*, *49*, 481–500.

Seligman, S. (2000). Clinical interviews with families of infants. In C. J. Zeanah, Jr. (Ed.), *Handbook of infant mental health* (2nd ed.). New York: Guilford Press.

Seligman, S. (2018). *Relationships in development: Infancy, intersubjectivity, and attachment*. London and New York: Routledge.

Seligman, S., & Pawl, J. (1984). Impediments to the formation of the working alliance in infant-parent psychotherapy. In J. D. Call, E. Galenson, & R. Tyson (Eds.), *Frontiers of infant psychiatry* (Vol. II). New York: Basic Books.

Shahmoon-Shanok, R. (2006). Reflective supervision for an integrated model: What, why and how? In G. Foley, & J. D. Hochman (Eds.), *Mental health in early intervention*. Baltimore, London, Sydney: Paul H. Brookes Publishing.

Shevrin, H., & Shechtman, F. (1973). *Bulletin of the Menninger Clinic*, *37*, 451–494.

Stern, D. N. (1985). *The interpersonal world of the infant*. New York: Basic Books.

Stern, D. N. (1995). *The motherhood constellation: A unified view of parent-infant psychotherapy*. New York: Basic Books.

Zeanah, C. J., Jr. (Ed.), (2000). *Handbook of infant mental health* (2nd ed.). New York: Guilford Press.

From autistic teenager to adult in decision-making—a parent's perspective

29

Check J. Tan

As a father of an autistic person with intellectual disability (ID), the teen years were challenging; trying to navigate between guiding and freedom. On one hand there is the desire to ensure little or no harm, both physical and psychological, will come to your child, yet on the other, there is the recognition that one must let the child to make mistakes and learn independence by doing it themselves. My son is now an adult and what I have learnt during those teenage years can be summarized into a few principles or strategies. Central to all of this is that the focus is his needs, how he learns, and how he communicates—a person-centered approach.

As my child approached his teenage years, my principal parenting objective for him was him to live an ordinary life. That said I had to define what ordinary meant—given his ID, he is unlikely to be able to define it himself. However I was keen to not fully prescribe a life for him. Instead I took on the strategy to support him in making a decision. This was when I encountered my first hurdle, how does he know the short- and long-term consequences of the decision he is making; what are his alternatives? Looking at my own life and those around me, I summarized a few broad areas with which I needed to assist him with decision-making.

1. An occupation of time during the weekdays
2. Leisure activities
3. A social life among people who accept him—his community
4. Physical and mental health
5. Financial security and financial well-being
6. His circle of supports

In his development from a child into his teenage years and adulthood, it was clear to me that I needed to help him learn and help him understand the world around him. When he was under 12 years of age, we (the parents) did almost everything for him, anticipated his thoughts and moods, and unknowingly at that time (in the early 2000s), we avoided many a meltdown. We observed and understood his triggering stimuli, his preferences, his special interests, what excited him, and what frightened him, and to some extent what made his tick—in short we tried as much as possible to understand him and set about to develop his training to suit his needs and personality. As such we understood how to manage his anxiety. We also noted that he mimicked our behavior albeit slower. So instead of just showing how to do and act, we became his role models and at all times we kept communicating with

Emerging Programs for Autism Spectrum Disorder. DOI: https://doi.org/10.1016/B978-0-323-85031-5.00017-7

him to help him understand how and why we acted the way we did. We were also quite accepting of his stimming, again unaware of how it helped him. More through ignorance than planning we accepted his behavior regardless of societal norms. For his part, he seemed to enjoy and learnt when he was calm and happy especially when we traveled both within our home city and outside. Travel being his extrinsic reward, we made it our aim to continue to take short trips to tourist sights and places of interests to continue to encourage his curiosity. We encouraged his collecting of tourist information and used such literature to talk to him, encourage him to read and discuss his items of interest which in his case were geographical facts, demographics, technology, cars, sports, different foods and cuisines, and live music.

What we established by age 12, before my son became a teenager, was a very curious boy with some speech (more echolalia), who was sociable and quite willing to interact with us. We also knew that he enjoyed playing games especially mini quizzes on various topics that were interesting to him. We knew innately that answering questions correctly gave him a sense of satisfaction which we now know as dopamine. So quite frequently on his various drives we would have quizzes on cars, sports, geography, current affairs—all of which would not only entertain him but also further got him to engage with us. It was at this point that we looked upon using his curiosity to initiate his ability to accept some changes in his life. We started out with simple routines such as wanting to ride on every escalator on every visit to any shopping center. We noticed that if we disallowed him, it would heighten his anxiety level almost to the point of a meltdown. So, we had to find ways to entice and distract him such that riding the escalator can perhaps be delayed until a later time—the concept of postponement. Later, we introduced other places of interest that were much more attractive to him such as a visit to a technology or gaming store—provision of alternatives. For both concepts (postponement and provision of alternatives) we always kept our promise to him in either delaying the ride on the escalator or, if we provided a better alternative, we ensured that he did visit the technology store and spent adequate time there. From that exercise he also learnt that we kept our promises and understood the concept of trust. In turn, we taught him that we trusted him by asking him to place his own preference on how much time he wanted to enjoy a console game. This reinforced his concepts of timing (how long he wanted to spend playing), decision-making (him telling us how long), negotiating and compromising (having to decide between riding an escalator and playing his console game), and empowerment (letting him decide how long to spend at the gaming place). To minimize misunderstandings and any conflict as a result of not wanting to finish a game at the allocated time, we would break down the time decided and agreed down to 10 minute blocks, reminding him at every block so that he was aware of when it was ending and continuously setting and meeting his expectations. So wherever possible we used daily activities to reinforce his learning and understanding of various concepts and skills we take for granted.

We used another area of my son's interest (sports) to help him with counting—simple arithmetic and multiplication. It turned out his favorite sport was Australian Football, which had minor and major goals with different points for each. As a result, we used this to teach him addition (major goals and minor goals to come up with the final score), subtraction (difference in the scores of the 2 teams), and multiplication (the major score was 6 points to 1 for the minor goal) starting with multiplication by 6. He also enjoyed shopping, especially at the checkout counter and so we encouraged him to unpack the shopping trolley and repack into our bags, At the same time, we would facilitate his understanding of money by getting him to pay for the groceries (we would ask him how much money we needed to give him), count the change and reward him with some of the change if it was a particularly good encounter. This consolidated his counting skills, money handling, interacting with sales staff, and also reading numbers from the cash registers.

By now, it was clear that we did not limit teaching him the skills he needed in life purely to the classrooms. Instead, we used daily activities and events to introduce and reinforce his skills and understanding. That meant that he learnt on the "job" rather than through a book or a verbal instruction, and we did not have to be concerned with generalization of skills. However, our next challenge was to increase his sphere of influence. To date, his principal tutors were teachers in his school in a more formal setting and his parents in an informal and much more ubiquitous setting. We realized that we had to transfer this willingness to learn to more people and so we introduced the concept of trust and relationship.

We noted that his willingness to accept our instructions and guidance was due to our reliability and us meeting his expectations—he trusted us in our undertaking as well as our commitments and promises to him. So in order for him to take instructions from others, we had to "transfer" that trust. This meant that we had guided these new tutors or carers on what he expected of each of them, his likes and dislikes, his triggering stimuli, and his expectations. We were also flexible such that if new tutors or carers could not complete their time sessions with him because he was not cooperative or was overanxious, we would cut short those sessions. At all times, we were guided by him and in turn our reward was he trusted us and the new tutors and carers even more. These trusting relationships enabled us to make changes to his routines albeit with frequent discussion/consultations similar to how we changed his routine of riding the escalator. Eventually, he trusted us (and his new tutors and carers) enough such that even though the final outcome was not clear or certain, our description of the possible outcomes in terms of Options A, B, or C was sufficient for him. We now know that having that trusting relationship with a carer or tutor was key in managing his need for certainty. In an ever-changing world, we cannot guarantee an outcome for any activity or event. My son's trust in his tutors and carers meant that he felt safe enough to depend on them to define the possible outcomes and one of those outcomes is likely to eventuate and that any of those outcomes is acceptable to him.

After the first hurdle of getting him to accept changes with a matter of fact attitude, we then worked on how to help him to make decisions. We started out with simple decisions such as deciding on his own meals when we eat out. Knowing his desire to taste new cuisines, we indulged and gave him the freedom to choose, initially this was only the main course. To make that transition from our choice to a supported decision-making, we would let him read the menu, and let him choose his main meal. Regardless of the choice we always allowed it, yet as the same time we ordered something safe just in case he did not like his choice. After some time, he gained confidence that he could make food decisions. Next, we chose cuisines which were new to him so that most items on the menu were new to him. Here, we reduced the uncertainty by limiting the range of decision-making by asking him to choose the type of protein he preferred. Based on that decision, we would point out the three to four meals that contained that protein and explained the ingredients, volume, and perhaps the taste associated with each of those meals. On the odd occasion that we knew it was a poor decision, we would order extra meals to supplement the shortfall but at the same time we would highlight how the meal was not suitable for the occasion after it had arrived and why it was not a good decision. This assessment of his decision-making was never about blame, but rather about learning why his initial decision was not a suitable choice. Ordering meals became a learning activity. Eventually, he learnt that he was able to make decisions by himself and that our discussion prior to the decision-making was to highlight any aspect that he was not familiar with. We aimed for a new level of independence and were able to achieve it. This concept I later learnt is called visualization, a technique I use almost every day to help his decision-making.

We then worked on his decision-making and independence to other aspects of his life—travel, handling money, budgeting, IT security, social events that he wanted to participate in, sporting events that he watched, and sports that he participated in. Each of these took similar strategies of small manageable steps and, most of all, we had to ensure that even though the decision made was not appropriate we used those as lessons to be learnt with minimal negative feedback. In short, we sacrificed some money and time in order to gain confidence and trust. We made decision-making similar to buying in a retail sales model, we would discuss the alternatives and likely outcomes and afterwards whether the outcomes were desired and how it could have been better off with an alternate decision without allocating guilt—post decision review. We also included planning and scheduling in the lessons—how much time did each activity take, time to travel, who was available to be his companion and the concept of limited resources. So in some instances when he wanted to participate in two activities, we would demonstrate by drawing a timeline with the two activities and their locations which clearly showed that he could not be in two places at the same time. Additionally, we involved him in the booking of various events that he wanted to join and demonstrated that it was sold out and therefore the activities were no longer available to him. Throughout the decision-making journey, we emphasized the concept of compromise and limited resources, something that we all have to live with in our society.

As a result of him understanding the concepts of compromise, limited resources and supported decision-making with trusted close circle of carers, we were able to assist him to decide on the various aspects of his future life. I would now go through each of the main areas below.

1. *An occupation of time during the weekdays*

   Whether my son worked, volunteered his time helping others or attending lifelong training programs, we knew we had to find something to occupy his weekday hours. Knowing that he prefers to be active and busy, part of the stoic nature he picked up from us, getting carers to plan his weekdays was not sustainable. As such, the alternatives were either work or volunteering. I did not have any preference but again knowing his stoic nature, working would have been his preferred option.

While he was still in high school, we encouraged various work options. We extended his home life to include chores that he was responsible for, which included laundry, vacuuming, table setting and clearing for meals, and his own breakfast preparation. This was the training we planned to prepare him for activities which would eventually become his work. We canvassed various options with the high school, one of which was working in the canteen. We also took him to our workplaces, getting him involved with simple tasks such as refilling of stationery and refreshments, and packing and unpacking under instructions. These excursions into the workplace helped him understand the work ethic, how to interact with colleagues, how to have discipline in the work environment, how long tasks took to complete, and how a collection of these responsibilities became a job. He was also exposed to retail activities during his senior high school days. Eventually working with food was his forte and his preference. Today he works as a kitchen hand in a café.

2. *Leisure activities*

Depending on the personality of the individual, options for leisure activities can be quite wide-ranging. Our strategy was to expose our son to as many activities as possible so that he could make his own choice as to which of these he enjoyed. The analogy I use is that if we have only introduced him to five leisure activities in total and he liked only one, then he is limited to that one. However if I introduced him to 20 activities in total, five activities at a time and he still only chose one out of five every time, he then has four different activities he can spend time on. Thus far, he has tried his hand at music, swimming, reading, movies, travel, tennis, squash, football, basketball, gymnastics, attending concerts and musicals, attending cultural festivals, martial arts, Pilates, and personal training among others. Our overriding guideline to him was to occupy 2–3 days per week of his time with after work activities and 2–3 weekends every month with special events. We sought to provide a balance between what he had to do at his own home and what he enjoyed. We were also conscious that without the exposure of many activities, he may not have enough choices to make his decisions.

Today his weekly activities are basketball with his friends, 1:1 Pilates training, squash on Sundays, and eating out on Fridays. His monthly events that he looks forward to are live music concerts and musicals which he enjoys in addition to cultural festivals and celebrations whenever these occur. Even though he now has a rather full calendar of events and activities we continue to explore new ones.

3. *A social life among people who accept him—his community*

While autism was diagnosed in the 1940s (Kanner, 1943) and the concept of neurodiversity came about in the late 1990s (Singer, 1999), having a social life for autistic young adults was still quite a novel concept while my son was growing up. During his teenage years he was in the company of other teens with ID, predominately teens with Down syndrome, who were more socially aware and adept. This frequently created issues around understanding and expectations. We encouraged him to create his own social life by incorporating anyone and everyone he came across either at his school, work (later in his life), or sporting field into his social world. As such he has created a network of acquaintances through Facebook and/or Instagram, many of whom are known to us and these people have become his circle of friends and guardians and acquaintances.

Lately, various nonprofit organizations and parents of autistic children have started organizing social events and activities for autistic kids and adults. These have provided an environment where autistic teens and adults can be accepted and socialize with their peers without the need to conform to societal norms. These have been very successful, and my son has enjoyed these to the extent that his outgoing nature made him stand out as a volunteer and a leader in such activities and events.

4. *Physical and mental health*

As a teen, we noticed that keeping him physically active helped to manage his moods. His first attempts at basketball was predictably uneventful; why would anyone want to throw a ball so high up into a small hoop, where the chance of getting the ball through the hoop is minimal. However we persisted and every time he ran and scored, the endorphins and dopamine kicked in and he started to enjoy the experience. Basketball and later playing squash was vital in teaching him to accept defeats and rejections in life. We celebrated wins and good plays/moves, and at the same time, did not criticize his poorly executed plays. Instead, we discussed what could be improved. We also had opportunities to teach him rules and how these rules can change depending on circumstances. In a rather interesting twist of fate, basketball taught us all a lesson in the autistic brain. When my son started becoming quite competent as a basketball player, he could dribble, defend, and shoot but he would never steal the ball because early in his life, he was taught stealing was not never permitted! Stealing in basketball was a way of winning a ball from the opposition based on one's ability to take the ball away whilst it is being bounced. This is move is known as stealing. However as stealing is not allowed under any circumstances, we had to explain the move and show various videos and live games played and especially highlighting when the ball was stolen and how it was entirely within the rules of basketball. It was in fact a desirable feature of basketball. With that extended coaching, watching, and reinforcement, my son did finally overcome this misunderstanding.

Throughout his teen, he discussed his routines and interests with a child psychologist. These were more informal chats, which allowed him discuss his interests with a friendly person who was able to help him overcome various challenges that he had been encountering. We continued to engage with psychologist who had specialized training with autistic individuals, one male psychologist and one female psychologist, as we noticed he would only discuss some topics with males and others with females—again we looked at my son's needs and tried to accommodate his preferences.

Lately, he has been under the guidance of a personal trainer to develop his balance and core muscle in a range of Pilates exercises. We have noticed a marked improvement in his posture as a result of these exercises.

5. *Financial security and financial well-being*

While my son is employed under a Supported Wage Scheme which meant that he receives some support to continue to work, his income is not adequate to support him. We have planned for this for some time now and we have established a trust (which has been facilitated by the Australian government) which meets his financial needs. However, it was his daily encounters with money that was more concerning for us. As previously mentioned, we introduced the concept of money during grocery shopping. Next, we introduced budgeting by giving him a weekly allowance and requiring him to enter every expenditure in a spreadsheet that he completed daily. This reinforced his understanding of his monetary limits and his budget, which was his weekly allowance. We were also able to demonstrate to him how much money he was spending and where it was being spent. These lessons were extended to credit cards, his own telephone expenses, and finally his weekly spending on food and entertainment. He now spends and pays his own way using his earned money if the expenditure is within an agreed amount. If it was above the agreed amount, he would discuss the reason for the expenditure and we would almost agree to the spending but we felt privileged and proud that he trust us and now uses us as his sounding board. He also shows his generosity as he has makes monthly donations to various charities.

6. *Circle of support*

We know that we cannot outlive our son and yet we do not have other children who may choose to support him in the future. Instead, we have initiated a group of friends and professionals who we see as his circle of support. This group will provide the guidance and, in some instances, emotional and social support that he may need. These are the people he can turn to should he need to discuss any issues. This circle of support includes his psychologists, two of his cousins, a few friends, and at least a few support workers. At this stage the setting is still informal as we have not needed to set up a set of rigid guidelines for his group to act within.

Central to this group workings is the acceptance that my son's needs and welfare is key—provided it is not illegal and does not hurt someone else, his preferences should prevail unless there are mitigating circumstances.

Conclusion

I hope that I have shown that learning important life skills for autistic teens is not only possible, but it can also be fun and not necessarily always occur in the classroom. The autistic person must always be front and center of any program of learning and support. Their needs and preference for learning, their feelings and their concerns and fears must guide our approach. We should help achieve their independence yet not lose their identity and their uniqueness. In the end I don't want to make my son to become a version of me, I want him to enjoy his life yet be able to navigate this world with his personality intact and in harmony with his community and society.

References

Kanner, L. (1943). Autistic disturbances of affective contact. *Nervous Child*, *2*, 217–250.

Singer, J. (1999). 'Why can't you be normal for once in your life?' From a 'problem with no name' to the emergence of a new category of difference. In M. Corker, & S. French (Eds.), *Disability discourse* (pp. 59–67). Buckingham: Open University Press.

Physical, sexual, and psychological child abuse of a 9-year-old autistic child

30

Patricia Sermabeikian
Bergen Evaluation and Counseling Associates, Fair Lawn, NJ, United States

Children and adolescents who are on the Autism Spectrum Disorder are vulnerable and unable to protect themselves from child abuse and neglect. Due to their disabilities and vulnerability, they frequently lack communication and self-protection skills. They require specialists who are trained to communicate with them (Sarris, 2018). The case presented is a Caucasian male, John, age 9, who was referred for a clinical trauma assessment due to his reports of sexual and physical abuse by his older biological brother, age 14.

The background information provided was that John was diagnosed at the age of 3 with autism. During that time period, he was living with his biological mother and father who divorced when he was 6 years old. Both biological parents have a history of mental illness and substance abuse. His father was deemed by the Family Court to be a more suitable parent than his mother. John's father remarried and had two children with John's stepmother. She was a stay-at-home mother. She was kind and loving toward John and would repeatedly tell John's father that he was being abused by his brother. She made every effort to protect John from his brother despite his father minimizing and ignoring her efforts. John's biological mother relocated to another state and maintained phone contact with John and her ex-husband. John would tell his mother and stepmother that he was being abused and hurt by his brother. His mother contacted Child Protective Services and reported allegations of abuse that were not taken seriously by the agency. The allegations were unsubstantiated as the case was considered to be in a divorce/custody problem. John made allegations of abuse by his older brother to the school officials. The school did not report the abuse to Child Protective Services because the parents were cooperative and assured the school that their children were supervised and never left alone with each other. The parents presented as cooperative but did not agree to attend counseling.

John continued to tell the school and his parents that his brother hit him and hurt him. The father was protective of his older brother but did not intervene to keep John safe. The father had an alcohol and drug problem but managed to convince the school and the Child Protective Service agency that there were no serious problems at home.

Emerging Programs for Autism Spectrum Disorder. DOI: https://doi.org/10.1016/B978-0-323-85031-5.00004-9

During the evaluation process, John verbalized that his stepmother said, "I love you. She's not mean. Mom is nice." His stepmother explained that she separated John to keep his brother from hitting him and from going into the bedroom with John. His stepmother explained to the evaluator that John's brother covered his mouth with his hand so that he could not call out for help or escape. John was being physically, sexually, and psychologically abused, terrorized, and trapped by his older brother.

John attended a special education school and received special services and education. He was diagnosed with Autism Spectrum Disorder-severity level two and had difficulties with communication and social interaction across multiple areas. The school reported that there was some improvement in his verbal communication skills but his social skills continued to be limited. He functioned at a preschool grade level. He was quiet and compliant at school. John disclosed vague information about his abuse to school officials. The school reported the concerns for sibling abuse to Child Protective Services.

John was referred for an evaluation at a center that specializes in child abuse and neglect. During the three-session evaluation process, John avoided eye contact and turned away from the evaluator when communicating with her. He repetitively drew pictures that were not specific in nature with a black magic marker and lined them up in front of him on the couch. He answered questions while engaging in repetitive drawing behavior. John smiled at the evaluator and sat on the couch with his back turned away.

His stepmother was able to explain the manner in which John related and spoke to others. She explained that he was easily intimidated and soft spoken. She explained to John that the evaluator would be talking to him about his brother. She told him the evaluator was "a nice person" to whom he could talk about being hit and hurt. John asked questions about the evaluator's toys. The evaluator was able to engage John by sitting behind her desk while John was sitting on a couch that did not face the evaluator. The evaluator told John that she was going to ask him to talk about his family. He was able to verbalize that his brother "hit" him and was "bad." He said, "My stepmother doesn't hurt me. She loves me. My brother's a big boy."

The evaluator showed him an anatomically detailed diagram of a naked male child with front and back views. He turned toward the evaluator and was curious and smiled. The evaluator pointed to the body parts. John was able to identify the body parts of the diagram and he provided the names for the private body parts. Upon inquiry, John pointed to the body parts at a simple and concrete level while he briefly described the abuse experiences. He said that his brother covered his mouth with his hand so he could not cry out. John explained that his brother put his pee pee (penis) in his mouth and put his pee pee (penis) in his booty (buttocks). He explained that his brother punched his stomach and it hurt. He said that his brother "peed" on his stomach and booty (buttocks). John was able to provide sensory information about being abused.

Given his developmental level, John's disclosure and details supported a clinical finding of sexual abuse, physical abuse, and psychological abuse. John was not able to say how many times the abuse occurred. However, he said, "A lot and it hurt. I am happy to talk." His information would not be considered legally reliable, consistent, or complete (Myers, 2002). John's testimony would be the most critical evidence (Myers, 2002), so there were no criminal or civil charges. Child Protective Services was able to contract with the father and brother to reside outside of the home. They agreed to no contact until the investigation was completed. Child Protective Services caseworkers did not substantiate child abuse because John refused to speak to them. His brother and his father were permitted to return to the home with the siblings not being left alone or unsupervised. John's stepmother explained to authorities that when their father came home from work, she would tell him that John and his brother were in the bedroom. John was being sexually abused and the stepmother was being pushed and hit by John's brother. She expressed fears of John's father and John's brother to agency members who were involved in the case. She explained that she always tried to keep John away from his brother but their father would ignore her concerns and permit the brother to return to the bedroom.

Child Protective Services initially separated John's brother and they resided with a friend, until the investigation was completed. The decision was that John and his stepmother would remain in one part of the home with her two children. John's brother and father agreed to live in another part of the home. The brothers were not permitted to have unsupervised contact, and in-home therapy was provided. The severity of the abuse was minimized to the point where John was not safe in the home. He was able to communicate fear of his brother as well as being happy that his brother was not in the home. He was able to tell the evaluator that his stepmother was nice to him and loved him. He explained, "She's nice. She loves me. My brother hits her too." He reported that his father did not stop the abuse. He further explained, "My mom takes care of me. She feeds me. She takes me to school." When he was asked how he knows that his stepmother loves him, he stated, "She loves me."

During the evaluation, John sat on the couch. He made no eye contact with the evaluator. He would draw repetitively and line the papers up on the couch. The examiner told him that she talks to kids about hurts, hits and being scared. She told him that she would talk to him about his brother. John was able to identify the private body parts on the anatomically detailed male diagram. He was able to identify mouth, pee pee (penis), bum (buttocks), stomach, hand, fingers, arms and legs. John was able to verbally express that his brother performed penile–oral sex, anal sex, and penile–penile sex. He demonstrated that his brother covered his mouth with his hand. He stated that his brother "peed" on his stomach and "bum" (buttocks). John said, "It hurt. I said it hurts." John told his stepmother, his father, and his teacher about different aspects of the abuse. This case is an example of how difficult it is to protect vulnerable autistic children. In this case John was able to communicate, so that finally the case was opened for services by Child Protective Services.

John's father initially convinced the school that there were no problems at home. John was compliant and unable to assert himself in school due to his fear and intimidation. Due to his communication problems, he was unable to provide specific details about the nature of the abuse to the degree that charges could be pressed.

The statistics suggest (Stop Abuse, 2020) that autistic children are often unprotected. Reports indicated that one in five autistic children have been physically abused and one in six have been sexually abused (Stop Abuse, 2020). John was overly compliant, passive, and withdrawn. He was not provided with the level of supervision to maintain his safety and protection. He did not receive attention or intervention and the level of primary or secondary prevention. His disclosures of abuse were considered to be unreliable and there was not sufficient evidence.

It is difficult to screen and treat autistic children who were traumatized or have PTSD (Sarris, 2018). If these children exhibit fear and tantrums, there continues to be problems with their symptoms or diagnosis not being fully understood. Although autistic children may not comprehend the nature of sexual acts, they may act out and have sexual behavior problems because of their experiences of sexuality and sexual abuse. They may exhibit or reenact aggressive behavior because they are being physically mistreated or abused. A sexual offender can manipulate an autistic child to remain silent, and instill fear and offer bribes in exchange for their cooperation. The conclusion suggests that the rates of abuse are higher than the abuse that is reported. Autistic children are vulnerable to being abused by their caretakers and family members or by others in school or in institutional settings. It is important that those of us who interact with autistic children become more aware of their vulnerabilities and behaviors that could indicate abuse and neglect. It is vital that we protect autistic children as the majority of them are not able to protect themselves.

It is important to teach autistic children boundaries, names of body parts, and good touch and bad touch. They need to be taught to tell someone if they are being hurt or sexually abused. Their parents and caretakers need workshops and education to teach them how to protect these children, and to be vigilant with supervision of those who are in caretaker roles. Identification of abuse and reporting, as well as protecting vulnerable children are imperative if the rights of autistic children are to be advanced. Education and awareness in the multiple professional disciplines of those who address child maltreatment have not sufficiently focused on the protection of autistic children. They remain an underserved and vulnerable population who are at risk of child maltreatment.

References

Myers, J. E. B. (2002). The legal system and child protection. In J. E. B. Myers, L. Berliner, L. Briere, C. T. Hendrix, & T. Reid (Eds.), *The APSAC handbook on child maltreatment*. Thousand Oaks, CA: Sage.

Sarris, M. (2018). *Abuse and PTSD among youth with autism*. Interactive Autism Network. Ian@kennedykrieger.org.

Stop Abuse. (2020). *The Maher Law Firm*.

Further reading

American Psychiatric Association. (2013). *Diagnostic and manual of mental disorders* (5th ed.). Washington, DC: American Psychiatric Association.

Garbarino, J., & Stott, F. M. (1992). *Faculty of Erikson Institute. What children can tell us.* San Francisco, CA: Jossey-Bass.

Intersubjectivity through dyadic states of consciousness

31

Alexandra Harrison[1] *and Ed Tronick*[2]
[1]Department of Psychiatry, Harvard Medical School, Boston Psychoanalytic Society and Institute, United States, [2]University of Massachusetts Boston, Developmental Brain Sciences Program, Department of Newborn Medicine, Harvard Medical School, Boston, MA, United States

Introduction

We will begin by unpacking our concept of intersubjectivity as an essentially nonlinear process in development. We contrast our more inclusive view of intersubjectivity as a messy and improvisational exchange of a wide range of meanings with the narrower use of the term by psychoanalysts in which the analyst gains insight into the patient's inner world through the exchange of verbal meanings and cognitive associations to these/their communications. The Still-Face paradigm is introduced as an instrument for exploring how meaning is made by mother and infant through nonverbal behavioral cues and vocalizations, and this model is elaborated to explain how humans of all ages create dyadic states of consciousness, which are the substrate from which individuals derive meanings to integrate into their own sense of self. We illustrate our points with a detailed clinical example of how a psychoanalyst and a gifted young child on the autistic spectrum communicate their implicit desire and intention to connect through the perceived but out of awareness movements of their bodies. This example concludes with the child putting into words the messy process by which he and the analyst finally succeeded in making a highly satisfying connection.

Intersubjectivity

We put forward a new conceptualization of intersubjectivity in which we refer to "intersubjectivity" as the exchange of meanings between two individuals in which cocreated new meanings are more complex and resource-enhancing than the meanings each individual had previously contributed to the exchange. This model fulfills Prigogene's first principle of open dynamic systems (Prigogine & Stengers, 1984): the system must gain resources to grow and develop or else dissipate. We hold that meanings are biopsychosocial or neurosomatic, by which we mean "bodily" and often out of awareness, and are made by polymorphic neurosomatic systems

Emerging Programs for Autism Spectrum Disorder. DOI: https://doi.org/10.1016/B978-0-323-85031-5.00040-2

operating at multiple levels in the individual. These polymorphic systems of meaning-making—of the conscious mind, the dynamic unconscious, the motor system, the endocrine system, the tactile sensory system, etc.—create qualitatively different forms of meaning that fit only messily together.

While derived from infant research, these ideas about meaning-making can be useful in apprehending developmental processes in older children and adults (Bruner, 1990; Tronick, 2007). In addition, this concept of developmental meaning-making can clarify the understanding of growth in psychotherapy, as well as in normal development (Harrison, 2014; Harrison & Tronick, 2007, 2011). Critically, meaning-making is most effective when occurring in interactions between two humans, in intersubjective experiences. That is because the meanings that are exchanged, and the potential cocreated new meanings, are more complex than those made by an individual alone. Moreover, intersubjectivity is not the end state of the process. Rather, achieving intersubjective states generates a connection to the other, a trust in oneself and in the other, and a more coherent sense of self in relation to the world (Tronick & Gold, 2020).

Psychoanalysis has embraced the concept of intersubjectivity as a way of explaining how one person gains access to another person's inner world. Although psychoanalysis has increasingly introduced ideas about nonverbal communication into psychoanalytic theory, the means of achieving intersubjectivity remains primarily through the exchange of verbal meanings. With few exceptions (Beebe & Lachmann, 2002; Harrison, 2014; Knoblauch, 2005; Seligman, 2018), analysts typically describe intersubjective experiences as the verbal trading of evocative images and metaphors in combination with astute self-reflection—again, in thoughts organized by language.

Still-Face experiment

The Face-to-Face Still-Face paradigm (FFSF; Tronick, Als, Adamson, Wise, & Brazelton, 1978) is a protocol in which the infant is positioned in an infant seat facing the mother, and the mother is instructed to play with her infant for 2 minutes, at which moment she receives a signal to assume an expressionless face. The "Still-Face" condition is maintained for a subsequent 2 minutes, after which the mother receives a second signal to resume her original responsive behavior towards her baby. During the Still-Face episode, infants typically attempt to engage the Still-Face mother by smiling, gesturing, and vocalizing. When that fails, the infants become distressed and experience physiological arousal—may drool, choke, and spit up. They avert their gaze from the mother and even turn their head away or arch their backs, communicating with their behavior their state of dysregulation and their attempt to manage the relationship through disengagement. In the reunion phase of the protocol, the infants generally regain their positive affect and reengage with their mothers, but often they display at least an initial hesitancy about resuming the social engagement. This experiment has been used to reliably assess infants' ability to regulate attentional and affective states, as well as qualities of the infant–caregiver relationship (Adamson & Frick, 2003; Mesman, van IJzendoorn, & Bakermans-Kranenburg, 2009; Provenzi, Giusti, & Montirosso, 2016). What can it tell us about intersubjectivity?

Infants and caregivers communicate their affect and intention through behavioral exchanges, using facial expression, gesture, and vocalization (Harrison, 2014; Harrison, in press). With these methods they create coordinated rhythms and other patterns of expression that constitute meanings about their relationship, and from which they also derive meanings about themselves. Some of these meanings will be organized by language, such as her assessments of her mothering behavior and her infant's responses, and these may become conscious memories. Many others will be out of her awareness. The infant is also making meanings with his mind and his body—meanings such as, "I like doing this with my mother," or "I do not want to do this anymore; I need a break," or meanings about contented satiety or discomfort in his gut. The infant communicates these meanings to his mother with his behavior. The cluster of meanings in mother and in infant at any particular moment constitutes the state of consciousness (SOC) of each partner (Tronick & Beeghly, 2011).

The infant demonstrates various SOCs in the Still-Face—from the enjoyment of playing in the first 2 minutes, to the eagerness to engage followed by distress during the Still-Face, and finally to the pleasure at reengagement in the reunion phase. The Still-Face offers a striking illustration of how the infant incorporates meanings from the exchange with his mother into his own sense of himself. Often the infant will initially hesitate before rejoining his mother in the reunion phase. It is as if he is asking himself, "Who is this new mother, so different from the one I have known from the beginning? Can I trust her to be there for me when I need her?"

We suggest that the Still-Face, among other things, demonstrates the interruption of intersubjectivity held by the infant and mother during the play episode before the signal for mother to become unresponsive. It may be that the mother and infant did not enjoy a relationship with a predominantly positive affective tone before they participated in the Still-Face experiment, but at least they shared meanings about a repertoire of relational patterns—generating SOCs—between them (Tronick, 2007). One of these patterns might have been, for example, that when mother is sad, the infant's smiles may cheer her up, and the infant sees her face relax. In the Still-Face, the infant may cycle through all the behaviors that belong to their way of reconnecting after a disruption, and none are successful (Banella & Tronick, 2019). Without her help, the infant cannot make meaning of the experience she just had with this vitally important person. Since these relational patterns in infant–caregiver relationships are associated with neurosomatic meanings to create complex SOCs, the infant is disrupted in multiple domains, making the infant's subjective experience all the more powerful.

The Still-Face experiment suggests the potential impact on the meaning-making process in the case of an infant on the autistic spectrum. Although all autistic individuals are unique, there are some general qualities of social exchange that can be identified in most people on the autistic spectrum. Among them are the difficulty meeting another person's direct gaze, qualitative differences in communication of affect in facial expression, and differences in the perception of high frequency sounds such as those that characterize motherese, the tone of voice that mothers use to comfort their infants (Porges et al., 2014). These differences create important challenges to the intersubjective process and suggest that individuals on the autistic spectrum may deviate from typical meaning-making with other humans and find creative alternative ways to populate their inner world through meanings they make with the inanimate world. This will be illustrated in our clinical case in which the child's atypical meaning-making served as a detour but one that resulted in a successful and innovative connection.

Dyadic states of consciousness

Tronick's (Tronick et al., 1998) concept of "dyadic state of consciousness" (DSC) resembles an "intersubjective state," although it is more inclusive than what is typically thought of as intersubjective experience. A DSC emerges between individuals when they use behavior to exchange intentions, affects, states of mind, and cognitive meanings—any neurosomatic meanings—with each other. The exchange has the potential to cocreate new meanings that in turn each individual can appropriate/assimilate into their own SOC, their private sense of self, their own inner worlds. Individuals overcome the limitation of self-organizing meaning-making by engaging in dyadic meaning-making, in that way creating intersubjectivity. When the cocreated meaning is assimilated an individual's SOC gains complexity and coherence, the individual undergoes an amplification of self-experience, a sense of emotional and cognitive expansion. Typically this is pleasurable, but not always. Pleasurable or not, the gaining of new meanings fulfills Priogene's first principle of systems.

One might consider that psychoanalysis supports developmental growth through an evolving process of creating a DOC between patient and analyst, which then gets disrupted before moving on to the cocreation of the next DOC (Harrison & Beebe, 2018). The potential for creating DOCs through intersubjectivity is greater in psychoanalysis than in a typical relationship because of the explicit knowledge and experience of the psychoanalyst, the implicit relational knowing of both psychoanalyst and patient, the motivation and capacities of the patient, and the frequency of the sessions—offering many opportunities to make meaning together. However, in contrast with most psychoanalytic thinking, our view of intersubjectivity includes neurosomatic meaning-making expressed with bodily movements, as well as verbal and symbolic communications.

Autism spectrum disorders

Clinical insights into intersubjective processes can be gained through the treatment of the highly heterogeneous group of autistic spectrum disorder (ASD) individuals because of their atypical processing of sensory perceptions and bodily experience. In this clinical vignette of an ASD child, we illustrate how intersubjective meaning was made between the child and the analyst through implicit and explicit awareness of bodily movements and rhythmic coordination, in concurrence with verbal meaning. Following Trevarthen, we emphasize the centrality of the body in our concept of "polysemic" meaning-making (Trevarthen, 2005, 2009, 2015). Though we do not have data on the neurosomatic processes making meaning in these cases, the literature documents atypical neurosomatic reactivity of individuals on the autistic spectrum, for example, oxytocin (functioning as anxiolytic) release (Hammock et al., 2012), response to human facial expressions (Nelson, 2012), and the sounds of the human voice (Porges et al., 2014, 2019). From this evidence we can assume that the child described below makes neurosomatic meaning of his encounter with the analyst in atypical ways. The correspondingly atypical and creative behavioral communications described in the example demonstrate the multiplicity of meanings taking part in intersubjective process more strikingly than if language and symbols alone were considered. In these examples, bodily movements used—both explicitly and implicitly—to make and convey meaning in the relationship illustrate how the "polysemic" bundles of evolving meaning-making occurring in the analytic sessions produce DOCs in an intersubjective process.

Clinical illustration

Our example is that of B, a 3-year old boy videoed and coded on a second-by-second basis. B had precocious language development, but his speech had the unmelodious quality of ASD individuals. He was interested in his peers but lacked the capacity for reciprocal play and had no real friends in his preschool class. When he had a plan in mind and had difficulty accomplishing it, he could become agitated and inconsolable. B also had unusual gifts. He taught himself to read at barely 3 years old and developed an interest in geography that allowed him to identify cities on the globe or in an atlas at lightning speed. Maps seemed to provide B with the comfort that was sometimes hard for him to find in human relationships. It was as if—the analyst came to learn—he was imaginatively placing himself in a familiar space (because all the cities were by now familiar to him and therefore comforting) and moving through that space without getting lost. As the analysis proceeded, B would explain to the analyst (A) that his lovey (stuffed animal) had a house in Guatemala City, and he showed her the route lovey took to get home. Through maps he and the analyst began to populate the cities of the world with human (or lovey) representations—though at a safe distance from where A and B as two humans were examining the atlas. In one session, B suggested that they "make a map" with a construction toy called "H-links."

In the beginning of the session, the A had just placed the construction toy, "H-links," on the floor of the playroom, and B had begun to organize the pieces. A walked around to a clear space next to B and in the first 6 seconds of the film, settled to the floor. At that moment B was gazing down at the H-links and had his back to her. He did not acknowledge her presence verbally or with his gaze. At second 6, A moved her hand to her chin. At second 8, she removed her hand from her chin, looked down, and began slowly to assemble a small pile of H-links near her. At second 10, B appeared to notice an H-link near A, and moved toward her. At second 11, A extended her right leg as if to balance herself. At second 15, B brought back the H-links to where he was originally working. As he leaned to the right, A also moved to the right, as she continued her slow, repetitive activity. At this moment, A and B assumed parallel body positions, leaning in the same direction with the same arch of their bodies, and with gaze down. Less than 1 second later, B spoke for the first time. He said, "These H-links don't go together at all." Not long after this statement, B slowly turned to A with a sustained direct gaze and a brilliant smile, which A returned.

In cocreating a polysemic intersubjective meaning, the two partners were moving forward microstep by microstep in time, implicitly assessing each other's behavior for fittedness in affect and intention: "Is this where I want to be in relation to the other? Is this how I want to feel in relation the other?"—but all implicit. Also, in the same process, they were explicitly considering what they thought about what is going on between them. A was thinking, "I must move slowly in order not to intrude and cause him to defensively withdraw." B may have been thinking, "I need this H-link in that pile." Clearly, there was no easy match between the two of them as they embarked on making-meaning together in this playtime. Instead, there was a layered organization of meanings made by the body and mind of each, and over time they moved toward a DSC and away from it, and closer to a DSC, and then at one point, the layers of different types and varieties of meanings—many of them partial and on the way to becoming a recognizable meaning—came together in a DSC. The Process of Change Group called this a moment of meeting, but we describe DSC as "polysemic" in order to capture the quality of multiplicity of type and origin.

As A sat down next to B, B is not consciously attending to A's body movements and did not signal an acknowledgment of her approach. The message from B was "My attention is focused on this toy, and information from the social world is not in my conscious awareness." A noticed B's lack of acknowledgment and settled into a comfortable position. Consciously, she wanted to respect B's agenda and prepared herself to wait until B initiated an interaction. However, she also made an unconscious gesture, touching her hand to her chin. This unconscious gesture appeared to indicate A's assessment of B's lack of preparedness for engagement. It was a communication both to B and to herself, indicating, "I will not intrude." Interestingly, the meaning of the communication related to both of them, although A is aware that B is not looking at her. This is a moment in an intersubjective process in which A is attempting to hold B in her mind. Two of the multiple domains of meaning-making here are B's bodily activity indicating unreadiness and A's conscious mental activity.

In the next few seconds, A consciously chose an alternative way of being with B rather than direct engagement. She was generating with her own body a rhythm that approximated his small repetitive movements, in that way creating a subjective sense of connection with him. Again, although she understood that he was not looking at her, she had the sense of communicating to him her readiness to engage but also her patience.

When B moved toward A, he again appeared not to notice her body positioned so closely to him in space. A moved away slightly to accommodate his proximity, throwing herself slightly off balance and causing her to extend her leg to stabilize her position. She had the impression that though B did not have her in mind at all at this point, though his body seemed to be making some kind of connection. Two seconds later, B moved away again, and A and B assumed symmetrical positions. It was as if their bodies were moving in relation to each other without making conscious or even dynamically unconscious meaning until they randomly achieved a "match" in symmetrical bodily positions at a distance. A DSC was formed between them by "match" in the shape of their bodies but not by their gaze.

There are two issues highlighted in this interaction. The first is that psychoanalysis—even with its concept of intersubjective—doesn't really have a way of making sense of this kind of interaction (Harrison, 2003, 2014; Harrison & Beebe, 2018). By contrast, our way of understanding it is through the idea of polysemic meaning-making. For us, A and B—as infant and mother, before language—were communicating affect and intention. Perhaps they were communicating a somewhat muted affect—mildly positive but tentative. A's intention was to make a connection with B, as was B's, though B was at least implicitly aware of how challenging it was for him to engage with another person. The "match" they made with their bodies assuming symmetrical positions seemed comfortable to B. A DSC was formed with neither verbal nor visual confirmation. With its cocreation B experienced a kind of engagement and initiated verbal communication for the first time.

The second issue highlighted by this interaction is the diversity and complexity of meaning-making activities. Perhaps it is a stretch to imagine that B's talent for finding his way—or making connections—in space through maps contributed to the mutual communication of their bodies outside of visual range. However, his stated intention at the beginning of the session was to "make a map out of H-links." Therefore, it does not seem like a stretch that making a connection with A, for whom he had affection and with whom he felt relatively safe, was on his mind. And perhaps it also does not seem like a stretch to imagine that he was bringing his particular method for making a meaningful connection through maps to the exchange with A. It is fascinating that the verbal communication he made was a symbolic confirmation of the atypical characteristics of their match and the difficulty they had making it: "These H-links don't go together that much." A and B now had cocreated a shared meaning, and the pleasure they both felt soon afterwards was indicated by their mutual gaze and smile. Though A thought she was not in B's mind until that moment, something about the interactive process of their bodies moving—perceiving the movement of their own and the other's body moving in space, in relation to each other—allowed them to cocreate that shared meaning. It is also a paradoxical meaning with an unexplainable complexity, in that they are together with their bodies and yet not with their minds until B made the statement of "these H links don't go together," at which point A took in the complex meaning of their being together and acknowledged the truth of what he said.

Conclusion

This example illustrates our point about intersubjectivity referring to an evolving and multifaceted process and not a "state." The process, following a nonlinear model, comprises a multiplicity of interactive meaning-making exchanges between two individuals—and simultaneously—within each individual. This bidirectionality is illustrated in the clinical example by A's bringing her hand to her chin after having settled her body to the floor next to B. This deceptively simple gesture is meaningful in many ways. First, it is a visual cue to the other person that she intends to "back off" or slow down. In this case, B was not looking at her, but it is clear that he was extremely sensitive to the movements of her body, so this meaning may have nonetheless been communicated. Second, A was out of her awareness, reminding herself to back off or slow down. Consciously, she was thinking about being careful not to "intrude" into the space around him that B needed to feel safe; she knew both from her experience with B and her experience with other ASD children, that anxiety about social engagement can be triggered by even a slight physical intrusion. This latter meaning may be called A's "implicit relational knowledge" about working with ASD children (BCPSG, 2002; BCPSG, 2005; Tronick, 2007). Finally, A's physical gesture of touching her face is self-regulating, calming her and relaxing her muscles of facial expression, which will via the vagus signal to the autonomic nervous system decrease her heart and respiration rates. In the case of B, his gaze aversion and lack of orientation of his body toward A communicated both to A and to himself his unreadiness to engage with A. However, his gift to the communicative exchange of "finding each other through a map" was appreciated by A in retrospect, and his astute comment, "These H-links don't go together that much"—confirming their difficulty making a connection in words—indicated that he had been working hard on preparing himself for a connection.

In conclusion, we would like to open up the concept of intersubjectivity to include an evolving process of multiple meaning-making activities, simultaneously occurring between two individuals and within each individual. In addition, we would like to introduce the study of autistic individuals' varied and creative methods of making meaning as a means of enhancing our understanding of the meaning-making process and intersubjectivity. We have said that another way of describing intersubjectivity is to talk about each individual's state of consciousness, SOC—as made up of many different meanings one is making of the self, including those in and out of awareness and of the body as well as of the mind—actively engaging with another's SOC, to create a DSC. In this case, B's meanings about a safe connection included finding the route from one place to another on a map. Autistic individuals provide the potential for considering the interplay or potential messiness of the meanings between individuals, the polysemic discord of meanings within the individual, and the potential dynamic conflicts engendered in the "within" and "between" or the inter- and intrasubjective meanings. Each individual receives the DSC as a subjective experience of enhancement, much as psychoanalysts describe intersubjective states. The warm smiles exchanged by A and B, accompanied by the sustained mutual gaze, is an example of that experience of the DSC. The DSC contributes meaning to each individual's SOC, but the subjective sense of enhancement does not last, because in the evolving intersubjective process each individual will exercise his or her own agency and the match with the other will be attenuated, until over time another DSC is created. There is a resemblance between the DSC and the "moment of meeting" described by Sander (2012), but in our inclusion of neurobiological, motoric, and endocrine processes—and our recognition of the unique qualities of meaning-making of the autistic individual—we have added significant complexity. Thus in our way of thinking, intersubjectivity is a term that describes the way humans grow in relationships, from the infant–caregiver relationship to all the other relationships—including in relationships with individuals who make meaning and communicate in uniquely different ways from us—throughout the lifetime.

References

Adamson, L. B., & Frick, J. E. (2003). The Still Face: A history of a shared experimental paradigm. *Infancy: The Official Journal of the International Society on Infant Studies*, *4*(4), 451–473. Available at:. Available from http://doi.wiley.com/10.1207/S15327078IN0404_01 >.

Banella, F. E., & Tronick, E. (2019). Mutual regulation and unique forms of implicit relational knowing. In G. Apter, E. Devouche, & M. Gratier (Eds.), *Infant psychopathology and early interaction* (pp. 35–55). Springer, 2019.

Beebe, B., & Lachmann, F. (2002). *Infant research and adult treatment*. Hillsdale, NJ: The Analytic Press.

Boston Change Process Study Group*. (2002). Explicating the implicit: the local level and the microprocess of change in the analytic situation. *The International Journal of Psychoanalysis*, *2002*(83), 1051–1062. (*Study Group members in alphabetical order: Bruschweiler-Stern, N., Harrison, A., Lyons-Ruth, K., Morgan, A., Nahum, J., Sander, L., Stern, D., Tronick, E.).

Boston Change Process Study Group*. (2005). The "something more" than interpretation revisited. *Journal of the American Psychoanalytic Association*, *53*, 693–730. (*Study Group members in alphabetical order: Bruschweiler-Stern, N., Harrison, A., Lyons-Ruth, K., Morgan, A., Nahum, J., Sander, L., Stern, D., Tronick, E.).

Bruner, J. (1990). *Acts of meaning*. Cambridge, MA: Harvard University Press.

Hammock, E., Veenstra-VanderWeele, J., Yan, Z., Kerr, T., Morris, M., Anderson, G., ... Jacob, S. (2012). Examining autism spectrum disorders by biomarkers: Example from the oxytocin and serotonin systems. *JAACAP*, *51*(7), 712–721.

Harrison, A. (In press). Insights into safety and connection in relationships provided by treatment of autistic individuals. *Psychoanalytic Inquiry*.

Harrison, A., & Beebe, B. (2018). Rhythms of dialogues in infant research and child analysis: Implicit and explicit forms of therapeutic action. *Psychoanalytic Psychology*, *35*(4), 367–381.

Harrison, A. M. (2003). Change in psychoanalysis: Change in psychoanalysis:Getting from A to B. *Journal of the American Psychoanalytic Association*, *51*(1), 221–257.

Harrison, A. M. (2014). The sandwich model: the 'music and dance' of therapeutic action. *The International Journal of Psychoanalysis*, *95*(2), 313–340.

Harrison, A. M., & Tronick, E. Z. (2007). Now we have a playground: Emerging new ideas of therapeutic action,". *Journal of the American Psychoanalytic Association, 2007*(55/3), 853–874.

Harrison, A. M., & Tronick, E. Z. (2011). "The noise monitor": A developmental perspective of verbal and non-verbal meaning-making in psychoanalysis. *Journal of the American Psychoanalytic Association, 59*(5), 961–983.

Knoblauch, S. (2005). Body rhythms and the unconscious: Toward an expanding of clinical attention. *Psychoanalytic Dialogues, 15*(6), 807–827.

Mesman, J., van IJzendoorn, M. H., & Bakermans-Kranenburg, M. J. (2009). The many faces of the Still-Face Paradigm: A review and meta-analysis. *Developmental Review, 29*(2), 120–162. Available from https://doi.org/10.1016/j.dr.2009.02.001.

Nelson, C. (2012). Facing autism: Eye tracking paves the way to underlying mechanisms. *JAACAP, 51*(3), 233–234.

Porges, S. (2019). Brain-body connection may ease autistic people's social problems, Viewpoint, Spectrum I Autism Research News, <https://www.specrumnews.org>

Porges, S., Bazhenova, O., Bal, E., Carlson, N., Sorokin, Y., Heilman, K., ... Lewis, G. (2014). Reducing auditory hypersensitivities in autistic spectrum disorder: preliminary fidings evaluatin the listening project protocol. *Frontiers in Pediatrics*. Available from https://doi.org/10.3389/fped.2014.00080.

Prigogine, I., & Stengers, I. (1984). *Order out of chaos: Man's new dialogue with nature*. Toronto, Ontario, Canada: Bantam New Age Books.

Provenzi, L., Giusti, L., & Montirosso, R. (2016). Do infants exhibit significant cortisol reactivity to the Face-to-Face Still-Face paradigm? A narrative review and meta-analysis. *Developmental Review, 42*, 34–55. Available from https://doi.org/10.1016/j.dr.2016.07.001.

Sander, L. (2012). Living systems, evolving consciousness, and the emerging person: A selection of papers from the life work of Louis Sander. <https://doi.org/10.4324/9780203837580>

Seligman, S. (2018). Relationships in development, infancy, intersubjectivity, attachment. In *Relationships in Development Book Series*. New York, NY: Routledge.

Trevarthen, C. (2005). First things first: Infants make good use of the sympathetic rhythm of imitation, without reason or language. *Journal of Child Psychotherapy, 31*(1), 91–113.

Trevarthen, C. (2009). The intersubjective psychobiology of human meaning: Learning of culture depends on interest for co-operative practical work—and affection for the joyful art of good company. *Psychoanalytic Dialogues, 19*(5), 507–518.

Trevarthen, C. (2015). Awareness of infants: what do they, and we, seek? *Psychoanalytic Inquiry, 35*(4), 395–416.

Tronick, E. (2007). *Neurobehavioral and social emotional development of the infant and young child*. Norton Press.

Tronick, E., & Beeghly, M. (2011). Infants' meaning-making and the development of mental health problems. *American Psychologist, 66*(2), 107–119. Available from https://doi.org/10.1037/a0021631.

Tronick, E., & Gold, C. (2020). *The power of discord: Why the ups and downs of relationships are the secret to building intimacy, resilience, and trust*. Sparks: Little Brown.

Tronick, E., Als, H., Adamson, L., Wise, S., & Brazelton, T. B. (1978). The infant's response to entrapment between contradictory messages in face-to-face interaction. *Journal of the American Academy of Child Psychiatry, 17*(1), 1–13. Available from https://doi.org/10.1016/S0002-7138(09)62273-.

Tronick, E. Z., Brushweller-Stern, N., Harrison, A. M., Lyons-Ruth, K., Morgan, A. C., Nahum, J. P., & Stern, D. N. (1998). Dyadically expanded states of consciousness and the process of therapeutic change. *Infant Mental Health Journal, 19*, 290–299.

Index

Note: Page numbers followed by "*f*" and "*t*" refer to figures and tables, respectively.

E

F

G

Kolibri 360 GmbH
Ferdinand-Jühlke-Straße 7
99095 Erfurt, Deutschland
produktsicherheit@kolibri360.de